Axial Spondyloarthritis

Axial Spondyloarthritis

PHILIP MEASE, MD, MACR
Director
Rheumatology Clinical Research
Swedish Medical Center
Providence St. Joseph Health
Seattle, WA, United States

Clinical Professor
Medicine
University of Washington
Seattle, WA, United States

MUHAMMAD ASIM KHAN, MD, FRCP, MACP, MACR
Professor Emeritus of Medicine
Medicine
Case Western Reserve University School of Medicine
MetroHealth Medical Center
Cleveland, OH, United States

ELSEVIER

Notices

Practitioners and researchers must always rely on their own experience and knowledge in evaluating and using any information, methods, compounds or experiments described herein. Because of rapid advances in the medical sciences, in particular, independent verification of diagnoses and drug dosages should be made. To the fullest extent of the law, no responsibility is assumed by Elsevier, authors, editors or contributors for any injury and/or damage to persons or property as a matter of products liability, negligence or otherwise, or from any use or operation of any methods, products, instructions, or ideas contained in the material herein.

Content Strategist: Nancy Duffy
Content Development Manager: Kathy Padilla
Content Development Specialist: Megan Ashdown
Publishing Services Manager: Shereen Jameel
Project Manager: Nadhiya Sekar
Designer: Gopalakrishnan Venkatraman

ELSEVIER

3251 Riverport Lane
St. Louis, Missouri 63043

Working together
to grow libraries in
developing countries

www.elsevier.com • www.bookaid.org

List of Contributors

Nurullah Akkoç, MD
Professor
Izmir, Turkey

Annelies Boonen, MD, PhD
Professor of Rheumatology
Professor
Internal Medicine, Rheumatology
Maastricht University Medical Center
Maastricht, The Netherlands
Chair Reseach Line
Care and Public Health Research Institute (CAPHRI)

Matthew A. Brown, MBBS, MD, FRACP, FAHMS, FAA
Distinguished Professor
Director of Genomics
Queensland University of Technology
Brisbane, Qld, Australia

Institute of Health and Biomedical Innovation
Translational Research Institute
Princess Alexandra Hospital
Brisbane, Australia

Carlo V. Caballero-Uribe, MD
Profesor Asociado de Medicina
Universidad del Norte
Barranquilla, Colombia

Philippe Carron, MD, PhD
Deputy Head-of-Clinic
Rheumatology
Ghent University Hospital
Ghent, Belgium

Francesco Ciccia, MD, PhD
Dipartimento Biomedico di Medicina Interna e
    Specialistica
University of Palermo
Palermo, Italy

Atul Deodhar, MD, MRCP
Professor of Medicine
Division of Arthritis & Rheumatic Diseases
Oregon Health & Science University
Portland, OR, United States

Jan Peter Dutz, MD, FRCPC
Professor
Dermatology and Skin Science
University of British Columbia
Vancouver, BC, Canada

Senior Scientist
BC Children's Hospital Research Institute
BC Children's Hospital
Vancouver, BC, Canada

Nigil Haroon, MD, PhD, DM
Assistant Professor
Medicine, Rheumatology
University of Toronto
Toronto, ON, Canada

Clinician Scientist
Medicine, Rheumatology
University Health Network
Toronto, ON, Canada

Scientist
Genes and Development
Krembil Research Institute
Toronto, ON, Canada

Muhammad Asim Khan, MD, FRCP, MACP, MACR
Professor Emeritus of Medicine
Medicine
Case Western Reserve University School of Medicine
MetroHealth Medical Center
Cleveland, OH, United States

Uta Kiltz, MD
Rheumazentrum Ruhrgebiet
Herne, Germany

Sonam Kiwalkar, MBBS
Fellow
Rheumatology
Oregon Health & Science University
Portland, OR, United States

Robert George William Lambert, MB BCh, FRCR, FRCPC
Professor
Radiology and Diagnostic Imaging
University of Alberta
Edmonton, AB, Canada

Rik Lories, MD, PhD
Professor
Skeletal Biology and Engineering Research Center
KU Leuven
Leuven, Belgium

Marina N. Magrey, MD
Associate Professor
Medicine
Case Western Reserve University School of Medicine
    at MetroHealth Medical Center
Cleveland, OH, United States

Walter P. Maksymowych, MD, FRCP(C), MRCP(UK), FACP
Professor in the Department of Medicine
Division of Rheumatology
University of Alberta
Alberta, Canada

Philip Mease, MD, MACR
Director
Rheumatology Clinical Research
Swedish Medical Center
Providence St. Joseph Health
Seattle, WA, United States

Clinical Professor
Medicine
University of Washington
Seattle, WA, United States

Victoria Navarro-Compán, PhD, MD
Rheumatology
University Hospital La Paz
IdiPaz
Madrid, Spain

Salih Özgöçmen, MD
Professor
Rheumatology
Istinye University
Medical Park Gaziosmanpasa Hospital
Istanbul, Turkey

Denis Poddubnyy, MD, MSc (Epi)
Professor of Rheumatology
Rheumatology Unit
Department of Gastroenterology
Infectiology and Rheumatology
Charité - Universitätsmedizin Berlin
Berlin, Germany

Head of the Spondyloarthritis liaison research group
Epidemiology
German Rheumatism Research Centre
Berlin, Germany

Fabian Proft, MD
Charité - Universitätsmedizin Berlin
Berlin, Germany

John D. Reveille, MD
Professor and Director
Rheumatology
University of Texas Health Science Center at
    Houston
Houston, TX, United States

James T. Rosenbaum, MD, PhD
Oregon Health & Science University
Legacy Devers Eye Institute
Portland, OR, United States

Sergio Schwartzman, MD
Doctor
Rheumatology
Hospital for Special Surgery, New York
Scarsdale, NY, United States

Joachim Sieper, MD, PhD
Professor of Rheumatology
Charité University Hospital
Berlin, Germany

Archita Srinath, BSc
Krembil Research Institute
Toronto, ON, Canada

Peter R. Sternes, PhD
Translational Genomics Group
Institute of Health and Biomedical Innovation
Translational Research Institute
Queensland University of Technology
Brisbane, QLD, Australia

Filip Van den Bosch, MD, PhD
Associate Professor
Rheumatology Ghent University
Ghent, Belgium

Head-of-Clinic
Rheumatology
Ghent University Hospital
Ghent, Belgium

Michael M. Ward, MD, MPH
Senior Investigator
National Institute of Arthritis and Musculoskeletal
    and Skin Diseases
National Institutes of Health
Bethesda, MD, United States

Casper Webers, MD
Research fellow
Maastricht University Medical Center and Care and
    Public Health Research Institute
Maastricht University
Maastricht, the Netherlands

Huji Xu, MD, PhD
Shanghai Changzheng Hospital
Second Military Medical University
Shanghai, China

Fanxing Zeng, PhD
Department of Medicine
University of Toronto
Toronto, ON, Canada

Contents

CHAPTER 1

Introduction

PHILIP MEASE, MD, MACR • MUHAMMAD ASIM KHAN, MD, FRCP, MACP, MACR

This textbook is a comprehensive review of axial spondyloarthritis (axSpA). Due to advances in our understanding of the genetics, pathogenesis, clinical features, assessment and therapeutics of axSpA, there has been an explosion of interest in this rheumatologic condition and related disorders. It is timely to have an updated textbook on axSpA highlighting our expanding knowledge as outlined below.

What is spondyloarthritis? Spondyloarthritis (SpA) is a group of inflammatory diseases which share a number of features including inflammation of the axial skeleton and occasionally peripheral joints, enthesial (tendon, ligament and joint capsule) insertion sites throughout the body, frequent association with the gene marker *HLA-B27*, and associated conditions including uveitis, inflammatory bowel disease (IBD), and psoriasis. Incidentally, in this book, *HLA-B27* gene is also shown as *HLA-B*27* gene to conform with the most current nomenclature. Historically, the SpA conditions have been subdivided into five subtypes: ankylosing spondylitis (AS), psoriatic arthritis (PsA), reactive arthritis (ReA), IBD-related arthritis, and undifferentiated spondyloarthritis (uSpA). AS, a male-predominant disease, presents in individuals in their 20 and 30s as back pain with characteristic inflammatory features such as worsening with rest, improvement with activity, and stiffness. With time, syndesmophytes bridge vertebral bodies and cause ankylosing of the spine in the most severely affected individuals. This may be accompanied by occasional inflammatory arthritis symptoms in peripheral joints and entheses, particularly in the lower extremity. As outlined by Navarro and Deodhar in Chapter 4, classification of SpA has evolved and the most recent classification criteria divide the condition into predominantly axial or peripheral manifestations. Although this division may seem to be somewhat arbitrary, since there can be overlap in many individuals, it is a simple categorization that may aid recognition of SpA, especially by non-rheumatologists. Ultimately, we may enter an era in which phenotypes and subphenotypes of patients are characterized by genetic profiling, which will allow for more precise classification and

treatment channeling - but for now this is only a future prospect.

What are the key clinical features of axSpA? How do we distinguish axSpA from other more common causes of back pain? As outlined by Khan in Chapter 2, disease manifestations can be quite diverse and no patient may exactly resemble another. A common denominator for the majority of patients is inflammatory back pain. As distinguished from more common forms of mechanical or degenerative back pain or fibromyalgia, inflammatory pain symptoms include a tendency to improve with activity, worsen with being still, e.g., while asleep, resulting in wakening with nocturnal and/or morning pain and stiffness, as well as having onset at a younger age. Typically the pain responds to non-steroidal anti-inflammatory drugs and effective immunomodulatory agents. Peripheral manifestations may include asymmetric joint inflammation, especially in the lower extremities. Enthesitis, wherein inflammation at tendon, ligament, or joint capsule fiber insertion sites, especially in lower extremities but also around the pelvic girdle and thorax causes persistent pain is an important feature which may be especially hard to diagnose correctly and may need advanced imaging approaches such as ultrasound and MRI to confirm. Dactylitis, swelling of a whole digit, can be an important extra-axial musculoskeletal clue to the diagnosis of axSpA. Non-musculoskeletal conditions which frequently are associated with axSpA include uveitis, IBD, and psoriasis. A few serum biomarkers may aid with diagnosis, including the presence of the genetic marker *HLA-B27* and elevation of inflammation blood tests such as C reactive protein. However, these are not absolutely diagnostic, may be absent, and need to be interpreted in the context of clinical symptoms and signs. With time, and especially in male patients, progressive osteoproliferation of syndesmophytes can lead to bridging calcification of vertebral bodies, resulting in severe spinal pain, deformity and difficulty with stance and gait. In addition to limitation of function, impairment of quality of life, adverse impact on work and family life, a patient's life may be foreshortened

Axial Spondyloarthritis. https://doi.org/10.1016/B978-0-323-56800-5.00001-1

due to a variety of factors such as spinal fracture due to ankylosis and associated osteoporosis, cardiovascular comorbidity leading to premature myocardial infarction and stroke, infection due to immunosuppressive therapy and impaired chest expansion, and so forth. Disease manifestations such as spinal ankylosis may be milder in females, leading to frequent delayed or lack of recognition of the condition, even though symptom burden may be as severe as in males. Variants of the condition may occur in children and adolescents.

How common is axSpA? As reviewed by Akkoc and Khan in Chapter 3, historically, we have considered ankylosing spondylitis (AS) to occur in 0.5% of the population of Western countries, less in Africa and some parts of Asia. Further, it has historically been considered a male-predominant disease, manifest in a 2:1 male:female ratio. With the advent of more frequent use of magnetic resonance imaging (MRI) technology to assess for inflammation rather than just damage as evidenced by X-rays, and the routine availability of the *HLA-B27* gene marker, we can now more sensitively diagnose a wider spectrum of patients with the newer category, axSpA. Using these more sensitive diagnostic approaches in patients presenting below the age of 45 with features of inflammatory back pain, axSpA may be seen in up to 1.4% of the population of the United States and in a similar frequency in Europe. Furthermore, many of these additional patients who do not display radiographic damage on X-ray of the sacroiliac joints and spine are female, making the male female ratio 1:1. Even though the prevalence of rheumatoid arthritis (RA) is 0.6%–1.0% of the North American and European population, i.e., less than axSpA, more RA is seen by rheumatologists. Indeed, many axSpA patients remain undiagnosed or misdiagnosed, presumably not seeking medical care because of the perception that back pain is common and not much can be done for it, or seeking medical care from primary care, orthopedic and chiropractic practitioners–never recognizing that this is a immunologic-inflammatory condition ideally managed with immunomodulatory therapy. There is a large unmet need to better educate non-rheumatologists about axSpA and increase public awareness about the disease in order to improve case finding.

How has axSpA been historically classified and how has this changed with increased understanding about the disease as well as increased recognition of it using advanced imaging and other approaches? Classification criteria are different than diagnostic criteria. The former are developed to try to identify a disease with a high degree of specificity so that when conducting a study of the disease (natural history, treatment,

etc.), we are confident that the correct disease is being investigated. On the other hand, diagnostic criteria are used for the purpose of identifying any individual who may have a disease in order not to miss the opportunity to treat them effectively, thus high sensitivity for identification purposes is the goal. In Chapter 4, Navarro and Deodhar trace the history of classification criteria for axSpA, beginning with the original New York Modified criteria for AS published in 1984 and taking us through the most recent classification criteria for axSpA developed by the Assessment of SpondyloArthritis international Society (ASAS) published in 2009. The 1984 criteria, utilizing objective imaging technology available at the time, required plain X-ray evidence of sacroiliitis for reliable classification of AS. We now know that symptoms of the disease may occur long before this finding is present, and that this requirement skews the classification toward males who tend to show more prominent radiologic changes than females. As the field has advanced, including the wider availability MRI and use of *HLA-B27* typing, we can now recognize the broader spectrum of disease not restricted to those solely with radiographic changes with minimal loss of specificity.

What causes axSpA? The pathogenesis of axSpA is a complex interplay of genetic factors, environmental and immunologic elements. AxSpA is one of the most heritable rheumatic diseases, as evidenced by the frequency of familial history of the disease or related diseases. The most prominent item in the genetic profile of axSpA is the *HLA-B27* gene, but increasingly we are recognizing other key genes, such as *ERAP1*, that play an important role. Indeed, the presence of both *HLA-B27* and *ERAP1* appears to have a synergistic effect in disease proclivity. Brown, Xu, and Reveille provide detail in Chapter 5 about our current understanding of the genetics of axSpA, including an explication of the geographic distribution of *HLA-B27* via historical pathways of population migration. These and other genes such as *IL-23R*, *TYK2*, and *TNFR1*, also give a hint about potential therapeutic pathways to target. The role of epigenetic alterations is also discussed.

Do alterations in the gut microbiome contribute to the pathophysiology of axSpA? Sternes and Brown in Chapter 6 contemplate the possible role of dysbiosis in the promulgation of axSpA, focusing on the gut microbiome. There has been a significant increase in study of the role of commensal bacteria and other organisms at interfaces such as the gut, skin and lung in the regulation or dysregulation of human physiology. There is clear evidence that both increase of pro-inflammatory and decrease of pro-anti-inflammatory bacteria occur in patients with axSpA. This appears to be influenced by the *HLA-B27* gene. A hypothesis is that local gut inflammation and alterations in gut permeability resultant from dysbiosis lead to immunologic stimulation that can become systemic. For example, increased cytokine production in the gut may lead to stimulation of resident immune cells at sites of bone, joint, eye and cardiac tissues, resulting in chronic inflammation at those sites. A significant amount of research is underway to further investigate these processes and determine if there is the possibility of modulation of the microbiome as a new therapeutic pathway.

Ciccia, Srinath, Zeng, and Haroon in Chapter 7 link our traditional understanding of the **pathogenesis of AxSpA/AS** to evolving concepts that are emerging as new scientific findings come to light. The chapter starts with the role of *HLA-B27* in AS followed by an introduction to aminopeptidases and other players in antigen processing and presentation. The gut-joint axis is discussed in some detail and finally bone-formation pathways in AS are explored. The hypotheses for the role of *HLA-B27* include an arthritogenic peptide mechanism, a potential role for natural killer cell and their receptors activation, unfolded protein response, and autophagy. The co-association of *HLA-B27* and endoplasmic reticulum aminopeptidases, *ERAP1* and *ERAP2*, which have a role in peptide clipping in preparation for antigen presentation may have a role in pathogenesis. The possibility that a newly discovered gene *Sec16a*, variants of which may lead to differences in *HLA-B27* trafficking to the cell surface may also have a role. It appears likely that intestinal lining pathology/inflammation contributes to axSpA pathophysiology, both due to gut dysbiosis as reviewed in this chapter and Chapter 6 on the gut microbiome, as well as activation of innate and adaptive immune mechanisms, especially involving the TH17 cell pathway and the IL23-IL17 axis. It is unknown at this time if manipulation of the microbiome or these immunologic pathways at the gut level could lead to improvement of axSpA, but these considerations are being researched. Complementing the chapter on bone pathophysiology, Lories' Chapter 8, this chapter provides additional perspective on the roles of bone morphogenetic proteins, the Wnt signaling, Hedgehog, macrophage migratory inhibitory pathways, as well as the role of IL23, IL17, and prostaglandin E2 and E4 in bone remodeling as a pathological process in axSpA.

Why and how does bone ankylosis occur in axSpA? In Chapter 8, Lories details our current understanding about bone pathophysiology. Key pathways for excessive bone formation are the Wnt signaling pathway, bone morphogenetic proteins (BMPs), and the Hedgehog signaling pathway. The balance of Wnt signaling proteins and antagonists such as sclerostin is important in normal bone remodeling; imbalance may contribute to excessive bone formation. BMPs are growth factors that are essential in the pathogenesis of enthesophytes in animal models. In axSpA, their excessive activity may have partly to do with autoantibodies directed against their natural antagonist, noggin. The Hedgehog pathway involves differentiation of chondrocytes into hypertrophic cells, essential for replacement of cartilage by bone. Lories proceeds to explicate the findings and controversies around the role of TNF and IL17 inhibition in controlling pathologic bone formation and ankyloses as well as recent observations about the crucial role that mechanical loading and microtrauma may play in pathologic bone formation.

How do we clinically assess patients with axSpA rigorously in clinical trials? Magrey and Kiltz address our assessment techniques in Chapter 9, starting with the ASAS-OMERACT core set summarization of the clinical domains of axSpA, published in 1999. These include the domains of physical function, pain, spinal mobility, patient global assessment, morning stiffness, fatigue, peripheral joints and entheses, and acute phase reactants. They then proceed to detail the specific measures, many of them patient reported questionnaires such as the Bath Ankylosing Spondylitis Disease Activity Index (BASDAI), and Bath Ankylosing Spondylitis Functional Index (BASFI), and the more recently developed Ankylosing Spondylitis Disease Activity Index (ASDAS), which includes an objective item, either a C-reactive protein (CRP) or Erythrocyte Sedimentation Rate (ESR) value. The patient questions in these composite measures ask about severity of the disease in relation to many of the items in the ASAS-OMERACT core set, including physical function and pain, both in the axial spine and periphery. Quantitative thresholds of disease severity have been defined, e.g., inactive or mild disease activity utilizing the ASDAS, which allows it to be used as a "treat-to-target" measure in clinical trials or clinical practice. Because axSpA can cause impaired mobility, e.g., when spinal ankyloses advances, specific measures of spine and hip mobility are utilized in clinical trials and to a certain extent in clinical practice to document progressive mobility impairment or (hopefully) lack thereof when patients are treated effectively. Specific measures for clinical domains such as enthesitis have been developed and are utilized in clinical trials to document changes in this domain. Newer measures which assess both quality of life and function, such as the ASAS Health Index, have been rigorously developed based on input from patient focus groups, guidance from psychometricians, and testing in patient populations for validation. As assessment tools become more reliable and validated, we can better rely on them to assess outcomes of interest in therapeutic clinical trials, long term observational registries, and to a certain extent, in clinical practice.

Maksymowych and Lambert provide in Chapter 10 an encyclopedic review of **imaging modalities for and findings in axSpA**, including plain radiography, computerized tomography (CT), and MRI. They also address the differential diagnosis from other mimicking conditions, including degenerative arthritis, infection, neoplasm, diffuse idiopathic skeletal hyperostosis, and osteitis condensans ilii. Whereas clearcut radiographic change of sacroiliac joints, including periarticular sclerosis and erosions can be virtually pathognomonic for AS, these findings are often absent or indistinct in early AS and in patients with axSpA who may never develop such changes, and so lack sensitivity for detecting the full spectrum of axSpA. CT scan provides more detailed features of bone anatomy, including cortical changes and erosive change, but is hampered by the problem of radiation exposure in its routine application. Newer CT applications with less radiation exposure hold promise. Advances in MRI scanning, along with generally greater access to this imaging modality have more significantly advanced our ability to diagnose and assess the impact of therapeutic intervention. MRI is able to distinguish soft tissue inflammation and inflammatory lesions in bone unlike any other imaging modality. In addition to standard MRI imaging of select areas such as the sacroiliac joints and spine, newer approaches such as whole body MRI which allows for a broader range of anatomic assessment and dynamic contrast enhanced MRI, allowing for greater detail that is digitally assessed. These advances broaden our imaging ability to assess disease activity and damage. Validated scoring methods for both plain radiography and MRI of the spine and sacroiliac joints are now routinely used in clinical studies to quantitate baseline damage, disease activity, and change with therapy.

Several non-musculoskeltal conditions display close association, both genetically and clinically, with axSpA, **uveitis, IBD and psoriasis.** Kiwalkar, et al., in Chapter 11, describe these conditions and this association both at a translational and clinical level. Such extra-articular manifestations (EAMs) may help with axSpA diagnosis, either because the patient presents to an ophthalmologist, gastroenterologist, or dermatologist respectively, and if musculoskeletal symptoms are also present, that clinician may be the first to suggest that AxSpA is present. Alternatively, a rheumatologist may hear a history or current evidence of one or more of these EAMs, thus increasing confidence that inflammatory back pain symptoms truly represent the presence of axSpA. The concomitant presence of these EAMs also may denote a more severe disease presentation, that leading to different considerations regarding relative intensity of treatment. The prevalence of acute anterior uveitis in axSpA is considered to be in up to a third of patients, varying with the cohort studied. IBD occurs overtly in approximately 5% and psoriasis in approximately 10% of axSpA patients. However, several studies have shown that subtle inflammatory changes can be seen in bowel biopsies of up to 60% of patients with axSpA. Genetic linkages are clearly present. Animal studies have also shown shared inflammatory pathologies in the eye, gut and skin, as well as the aortic root, suggesting a link to another less common EAM, aortic valve dysfunction and cardiac conduction abnormalities in axSpA. Clinical presentation of these EAMs is reviewed as is treatment. Regarding a number of medications, there is overlap between efficacy for both axSpA and the EAM. However, it appears that regarding TNF inhibitor agents, that the monoclonal antibody constructs (infliximab, adalimumab, golimumab, and certolizumab) have superior efficacy compared to the soluble receptor antibody construct (etanercept) in the treatment of these EAMs.

What are the key comorbidities of AxSpA? In Chapter 12, Ward describes comorbidities which are not the more common associated conditions of uveitis, IBD, and psoriasis. Numerous forms of cardiovascular disease may occur, ranging from mildly increased frequency of atherosclerotic vascular disease with attendant myocardial infarction and stroke, to specific conditions such as aortitis, other valvular disorders, conduction abnormalities, and myocardial dysfunction. Animal models of SpA (Chapter 7) demonstrate the model in which resident T cells, influenced by IL23, cause inflammation in enthesial, aortic, and ciliary body tissue, thus predicting valvular and conduction system abnormalities. In the lung, restrictive lung disease and apical fibrosis may occur, as well as obstructive sleep apnea. In the kidney, signs of amyloidosis, IgA nephropathy, and urolithiasis may be present. Osteoporosis is common and may predispose to fractures. Post-traumatic displaced spinal fractures can result in severe neurologic compromise and even death, especially if it occurs in the cervical spine. Neurologic manifestations such as cauda equina syndrome should be considered with atypical neurologic presentations. Fibromyalgia can co-exist with axSpA more frequently than in the general population, possibly related to the influence of chronic pain and inflammation on the pathogenesis of central sensitization. Not only does concomitant fibromyalgia contribute to the overall symptom burden of disease, but it can also distort a patient's subjective evaluation of disease activity, rendering unreliable standard measures of disease activity which include multiple patient-reported elements. These may be falsely amplified, leading the clinician desiring to "treat to target" of remission or of low disease activity to inappropriately switch from one immunomodulatory drug to another, when indeed it is a neuromodulatory treatment for central sensitization which might be more ideally brought to bear on the condition.

Frequently patients ask "What can I do myself, other than medications, to help my condition?". In Chapter 13, Ozgocmen reviews the evidence for **non-pharmacologic therapeutic approaches** to axSpA. Although this is an area less amenable to carefully controlled research, there is a substantial evidence base for the benefits of physical therapy, exercise, patient education, and other approaches that should be part of all multidisciplinary therapeutic programs. In general, when comparing outcomes of patients involved in either group or individual education and exercise programs are compared with patients not involved in these modalities, the former have better functional and disease activity measures than those not receiving such treatment. These non-pharmacologic therapies constitute an important pillar of treatment in all sets of treatment recommendations for axSpA.

Although much of the focus on treatment of axSpA is on the efficacy and safety of biologic therapies, there remains an important role for older, simpler, and less costly medicines such as **non-steroidal anti-inflammatory durgs (NSAIDs), as well as a potential emerging role for newer non-biologic medications** that target specific molecular pathways operant in axSpA, such as the Janus Kinase (JAK) inhibitors. In Chapter 14, Proft and Poddubnyy, review the evidence for and role of non-biologic pharmacologic agents in AxSpA treatment. A cornerstone of various treatment recommendations is an adequate trial of NSAIDs, since these may be helpful for treating symptoms, either as monotherapy or ultimately in combination with other medicines. Although inexpensive and widely available, NSAID therapy does need to be monitored for gastrointestinal and renal adverse effects, and a small cardiovascular risk profile must be kept in mind in assessing the patient's overall cardiac risk (blood pressure, lipid profile, weight, family history, etc.). There is controversy about whether NSAIDs may have a disease-modifying effect for axSpA radiographic progression, with one studiy suggesting such benefit and another not. Although widely used for symptom and disease modifying treatment in RA, the traditional oral immunomodulatory medicines methotrexate, sulfasalazine, and leflunomide are not effective for the axial manifestations of axSpA. There is some evidence for potential benefit of sulfasalazine in peripheral manifestations. Newer "targeted synthetic" drugs such as apremilast, a PDE4 inhibitor, and tofacitinib, a JAK inhibitor, which are effective in PsA/psoriasis and RA/PsA respectively, have been studied. Apremilast failed to show benefit in a phase 3 AS study. Tofacitinib showed benefit in AS and is now being studied in phase 3. Other JAK inhibitors with differing targeted specificities will also be studied. There is little role for sustained oral glucocorticoid use, but selective glucocorticoid injections can be useful for peripheral joints and entheses as well as the sacroiliac joint.

The advent of **"biologic" immunotherapy** for immunologic diseases such as RA, PsA and psoriasis, axSpA, and IBD clearly revolutionized our ability to achieve more substantial responses, including sustained remission and low disease activity. However, potentially significant safety issues require close monitoring of therapy and the cost of these medicines has created a challenge of affordability for health care systems globally. Van den Bosch, Carron and Mease review the history of studies and application of these drugs in practice for axSpA in Chapter 15. The term "biologic" has been coined because these drugs are complex proteins, typically manufactured in mammalian cells such as Chinese Hamster Ovary (CHO) cells, which mimic our own immunologic proteins, immunoglobulins, which bind to specific pro-inflammatory molecules or their receptors, thus blocking their activity and down-regulating immune cell activation. Building on the knowledge that certain cytokines and cellular pathways, particularly TNF and IL17 have been implicated in driving inflammation in conditions such as axSpA, inhibitors of these cytokines have been developed for subcutaneous or intravenous administration. Clinical studies have shown consistently positive results in improving measures of disease activity, function and quality of life in treated groups relative to placebo sometimes within weeks but typically by 12–24 weeks of initiation. Although serious adverse events can occur with these therapies, particularly serious infection, including opportunistic infection such as tuberculosis, these adverse effects can often be adequately treated and mitigated, yielding an overall positive benefit to cost balance. Less clear is whether these drugs can alter gradual spinal ankylosis as measured radiographically. These changes are typically gradual enough that a difference between treatment and placebo cannot be discerned in the placebo-controlled phase of a trial, which ethically is limited in time to between 12 and 24 weeks. On the other hand, long term registry studies suggest that if intervention with a TNF inhibitor is utiliized early in disease course that some inhibition of structural damage may be achieved. In addition to TNF inhibitors, an emerging class of IL17 inhibitors has also been shown to be effective in treating axSpA. Most of the studies documenting efficacy have been conducted in patients with AS. More recently, studies in patients with non-radiographic axSpA, i.e., those without evidence of damage in the sacroiliac joints, have demonstrated similar efficacy as in AS. Approvals of these agents for this latter indication have already occurred in Europe and some of the other parts of the world; approval in the United States is pending. Because these agents are proteins, it is possible that a treated patient may develop anti-drug antibodies to the therapeutic agent, sometimes resulting in blocking the ability of the drug to achieve full effect. Fortunately, this phenomenon is uncommon. Some agents, such as infliximab, are more likely to have neutralizing antibodies develop, leading to recommendation to use methotrexate with the drug to reduce antibody formation. Studies regarding this phenomenon in axSpA have been mixed and at the moment, it is not routinely recommended that any of these agents need to be given with methotrexate to avoid immunogenicity. Strategic trials to determine the value of "treat-to-target" of remission or low disease activity are underway as are studies to determine if drug tapering or cessation may be considered for patients who have achieved remission.

Treatment recommendations for diseases are important for aiding clinicians seeking expert advice on optimal treatment approaches to axSpA, as well as providing an evidence-based framework to inform payors such as government agencies and insurers. Kiwalkar, Deodhar and Sieper in Chapter 16 discuss the methodology behind development of treatment recommendations and then detail the two major sets of such recommendations for axSpA. The ASAS-EULAR recommendations have been long-standing and have been updated as new therapy options as well as more evidence for older therapies have emerged. More recently, the American College of Rheumatology (ACR) teamed with the Spondyloarthritis Research and Treatment Network (SPARTAN) and Spondyloarthritis Association of America (SAA) to generate a set of treatment recommendations. Both

sets of treatment recommendations are overall similar, since the same evidence base was used for both. Subtly different methodologies result in subtle differences in presentation of recommendations. Both recommend a background of patient education, physical therapy and exercise in addition to pharmacologic treatment. Both recommend initiation of therapy with a trial of NSAIDs. Both do not recommend use of conventional synthetic drugs such as methotrexate, sulfasalazine or leflunomide for axial manifestations. Both recommend treatment with TNF inhibitors for those with inadequate response to NSAIDs. The updated ASAS-EULAR guidelines (2016) suggest moving on to an IL-17 inhibitor after inadequate response or toxicity with TNF inhibitors. The ACR-SPARTAN-SAA recommendations (2015) do not mention IL-17 inhibitors since the evidence for these was not published in time for their inclusion in the recommendations. There are specific call-outs for issues such as concomitant uveitis and IBD, notation of when glucocorticoid injections may be utilized, and sections wherein specific drugs are not recommended. The updated ASAS-EULAR recommendations address emerging "treat-to-target" strategies of aiming for a quantized (by disease activity measure) state of remission, or low disease activity if remission cannot be achieved. Additionally, these updated recommendations address cost-containment and the potential for tapering therapy. Both sets of recommendations stress the importance of shared decision-making between clinician and patient regarding therapy options and discussion about risk and cost considerations. It should be emphasized that these are not rigid guidelines, since depending on a variety of factors including differences in access due to differences in country or individual insurance programs, socioeconomic factors, differences in patient preferences vis a vis risk, mode of administration, and other factors, these should be considered as flexible recommendations based on available evidence. Furthermore, given the pace of advance in our understanding of disease and drug discovery, recommendations are typically out of date when they are published, so periodic updates with appropriate changes are to be expected. In fact, the updated ACR-SPARTAN-SAA recommendations have just been submitted for publication.

Treatments for AxSpA, especially biologic therapies, are expensive. Such treatment constitutes an increasing percentage of the health care budgets for governments, insurers, and individuals. Is this cost justified? In Chapter 17, Boonen and Webers address this question by introducing the increasingly sophisticated methodology of **cost-benefit analysis of treatments** and describing the efforts to provide this analysis for axSpA. A standard clinical trial establishes the immediate "cost" (safety considerations) and "benefit" (reduction of symptoms, improved function and quality of life, including work productivity and participation in meaningful life activities). But this does not address the broader question of societal financial cost and benefit of individual treatments to society. Boonen and Webers introduce the field of broad economic evaluation and quantitative assessment of benefit using Quality Adjusted Life Year (QALY) analysis which takes into account financial cost of treatment, benefit as measured by improved function and quality of life, work productivity, and if possible, health care cost savings realized by better disease outcomes. She then reviews studies done in axSpA with individual medications, which generally show a positive benefit, especially when societal benefits are weighed, relative to cost. Such evidence and research is critical as an increasing number of patients are being diagnosed with axSpA due to improved understanding about the spectrum of disease, growing awareness of previously undiagnosed patients, increased access to drugs in parts of the world with expanding economies, and more therapeutic options becoming available, leading to increased treatment and its attendant costs. Cost containment will arise from increasing use of biosimilars and other methods of competitive drug price reduction, and utilization of treatment strategies such as dose reduction or discontinuation once remission is achieved. It will be important that payors have access to quantitative cost-benefit research to make informed decisions about treatment access.

Patient education and self-management are important components of axSpA care. Numerous studies have shown that the more educated the patient is about their condition, the better the outcomes. Caballero-Uribe and Khan in Chapter 18 espouse this concept and speak to (1) the role of traditional patient service organizations to promote awareness and education about axSpA both through internet-based education and in person educational activities, and (2) the increasing role of social media and "digital health" methodologies in raising educational awareness about axSpA. Along with increased online educational content and patient-interactive options comes the potential for promulgation of misinformation about unsubstantiated remedies which confuse the patient and can lead to distrust between patients and clinicians when the latter discredit such misinformation. These exchanges take time and sensitivity, which may be in short supply in today's busy clinical care environment. It seems unlikely that the patient-clinician relationship based on trust and ongoing care will be replaced by "Dr. Google" in the near future.

Science doesn't stand still. Although we hope that this textbook provides a comprehensive overview of all aspects of axSpA, from clinical features to diagnosis, to epidemiology, to pathophysiology, to assessment and treatment, we humbly recognize that new observations about disease state, immunology, and treatment will be forthcoming. For now, we trust that these chapters will fulfill a current educational need for understanding about this important condition.

CHAPTER 2

Clinical Features, Physical Findings, and Diagnosis of Axial Spondyloarthritis

MUHAMMAD ASIM KHAN, MD, FRCP, MACP, MACR

INTRODUCTION

The term spondyloarthritis (SpA), previously called spondyloarthropathy, defines a group of interrelated chronic inflammatory rheumatic disorders that share several clinical features, as well as genetic predisposing factors, especially *HLA-B*27*, a normal gene that is also present in a small percentage of the general population.[1,2] Its epidemiology is discussed in Chapter 3. The primary underlying pathologic process is enthesitis, defined as inflammation at the sites of bony insertions of tendons and ligaments,[3–5] and associated osteitis and, to a lesser extent, synovitis (see Fig. 2.1). Enthesis is now more broadly defined as "enthesis organ" that also includes the adjacent fibrocartilage, bursa, fat pad, deeper fascia, and trabecular bone because they all function collectively to carry out a common task, namely anchorage and resistance to physical stress.[5,6] Because of the ubiquitous nature of enthesis organs, there is a diversity of resultant clinical manifestations that range from enthesitis, on one hand, to full ankylosis (see Fig. 2.1). The pathogenesis is driven by interaction between a genetically primed host immune system and the gut microbiome, as detailed in Chapters 5 and 6.

As explained further in Chapter 4, SpA patients have now been subclassified, based on their predominant symptoms, into two broad subgroups (see Fig. 2.2):

- A predominantly axial form called "axial SpA" (abbreviated as "axSpA"), best exemplified by patients suffering from ankylosing spondylitis (AS), the prototype of SpA that has afflicted mankind since antiquity. The term AS is a more restrictive form of axSpA that requires X-ray evidence of sacroiliitis.
- A predominantly peripheral form called peripheral SpA (abbreviated as "pSpA") that includes psoriatic arthritis (PsA), enteropathic arthritis (inflammatory arthritis associated with Crohn disease or ulcerative colitis), reactive arthritis, and undifferentiated forms of SpA (abbreviated as "uSpA").

Axial Spondyloarthritis

This book, as its title indicates, deals primarily with axSpA, and the patients suffering from this clinical entity have been further subclassified into two subgroups:

- Patients that show X-ray evidence of sacroiliitis have been termed "radiographic axSpA" (abbreviated as "r-axSpA"), a term that is largely synonymous with AS, as defined by the modified New York criteria.[10] Most of the existing knowledge about axSpA as an entity comes from the long-standing literature primarily based on patients suffering from AS.[1,7–9]
- Patients with "spondylitis disease without radiographic evidence of sacroiliitis,"[11] currently renamed as "nonradiographic axSpA'" (abbreviated as "nr-axSpA") (Figs. 2.2 and 2.3). These patients tend to have less pronounced inflammatory signs and predominance of females.[12–15] Not all of them progress to r-axSpA/AS.

This concept of the two subtypes of axSpA has helped in its earlier recognition and treatment, emphasized the wider disease spectrum, and enhanced clinical research.[12–15] It has been proposed that for diagnostic purposes the term axSpA be used, whereas the terms nr-axSpA and AS be used for disease classification and not as separate diagnoses, unless there is a meaningful medical reason to do so.[15]

CLINICAL PRESENTATION

This chapter is based, in part, on the author's earlier publications on this subject.[1,2,7,16–18] The disease symptoms usually start insidiously at young age (late adolescence and early adulthood), ranging from childhood (age 9 years and older) to age 45 years, with the mean age of onset in developed countries hovering around age 23 years. There are rare occurrences of onset of symptoms

Axial Spondyloarthritis. https://doi.org/10.1016/B978-0-323-56800-5.00002-3

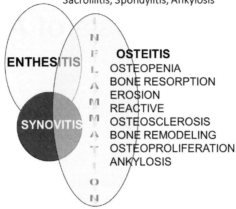

Clinical and Pathological Features of SpA

Enthesitis, Arthritis, Tendonitis, Tenosynovitis, Periostitis, Dactylitis, Sacroiliitis, Spondylitis, Ankylosis

ENTHESITIS

SYNOVITIS

INFLAMMATION

OSTEITIS
OSTEOPENIA
BONE RESORPTION
EROSION
REACTIVE
OSTEOSCLEROSIS
BONE REMODELING
OSTEOPROLIFERATION
ANKYLOSIS

FIG. 2.1 Clinical and pathologic features of SpA.

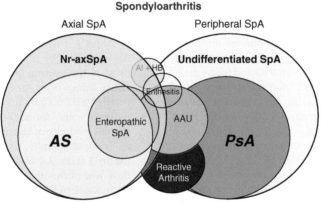

Spondyloarthritis

Axial SpA   Peripheral SpA

Nr-axSpA   **Undifferentiated SpA**

AI+HB

Enthesitis

Enteropathic SpA   AAU

AS   **PsA**

Reactive Arthritis

SpA = Spondyloarthritis, Nr-axSpA = non-radiographic axial SpA, PsA = psoriatic arthritis, AAU = acute anterio uveitis, AI+HB = aortic incompetence plus heart block.

Ozgocmen S, Khan MA. *Curr Rheum Report.* 2012;14(5):409-14

FIG. 2.2 The various forms of SpA have been divided into predominantly axial and predominantly peripheral subgroups. (From Elyan M, Khan MA. Diagnosing ankylosing spondylitis. *J Rheumatol Suppl.* 2006;78:12–23.)

after age 45 years.[19] The patients typically present to their healthcare provider with chronic low back pain and stiffness resulting from inflammation of their sacroiliac joints and/or lumbar spine. However, these symptoms at onset can sometimes be subtle or fleeting.[1,16] Other patients may first present with symptoms resulting from enthesitis, synovitis, and/or involvement of extraskeletal organs, such as the eye, gut, or skin.

Constitutional Symptoms

These include malaise, anorexia, weight loss, or low-grade fever; and they are relatively more commonly observed among patients with more severe disease, childhood onset, and especially in developing countries.[1,7,16] Moreover, fatigue can be a common complaint; it can sometimes be severe and is usually due to active disease and/or inadequate and interrupted sleep as a result of back pain and stiffness.

Axial Pain

The back pain is usually insidious in onset, dull in character, difficult to localize, and initially felt deep in the gluteal region. It can be intermittent and may affect one side or alternate from one side to the other

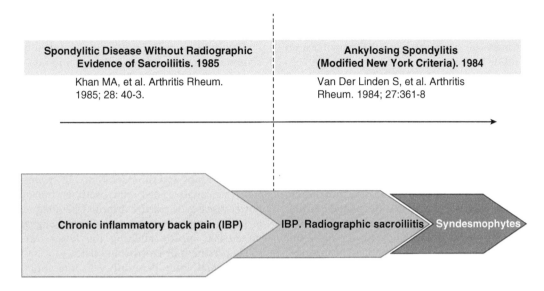

Spondylitic Disease Without Radiographic Evidence of Sacroiliitis. 1985	Ankylosing Spondylitis (Modified New York Criteria). 1984
Khan MA, et al. Arthritis Rheum. 1985; 28: 40-3.	Van Der Linden S, et al. Arthritis Rheum. 1984; 27:361-8

Chronic inflammatory back pain (IBP) | IBP. Radiographic sacroiliitis | Syndesmophytes

Axial Spondyloarthritis

Rudwaleit M, Khan MA, Sieper J. The challenge of Diagnosis and classification of early AS. Do we need new criteria? Arthritis Rheum 2005 Apr;52(4):1000-8

FIG. 2.3 The spectrum of predominantly axSpA: subdivided into "spondylitic disease without radiographic evidence of sacroiliitis," now called nr-axSpA, and r-axSpA that is virtually identical with AS. Not everyone suffering from nr-axSpA progresses to AS, and not every patient with r-axSpA/AS develops syndesmophytes and spinal ankylosis. (Adapted from Khan MA. *Ankylosing Spondylitis—Axial Spondyloarthritis*. West Islip, NY: Professional Communications Inc.(PCI); 2016:1–333.)

in the very early stages before becoming bilateral and/or persistent. Such alternating buttock pain, if present, is a helpful clue in early disease and reflects the fluctuating nature of early inflammation of sacroiliac joints in axSpA.[1,16] Symptoms gradually spread to involve the lumbar spine. Pain and stiffness in thoracic and cervical spine tend to develop later, but they may occasionally be the presenting complaint, especially in women. Tenderness and stiffness of the paraspinal muscles may also be a prominent symptom.

This inflammatory back pain (IBP) has been defined by ASAS criteria as chronic back pain (i.e., duration longer than 3 months) that has at least four of the following five features: an onset before the age of 40 years, insidious onset, improvement with physical activity, no improvement with rest, and night pain that improves upon getting up from bed in the morning and moving about or exercising[20,21] (Table 2.1). It must be kept in mind that among patients with undiagnosed chronic back pain, this definition of IBP does not always mean that an underlying inflammatory condition exists because it has roughly 80%

TABLE 2.1
Features That Suggest Inflammatory Back Pain

Insidious onset	Odds ratio = 12.7
Pain at night (with improvement on getting up)	Odds ratio = 20.4
Age at onset <40 years	Odds ratio = 9.9
Improvement with exercise	Odds ratio = 23.1
No improvement with rest	Odds ratio = 7.7

If at least four out of the above five parameters are met, the criteria had a sensitivity of 77% and specificity of 91.7% in the patients participating in the initial analysis, and 79.6% sensitivity and 72.4% specificity in the validation cohort. Note that these sensitivity and specificity values refer to the presence of IBP, not to the diagnosis of axSpA. Please note that the five parameters are listed in a sequence so that the use of their initial (bold) letter results in a mnemonic IPAIN (or iPAIN to go along with the popular names iPHONE or iPAD) to help recall the five features of inflammatory back pain[107]. The odds ratios of the five parameters are listed to show that pain at night that improves on getting up from bed in the morning and improvement with exercise are the most useful. From Sieper J, et al. The Assessment of SpondyloArthritis international Society (ASAS) handbook: a guide to assess spondyloarthritis. *Ann Rheum Dis.* 2009;68(suppl II):ii1–ii44.

sensitivity and 74% specificity (Table 2.1). This means that approximately 20% (100 – 80) of axSpA patients may not meet the criteria because they may have no or only subtle back symptoms. Conversely, some 26% (100 – 74) of patients with noninflammatory spinal conditions, such as degenerative disc disease and facet joint osteoarthritis, may label their chronic back pain with inflammatory descriptors.

Some patients may primarily complain of pain, stiffness and tenderness of their back, chest and/or shoulder girdles, which may worsen on exposure to cold or humidity, often accompanied by fatigue, and disturbed sleep.[1,7,16] Women are two to three times more likely to have widespread axial and peripheral articular pain than men.[22,23] Such clinical presentations may sometimes be confused with fibromyalgia and result in delayed diagnosis and inappropriate treatment.[23] Depression and anxiety are not uncommon among patients with more severe and active disease with chronic pain, declining functional capacity, worsening deformity, and sleep disturbance.[7,17,24]

Chest pain that worsens on coughing, sneezing, or deep inspiration can sometimes be the presenting complaint. It should be differentiated from the pain of pleuritis and pericarditis, and it results from inflammation of the facet, costovertebral, and costotransverse joints, which can slowly, over many years, diminish chest expansion. Anterior chest wall can become painful and tender due to enthesitis of sternoclavicular, manubriosternal, and costosternal junctions.[25]

Hip and Shoulder Joint Involvement

The hip and shoulder joints are affected in some stage of the disease in one-third of the patients and occasionally may be the presenting location of symptoms.[1,16] Involvement of these joints has not been systematically evaluated in patients with nr-axSpA but seems to be less common and less severe. The hip joint involvement is typically bilateral and progressive, leading to concentric joint space narrowing. It is relatively more common among those with juvenile AS. The pain is felt in the groin, but sometimes in the anterior or medial thigh or the knee (referred pain). It leads to severe functional impairment and worse overall prognosis because of progressive limitation of motion and development of fixed flexion contracture of the hip joints. Such patients have a characteristic rigid gait, with the knees somewhat bent as the patient tries to maintain an upright posture.[16] In advanced stages, there is severe disuse atrophy and weakness of thigh and buttock muscles. If hip joint involvement has not occurred within the first 10 years of the disease, it is quite unlikely that it will occur later,

although some degree of flexion contracture of the hip joints may be noted at later stages of the disease.

Enthesitis at the shoulder girdle (glenohumeral, acromioclavicular, and sternoclavicular joints) tends to result in relatively milder limitations as compared with involvement of the hip joints.[16] Inflammation primarily of the glenohumeral joint is rare but can lead to progressive loss of motion and ankylosis.

Peripheral Arthritis

Involvement of peripheral joints (defined as limb joints other than hips and shoulder joints) in "primary" disease (i.e., unassociated with psoriasis, inflammatory bowel disease, or reactive arthritis) is infrequent. It is usually asymmetric, monoarticular or oligoarticular, nonerosive, mostly affecting the lower extremities, rarely persistent or erosive, and tends to resolve without residual joint deformity.[16,26] Intermittent knee effusions may occasionally be the presenting manifestation, especially in patients with juvenile SpA. Persistent inflammation of the knee joint is rare but can lead to progressive loss of motion and ankylosis.

Enthesitis, Dactylitis, Tendinitis, and Tenosynovitis

Peripheral enthesitis is most common at sites that are subject to greater physical stress, and it usually manifests with localized pain, stiffness, and/or tenderness with or without swelling.[16] Patients with axSpA of juvenile onset or those who have concomitant psoriasis, inflammatory bowel disease, or reactive arthritis tend to have more often or more prominent peripheral arthritis, enthesitis, tendinitis, bursitis, tenosynovitis, or dactylitis, as compared with patients with "primary" axSpA.[7,16,26-28] Enthesitis involving the feet, including Achilles tendinitis and plantar fasciitis, is a very helpful clinical finding observed in approximately one-third of patients with axSpA, is even more common in Mexico and some of the other developing countries.[7,16]

Enthesitis can also cause pain and tenderness over the spinous processes, costochondral and chondrosternal junctions, the manubriosternal and sternoclavicular joints, iliac crests, ischial tuberosities, greater trochanters, anserine bursae, patellae, and the infrapatellar tendon insertion into the tibial tubercles. Some patients, especially those with juvenile onset of SpA, can present with enthesitis (called enthesitis-related arthritis or ERA) before the onset of inflammatory back pain.

Dactylitis describes the diffuse swelling of one or more of the fingers and/or toes resulting in the classical appearance of "sausage digit." It is usually caused by the

TABLE 2.2 Features That Suggest axSpA
Inflammatory back pain
Alternating buttock pain
Enthesitis
Acute anterior uveitis
Peripheral arthritis (usually asymmetric and in lower extremities)
Family history of SpA
Psoriasis
Dactylitis
Inflammatory bowel disease (Crohn disease or ulcerative colitis)
Good symptomatic response to NSAIDs
Elevated CRP and/or ESR
HLA-B27 positivity
Imaging features

The abovementioned features[29, 52] can be rearranged as shown below to create a mnemonic SPINEACHE[107] to help easily recall these features that suggest axSpA.

- Sausage digits (dactylitis)
- Psoriasis-positive family history of SpA
- Inflammatory back pain
- NSAID good response
- Enthesitis (heel)
- Arthritis
- Crohn/colitis—CRP elevation
- HLA-B27
- Eye (uveitis)

combination of synovitis, tenosynovitis, and enthesitis of the fingers and toes. It may occur in all forms of SpA but is more common in psoriatic arthritis, and can rarely be observed in patient suffering from other illnesses, such as infection, sarcoidosis, and gouty arthritis.

The clinical tools to assess and monitor the various clinical features discussed above have been published elsewhere[29–32] and further discussed in Chapter 9. The clinical features that suggest the presence of axSpA are listed in Table 2.2.

PHYSICAL FINDINGS

A careful and thorough physical examination is essential to look for signs that support the diagnosis and also to determine the disease extent and severity.[28] They may, however, provide only imprecise clues at early

disease state but are very much aided by imaging of sacroiliac joints and spine. A detailed, well-illustrated handbook to assess physical examination and imaging, has been published by ASAS.[29] The examination should include observation of the patient's posture and gait, before examining the sacroiliac joints and the spine. Clinical detection of enthesitis and dactylitis in the feet requires examining the feet (with shoes and socks removed) for local swelling and tenderness and also making the patient walk on tip toes and then heels on a hard floor, while holding the patient to prevent fall.[7,28]

The typically involved sites in axSpA are deep structures that do not often demonstrate visible clinical signs of inflammation. Abnormalities on physical findings may be subtle or absent in early stages of the disease. However, inflamed sacroiliac joints and spine may often show tenderness on direct pressure. One may also elicit pain in the sacroiliac area indirectly by maneuvers that physically stress these joints, as shown in Fig. 2.4. The patient is asked to lie supine on a firm examination table, and the examiner applies downward pressure on flexed knee, with the hip joint flexed, abducted, and externally rotated (forms a "number 4" by placing the ankle on the contralateral knee as shown in A.1 segment of this figure). This test is called Patrick test and also FABERE test (because it involves flexion, abduction, external rotation, and extension of the hip joint). A positive test will elicit pain in the ipsilateral sacroiliac area. This test also evaluates the hip joint because pain in the groin or limited range of motion may indicate hip joint involvement. The test is then repeated on the contralateral side. Non-inflammatory sacroiliac disease and iliopsoas spasms may produce a false-positive result.

The sacroiliac joints can also be stressed by lateral pelvic compression test (A.2 segment of Fig. 2.4); the patient lying on his/her side on a firm examining table and the examiner presses down on the iliac crest on the iliac crest. Occurrence of sacroiliac area pain on both or either side suggests presence of sacroiliitis. Another way to elicit sacroiliac pain is by applying downward pressure over anterior superior iliac spine bilaterally with the patient lying on his/her back.

Gaenslen test, as shown in B segment of Fig. 2.4, involves forced maximal flexion of one hip joint, with hyperextension of the other, while the patient is lying on his/her back with the hip joints resting at the end of the examining table. Occurrence of sacroiliac area pain suggests presence of sacroiliitis. The test is then repeated on the contralateral side.

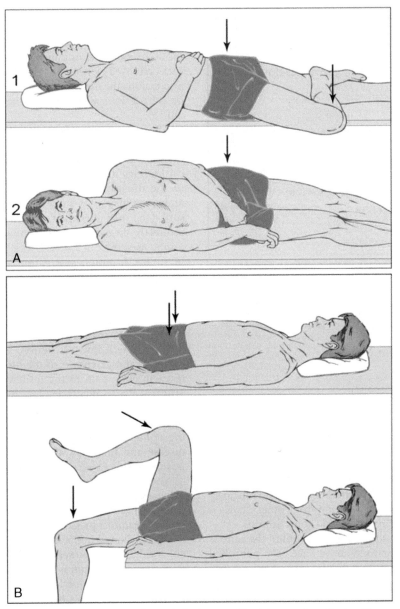

FIG. 2.4 Physical maneuvers that may elicit pain in the sacroiliac joint area in patients with sacroiliitis. Details are discussed in the text. (From Khan MA, Spondyloarthropathies. In: Hunder G, ed. *Atlas of Rheumatology*. Philadelphia: Current Medicine; 2005:151–180.)

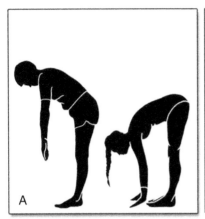 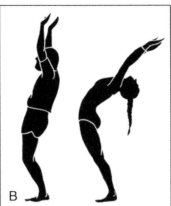 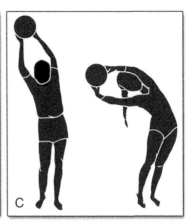

FIG. 2.5 Spinal mobility of an AS patient is compared with that of a healthy physical therapist (Courtesy Heinz Baumberger). (From Khan MA. *Ankylosing Spondylitis—Axial Spondyloarthritis*. West Islip, NY: Professional Communications Inc.(PCI); 2016:1–333.)

Clinical measures of spinal mobility are discussed in Chapter 9 and are well described and illustrated in the ASAS handbook.[29] The spine should be examined to look for flattened lower back due to loss of the lumbar lordosis and for any impaired spinal flexibility. Loss of hyperextension and lateral flexion (Fig. 2.5) is generally noticeable earlier than loss of forward flexion. Pain and stiffness in the cervical spine are generally a late finding, but occasionally they can occur in the early stages of the disease, especially in women. A few patients may have recurrent severe episodes of stiff neck (torticollis) in early stages. Maximal forward flexion of normal cervical spine should result in the chin almost touching the anterior chest, whereas full cervical extension should result in the chin becoming higher than the ear (Fig. 2.5). Involvement of the cervical spine results in a gradual and progressive decrease of these movements. The tests for checking limitation of axial rotation and lateral flexion and for measuring forward stooping of the cervical spine are discussed in Chapter 9.

Limitation of chest expansion resulting from involvement of costovertebral and costotransverse joints can be an early physical finding in some patients, but severe limitation is typically a late physical finding along with exaggerated thoracic kyphosis. Limitation of spinal mobility is a better clinical indicator of axSpA than limitation of chest expansion. Although both of these abnormalities are not specific for axSpA, they are very useful for assessing the extent of disease after the diagnosis has been established, and for long-term monitoring.[31]

Range of motion of the hip and shoulder joints should be measured. Flexion contracture of the hip joint can be easily detected by having the patient lie on a firm examining table and flexing one hip joint maximally to bring out the contracture in the contralateral hip joint (Fig. 2.6). Shoulder joint involvement is often relatively mild, and any resulting limitation of motion can be easily detected by asking the patient to reach upto upper back, as explained in the legend for Fig. 2.7. Extremities should be examined for synovitis of peripheral joints, and enthesitis in the feet[32], and at other sites, such as the spinal processes, iliac crests, ischial tuberosities, greater trochanters, patellar insertions, and tibial tubercle. Fingers and toes should be inspected for nail changes and also for tenosynovitis and dactylitis that can result in "sausage digits."

Examination should also include evaluation of the temporomandibular, acromioclavicular, and sternoclavicular joints. Temporomandibular joint involvement may manifest with jaw pain, stiffness, tenderness, and inability to fully open the mouth. It is usually associated with more severe disease, and milder degrees of involvement may be underrecognized.[33]

Skin should be examined thoroughly for signs of psoriasis (in any of its forms: plaque, guttate, pustular, inverse, and erythrodermic) and other skin lesions, such as erythema nodosum, hidradenitis suppurativa, and acne conglobata. Common sites of psoriatic lesions include the scalp, elbows, knees, and gluteal cleft, but palms and nails can be also involved. "Hidden psoriasis" should be looked for in the intertriginous areas,

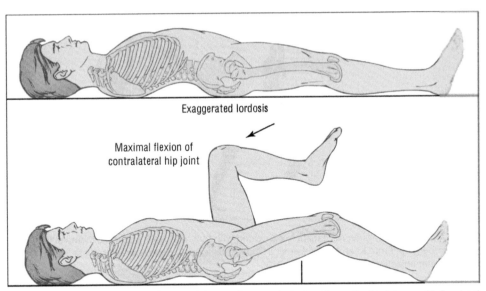

FIG. 2.6 Fixed flexion deformity of the hip joint can be revealed when the patient is lying on his/her back on a firm examining table, and the contralateral hip joint is maximally flexed to eliminate the effect of any compensatory exaggeration of lumbar lordosis. (From Khan MA, Spondyloarthropathies. In: Hunder G, ed. *Atlas of Rheumatology*. Philadelphia: Current Medicine; 2005:151–180.)

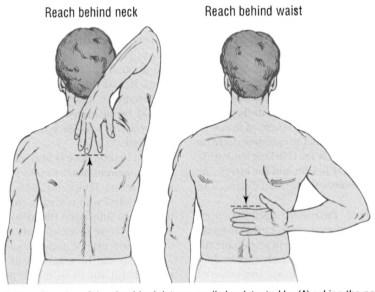

FIG. 2.7 Limitation of motion of the shoulder joint can easily be detected by (A) asking the patient to raise the arm up and maximally reach down behind the neck and (B) internal rotation of the shoulder joint and reach up along the spine as high as possible. In individuals with normal range of motion of the shoulder joint, these points overlap, but not in those with limited range of motion, as shown in this figure. (From Khan MA, Spondyloarthropathies. In: Hunder G, ed. *Atlas of Rheumatology*. Philadelphia: Current Medicine; 2005:151–180.)

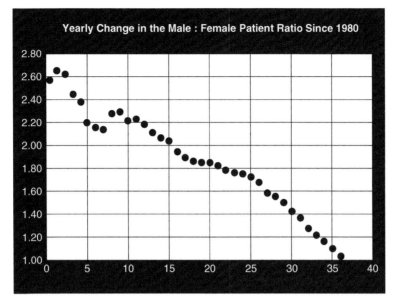

FIG. 2.8 Gradual progressive improvement in recognition of axSpA since 1980 in Switzerland, resulting in equal ratio between males and females by December 2016. (From Baumberger H, Khan MA. SAT0417 Gradual progressive change to equal prevalence of ankylosing spondylitis among males and females in Switzerland: data from the swiss ankylosing spondylitis society (SVMB). *Ann Rheum Dis*. 2017;76(suppl 2):929.)

ear canals, and umbilicus. Nail pitting, discoloration, and onycholysis also suggest psoriasis. Patients with chronic diarrhea or other gastrointestinal symptoms would need gastrointestinal evaluation for chronic inflammatory bowel disease.

The eyes should be examined for signs that may suggest current or past evidence of anterior uveitis. Patients with acute anterior uveitis require prompt referral to an ophthalmologist for evaluation (slit lamp examination) and treatment. Patients with recurring uveitis, especially those who receive no or inadequate treatment, may develop cataracts and synechiae (adhesions of iris anteriorly to the cornea or posteriorly to the lens that may become more noticeable on dilatation of the pupils). See Chapter 11 for further discussion about uveitis.

Cardiopulmonary, neurologic, and other nonrheumatologic involvements and co-morbidities listed in Table 2.3 are discussed in detail in Chapter 12.

Disease Occurrence in Women

Historically, AS/axSpA was wrongly considered to be a predominantly male disease and was underrecognized in women.[34] However, more recent data and epidemiologic studies show almost equal prevalence, especially among patients with nr-axSpA.[35] A very recent study from Switzerland observed that over the past four decades, the estimated disease prevalence in males and females has gradually equalized[36] (Fig. 2.8).

There is no difference in the age of onset, but women generally suffer from a longer delay in diagnosis.[37] They are more likely to present with "atypical" features, such as pain and stiffness along with tenderness due to enthesitis in the upper back (and interscapular and shoulder regions), chest, and neck, which can sometimes precede the onset of typical inflammatory low back pain, and are also a little less likely to possess *HLA-B*27* than men.[7,29,34,38] For all these reasons and also because of a higher frequency of enthesitis, women with axSpA may often be misdiagnosed to be suffering from fibromyalgia. No gender-specific diagnostic algorithm has yet been proposed.[39]

Despite the fact that axSpA is generally more severe in males (higher Bath Ankylosing Spondylitis Radiology Index (BASRI) and modified Stoke Ankylosing Spondylitis Spine Scores (mSASSS)), the overall disease burden and functional outcome (as analyzed by studying disease activity (BASDAI) and quality of life (AsQol) scores are significantly higher in women.[34] This is possibly due to a longer delay in their diagnosis, slower spinal fusion, and significantly less responsiveness and/or adherence to the prescribed treatment.[34] Moreover, women more often have associated psoriasis,

---

TABLE 2.3
Rheumatological and extra-rheumatological manifestations and comorbidities of AS/axSpA

- The wide spectrum of rheumatological manifestations includes enthesitis, arthritis, tendonitis, tenosynovitis, periostitis, dactylitis, sacroiliitis, spondylitis, ankylosis, and osteopenia/osteoporosis. Spinal ankylosis is associated with a high risk of fracture, with or without associated neurological complications. Atlantoaxial subluxation is a rare complication.

- The most common extra-rheumatological manifestation is acute anterior uveitis; one or more episodes occur in anywhere from 25% to 45 % of patients.

- Other extra-rheumatological manifestations include psoriasis, chronic inflammatory bowel disease (ulcerative colitis and Crohn's disease), and subclinical gut inflammation.

- Restrictive chest expansion is very common. It can impair pulmonary function and can be associated with interstitial pulmonary fibrosis and very rarely apical fibrocystic disease. There is diminished quality of sleep, and obstructive sleep apnea is more common than in the general population.

- Impairment of cardiovascular function as a result of arthrosclerosis, coronary artery disease, cardiac diastolic dysfunction, ectopic beats, aortic insufficiency with or without partial or complete heart block can occur. There is an increased risk of hypertension and possible other NSAID-associated side effects.

- IgA nephropathy has rarely been reported, renal amyloidosis has become very uncommon, and renal toxicity can rarely occur in association with NSAID therapy.

- Subarachnoidal cysts with or without associated neurological symptoms, in extreme cases, cauda equina syndrome can occur as a rare and late complication.

Data from Refs 7 and 17.

and inflammatory bowel disease, whereas acute anterior uveitis is more prevalent in male patients.[34] There are also differences in levels of some of the cytokines (such as TNF, IL-6, IL-17, and IL-18), and immunologic and genetic responses.[34] Hormonal status and fertility are normal, and pregnancy does not improve the symptoms of axSpA (there is either no change or only temporary aggravation). Childbirth is normal in the absence of severe hip disease.

Juvenile SpA

Juvenile SpA (onset before the age of 16 years) mostly occurs in boys aged 9 years or above, and the common presentation is that of a seronegative oligoarthritis of the lower extremities, frequently with enthesitis.[40,41] Recent epidemiologic studies suggest that this disease may be much more prevalent than previously realized, and the clinical presentations may be defined as uSpA, ERA, seronegative enthesitis and arthritis (SEA), or juvenile axSpA.[42,43] These patients show strong association with HLA-B*27, and they frequently have a positive family history for SpA. In early stages, there may not be clinically or roentgenographically identifiable involvement of the sacroiliac joints or the spine in most of these patients. They may also lack inflammatory back pain and extraarticular symptoms in early stages and may get misclassified as having a late-onset form of pauciarticular juvenile chronic arthritis.[44] Enthesitis and hip joint involvement are more frequent

in children than adults with SpA, and therefore, some modification of their imaging protocol may be needed, as discussed in Chapter 10. Juvenile AS/axSpA is generally associated with worse functional outcomes than adult-onset disease.[45] Rarely PsA, reactive arthritis, or enteropathic arthritis can also occur in childhood.

HLA-B*27-Positive versus HLA-B*27-Negative AS/axSpA

There is a high degree of similarity of the disease between these two groups, except that the patients possessing HLA-B*27 have a younger age of onset, a shorter delay in diagnosis, a better clinical response to TNF inhibitors, a greater familial occurrence, a greater risk for occurrence of acute anterior uveitis, and a relatively lower risk for occurrence of psoriasis, ulcerative colitis, and Crohn disease.[37,46–48] Moreover, it is unusual to observe occurrence of "primary" AS among families of AS patients of northern European extraction that lack HLA-B*27 and familial occurrence of colitis or psoriasis. At the genetic level, the two groups are also quite similar, with few exceptions, such as ERAP1 association, which is observed only among AS patients that possess HLA-B*27 or HLA-B*40.[49] See Chapter 5 for detailed discussion of the genetic aspects of axSpA.

Extraarticular Features and Comorbidities

AxSpA is associated with many extraarticular (extrarheumatologic) features and comorbidities that are listed in Table 2.3.[7,17,26] The most common is the occurrence of one or more episodes of acute anterior uveitis, observed in up to 40% of *HLA-B*27*-positive AS patients with long disease duration.[50,51] See Chapters 11 and 12 for detailed discussion of this and the other extraarticular manifestations and comorbidities. These associated conditions can further markedly affect the overall well-being of the patients with axSpA, as well as the overall socioeconomic burden associated with it. This subject is reviewed in detail in Chapter 17.

DIAGNOSIS

The earliest clinical symptoms and signs can often be minimal, fleeting, subtle, and nonspecific. Moreover, symptoms, in isolation, are very often insufficient to help establish a diagnosis. A teenager or a young adult presenting with chronic back pain is a common presentation of axSpA, but back pain as a whole is very prevalent in the general population, and axSpA is not its most common cause. Therefore, when clinically evaluating a patient with symptoms that could potentially be due to axSpA, a thorough history is needed, including inquiry about acute anterior uveitis, psoriasis and inflammatory bowel disease, and occurrence of SpA in first- or second-degree relatives, cigarette smoking, and use of over-the-counter and herbal medications.[16,27,28,52]

As discussed earlier in this chapter, a thorough physical examination should include assessment of the patient's spinal, hip and shoulder range of motion, chest expansion, and looking for enthesitis and synovitis. Important physical findings resulting from enthesitis are present in many patients but are often overlooked; these include pain and tenderness over sacroiliac joints (by direct or indirect pressure), vertebral spinal processes, iliac crests, anterior chest wall, calcaneum (plantar fasciitis and/or Achilles enthesitis/tendinitis), ischial tuberosities, greater trochanters, patellae and tibial tubercles, and the feet.[16,27,28,52]

Clinicians must use their clinical judgment based on such clinical information, aided by laboratory and imaging tests, and exclusion of other disease that may share some or many features ("look-alikes").[16,52] Table 2.2 lists the clinical parameters or "red flags" that aid in disease recognition when used in the clinical context.[16,52] It is worth noting that elevation of acute phase reactants (ESR and CRP) is only observed in approximately 50% of patients with axSpA, and even less often among those with nr-axSpA.

Imaging

The musculoskeletal imaging strategies are discussed in Chapter 10, including the potential risks of misreading and overinterpreting some nonspecific findings because of lack of knowledge or inappropriate use of the proposed definition of a positive finding.[53,54] Low-grade bone marrow edema on sacroiliac MRI, fulfilling the ASAS definition, is seen in roughly 25% healthy individuals and those with nonspecific mechanical low back pain.[54] There is an urgent need to come up with a data-driven threshold definition of sacroiliitis on MRI in young adults to prevent overdiagnosis of axSpA.[54] The presence of axSpA is much more likely if there is concomitant erosion or other structural damage, as discussed in Chapter 10. It needs to be emphasized that sacroiliitis is not unique to axSpA and does occur in some of the other forms of SpA.[16,53] Low-dose CT is now emerging as a new promising tool to detect early sacroiliitis.

*HLA-B*27* Test

It can be very helpful as an aid to diagnosis in certain clinical situations, but the following aspects are important to keep in mind[16,55–58]:

- The sensitivity and specificity of this test depend on the racial and ethnic background of the patient.
- The clinical usefulness of this test, like any other "imperfect" test, depends on the clinical setting, in which it is performed, and requires Bayesian analysis to correctly interpret the clinical meaning of positive or negative test results, based on a priori likelihood.[56]
- It is not a "routine" or "diagnostic" or "confirmatory" test and cannot be used as a screening test for axSpA or related forms of SpA in the general population.
- Most patients with axSpA can be diagnosed clinically, and so they do not need this test, but it may be more often needed in cases of nr-axSpA.
- The test does not help distinguish axSpA from other *HLA-B*27*-associated forms of SpA; however, it can provide some help in their differential diagnosis or subclassification.

NEED FOR EARLY DIAGNOSIS

The diagnosis of axSpA/AS is often delayed, usually by 5 or more years.[16] A relatively recent US-based study demonstrated that patients with AS experience on average 14 years of delay in their diagnosis from symptom onset.[59] Such a delay puts a very high clinical and economic burden on these patients and their caregivers, even when it is followed by initiation of appropriate and more effective treatment.[60] Healthcare providers need to keep axSpA on their mental list of differential diagnoses when evaluating patients with chronic back pain starting at young age, both among males and females.[60–63] Some specific clinical, laboratory, or imaging biomarkers are sorely needed, especially for nr-axSpA.

The need for early diagnosis and effective management is becoming increasingly important because of the availability of very effective therapies (especially when started early) that have even raised hopes that disease remission might be feasible.[60–65] Early diagnosis also helps early initiation of lifestyle modification at home and at work, and appropriate lifelong physical exercise programs.[62–65] Surveys conducted in the United States have suggested that approximately 20 out of 100 subjects in the general population report chronic axial pain, and 5 of these 20 meet the criteria for IBP, but only 1 of these 5 subjects can be classified as suffering from axSpA.[66,67] This means that the likelihood of axSpA among subjects with chronic back pain is approximately 5% (1 out of 20 as detailed above). If the chronic back pain meets the ASAS definition of IBP, this likelihood increases from 5% to only 14%–16%.[52] Nevertheless, IBP is a useful screening tool when entertaining the possibility of axSpA in a younger patient with chronic low back pain. If such a patient responds well (50% or more improvement) to regular use of full-dose prescription-strength NSAIDs, the back pain is more likely to be inflammatory than the usual mechanical back pain.[68,69]

In the absence of any universally agreed-upon and validated diagnostic criteria, two diagnostic algorithms have been proposed to help facilitate early recognition of axSpA in daily practice.[52,69] The first of them named Berlin algorithm was developed for physicians less experienced in handling rheumatologic problems (such as primary care physicians) (Fig. 2.9). It advised early referral of young patients with IBP to a rheumatologist, especially if the patient has one or more other features suggesting SpA, including a prior report in the patient's chart of a positive *HLA-B*27* test and/or sacroiliitis.[52] The referring physician ideally should not order imaging or the HLA-B*27 test and leave it for the rheumatologist to decide.[16,68] However, the recognition of IBP is quite challenging for health care professionals in non-specialist settings who mistakenly attributed spinal symptoms to other vastly more common causes of back pain.[16,52,62–77] This diagnostic algorithm was subsequently modified by ASAS for physicians experienced in taking care of patients with rheumatologic problems, and is discussed further in Chapter 4 (see Figure 4.2). In this modified algorithm IBP as obligatory entry criterion was removed and added as an additional SpA feature.[73] Newer strategies are needed to assist primary care physicians in screening for axSpA so that they can be referred to a rheumatologist when the disease is in its early stages.

It is the presence of various combinations of clinical features ("pattern recognition") of axSpA that helps establish the diagnosis with various levels of certainty, based on the clinical judgment of an experienced rheumatologist after exclusion of other "look-alike" conditions.[16,52,60–63] The use of the positive likelihood ratio approach needs three to four SpA features listed in Table 2.2 for a high likelihood of early axSpA. For example, the diagnosis of axSpA should be relatively easy in a young patient with acute anterior uveitis who has IBP, tenderness over sacroiliac joints, and an elevated ESR.[52] One would, of course, need to exclude "look-alike" conditions.[16,70–77] Presence of *HLA-B*27* and/or positive MRI would further assure the diagnosis in some other patients lacking enough clinical features and X-ray evidence of sacroiliitis.[16,27,52,60,61]

DIFFERENTIAL DIAGNOSIS
Chronic Low Back Pain

Back pain, in its acute and chronic forms, is one of the most common health problems in the general population, resulting from multiple possible causes, most commonly mechanical (degenerative and discogenic) factors, fractures and axial skeletal infections or malignancies.[69] Because chronic back pain is the most common presenting symptom of patients with axSpA, it necessitates organized clinical and imaging strategies for its differential diagnosis.[16,52,69–77] These are further discussed in Chapter 10. European radiologists have published their recent perspective/consensus regarding imaging strategies for differentiating axSpA from such conditions.[77]

SAPHO Syndrome

It is an eponym for synovitis-acne-pustulosis-hyperostosis-osteitis syndrome used to encompass multifocal and often recurrent osteoarticular manifestations that include sternocostoclavicular hyperostosis and chronic aseptic osteomyelitis in association with acne and palmoplantar pustulosis.[78] Inflammatory back pain and sacroiliitis can be seen in some of these patients and also among those who suffer from another similar seronegative asymmetric recurrent oligoarthritis/enthesitis in association with hidradenitis suppurativa, dissecting cellulitis of the scalp and severe forms of acne (acne conglobata and acne fulminans).[79] All of these clinical conditions lack any association with *HLA-B*27* and lack familial aggregation.

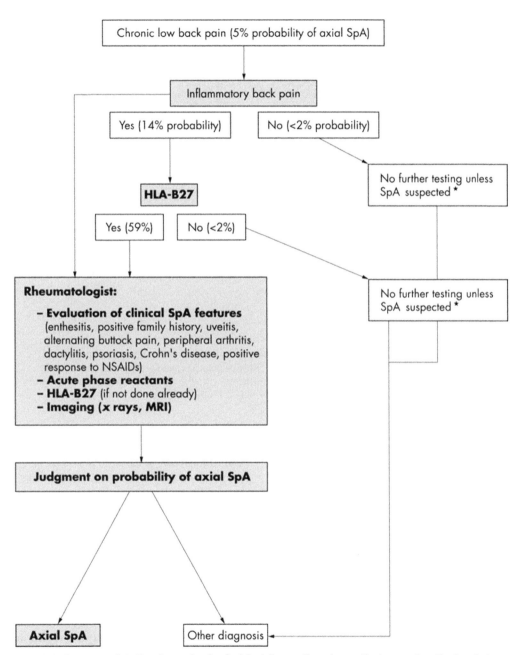

FIG. 2.9 An approach to the diagnosis of axSpA in daily practice when patient presents with chronic low back pain. Percentages in brackets indicate the probability of axSpA before (pretest probability) and after the test has been performed (posttest probability). The asterisk (*) indicates suspicion that SpA could be present because of the presence of some other clinical features of SpA (other than IBP). (From Rudwaleit M, et al. How to diagnose axial spondyloarthritis early. *Ann Rheum Dis*. 2004;63(5):535–543.)

Feature	Ankylosing hyperostosis	Ankylosing spondylitis
Usual age of onset (years)	>50	<40
Thoracolumbar kyphosis	±	++
Limitation of spinal mobility	±	++
Pain	±	++
Limitation of chest expansion	±	++
Radiographic features:		
Hyperostosis	++	+
Sacroiliac joint erosion	– –	++
Sacroiliac joint (synovial) obliteration	±	++
Sacroiliac joint (ligamentous) obliteration	±	++
Apophyseal joint obliteration	– –	++
Anterior longitudinal ligament ossification	++	±
Posterior longitudinal ligament ossification	+	?
Syndesmophytes	– –	++
Enthesopathies (whiskerings) with erosions	– –	++
Enthesopathies (whiskerings) without erosions	++	+

FIG. 2.10 Features that differentiate ankylosing hyperostosis from AS. (From Khan MA, Spondyloarthropathies. In: Hunder G, ed. *Atlas of Rheumatology*. Philadelphia: Current Medicine; 2005:151–180 and Olivieri I, et al. Diffuse idiopathic skeletal hyperostosis may give the typical postural abnormalities of advanced ankylosing spondylitis. *Rheumatology*. 2007;46(11):1709–1711.)

Ankylosing Hyperostosis

It is also called Forestier disease or diffuse idiopathic skeletal hyperostosis (DISH) and results from idiopathic ossifying enthesopathies of the axial as well as the appendicular skeleton.[70] Its most characteristic finding is roentgenographically evident flowing ossification of the anterior longitudinal ligament and relatively well-preserved intervertebral disc spaces.[80] This may or may not be associated with large anterior spurs at disc levels. It usually occurs in elderly individuals, becoming evident on spinal X-rays after 50 years of age.[80] Some patients with advanced disease can have the typical postural abnormalities of advanced AS and can even be confused with AS on X-ray findings.[80,81] The sacroiliac joints, however, are typically unaffected, and there is no association with *HLA-B*27*. A very recent study of 53 patients with DISH has reported frequent presence of MRI evidence of inflammatory lesions in the spine, as defined by the ASAS criteria for axSpA.[82] However, only six patients (15.8%) with an available sacroiliac joint MRI had sacroiliitis according to the ASAS criteria, and only one patient (3.3%) had more than three erosions in the sacroiliac joint.

Occasionally, hyperostotic and degenerative changes of the sacroiliac joints, often restricted to the upper one-third (ligamentous) part of the joint, can occur. This can result in capsular ossifications, joint space narrowing, and subchondral bone sclerosis that can give an appearance superficially resembling sacroiliitis or fused sacroiliac joints on pelvic X-ray but not on CT.[80,81] The differentiating features of the two diseases are listed in Fig. 2.10. Chronic treatment with retinoids (synthetic derivatives of vitamin A) for skin diseases such as acne and psoriasis can sometimes cause bone abnormalities mimicking axSpA or DISH.[83,84]

Osteitis Condensans Ilii

It is characterized by benign dense sclerosis of the lower part of the ilium and adjacent to the sacroiliac joint, typically bilateral and triangular in shape, lacking sacral involvement or joint space narrowing, and is usually self-limiting and often asymptomatic.[70,85] It is most often seen in young multiparous women and is thought to be due to mechanic stress across the sacroiliac joint. It can sometimes occur in men and nulliparous women. It shows no association with *HLA-B*27* and should not be confused with sacroiliitis.[16,85]

Characteristic	Ankylosing Spondylitis	Reactive Arthritis (Reiter's Syndrome)	Juvenile Spondyloarthropathy	Psoriatic Arthropathy*	Enteropathic Arthropathy†
Usual age at onset	Young adult age < 40	Young to middle-age adult	Childhood onset, ages 8–18	Young to middle-age adult	Young to middle-age adult
Sex ratio	3× more common in males	Predominantly males	Predominantly males	Equally distributed	Equally distributed
Usual type of onset	Gradual	Acute	Variable	Variable	Gradual
Sacroiliitis or spondylitis	Virtually 100%	< 50%	< 50%	~ 20%	< 20%
Symmetry of sacroiliitis	Symmetric	Asymmetric	Variable	Asymmetric	Symmetric
Peripheral joint involvement	~ 25%	~ 90%	~ 90%	~ 95%	15%–20%
HLA-B27 (in whites)	> 90%	~ 75%	~ 85%	< 50%‡	~ 50%
Eye involvement§	25%–30%	~ 50%	~ 20%	~ 20%	~ 15%
Cardiac involvement	1%–4%	5%–10%	Rare	Rare	Rare
Skin, mucosal, or nail involvement	None	~ 40%	Uncommon	Virtually 100%	Uncommon

*About 5%–7% of patients with psoriasis develop arthritis, and psoriatic spondylitis accounts for about 5% of all patients with psoriatic arthritis.
†Associated with chronic inflammatory bowel disease.
‡B27 prevalence is higher in those with spondylitis or sacroiliitis.
§Predominantly conjunctivitis in reactive and psoriatic arthritis, and acute anterior uveitis in the other disorders listed above.

FIG. 2.11 Comparison of clinical features of AS and related forms of SpA. (From Khan MA, Spondyloarthropathies. In: Hunder G, ed. *Atlas of Rheumatology*. Philadelphia: Current Medicine; 2005:151–180.)

Fibromyalgia

AxSpA and fibromyalgia (chronic widespread pain syndrome) are two different conditions, although they can cooccur in 4%–18% of men and a much higher percentage of women[22,23,87,88] (see Chapter 11). Fibromyalgia can sometime cause diagnostic confusion with axSpA, especially in women, as explained earlier in this chapter. However, fibromyalgia patients without any concomitant axSpA rarely fulfill the ASAS classification criteria.[86,87]

Differentiation From Other Forms of SpA

This is summarized in Fig. 2.11.

Psoriatic Arthritis

Among patients suffering from psoriasis, more than 10% (range, 5%–42%) have associated inflammatory arthritis, including sacroiliitis and/or spondylitis.[88–90] Psoriatic arthritis (PsA), defined as an inflammatory arthritis in patients with psoriasis that is unassociated with rheumatoid nodules and serum rheumatoid factor, usually begins between 30 and 50 years of age, usually preceded by psoriasis by one to two decades. Presence of axial involvement is associated with a higher likelihood of moderate/severe psoriasis, with higher disease activity and greater effect on quality of life.[90] A subset of patients with psoriasis may show peripheral enthesitis without arthritis. Isolated spondylitis is rare among patients with PsA, occurring in less than 5% of patients, but many PsA patients have axial disease quite similar to AS concurrent with peripheral arthritis.[89] At the other end of the SpA spectrum, psoriasis is observed in 10% of patients with AS.[89] A search for psoriasis in an arthritis patient suspected to have PsA should not be limited to the extremities (including palms, soles, and nails) but also include the scalp, ears, umbilicus, and pelvic, perianal, and genital areas.

Reactive Arthritis

Reactive arthritis is defined as an episode of aseptic asymmetric peripheral arthritis, predominantly of the lower limbs, occurring within a month of a primary infection elsewhere in the body, usually genitourinary infection with *Chlamydia trachomatis* or an enteritis due to certain gram-negative enterobacteria, such as *Shigella*, *Salmonella*, *Yersinia*, or *Campylobacter*.[91-93] Some patients may not demonstrate any recognized antecedent infection or may have asymptomatic triggering infection. In about one-quarter of all cases, the triggering organism remains unknown. The sexually acquired postchlamydia reactive arthritis is most commonly seen in sexually active young men and may be underrecognized in women (because chlamydial infection is frequently asymptomatic in females, and pelvic examinations are very infrequently performed by physician). Postenteritic reactive arthritis affects children and adults, including the elderly, both males and females. There are few reports of reactive arthritis or undifferentiated SpA following infection with atypical organisms such as *Clostridium difficile* and *Giardia lamblia*, and after local injection of Bacille Calmette-Guérin (BCG) into cancerous tissues in the bladder.[91-94]

The arthritis is frequently associated with one or more characteristic extraarticular features. Conjunctivitis occurs in one-third of patients, usually in synchrony with flares of arthritis, and some patients experience one or more episodes of acute anterior uveitis. The triad of arthritis, conjunctivitis, and urethritis has been called Reiter syndrome, but most patients with reactive arthritis do not present with this classic triad. The full clinical spectrum of reactive arthritis has been broadened considerably, and "incomplete" forms are much more common.[93]

The other extraarticular features include enthesitis (Achilles tendonitis and plantar fasciitis), dactylitis ("sausage" digits), tenosynovitis, superficial buccal mucosal ulcers, psoriasiform lesions and nail changes, keratoderma blennorrhagica, urethritis, prostatitis, circinate balanitis or cervicitis and vulvitis, and, on rare occasions, carditis.[16,91–93] It is worth noting that urethritis, cervicitis, and/or balanitis can sometimes occur in postenteritic reactive arthritis and do not directly imply a sexually acquired infection. A history of a preceding or associated diarrhea, urethral discharge, urinary frequency, dysuria, lower abdominal discomfort, tender enlarged prostate, or the abovementioned mucocutaneous lesions should suggest the possibility of reactive arthritis. Septic arthritis should be ruled out by joint aspiration, Gram stain, and culture of any accessible joint fluid.

The average duration of the arthritis is 4–5 months, but many patients have mild musculoskeletal symptoms persisting for more than a year. HLA-B*27-positive patients tend to have more severe and more prolonged joint symptoms. Recurrent attacks are more common in those with chlamydia-induced reactive arthritis. Approximately 15%–30% develop chronic or recurrent arthritis or sacroiliitis and axSpA, and these patients are mostly those who are positive for HLA-B*27 and often have severe and more chronic disease.

Severe arthritis, or an illness resembling typical reactive arthritis, psoriasis with progression to widespread erythrodermic form, psoriatic arthritis, or undifferentiated SpA can occur in some patients infected with HIV,[95] but it is now very uncommonly observed in developed countries because of the availability of more effective antiviral therapies.

Enteropathic Arthritis

The term enteropathic arthritis implies the occurrence of inflammatory arthritis in patients with ulcerative colitis and Crohn disease. It is more common than previously reported. In one series, 39% of 103 patients with ulcerative colitis or Crohn disease, irrespective of the extent of the bowel disease, had enteropathic arthritis.[96] Inflammatory back pain was present in 30% of these 103 patients, and 10% fulfilled the criteria for AS. Examination of the sacroiliac joints on abdominal CT scans has found structural changes of sacroiliitis in up to 35% of patients with inflammatory bowel disease.[97]

Peripheral arthritis that tends to be self-limited and nondeforming occurs much more frequently in enteropathic arthritis than with primary AS and correlates with flare-up of bowel disease, especially in the case of ulcerative colitis. The axial disease (sacroiliitis alone or with classic clinical and radiographic features of AS) does not fluctuate with bowel disease activity.

An increased frequency of subclinical inflammatory lesions in the gut (20%–70%) is observed on colonoscopic mucosal biopsy in patients with AS/axSpA who have no gastrointestinal symptoms or clinically obvious inflammatory bowel disease.[98] Follow-up studies of such patients have shown that 6% of them will develop inflammatory bowel disease, and among those with histologically "chronic" inflammatory gut lesions, 15%–25% will develop clinically obvious Crohn disease.[99]

DISEASE COURSE

The course of the early stages of axSpA is highly variable. Some patients can be minimally symptomatic or have almost a pain-free disease for long periods of time, and can be characterized by exacerbations and remissions. Most of the studies indicate that anywhere between 10% and 40% of patients with nr-axSpA go on to develop r-axSpA/AS over a period of 2–10 years, but the clinical burden of the disease may not be significantly different between these two entities.[100,101] As discussed in detail in Chapter 3, a large proportion of these patients do not progress to AS, just like not all patients with established AS develop spinal ankylosis, and instead some have a disease course that remains primarily confined to the sacroiliac joints with little impact elsewhere. However, most patients with AS show a slow but progressive diminution of spinal mobility resulting from syndesmophyte formation, usually evolving over at least 10 years[100–103] (Fig. 2.4).

A recent study reported that approximately 70% of a select group of AS patients, who at baseline had radiographic evidence of at least one syndesmophyte and at least one inflammatory lesion on MRI, developed detectable growth in syndesmophyte by volume or height as assessed by CT.[104] These syndesmophytes are not randomly distributed around the vertebral rim but have preferred locations, which vary with the vertebral level and may be related to biomechanics.[97,104] They start more often at posterolateral and anterolateral aspects of the thoracolumbar spine segment and spreads higher up in the thoracic and downward in the lumbar spine.[104] Although it is difficult to predict the ultimate outcome for an individual patient, factors

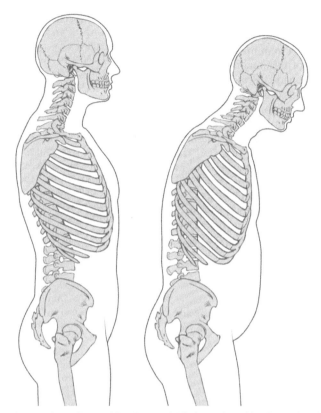

FIG. 2.12 Postural changes in patients with advanced AS: flattening of lumbar spine, forward stooping of the thoracic and cervical spine, flattening of the anterior chest, prominence of the abdomen, mild flexion contracture of the hip joints, and diminution of vertical height after many years of the disease process. (From Khan MA, Spondyloarthropathies. In: Hunder G, ed. *Atlas of Rheumatology*. Philadelphia: Current Medicine; 2005:151–180.)

increasing the likelihood of worse disease include male sex, presence of HLA-B27, positive MRI, radiographic evidence of at least one syndesmophyte, elevated CRP, hip joint involvement, and smoking.[100,104]

More than 30% of patients with r-axSpA/AS develop severe spinal ankylosis ("bamboo spine") with worsening spinal osteoporosis. This aspect and the bone pathophysiology in axSpA are discussed in Chapters 8 and 11. These patients develop progressive spinal kyphosis, decreased chest expansion, flattening of the anterior chest wall, prominence of the abdomen, forward stooping of neck and shoulders, and loss of height, as shown in Fig. 2.12.[16] The breathing becomes increasingly diaphragmatic, and severe diminution of inspirational capacity can lead to dyspnea on exertion. Those patients who also have hip joint involvement are more severely incapacitated, with more severe limitations in their self-care and activities of daily living. Patients with AS have a fivefold higher risk of

clinical spinal fracture and a 35% increased risk of nonvertebral fracture.[105]

The possibility of spinal fracture should be considered in any new onset of neck or back pain in patients with advanced AS, even in the absence of a history of physical trauma.[17] Particular caution must be taken during neck/spine immobilization, transportation, and imaging to avoid further displacing the fracture. Lower cervical spinal fractures are often difficult to visualize on X-ray, and neurologic deficit can be subtle. Transverse displaced fractures, especially of the neck, are associated with significant morbidity and mortality because of resulting paraplegia or quadriplegia. Spontaneous atlantoaxial and upward subluxations of the axis are rare and late complications.[17] The impact of axSpA/AS on family life and work ability and the socioeconomic aspects are discussed in Chapter 17.

LIFE SPAN

Many studies have reported shortening of the life span of patients with axSpA, resulting from many causes that include duration and intensity of inflammation (increased levels of CRP), cardiopulmonary diseases, smoking, accidental fall and trauma, spinal fractures, presence of comorbidities, diagnostic delay, previous hip replacement surgery, work disability, amyloidosis, lower level of education, not using any NSAIDs or biologics, gastrointestinal bleeding, and other treatment-related side effects.[7,17] This subject is reviewed in Chapter 3. There is a very illustrative case report of a patient with AS for 72 years, who has experienced many disease- and treatment-related life-threatening experiences.[106] It is hoped that as a result of earlier diagnosis and more effective treatment, life span of patients with severe axSpA/AS will one day approach and equal that of the general population.

ACKNOWLEDGMENTS

The author is very grateful to Prof. Nurullah Akkoc and Dr. Mazen Elyan for their critical review of the manuscript and many helpful suggestions.

REFERENCES

1. Khan MA. Update on spondyloarthropathies. *Ann Intern Med.* 2002;136(12):896–907.
2. Khan MA. Clinical features of ankylosing spondylitis. In: Hochberg MH, et al., ed. *Rheumatology.* Philadelphia: Mosby/Elsevier; 2003:1161–1181.
3. McGonagle D, et al. Enthesitis in spondyloarthropathy. *Curr Opin Rheumatol.* 1999;11(4):244–250.
4. Francois RJ, Braun J, Khan MA. Entheses and enthesitis: a histopathologic review and relevance to spondyloarthritides. *Curr Opin Rheumatol.* 2001;13(4):255–264.
5. Watad A, et al. Enthesitis: much more than focal insertion point inflammation. *Curr Rheumatol Rep.* 2018;20(7):41.
6. Jacques P, et al. Proof of concept: enthesitis and new bone formation in spondyloarthritis are driven by mechanical strain and stromal cells. *Ann Rheum Dis.* 2014;73(2):437–445.
7. Khan MA. *Ankylosing Spondylitis—Axial Spondyloarthritis.* West Islip, NY: Professional Communications Inc.(PCI); 2016:1–333.
8. Taurog JD, Chhabra A, Colbert RA. Ankylosing spondylitis and axial spondyloarthritis. *N Engl J Med.* 2016;374(26):2563–2574.
9. Sieper J, Poddubnyy D. Axial spondyloarthritis. *Lancet.* 2017;390(10089):73–84.
10. van der Linden S, Valkenburg HA, Cats A. Evaluation of diagnostic criteria for ankylosing spondylitis. A proposal for modification of the New York criteria. *Arthritis Rheum.* 1984;27(4):361–368.
11. Khan MA, et al. Spondylitic disease without radiologic evidence of sacroiliitis in relatives of HLA-B27 positive ankylosing spondylitis patients. *Arthritis Rheum.* 1985;28(1):40–43.
12. Kiltz U, et al. Do patients with non-radiographic axial spondylarthritis differ from patients with ankylosing spondylitis? *Arthritis Care Res.* 2012;64(9):1415–1422.
13. Robinson PC, et al. Axial spondyloarthritis: a new disease entity, not necessarily early ankylosing spondylitis. *Ann Rheum Dis.* 2012;72(2):162–164.
14. Akkoc N, Khan MA. ASAS classification criteria for axial spondyloarthritis: a look at the unfilled part of the glass. *Clin Exp Rheumatol.* 2014;32(6 suppl 87):14–15.
15. Deodhar A, et al. The term 'non-radiographic axial spondyloarthritis' is much more important to classify than to diagnose patients with axial spondyloarthritis. *Ann Rheum Dis.* 2016;75(5):791–794.
16. Khan MA. Spondyloarthropathies. In: Hunder G, ed. *Atlas of Rheumatology.* Philadelphia: Current Medicine; 2005:151–180.
17. Khan MA. Clinical features of axial spondylorthritis. In: Inman R, Sieper J, eds. *Oxford Textbook of Axial Spondyloarthritis.* Oxford, UK: Oxford University Press; 2016:91–100.
18. Khan MA. In: Rheumatology JHK, Dieppe PA, eds. *Ankylosing Spondylitis: Clinical Features.* London: Mosby-Wolfe; 1998:6.16.1–6.16.10.
19. Olivieri I, et al. Spondyloarthritis with onset after age 45. *Curr Rheumatol Rep.* 2013;15(12):374.
20. Rudwaleit M, et al. Inflammatory back pain in ankylosing spondylitis: a reassessment of the clinical history for application as classification and diagnostic criteria. *Arthritis Rheum.* 2006;54(2):569–578.
21. Sieper J, et al. New criteria for inflammatory back pain in patients with chronic back pain: a real patient exercise by experts from the Assessment of SpondyloArthritis international Society (ASAS). *Ann Rheum Dis.* 2009;68(6):784–788.
22. Swinnen TW, et al. Widespread pain in axial spondyloarthritis: clinical importance and gender differences. *Arthritis Res Ther.* 2018;20(1):156.
23. Mease PJ. Fibromyalgia, a missed comorbidity in spondyloarthritis: prevalence and impact on assessment and treatment. *Curr Opin Rheumatol.* 2017;29(4):304–310.
24. Zhao S, et al. The prevalence of depression in axial spondyloarthritis and its association with disease activity: a systematic review and meta-analysis. *Arthritis Res Ther.* 2018;20(1):140.
25. Rennie WJ, et al. Anterior chest wall in axial spondyloarthritis: imaging, interpretation, and differential diagnosis. *Semin Musculoskelet Radiol.* 2018;22(2):197–206.
26. de Winter JJ, et al. Prevalence of peripheral and extra-articular disease in ankylosing spondylitis versus non-radiographic axial spondyloarthritis: a meta-analysis. *Arthritis Res Ther.* 2016;18:196.

27. Rudwaleit M, Feldtkeller E, Sieper J. Easy assessment of axial spondyloarthritis (early ankylosing spondylitis) at the bedside. *Ann Rheum Dis.* 2006;65(9):1251–1252.

28. Elyan M, Khan MA. Diagnosing ankylosing spondylitis. *J Rheumatol Suppl.* 2006;78:12–23.

29. Sieper J, et al. The Assessment of SpondyloArthritis international Society (ASAS) handbook: a guide to assess spondyloarthritis. *Ann Rheum Dis.* 2009;68(suppl II):ii1–ii44.

30. Landewe R, van Tubergen A. Clinical tools to assess and monitor spondyloarthritis. *Curr Rheumatol Rep.* 2015;17(7):47.

31. Ramiro S, et al. Reference intervals of spinal mobility measures in normal individuals: the MOBILITY study. *Ann Rheum Dis.* 2015;74(6):1218–1224.

32. Gladman DD, et al. International spondyloarthritis interobserver reliability exercise--the INSPIRE study: II. Assessment of peripheral joints, enthesitis, and dactylitis. *J Rheumatol.* 2007;34(8):1740–1745.

33. Ramos-Remus C, et al. Temporomandibular joint osseous morphology in a consecutive sample of ankylosing spondylitis patients. *Ann Rheum Dis.* 1997;56(2):103–107.

34. Rusman T, van Vollenhoven RF, van der Horst-Bruinsma IE. Gender differences in axial spondyloarthritis: women are not so lucky. *Curr Rheumatol Rep.* 2018;20(6):35.

35. Tournadre A, et al. Differences between women and men with recent-onset axial spondyloarthritis: results from a prospective multicenter French cohort. *Arthritis Care Res.* 2013;65(9):1482–1489.

36. Baumberger H, Khan MA. SAT0417 Gradual progressive change to equal prevalence of ankylosing spondylitis among males and females in Switzerland: data from the swiss ankylosing spondylitis society (SVMB). *Ann Rheum Dis.* 2017;76(suppl 2):929.

37. Feldtkeller E, et al. Age at disease onset and diagnosis delay in HLA-B27 negative vs. positive patients with ankylosing spondylitis. *Rheumatol Int.* 2003;23(2):61–66.

38. Magrey M, Khan MA. Do validated tools of disease activity in ankylosing spondylitis measure fibromyalgia pain? (Abstract). *Arthritis Rheumatol.* 2018;68 (suppl. 10).

39. Ortolan A, et al. OP0323 Are gender-specific approaches needed in diagnosing early axial spondyloarthritis? data from the spondyloarthritis caught early cohort. *Ann Rheum Dis.* 2018;77:207–208.

40. Burgos-Vargas R. The juvenile-onset spondyloarthritides. *Rheum Dis Clin N Am.* 2002;28(3):531–560 (vi).

41. Tse SM, Laxer RM. New advances in juvenile spondyloarthritis. *Nat Rev Rheumatol.* 2012;8(5):269–279.

42. Weis PF, Colbert RA. Juvenile spondyloarthritis: a distinct form of juvenile arthritis. *Pediatr Clin N Am.* 2018;65(4):675–690.

43. Petty RE, et al. Juvenile spondyloarthropathies. In: Cassidy JT, et al., ed. *Textbook of Pediatric Rheumatology.* Philadelphia: Saunders Elsevier; 2010.

44. Colbert RA. Classification of juvenile spondyloarthritis: enthesitis-related arthritis and beyond. *Nat Rev Rheumatol.* 2010;6(8):477–485.

45. Stone M, et al. Juvenile-onset ankylosing spondylitis is associated with worse functional outcomes than adult-onset ankylosing spondylitis. *Arthritis Rheum.* 2005;53(3):445–451.

46. Khan MA, Kushner I, Braun WE. Comparison of clinical features in HLA-B27 positive and negative patients with ankylosing spondylitis. *Arthritis Rheum.* 1977;20(4):909–912.

47. Reynolds TL, et al. Differences in HLA-B27 positive and negative patients with ankylosing spondylitis: study of clinical disease activity and concentrations of serum IgA, C reactive protein, and haptoglobin. *Ann Rheum Dis.* 1991;50(3):154–157.

48. Akkoc N, et al. Ankylosing spondylitis: HLA-B*27-Positive versus HLA-B*27-Negative disease. *Curr Rheumatol Rep.* 2017;19(5):26. https://doi.org/10.1007/s11926-017-0654-8.

49. Cortes A, et al. Major histocompatibility complex associations of ankylosing spondylitis are complex and involve further epistasis with ERAP1. *Nat Commun.* 2015;6:7146.

50. Zeboulon N, Dougados M, Gossec L. Prevalence and characteristics of uveitis in the spondyloarthropathies: a systematic literature review. *Ann Rheum Dis.* 2008;67(7):955–959.

51. Khan MA, Haroon M, Rosenbaum JT. Acute anterior uveitis and spondyloarthritis: more than meets the eye. *Curr Rheumatol Rep.* 2015;17(9):59. https://doi.org/10.1007/s11926-015-0536-x.

52. Rudwaleit M, et al. How to diagnose axial spondyloarthritis early. *Ann Rheum Dis.* 2004;63(5):535–543.

53. Barozzi L, et al. Seronegative spondylarthropathies: imaging of spondylitis, enthesitis and dactylitis. *Eur J Radiol.* 1998;27(suppl 1):S12–S17.

54. Weber U, et al. Frequency and anatomic distribution of magnetic resonance imaging features in the sacroiliac joints of young athletes: exploring "background noise" toward a data-driven definition of sacroiliitis in early spondyloarthritis. *Arthritis Rheumatol.* 2018;70(5):736–745.

55. Khan MA. Clinical application of the HLA-B27 test in rheumatic diseases. A current perspective. *Arch Intern Med.* 1980;140(2):177–180.

56. Khan MA, Khan MK. Diagnostic value of HLA-B27 testing ankylosing spondylitis and Reiter's syndrome. *Ann Intern Med.* 1982;96(1):70–76.

57. Mustafa KN, Hammoudeh M, Khan MA. HLA-B27 prevalence in arab populations and among patients with ankylosing spondylitis. *J Rheumatol.* 2012;39(8):1675–1677.

58. Khan MA. *Ankylosing Spondylitis Oxford American Rheumatology Library.* Oxford University Press; 2009.

59. Deodhar A, et al. Frequency of axial spondyloarthritis diagnosis among patients seen by US rheumatologists for evaluation of chronic back pain. *Arthritis Rheumatol.* 2016;68(7):1669–1676.

60. Khan MA. Thoughts concerning the early diagnosis of ankylosing spondylitis and related diseases. *Clin Exp Rheumatol.* 2002;20(6 suppl 28):S6–S10.

61. Rudwaleit M, Khan MA, Sieper J. The challenge of diagnosis and classification in early ankylosing spondylitis: do we need new criteria? *Arthritis Rheum.* 2005;52(4):1000–1008.

62. Ozgocmen S, Khan MA. Current concept of spondyloarthritis: special emphasis on early referral and diagnosis. *Curr Rheumatol Rep.* 2012;14(5):409–414.

63. Wendling D, Claudepierre P, Prati C. Early diagnosis and management are crucial in spondyloarthritis. *Joint Bone Spine.* 2013;80(6):582–585.

64. van Tubergen A. The changing clinical picture and epidemiology of spondyloarthritis. *Nat Rev Rheumatol.* 2015;11(2):110–118.

65. Terenzi R, et al. One year in review 2017: spondyloarthritis. *Clin Exp Rheumatol.* 2018;36(1):1–14.

66. Weisman MH, Witter JP, Reveille JD. The prevalence of inflammatory back pain: population-based estimates from the US National Health and Nutrition Examination Survey, 2009-10. *Ann Rheum Dis.* 2013;72(3):369–373.

67. Weisman MH. Inflammatory back pain: the United States perspective. *Rheum Dis Clin N Am.* 2012;38(3):501–512.

68. Braun J, et al. Assessment of spinal pain. *Best Pract Res Clin Rheumatol.* 2014;28(6):875–887.

69. Borenstein D. Mechanical low back pain--a rheumatologist's view. *Nat Rev Rheumatol.* 2013;9(11):643–653.

70. Slobodin G, Lidar M, Eshed I. Clinical and imaging mimickers of axial spondyloarthritis. *Semin Arthritis Rheum.* 2017;47(3):361–368.

71. Hetem SF, Schils JP. Imaging of infections and inflammatory conditions of the spine. *Semin Musculoskelet Radiol.* 2000;4(3):329–347.

72. Antonelli MJ, Magrey M. Sacroiliitis mimics: a case report and review of the literature. *BMC Musculoskelet Disord.* 2017;18(1):170.

73. van den Berg R, et al. ASAS modification of the Berlin algorithm for diagnosing axial spondyloarthritis: results from the SPondyloArthritis Caught Early (SPACE)-cohort and from the Assessment of SpondyloArthritis international Society (ASAS)-cohort. *Ann Rheum Dis.* 2013;72(10):1646–1653.

74. van Hoeven L, et al. Identifying axial spondyloarthritis in Dutch primary care patients, ages 20-45 years, with chronic low back pain. *Arthritis Care Res.* 2014;66(3):446–453.

75. Chou R, et al. Diagnosis and treatment of low back pain: a joint clinical practice guideline from the American College of Physicians and the American Pain Society. *Ann Intern Med.* 2007;147(7):478–491.

76. Chou R, et al. Imaging strategies for low-back pain: systematic review and meta-analysis. *Lancet.* 2009;373(9662):463–472.

77. Schueller-Weidekamm C, et al. Imaging and interpretation of axial spondylarthritis: the radiologist's perspective--consensus of the Arthritis Subcommittee of the ESSR. *Semin Musculoskelet Radiol.* 2014;18(3):265–279.

78. Kahn MF, Khan MA. The SAPHO syndrome. *Bailliere's Clin Rheumatol.* 1994;8(2):333–362.

79. Lim DT, et al. Spondyloarthritis associated with acne conglobata, hidradenitis suppurativa and dissecting cellulitis of the scalp: a review with illustrative cases. *Curr Rheumatol Rep.* 2013;15(8):346.

80. Yagan R, Khan MA. Confusion of roentgenographic differential diagnosis between ankylosing hyperostosis (Forestier's disease) and ankylosing spondylitis. *Clin Rheumatol.* 1983;2(3):285–292.

81. Olivieri I, et al. Diffuse idiopathic skeletal hyperostosis may give the typical postural abnormalities of advanced ankylosing spondylitis. *Rheumatology.* 2007;46(11):1709–1711.

82. Latourte A, et al. Imaging findings suggestive of axial spondyloarthritis in diffuse idiopathic skeletal hyperostosis. *Arthritis Care Res.* 2018;70(1):145–152.

83. Silverman AK, Ellis CN, Voorhees JJ. Hypervitaminosis A syndrome: a paradigm of retinoid side effects. *J Am Acad Dermatol.* 1987;16(5 Pt 1):1027–1039.

84. Kaplan G, Haettich B. Rheumatologic symptoms due to retinoids. *Baillier's Clin Rheumatol.* 1991;5:77–97.

85. Olivieri I, et al. Differential diagnosis between osteitis condensansilii and sacroiliitis. *J Rheumatol.* 1990;17(11):1504–1512.

86. Rudwaleit M. *Fibromyalgia Is Not Axial Spondyloarthritis: Towards an Appropriate Use of the ASAS Classification Criteria for Axial SpA.* Rheumatology (Oxford); 2017.

87. Baraliakos X, et al. *Patients with Fibromyalgia Rarely Fulfil Classification Criteria for Axial Spondyloarthritis.* Rheumatology (Oxford); 2017.

88. Gladman DD. Clinical features and diagnostic considerations in psoriatic arthritis. *Rheum Dis Clin N Am.* 2015;41(4):569–579.

89. Feld J, et al. Axial disease in psoriatic arthritis and ankylosing spondylitis: a critical comparison. *Nat Rev Rheumatol.* 2018;14(6):363–371.

90. Mease P, et al. Influence of axial involvement on clinical characteristics of psoriatic arthritis: analysis from the Corrona Psoriatic Arthritis/Spondyloarthritis registry. *J Rheumatol.* July 1, 2018:pii: jrheum.171094. https://doi.org/10.3899/jrheum.171094.

91. Morris D, Inman RD. Reactive arthritis: developments and challenges in diagnosis and treatment. *Curr Opin Rheumatol.* 2012;14(5):390–394.

92. Zeidker H, Hudson AP. Causality of Chlamydiae in arthritis and spondyloarthritis: a plea for increased translational research. *Curr Rheumatol Rep.* 2016;18(2):9. https://doi.org/10.1007/s11926-015-0559-3.

93. Khan MA, Sieper J. Reactive arthritis. In: Koopman WJ, ed. *Arthritis and Allied Conditions: A Textbook of Rheumatology.* Baltimore: Lippincott Williams & Wilkins; 2004.

94. Schwartzenberg JM, Smith DD, Lindsley HB. Bacillus Calmette-Guerin associated arthropathy mimicking undifferentiated spondyloarthropathy. *J Rheumatol.* 1999;26(4):933–935.

95. Mody GM, Parke FA, Reveille JD. Articular manifestations of human immunodeficiency virus infection. *Best Pract Res Clin Rheumatol.* 2003;17(2):265–287.

96. de Vlam K, et al. Spondyloarthropathy is underestimated in inflammatory bowel disease: prevalence and HLA association. *J Rheumatol.* 2000;27(12):2860–2865.

97. Tan S, Ward MM. Computed tomography in axial spondyloarthritis. *Curr Opin Rheumatol.* 2018;30(4):334–339.

98. De Keyser F, et al. Gut inflammation and spondyloarthropathies. *Curr Rheumatol Rep.* 2002;4(6):525–532.

99. Queiro R, et al. Subclinical sacroiliitis in inflammatory bowel disease: a clinical and follow-up study. *Clin Rheumatol.* 2000;19(6):445–449.

100. Protopopov M, Poddubnyy D. Radiographic progression in non-radiographic axial spondyloarthritis. *Expert Rev Clin Immunol.* 2018;14(6):525–533.

101. Burgos-Varga R, et al. The prevalence and clinical characteristics of nonradiographic axial spondyloarthritis among patients with inflammatory back pain in rheumatology practices: a multinational, multicenter study. *Arthritis Res Ther.* 2016;18(1):132.

102. Brophy S, et al. The natural history of ankylosing spondylitis as defined by radiological progression. *J Rheumatol.* 2002;29(6):1236–1243.

103. Costantino F, et al. Radiographic sacroiliitis develops predictably over time in a cohort of familial spondyloarthritis followed longitudinally. *Rheumatology.* 2017;56(5):811–817.

104. Ward MM, Tan S. Better quantification of syndesmophyte growth in axial spondyloarthritis. *Curr Rheumatol Rep.* 2018;20(8):46.

105. Prieto-Alhambra D, et al. Ankylosing spondylitis confers substantially increased risk of clinical spine fractures: a nationwide case-control study. *Osteoporos Int.* 2015;26(1):85–91.

106. Khan MA. Accomplishments of Heinz Baumberger PhD: a remarkable patient with ankylosing spondylitis for 72 years. *Clin Rheumatol.* 2016;35(6):1637–1641.

107. Ozgocmen S, Akgul O, Khan MA. Mnemonic for assessment of the spondyloarthritis international society criteria. *J Rheumatol.* 2010;37(9):1978.

CHAPTER 3

Epidemiology of Axial Spondyloarthritis

NURULLAH AKKOÇ, MD • MUHAMMAD ASIM KHAN, MD, FRCP, MACP, MACR

INTRODUCTION

Epidemiology is very broadly defined as "the study of the occurrence and distribution of health-related events, states, and processes in specified populations, including the study of the determinants influencing such processes, and the application of this knowledge to control relevant health problems".[1] In this definition the health-related events, states, and processes refer to "outbreaks, diseases, disorders, causes of death, behaviors, environmental and socioeconomic processes, effects of preventive programs, and use of health and social services."[1] The scope of epidemiology can therefore be defined by two overlapping perspectives: a biomedical perspective and a public health perspective.[2] The biomedical perspective focuses mainly on disease etiology and disease process, which include the description of the disease spectrum, the natural history, investigation of the physiologic or genetic factors that influence the disease outcome, and early disease markers or indicators. The final aim of all epidemiologic research is to promote, protect, and preserve the health of a population. Study designs for epidemiologic research are mainly of descriptive and analytical types; the former describes disease occurrence and distribution in terms of time, persons, and place without much regard to causal relationships, whereas the latter type mostly deals with identifying or measuring the effects of risk factors contributing to disease. Many of these epidemiologic aspects are covered extensively elsewhere in this book. So, in this chapter, we review primarily the descriptive epidemiology (incidence, prevalence, and survival), and to a lesser extent the risk factors associated with occurrence of axial spondyloarthritis (axSpA) and its progression.

DISEASE DEFINITION

Standard case definitions are crucially important for interpretation and comparison of epidemiologic studies conducted at different places and at different time points. Case definitions based on validated classification criteria are much more reliable than clinical diagnosis for better standardization of case verification in epidemiologic

research. The classification criteria for spondyloarthritis (SpA) are discussed in detail in Chapter 4. A major challenge in reviewing epidemiologic research on axSpA is the use of different classification criteria for case definition. Most of the studies have included patients with ankylosing spondylitis (AS) according to the modified New York criteria,[3–5] whereas some recent studies have also included patients with axSpA based on the recent ASAS classification criteria for axSpA.[6] The 1961 Rome classification criteria for AS were particularly useful for epidemiologic studies because they allowed inclusion based on clinical components, even in the absence of radiographic sacroiliitis. However, one of the clinical components (thoracic pain) had low specificity and the other (uveitis) had low sensitivity. In 1966, these two components were excluded, and radiographic sacroiliitis was included as a mandatory component, resulting in the New York criteria. A modification of these criteria was proposed in 1983[3] and published a year later.[5] The modification involved improvement of dorsolumbar pain definition and adjustment of the chest expansion by basing it on age and sex. The ASAS criteria for axSpA define a broader disease spectrum that encompasses AS and "spondylitic disease without radiographic evidence of sacroiliitis,"[7] now called nonradiograhic axSpA (nr-axSpA).[6,8] According to the ASAS criteria, patients with chronic back pain with age at onset of <45 years can be classified as having axSpA if they have evidence of sacroiliitis by either X-ray or MRI and at least one SpA feature, or if they possess *HLA-B*27* and at least two SpA features (see Chapter 4).

DISEASE OCCURRENCE

There are two approaches to define occurrence of a disease in a defined population: *incidence* and *prevalence*. The incidence of a disease is the number of new cases that occur within a given period of time and generally reported as the number of cases per 100, 000 people, whereas the prevalence refers to the proportion of diseased individuals in a population at a specific time and is often expressed as percentage.

Axial Spondyloarthritis. https://doi.org/10.1016/B978-0-323-56800-5.00003-5

Epidemiologic studies on disease occurrence use different methods for data collection. Population-based cross-sectional studies attempt to identify cases in a defined population at a specific time period through different types of surveys and interviews followed by a detailed clinical evaluation of the screening-positive individuals. This type of study has the potential of capturing all the cases in the community, including those who were previously undiagnosed, and allows for the use of classification criteria for a standardized diagnosis. Sample sizes of population-based cross-sectional studies are limited by financial and time constraints, but they can provide reliable prevalence estimates with modest sample sizes. Many of the studies assessing the prevalence of AS have used this design. However, it is not suitable for incidence studies, which require large source populations and a long period of observation time to estimate reliable and stable rates. This can be done by using a hospital-based study design. In this method, cases are identified through the search of healthcare databases and/or medical records of hospitals and/or clinics, providing health service to the population in a catchment area. Because of the ease of collecting data with this approach, it has been increasingly used for epidemiologic studies examining the prevalence or incidence of axSpA/AS. However, studies with this design are more likely to underestimate the true disease occurrence rates because of its inability to identify undiagnosed cases. Such studies carry the likelihood of overestimating the disease severity because of referral bias. Moreover, reliability of the derived estimates depends on the completeness of medical records, accuracy of clinical diagnoses, and their proper registration. Notably, current classification systems used in healthcare, such as the International Classification of Diseases issued by the World Health Organization, have a specific code only for the AS subset of axSpA. This creates a major challenge in using electronic healthcare data for epidemiologic research on axSpA.

Prevalence Studies

Prevalence of axSpA and of its subsets, AS and nr-axSpA, around the globe are comprehensively listed in Table 3.1. A recent systematic review assessed all the published studies on the prevalence of AS until May 2012.[9] The authors calculated mean and weighted mean (based on study sample size) prevalence estimates of AS for different continents. Notably, they excluded hospital-based studies from their calculations, because of their potential bias. They also excluded a study from Germany because it used MRI scanning during the process of diagnosis.[9] They calculated mean prevalence of AS

to be 0.24% (weighted mean: 0.18%) within Europe, 0.17% (mean weighted mean 0.18%) within Asia, and 0.10% (weighted mean 0.12%) within Latin America.[9] Single population–based studies from North America and Africa reported the prevalence of AS, as 0.32% and 0.07%, respectively.[10,11] A subsequent systematic review and metaanalysis, which covered the literature up until July 2014 reported roughly similar continent-specific prevalence estimates for Europe (0.25%), East Asia (0.16%), Latin America (0.14%), North America (0.20%), and sub-Saharan Africa (0.02%). The highest AS prevalence (0.35%) was found in Northern Arctic Communities. This analysis included both population-based and hospital-based studies.[12] Newer studies have reported prevalence of AS in the United States, Canada, Sweden, Norway, Scotland, and Turkey. All of these studies, as well as the older ones,[13–35,36–55,56–79] are summarized in Table 3.1.

A US study performed in a nationally representative sample of 5013 US adults participating 2009–10 National Health and Nutritional Examination Survey (NHANES) reported the prevalence of SpA, as 1.4% and 0.9%, according to the ESSG and the Amor criteria, respectively.[62] Data collection for this survey included items needed for the case definition of inflammatory spinal pain component of the ESSG criteria and the pain/stiffness component of the Amor criteria, whereas no data were collected on peripheral arthritis. Therefore, these figures were pronounced to refer to axSpA in the title of the original article[62] and also in a later review article by the same authors.[80] However, it should be emphasized that the cases in this study had no data pertaining to the HLA-B*27 status, pelvic radiographs, or sacroiliac MRI examination, which are the key elements for classification of axSpA according to the ASAS criteria. Moreover, it should be noted that the ESSG and Amor criteria have shown only 64% and 78% specificity for axSpA, respectively, in the validation set of ASAS cohort.[6] Lastly, the 0.55% prevalence of AS based on patients "reporting as having a diagnosis of AS" in the NHANES survey[80] should also be taken with caution, because of the 86% false positivity rate when patients self-reported as having a diagnosis of AS in a Norwegian study.[79]

Strand et al.[64] reviewed medical records of 861 randomly selected patients aged 18–44 years with chronic back pain, who were representative of 101 participating rheumatology practices in the United States, and reported a national prevalence estimate of axSpA to be 0.7%, based on ASAS classification criteria, and 0.67%, based on clinical diagnosis. These values were obtained by estimating the observed local prevalence estimates of axSpA and projecting that to a total at-risk population of US rheumatology practices in general, and then applying that estimate to the US census data for individuals aged 18–44 years. The investigators found identical prevalence estimates of 0.35% for AS (as defined by the modified New York criteria) and 0.35% for nr-axSpA (as defined by the ASAS criteria). It is worth pointing out that although the two figures for national prevalence of axSpA (0.7% and 0.67%), based on the two case definitions discussed above look quite similar, the agreement between them was low to moderate. About one-fourth of the patients classified as axSpA did not have a clinical diagnosis.[64] Most notably, this study has also shown that it is not uncommon for American rheumatologists to make a diagnosis of AS in the absence of the needed radiographs or in the presence of negative radiographic findings. An additional limitation is that the study may have underestimated prevalence because patients with axSpA may not have been referred for rheumatologic care.

Another US study utilized the computerized International Classification of Diseases, Ninth Revision (ICD-9), of a nonprofit health delivery system serving over 3 million people in North California, to assess the diagnostic prevalence of axSpA. The authors assumed that, in the absence of a unique ICD-9 code, all axSpA cases would possibly be recorded by physicians with the code of 720.X (including 720.0 specifically for AS, 720.1 for spinal enthesopathy, 720.2 for sacroiliitis, 720.8 for other inflammatory spondylopathies, and 720.9 for unspecified spondylopathies). Using their most sensitive case finding strategy based on a single physician diagnosis code for ICD-9 720.X, they found quite a low prevalence estimate for axSpA (0.23%).[76] These authors did not attempt to validate this case definition because their study included patients enrolled in the database between 1996 and 2009, before the publication of the ASAS classification criteria for axSpA. When they tried a more specific case definition based on ≥ 2 diagnoses by a primary care specialist or ≥1 diagnosis by a rheumatologist, the prevalence figure fell by almost half (0.11%), of which 80% had AS. Of note, even this somewhat more specific diagnostic algorithm had a low positive predictive value (PPV) for AS (62%). A study in a general practice setting from Norfolk, UK, identified individuals who consulted their general practitioner for low back pain (LBP) through a READ code search of electronic health records. A validated questionnaire for axSpA was mailed to a sample of 971 potential participants, randomly selected from the eligible patients.[72] Among the respondents (response rate 51.6%) those with a prior diagnosis of axSpA or AS were

considered as positive cases, after the review of their medical records for verification, whereas those meeting the ASAS IBP criteria were invited for a detailed clinical evaluation including MRI scanning and *HLA-B*27* testing. This study also reported low prevalence rates for axSpA (0.3%) and AS (0.15%), according to ASAS and modified New York criteria, respectively.

A recent smaller sized Turkish study assessing the frequency of IBP among the 381 university employees with a mean age of 38 identified 115 subjects with chronic back pain with an onset before the age of 45 years in the study population.[73] These patients underwent pelvic X-ray and/or MRI examination, if they had at least one SpA feature and were tested for *HLA-B*27* if they had at least two SpA features. This study reported a prevalence of 6.6% and 1.3% for IBP and axSpA, respectively, according to ASAS criteria, and a prevalence of 0.5% for AS according to modified New York criteria.

Another institutionally defined population study aimed to assess the prevalence of SpA in reference to *HLA-B*27* among employees of a French national electricity and gas company.[70] Among the respondents to a validated questionnaire for SpA sent by mail, 6556 subjects with available DNA samples constituted the source population. All screening-positive patients underwent a plain anterior-posterior pelvic radiograph and *HLA-B*27* testing. This study estimated a standardized prevalence of SpA of 0.43%, with 75% of the cases fulfilling the ASAS criteria for axSpA. In the same cohort, the prevalence of AS was found to be 0.31 based on the modified New York criteria. All subjects included in this study were ≥57 years old.

A Dutch group aimed to determine the prevalence of axSpA based on ASAS criteria in patients with chronic low back pain. Although they did not present any prevalence estimate for the prevalence of axSpA, AS, and nr-axSpA in the general population, they can be calculated from the data provided in their article, and these values are 0.69, 0.12, and 0.57%, respectively.[69] It should be underlined that these estimates refer to only the undiagnosed cases in the population. The same group, using the same methodology and partly in the same population, reported almost 50% lowered rates for each entity[75] (Table 3.1). Notably, only about 20% of the patients in these studies were typed to be *HLA-B*27* positive, indicating that different classification criteria may identify different patient populations. A very recent publication has pointed out methodologic challenges in conducting epidemiologic studies in axSpA and explained potential reasons for disparate disease occurrence estimates (i.e., geographic

TABLE 3.1   Prevalence of Axial Spondyloarthritis (axSpA) and of Its Subsets, Ankylosing Spondylitis (AS) and Nonradiographic axSpA (nr-axSpA) Around the Globe

Author, Publication Year	Years of Study	Country/Region	Mean Age	Total Population	Source of Data
(Gofton, 1972)[13]	NR	BC, Haidans	≥20	175	Males >15 years from two villages
		BC, Bella Bella		158	Males >20 years from a village
		BC, Bella Coola		109	Males >15 years from a village
		US, Pima		166	Age stratified random sample
(Gomor, 1977)[14]	1971–1975	Hungary	>15	6,469	Seven samples of general population.
(Atkins, 1988)[15]	1971–1986	Canada, Vancouver Island (Nootka Indians)	NR	2,300	Patients referred to rheumatologist
(Carter, 1979)[16]	1950–1973	USA, Rochester, Minnesota	≥15	33,000 (1950); 52,000 (1973)	Centralized computer record system at the Mayo clinic also linked to other health facilities
(Gran, 1985)[17]	1979–1980	Norway, Tromso	20–54	14,539	Responders to an epidemiologic survey on cardiovascular health, who answered the questions concerning back pain
(Lutalo, 1985)[18]	NR	Zimbabwe, Gwery city, and its surrounding		100,000	Register of chronic diseases at the only hospital in the area
(Oen, 1986)[19]	1972–1982	Canada, Northwest Territories (Inuit Eskimos)	≥15	2,055	Medical records kept at the primary, secondary or tertiary care centers serving the area
(Boyer, 1988)[20]	1970–1982	USA, Alaska, (Inupiat Eskimos)	≥20	2,419	Computerized patient care database
(Boyer, 1990)[21]	1970–1982	USA, Western Alaska (Yupik Eskimos)	≥20	7,052	Computerized patient care database
(Boyer, 1991)[22]	1970–1984	USA, Alaska (Tlingit, Haida, and Tsimshian)	≥20	5,223	Computerized patient care database
(Boyer, 1994)[23]	1990	USA, Alaska, (Inupiat and Yupik Eskimos)	≥20	3,786	Pre-existing rheumatic disease registries, computerized patient care database, reports from healthcare providers
(Wigley, 1994)[24]	NR	China, Beijing and Shantou	≥20	9,249	Subjects were selected from the village registers

Screening Strategy for Case Finding	Method for Case Ascertainment	Case Definition/ Criteria	Prevalence of AS (%)	Male/ Female Ratio	Mean Age at Onset	HLA-B*27 Prevalence (N-Tested)
Survey (Clinical +pelvic X-ray exam)	Clinical data + radiographs in all cases	NY	6 6.3 2.7 5.4	No females	NR	NR
Interview and examination by a physician team	Radiographic assessment when AS suspected	NY	0.23	5	NR	93% (n=55)
Medical records and interviews	Review of all clinical and laboratory details reviewed by two rheumatologists (radiographs if available)	NY	0.00	0/0	Not relevant	Not relevant
Search for cases with a diagnosis of AS in the electronic record system	Review of medical records	Definite radiographic sacroiliitis required	0.13	2.7	NR	NR
Selection of a random sample from responders who reported back pain and/or stiffness	Clinical examination + radiographic findings	NY	1.1-1.4	3.9-6.1	NR	89% (n=25)
Analysis of medical records from last 10 years	Case review based on medical records	Clinical	0.001	0/1	NR	NR
Review of medical records for a coded diagnosis of AS or low back pain	Interview and examination by a rheumatologist, radiography, when indicated	NY	0.19	5/0	NR	NR
ICD-9-CM for AS	Review of medical records + consultation with clinicians following the cases	Rome	0.12	2/0	NR	NR
At least one time diagnosis of AS	Review of medical records, including radiographs if available	Rome	0.21	3	NR	NR
At least one time diagnosis or suspected of having AS	Review of medical records, including radiographs if available	Rome	0.36	5.2	NR	NR
Preliminary review of medical records for possible cases	Clinical evaluation at the clinic, including radiographs when indicated	NY	0.4	1	NR	NR
COPCORD questionnaire	Clinical evaluation by study committee members; including radiographs when indicated	Clinical	0.26	NR	NR	NR

Continued

TABLE 3.1 Prevalence of Axial Spondyloarthritis (axSpA) and of Its Subsets, Ankylosing Spondylitis (AS) and Nonradiographic axSpA (nr-axSpA) Around the Globe—cont'd

Author, Publication Year	Years of Study	Country/Region	Mean Age	Total Population	Source of Data
(Chou, 1994)[25]	NR	Taiwan, rural Taiwan, suburban Taiwan, urban	>20	8,998	A random sample stratified by age and sex from 3 districts
(Benevolens-kaya, 1996)[26]	1989–1990	Russia, Siberia (Chuckis) and USA, Alaska (Inupiat & Yupik Eskimos)	≥20	731 (Siberia) 3786 (Alaska)	Residents of four villages in Siberia As in Ref. [23] in Alaska
(Brown, 1997)[27]	NR	Gambia, Fula ethnic group	25+	1,115	Family members of HLA-B*27 (+) twin pairs and randomly selected males
(Dans, 1997)[28]	NR	Philippines, Manilla (Urban)	≥15	3,065	670 households selected with multistage cluster sampling
(Kaipiainen-Seppanen, 1997)[29]	1978–1980	Finland	≥30	7,217	Participants of Mini-Finland Health Survey
(Braun, 1998; Akkoc, 2005)[30,31]	NR	Germany, Berlin	NR	348	HLA-B*27 positive blood donors from five blood banks, matched with HLA-B*27 negative blood donors
(Hukuda, 2001)[32]	1985–1996	Japan	>15	101,100, 000	All SpA patients seen at clinics and hospitals in nine districts
(Bruges-Armas, 2002)[33]	1994	Portugal, Azores Island, Terceira	>50	450	A randomly selected sample stratified by age and sex from the participants of a previous osteoporosis survey
(Cardiel, 2002)[34]	NR	Mexico, Mexico City	≥18	2,500	Stratified sample of subjects from census
(Dai, 2003)[35]	1997–1998	China, Shanghai	>15	6,584	All persons in the selected communities
(Minh Hoa, 2003)[36]	September–December, 2000	Vietnam, Hanoi City	≥16	2,119	Residents of Trung Liet Commune
(Alamanos, 2004)[37]	1983–2002	Greece, North-west	≥16	488,435	Patients referred to rheumatology clinics of hospitals or to private rheumatologists in the study area
(Al-Awadhi, 2004)[38]	NR	Kuwait, country-wide	≥15	7,670	Nationally representative random sample of households of Kuwaiti nationals

Screening Strategy for Case Finding	Method for Case Ascertainment	Case Definition/ Criteria	Prevalence of AS (%)	Male/ Female Ratio	Mean Age at Onset	HLA-B*27 Prevalence (N-Tested)
Questionnaire for detecting potential rheumatic disorders	Clinical evaluation by rheumatologists; radiography in all subjects with back pain	NY	0.54 0.19 0.4	0.9 0.7 4.6	NR	NR
Community survey + examination in Siberia As in Ref. [23] in Alaska	Clinical evaluation by rheumatologists; radiography in all subjects with back pain in Siberia; only when indicated in Alaska	NY	0.53	NR	NR	NR
Interview	Examination + sacroiliac X-ray if indicated	Radiographic findings	0.0	0/0	Not relevant	Not relevant
COPCORD questionnaire	Examination + evaluation by rheumatologists	Clinical	0.03	NR	NR	NR
Interview and examination by trained nurses	Examination by trained physicians (+radiography if available)	Clinical	0.15	2.3	28.4	92% (n=51)
Postal questionnaire for SpA features including IBP	Clinical evaluation including pelvic X-rays and sacroiliac MRI	mNY	0.55	1.7	NR	100% (n=9)
Questionnaire forms for medical record abstracts	Diagnosis made by physicians at institutes; radiography required for diagnosis	Rome or NY	0.007	5.4	NR	NR
Interview	Clinical evaluation including pelvic and spinal radiograph and CT if needed	mNY	0.6	3/0	NR	100% (n=3)
COPCORD questionnaire	Examination (mostly same day of interview)	Clinical	0.08	NR	NR	NR
COPCORD questionnaire	Examination by rheumatologist (same day of interview)	mNY	0.12	8/0	NR	NR
COPCORD questionnaire	Clinical evaluation by rheumatologists, including radiography and blood tests	Clinical	0.10	NR	NR	NR
Review of medical records for a clinical diagnosis of AS	Diagnosis confirmed by the study group based on medical records	mNY	0.02	4.7	31	81% (n=113)
COPCORD questionnaire	Clinical evaluation by rheumatologists, including laboratory tests	Clinical	0.01	NR	NR	NR

Continued

TABLE 3.1   Prevalence of Axial Spondyloarthritis (axSpA) and of Its Subsets, Ankylosing Spondylitis (AS) and Nonradiographic axSpA (nr-axSpA) Around the Globe—cont'd

Author, Publication Year	Years of Study	Country/Region	Mean Age	Total population	Source of Data
(Zeng, 2004)[39]	February–June, 1995	China, Chenghai City	≥16	2,040	All residents in a rural area of the East administration
(Bakland, 2005)[40]	1960–1993	Norway, Northern Norway	≥16	217,000	Hospital diagnostic database
(Haq, 2005)[41]	January–February, 2001	Bangladesh, Dhaka	≥15	5,160	All inhabitants of three localities
(Saraux, 2005)[42]	2001	France, country-wide	>18	9,395	A nationally representative sample selected with multistage random sampling
(Trontzas, 2005)[43]	NR	Greece, country-wide	≥19	8,740	All residents in seven areas in mainland Greece + randomly selected subjects from one rural and one suburban area
(De Angelis, 2007)[44]	April–June, 2004	Italy, Marche	>18	2,155	Random sample of individuals, selected from list of 16 general practices
(Veerapen, 2007)[45]	February–November, 1988	Malaysia, Banting	>15	2,594	All members of a community
(Davatchi, 2008)[46]	2004–2005	Iran, Tehran	≥15	10,291	Randomly selected clusters from 22 districts
(Onen, 2008)[47]	2001–2002	Turkey, Izmir	≥20	2,835	Households of randomly selected 26/845 clusters
(Adomaviciute, 2009)[48]	September–October, 2004	Lithuania, Vilnius, and Kaunus	≥18	4,244	Random sample of individuals selected from local telephone books
(Joshi, 2009)[49]	May–September, 2004	India, Pune	>16	8,145	All residents in Narayan Peth
(Liao, 2009)[50]	January–May, 2006	China, Dalang Town	>16	10,921	All officially registered residents

Screening Strategy for Case Finding	Method for Case Ascertainment	Case Definition/ Criteria	Prevalence of AS (%)	Male/ Female Ratio	Mean Age at Onset	*HLA-B*27 Prevalence (N-Tested)
COPCORD questionnaire	Examination at a health center; including radiography and blood tests	mNY	0.2	NR	NR	NR
ICD-9: 720, ICD-10:M45	Review medical records + reexamination	mNY (primary AS)	0.04	3.1	24	93% (n=534)
COPCORD questionnaire	Examination by internists and by rheumatologists, when needed	Clinical	0.06	NR	NR	NR
Telephone survey to detect possible cases of SpA first by patient interviewers and then rheumatologists	Confirmation by local rheumatologist or examination at closest study center	Clinical	0.15	NR	NR	NR
Face-to-face interview by rheumatologists	Evaluation by rheumatologists (at the same visit); laboratory tests, X-ray when appropriate	mNY	0.20	6.1	26	NR
Postal questionnaire	Evaluation by rheumatologists; laboratory tests, X-ray, and MRI, when appropriate	mNY	0.37	7	31	63% (n=8)
COPCORD questionnaire	Examination by rheumatologist, including X-ray	Clinical	0.08	4/0	NR	NR
COPCORD questionnaire	Examination by rheumatology fellows (same day) + X-ray if requested → confirmation by senior rheumatologists	Clinical	0.12	2.4	NR	NR
Face-to-face interview → phone interview	Examination by rheumatologists; including X-ray, CT, or MRI as appropriate	mNY	0.47	1.2	NR	80% (n=10)
Validated telephone questionnaire	Phone interview by a rheumatologist → medical examination, in case of uncertain diagnosis	Clinical	0.09	NR	NR	NR
COPCORD questionnaire	Examination by rheumatologist; radiography in very suspicious cases	Clinical	0.06	NR	NR	NR
A validated questionnaire for detection of SpA (face-to-face)	Examination of cases with spinal pain by rheumatologist; *HLA-B*27 testing and radiography in all suspected cases	ESSG for axSpA	0.50	1.3	34	83 (n=75)
		mNY for AS	0.25	NR	NR	NR

Continued

TABLE 3.1   Prevalence of Axial Spondyloarthritis (axSpA) and of Its Subsets, Ankylosing Spondylitis (AS) and Nonradiographic axSpA (nr-axSpA) Around the Globe—cont'd

Author, Publication Year	Years of Study	Country/Region	Mean Age	Total Population	Source of Data
(Reyes-Llerena, 2009)[51]	NR	Cuba, Havana	≥15	3,155	Random sample
(Anagnostopoulos, 2010)[52]	2007–2008	Greece, Magnesia	>18	1,705	Random sample of poll catalogs
(Eaton, 2010)[53]	1977–2006	Denmark, country-wide	All ages	5,506,574	Identification from Danish Civil Registration system and National hospital register
(Geirsson, 2010)[54]	1947–2005	Iceland, country-wide	≥18	220,441	A genetic studies database for AS and IBD, Electronic records of two major hospitals, reports from private rheumatology services
(Hanova, 2010)[55]	2002–2003	Czechia, Ceske Budejovice and the district of Cheb	≥16	154,374	Patients registered with a diagnosis of AS by a rheumatologist
(Alvarez-Nemegyei, 2011)[56]	NR	Mexico, Yucatán region	≥18	3,915	Subjects selected through a multistage, stratified (by region), randomized method
(Haglund, 2011)[57]	2003–2007	Sweden, Skane	≥15	849,253	Skane healthcare register
(Karkucak, 2011)[58]	2002–2004	Turkey, Eastern Black Sea Region	≥20	4,031	A random sample of households from five cities
(Pelaez-Ballestas, 2011)[59]	NR	Mexico, five regions	>18	19,213	Subjects selected through multistage random probability sampling, stratified by region
(Rodriguez-Amado, 2011)[60]	2008–2009	Mexico, State of Nuevo Leon	≥18	4,713	A random sample stratified by region representing the whole state
(Cakir, 2012)[61]	NR	Turkey, Havsa region	≥20	12,500	Every household in Havsa administered a structured questionnaire

Screening Strategy for Case Finding	Method for Case Ascertainment	Case Definition/ Criteria	Prevalence of AS (%)	Male/ Female Ratio	Mean Age at Onset	*HLA-B*27* Prevalence (N-Tested)
COPCORD questionnaire	Examination by family physicians (on the same day) → confirmation by rheumatologists; radiologic tests when appropriate	Clinical	0.19	3	NR	NR
Postal questionnaire for self-reporting of a physician diagnosis	Clinical evaluation by a rheumatologist	Clinical	0.29	4	NR	NR
ICD-8: 712.49 ICD-10: M45.9	Admission to hospital or a clinic with an ICD code for AS	Clinical	0.07	1.2	NR	NR
ICD 10 codes of M45, M45.5, M45.9, M46, and M 6.9 for search of hospital records	Clinical evaluation of all identified cases by a rheumatologist	mNY	0.10	1.9	24	84% (n=223)
Medical records; search strategy for case finding not clearly explained	Diagnosis by rheumatologist	mNY	0.1	4.8	24	62% (n=50)
COPCORD questionnaire → examination of patients reporting MSK pain	Examination by certified rheumatologists in case of uncertainty	mNY	0.02	NR	NR	NR
ICD10: M45	≥1 M45 code assigned by a rheumatologist/internist or ≥two clinic visits with the same code by any other physician	NY	0.12	2.1	NR	NR
Face-to face interview for CBP → telephone interview for confirmation	Clinical evaluation, including pelvic X-rays	mNY	0.25	8.8	28	80% (n=10)
COPCORD questionnaire → examination of patients reporting MSK pain	Examination by certified rheumatologists in cases suspected to have rheumatic disease	mNY	0.15	NR	NR	NR
COPCORD questionnaire → examination of patients reporting MSK pain	Examination by certified rheumatologists	mNY	0.04	NR	NR	NR
Clinical evaluation at the nearest healthcare center for a possible diagnosis of AS	Examination of possible AS cases, at the university hospital	Rome	0.12	3.0	NR	NR

Continued

TABLE 3.1 Prevalence of Axial Spondyloarthritis (axSpA) and of Its Subsets, Ankylosing Spondylitis (AS) and Nonradiographic axSpA (nr-axSpA) Around the Globe—cont'd

Author, Publication Year	Years of Study	Country/Region	Mean Age	Total Population	Source of Data
(Reveille, 2012)[62]	2009–2010	USA	20-69	5,103	Data from NHANES survey administered to a nationally representative sample
(Pelaez-Ballestas, 2013)[63]	2009–NR	Mexico, Cuajimalpa, Mexico City	>18	4,059	Individuals listed in a primary health clinic
(Strand, 2013)[64]	1985–2011	USA	18–44	109,377,973	Medical records of randomly selected patients with CBP from randomly selected rheumatology practices
(Haroon, 2014)[65]	1995–2010	Canada, Ontario	≥15	11,016,692	Provincial administrative health databases, core sets
(Kassimos, 2014)[66]	1989–1995	Greece	18–30	347,184	Medical records of General Military Hospital of Athens
(Koko, 2014)[67]	1995–2011	Albania, Region of Gjirokaster	≥14	82,567	Regional hospital, healthcare clinics, and family practitioners and work disability records
(Munoz-Ortego, 2014)[68]	2006–2011	Spain, Catalonia	NR	4,920,353	Public healthcare system for primary care
(van Hoeven, 2014)[69]	January–July, 2010	Netherlands, Rotterdam	20–45	12,477	Primary care records
(Costantino, 2015)[70]	2010	France	≥57	6,556	Respondents to a survey among the employees of a French company who had DNA samples for HLA-B*27 testing
(Exarchou, 2015)[71]	1967–2009	Sweden	16–64	5,982,237	National Patient Register

Screening Strategy for Case Finding	Method for Case Ascertainment	Case Definition/ Criteria	Prevalence of AS (%)	Male/ Female Ratio	Mean Age at Onset	*HLA-B*27* Prevalence (N-Tested)
Data collection for ESSG and Amor criteria, including items for CBP, but not for peripheral arthritis	Review of survey data by expert rheumatologists	ESSG for axSpA	1.4	0.6	NR	NR
		Amor for axSpA	0.9	0.3		
COPCORD questionnaire → evaluation of individuals for IBP at the clinic by general physicians and rheumatology fellows	Examination of subjects with possible IBP by two expert rheumatologists	mNY	0.09	NR	NR	NR
Extraction of patient data including SpA features specific to the ASAS criteria	Review of medical records by a central analytics organization	ASAS for axSpA	0.35	2.1	NR	NR
		mNY for AS	0.17	NR	NR	NR
		ASAS for nr-axSpA	0.17	NR	NR	NR
ICD-9-CM: 720 ICD-10-CA: M45	≥ 2 physician billing claims for over 2 years; or one relevant ICD code for hospitalization discharge diagnosis	Clinical	0.21	1.2-1.7	NR	NR
Examination before military training → admission to hospital	Review of medical records	mNY	0.08	No female included	NR	90 (n=285)
A recorded diagnosis of AS	Confirmation by tertiary university medical center	mNY	0.06	8	30	NR
ICD-10 code: M45	≥1 record of ICD code for AS	Clinical	0.13	NR	NR	NR
ICPC code: L03 (low back pain)	Clinical evaluation; including X-ray, MRI, and *HLA-B*27* testing	ASAS for axSpA	0.69	0.6	NR	20% (n=86)
		mNY for AS	0.12	0.6	NR	NR
		ASAS for nr-axSpA	0.57	0.8	NR	NR
Postal survey for a self-report of SpA and SpA features	Telephone interview → *HLA-B*27* testing and radiographs in all self-reporting cases of SpA	ASAS for axSpA	0.43	NR	NR	80% (n=20)
		mNY for AS	0.31			
S-ICD8: 712.40, 726.99 S-ICD9: 720A S-ICD10:M45	≥1 record of ICD code for AS	Clinical	0.18	1,6	39	NR

Continued

TABLE 3.1 Prevalence of Axial Spondyloarthritis (axSpA) and of Its Subsets, Ankylosing Spondylitis (AS) and Nonradiographic axSpA (nr-axSpA) Around the Globe—cont'd

Author, Publication Year	Years of Study	Country/Region	Mean Age	Total Population	Source of Data
(Hamilton, 2015)[72]	NR	UK, Norfolk	18–80	13,387	Electronic health records (general practice)
(Onen, 2015)[73]	2012	Turkey, Izmir (hospital employees)	38	2,894	A randomly selected sample from hospital employees (n= 395)
(Sliwczynski, 2015)[74]	2008–2013	Poland	NR	NR	National Health Fund-National payer database
(van Hoeven, 2015)[75]	2011–2012	Netherlands, Rotterdam and Hague	20–45	28,842	Primary care records
(Curtis, 2016)[76]	1996–2009	USA, North California	≥18	>3 million	Computerized clinical data of a nonprofit health delivery system
(Dean, 2016)[77]	2000–2011	Scotland, PC population	≥16	1,469,688	Scottish Primary Care Clinical Informatics Unit Research
	2010–2013	SC population countrywide, two regions excluded		3,620,405	Scotland Registry for Ankylosing Spondylitis
(Barnabe, 2017)[78]	1993–2011	Canada, Alberta, First Nations and non-First Nations	NR	NR	Provincial administrative health databases
(Videm, 2017)[79]	1995–1997/2006–2008	Norway, Nord-Trøndelag	≥20 years	70,805	Participants of HUNT2/HUNT3 surveys

NR, not reported; *NY*, New York; *USA*, United States of America; *mNY*, modified New York; *ASAS*, Assessment of SpondyloArthritis International Society; *ICD-9*, International Classification of Diseases, Ninth Revision; *CM*, Clinical Modification; *HLA-B*27*, human leukocyte antigen *HLA-B*27*; *COPCORD*, Community Oriented Program for the Control of Rheumatic Disease; *IBP*, inflammatory back pain; *SpA*, spondyloarhritis; *MRI*, magnetic resonance imaging; *ICD-10*, ICD Tenth Revision; *ESSG*, The European Spondylarthropathy Study Group; *ICD-8*, ICD Eighth Revision; *CT*, computerized tomography; *MSK*, musculoskeletal; *NHANES*, National Health and Nutrition Examination Survey; *CA*, Canadian adaptation; *ICPC*, International Classification of Primary Care; *S-ICD*, Swedish version of the ICD; *PC*, Primary Care; *HUNT*, Nord-Trøndelag Health Study.

Screening Strategy for Case Finding	Method for Case Ascertainment	Case Definition/ Criteria	Prevalence of AS (%)	Male/ Female Ratio	Mean Age at Onset	HLA-B*27 Prevalence (N-Tested)
Two step: Read Code for back pain → questionnaire for IBP or prior diagnosis of axSpA or AS	Verification of self-reported diagnosis from medical records and clinical evaluation for others	ASAS for axSpA	0.3	NR	NR	NR
		mNY for AS	0.15*	NR	NR	NR
Questionnaire for IBP	Clinical evaluation; *HLA-B*27* testing, radiography, CT and MRI, when indicated	ASAS for axSpA	1.3	1.3	NR	NR
		mNY for AS	0.5	2	NR	NR
		ASAS for nr-axSpA	0.8	1	NR	NR
ICD-10 code: M45	≥1 record of ICD code for AS, as main or coexisting diagnosis	Clinical	0.07	NR	NR	NR
ICPC code: L03 (low back pain)	Clinical evaluation; including X-ray, MRI, and *HLA-B*27* testing	ASAS for axSpA	0.33	0.6	NR	22% (n=95)
		mNY for AS	0.08	NR	NR	NR
		ASAS for nr-axSpA	0.25	NR	NR	NR
ICD-9: 720.x axSpA ICD-9: 720.0 AS	≥1 record of 720.x for axSpA;	Clinical	0.23	NR	NR	34% (n=35)
	≥2 records of 720.0 in primary care or ≥1 diagnosis of AS by rheumatologist	Clinical	0.17			
Read Codes (N100) relating to AS	≥1 record of Read Code in the PC database	Clinical	0.13	3.3	38	NR
Cases in the AS registry	Enrollment in the AS registry		0.05	3.2	35	
ICD-9-CM: 720.x ICD-10-CA: M45.x	≥ 2 physician billing claims for a relevant ICD code over 2 years; or 1 relevant ICD code for hospitalization discharge diagnosis	Clinical	0.6 (First Nations) 0.2 (non-First Nations)	NR	NR	NR
Self-reported cases of AS	Verification of diagnosis by review of hospital case files	mNY	0.32	2.5	39	88% (n=172)

or ethnic differences, use of different classification criteria, reporting crude or standardized rates).[81] We can add that *it has become quite difficult to interpret the data and review papers with increasing misuse of the term axSpA as equivalent to AS in the original articles or sometimes in the citing manuscripts.*

Incidence Studies

There are fewer incidence studies of AS than those dealing with prevalence, and many of them[16,19,29,32, 37,40,54,55,67,78,79] are also listed in Table 3.1, along with short descriptions of their study designs. There are no published studies that deal with the full spectrum of axSpA or its nr-axSpA subset. The incidence studies of AS mostly come from North America and Europe. A US study from Rochester, the main city in Olmsted County of Minnesota, which at the time of the study had a 99% white population of mostly Scandinavian descent, estimated an (age- and sex-adjusted) annual incidence of 6.6 per 100,000 among persons aged ≥15 years for the study period between1935 and 1973.[16] The case ascertainment included presence of chronic back pain and roentgenographically documented sacroiliitis in the absence of other diseases or causes to explain the symptoms. A subsequent analysis covering a longer period until 1989 reported a similar annual incidence at 7.3 per 100.000 (95% CI: 6.1–8.4) for primary AS, using the modified New York criteria for the case definition.[82]

Three studies from Finland have also reported comparable incidence rates, as reported in the above-mentioned US studies. The first of these three studies covered 5 of 21 hospital districts serving about 1 million adults aged 16 years and above.[29] The authors searched the register of the Social Insurance Institution to identify cases based on an issuance of a drug reimbursement certificate for AS by their physicians in the years of 1980, 1985, and 1990. Case ascertainment was based on the information available on the medical certificate, which was supplemented by review of hospital records when needed. They calculated the annual incidence of AS for the study period to be 6.9 per 100,000 (95% CI: 6.0–7.8). The second study using the same methodology in the same population in 1995 recorded a very similar incidence, 6.3 per 100,000 (95% CI: 4.9–7.9).[83] The last one was a hospital-based study from Kuopio, a city in central Finland, which noted an annual incidence comparable with the other Finnish studies, 5.8 per 100,000 (95% CI: 1.6–14.8).[84] Case definition in these studies were not based on any classification for AS.

A hospital-based study from Northern Norway estimated an incidence of 7.26 per 100,000 (95% CI: 5.30–9.22) for primary AS (in the absence of psoriasis or inflammatory bowel disease) and 8.71 per 100,000 (95% CI: 6.38–11.04) for secondary AS (secondary to psoriasis or inflammatory bowel disease) in those aged ≥16 years for the period from 1960 and 1993.[40] The database of the Northern Norway University Hospital, which is the only rheumatology department in the catchment area, was searched to find cases registered in the system with an ICD-9 or ICD-10 code for AS. Records and radiographs of the SI joints of all identified patients were reviewed for fulfillment of the modified New York criteria. A new radiologic examination of the SI joints was performed, if needed. A very recent Norwegian study reported a crude incidence of 19 per 100,000 (95% CI: 15–24) for those aged ≥ 20 years.[79] Cases, with at least one record of ICD-9 or ICD-10 code for a diagnosis of AS in the registries of the hospitals with rheumatology clinics in Central Norway, were identified, and the diagnosis was ascertained according to modified New York criteria using the hospital case files. Notably, 168 of the 187 cases with the confirmed diagnosis of AS were among the 70,805 participants of the survey, leaving only 19 cases for the nonparticipants who can be estimated to be about 24,000 people. The authors calculated both the prevalence and incidence based on the number of participants, rather than the whole survey population, and therefore both are likely to be overestimates considering that only few cases existed among the nonparticipants.

A study from Iceland reported an annual incidence rate ranging from 0.44 to 5.48 per 100,000 for the period from 1947 to 2005.[54] Most notably, this study was designed to determine the nationwide prevalence of AS in Iceland. The crude annual incidence was calculated based on the year of diagnosis as reported by patients. The cross-sectional design of the study would not allow for capturing AS patients who died over the study period of 58 years.

Incidence estimates in Czech Republic have been reported to be 6.4 per 100,000 (95%CI: 3.3–11.3) and in Albania to be 6 per 100,000 (95% CI: 3.3–11.3).[55,67] A study from Greece reported the lowest annual incidence at 1.5 per 100.000 (95% CI: 0.4–2.5),[37] probably because of its methodology, which involved manual search of medical records from two hospitals and eight private practices in the northwestern part of the country.

Similar to the recent study from Central Norway discussed above,[79] another recent study,[65] this one from Canada, reported a standardized annual incidence of AS to be 15 per 100,000 for those aged ≥15 years for the period from 1985 through 2010, based on cases found in the administrative health databases in Ontario. The diagnosis was established on the basis of at least two records of the ICD-9 code of 720 over a period of 2 years in the Ontario Health Insurance Plan Claims History Database registered by two physicians, at least one being a rheumatologist or at least one record of an ICD-9 code of 720 or ICD-10 code of M45 in the Canadian Institute for Health Information Discharge Abstract Database. The major weakness of this study is that no case verification was done, and no data were provided for the validity of this diagnostic algorithm in their setting. Importantly, the diagnosis code of 720 does include AS and other inflammatory spondylopathies.

Besides the methodologic issues pointed out above, there may be other reasons to explain the high incidence figures for AS, relative to those reported by previous studies. They may be just a reflection of the increasing awareness of the disease over the years by physicians, particularly after the introduction of anti–tumor necrosis factor (TNF) agents into clinical practice for the treatment of AS, as well as the changing attitude of physicians for the diagnosis of AS after the introduction of MRI as a sensitive tool for detecting sacroiliitis. A recent epidemiologic study of axSpA from US rheumatology practices showed that it is not uncommon for physicians to make a diagnosis of AS, in the absence of any radiographic exam or despite the presence of negative radiographic findings for definite sacroiliitis.[64] Moreover, physicians may be prone to making a diagnosis of AS in some patients with equivocal findings on pelvic radiographs and only chronic (not active or acute) osteitis of the sacroiliac joints (SIJs) on MRI. Some healthcare providers may be particularly inclined to do so to meet insurance coverage criteria, when nr-axSpA is not an approved indication for anti-TNF treatment.

Information on the incidence of AS in nonwestern populations is scarce. A Japanese study reported a very low incidence of AS of 0.48 per 100.000 for those aged >15 years, based on the data obtained from two nationwide surveys administered to physicians in 1990 and 1997.[32] Physicians selected from hospitals with a high potential of admitting patients with SpA were asked to complete the questionnaires by reviewing the medical records of SpA patients who attended their institutions within the preceding 5 years. Although a low incidence estimate of AS is not unexpected in the Japanese population, which has a very low prevalence of HLA-B*27 (0.5%) in the general population,[85] the case finding

strategy used in this study may have led to underestimation of the true incidence, because of its likely inability to capture all diagnosed AS patients in the whole country. The only other incidence study in a nonwestern population was conducted in Inuit Eskimos located in Northwest territories of Canada.[19] Annual incidence in this population that has a high HLA-B*27 prevalence (25%) was estimated to be 5.1 per 100,000 for the period between 1975 and 1986.

RISK FACTORS

Age and Sex

AS had traditionally been known to be a disease of young people with range of onset of symptoms between 12 and 45 years, both among males and females. The median age of onset of symptoms was reported to be 18 years in the 1930s, which steadily increased up to 28 years in the early 1980s.[86] The mean age at onset now ranges between 23 and 31 years among recent cohorts from the Netherlands, Belgium and France (OASIS),[87] Germany (GESPIC),[88] Switzerland (SCQM),[89] Spain (REGISPONSER),[90] Ibero-America (RESPONDIA),[91] and Turkey (TRASD-IP)[92] (Table 3.2). Younger mean ages at onset have been reported from US and Korean cohorts (PSOAS and OSKAR, respectively), probably because of their inclusion of relatively higher percentage of juvenile onset cases, 19% and 29%, respectively.[93,94]

Whereas the age of onset has gradually increased over the years, especially in developed countries, there has been a progressive decrease in the reported male predominance in AS. Thus, for example, male to female ratio of 9:1 reported in the 1940s[95] has declined to 2–3:1 in recent cohorts.[87–92,96,97] The most current study reports a steady decline in the male to female ratio among patients with AS/axSpA in Switzerland from 2.6:1 in 1980, down to 1:1 by the end of 2016.[98] In contrast to AS, nr-axSpA patients show hardly any difference in its prevalence among males and females.[99] Data from national registries involving both subsets of axSpA, that is, AS and nr-axSpA, suggest that patients with nr-axSpA are likely to be slightly older and more frequently females, when compared with those suffering from AS.[88,89,100,101] Results from a very recent multinational large prospective cohort (PROOF) of recently diagnosed axSpA (≤1 year) patients who were classified into AS or nr-axSpA after central assessment of radiographs seem to support these findings[102] (Table 3.2). Spondyloarthritis Caught Early (SPACE) cohort is included in Table 3.2, but it should be noted that it is

TABLE 3.2   Age and Sex Characteristics and *HLA-B*27* Prevalence of Patients With Ankylosing Spondylitis (AS) and Axial Spondyloarthritis (axSpA) in Several Registries

Cohort	Years of Recruitment	Target Population	SpA Subtype	Classification Criteria	Number of Enrollment	Mean Age of Onset	Male to Female Ratio	HLA-B*27 Prevalence (%)
OASIS[87]	1996–2006	AS	AS	mNY	216	23	2.5	85
PSOAS[96]	2002–2005	AS	AS	mNY	402	23	3.0	87
SPARCC[97]	2006–2010	SpA	AS	mNY + ASAS	1108	31	2.8	79
OSKAR[94]	2006–2007	AS	AS	mNY	830	21	7.3	98
REGISPON-SER[90]	2004–2005	SpA	AS	mNY	842	26	3.2	85
RESPON-DIA[91]	2010–2011	SpA	AS	mNY	1083	28	3	71
TRASD-IP[92]	2007–2009	AS	AS	mNY	1381	28	3	73
GESPIC[88]	2000–2004	axSpA	AS (DD ≤10 years)	mNY	226	30	1.8	82
			Nr-axSpA (DD ≤5 years)	ESSG*	236	33	0.8	75
SCQM[89]	2005–2011	SpA	AS	mNY	1199	27	2.2	79
			Nr-axSpA	ASAS*	333	28	0.9	78
DESIR[100,101]	2007–2010	SpA + CBP (>3 months ≤3 years)	AS	mNY	181	30†	1.4	72
			Nr-axSpA	ASAS	259‡	32†,‡	0.9‡	90‡
PROOF[102]	2014–2016	axSpA (diagnosis ≤1 year)	AS	mNY	1039	29†	2.4	69
			Nr-axSpA	ASAS	544	31†	0.9	55
SPACE[103]	2012–ongoing	CBP (>3 months ≤2 years)	AS	mNY	11	27†	2.7	55
			Nr-axSpA	ASAS	49	29†	0.8	84

OASIS, Outcome Assessments in AS International Study; *PSOAS*, Prospective Study of Outcomes in Ankylosing Spondylitis; *SPARCC*, Spondyloarthritis Research Consortium of Canada; *REGISPONSER*, Registry of Spondyloarthritis of the Spanish Society of Rheumatology; *RESPONDIA*, Ibero-American Registry of Spondyloarthritis; *DESIR*, Devenir dEs SpondyloarthropathIes Récentes; *GESPIC*, German Spondyloarthritis Inception Cohort; *PROOF*, Patients with axial spondyloaRthritis: Multi-cOuntry Registry OF clinical characteristics, including radiographic progression, and burden of disease over 5 years in real-life setting; *SPACE*, Spondyloarthritis Caught Early (SPACE) cohort; *NR*, not reported; *CBP*, chronic back pain; *mNY*, modified New York; *ASAS*, Assessment of SpondyloArthritis International Society; *ESSG*, European Spondylarthropathy Study Group; *DD*, disease duration; *Nr-axSpA*, nonradiographic axial spondyloartritis
*with minor modifications
†calculated from age of inclusion and disease duration;
‡calculated from data provided by Ref. 101.

an early chronic back pain cohort.[103] Because nr-axSpA and AS represent the two ends of the axSpA spectrum, one can speculate that male sex exerts either a permissive or an enhancing effect for progression to AS. On the contrary, female sex may have a relatively protective effect against progressive ankylosis.

HLA-B*27 and Family History

This aspect and the other genetic predisposing factors and biomarkers are discussed in detail in Chapter 5. In brief, the remarkable association between AS and *HLA-B*27* was first published by investigators from London[104,105] and Los Angeles, the United States, in

1973.[106] After 45 years, the precise role of *HLA-B*27* in genetic predisposition to AS and related forms of SpA is still an enigma. *HLA-B*27* prevalence among patients with AS and AxSpA in several registries is listed in Tables 3.1 and 3.2. *HLA-B*27* seems to be less strongly associated with nr-axSpA than with AS.

The role of heredity in AS has long been known. More than 65 families with multiple affected cases were reported in the literature from 1918 through 1950.[107] A recent study from Iceland quantitated the risk of developing AS among the first- through fourth-degree relatives of AS cases and found an increased risk extending to the third-degree relatives, but not any further. The estimated relative risks (RRs) for the first-, second-, and third-degree relatives were 75.5, 20.2, and 3.5, respectively (all P values < 0.0001).[108] The impact of sex on disease inheritance has been noted since early times. An analysis of 50 affected family pedigrees noted an equal sex distribution among the family cases and an increased risk for disease inheritance in sibships containing at least one affected female, especially when the affected case is a mother.[107] Many years later a British study confirmed these findings in a much larger population.[109] In this study, when analysis was restricted to the relatives aged ≥39 years, inheritance of AS from fathers to sons (12%) occurred more frequently than to daughters (5%). Similarly, rate of disease inheritance from affected males to brothers (9.5%) of affected males was significantly higher than to their sisters (5.8%). No significant differences were observed between the inheritance rates from mothers to sons (20%) and to daughters (15%) or between the rates of inheritance to brothers (12.6%) of affected females and to their sisters (9.3%). A similar analysis was performed for parental inheritance of SpA in a French cohort of multiplex SpA families, and about one-third of them did not have AS phenotype.[110] However, when the analysis was limited to offsprings with AS, there was a trend for a higher inheritance rate from mothers to sons (45%) than to daughters (27%). More frequent disease inheritance by women has been explained by greater genetic load. A later study from Britain reported higher disease prevalence among second-degree relatives of children with affected mothers than those with affected fathers (20 vs. 9%) and provided further support to increased heritability by female patients.[111] A study conducted in Mexican Mestizos found no correlation between the inheritance of AS and the sex of the affected parent. However, in this study, the parents were healthy but considered affected because of their family history.[112]

Infections

This aspect is covered in detail in Chapters 5–8. In brief, recent studies examining the gut flora have demonstrated a discrete microbial signature in the bowels of patients with AS or SpA compared with controls. They did not confirm the previous reports that Klebsiella infection is a triggering factor for AS.[113,114] There is evidence that diet has a strong impact on the composition of the gut microbiota,[115] but no specific dietary components have, as yet, been identified that can impact the risk of development of AS. A report suggesting that non–breast-fed babies are more likely to develop AS than their breast-fed siblings or healthy controls[116] needs further verification. Infections encountered in childhood may also influence the risk, and a Swedish study reported higher rates of hospitalizations during childhood because of respiratory tract infections, particularly tonsillitis, among patients with AS than in controls matched for sex, birth year, and country.[117] Reactive arthritis, which can sometimes lead to AS,[118] is usually triggered by enteric or urogenital infections, which include but not limited to *Chlamydia trachomatis*, *Yersinia*, *Salmonella*, *Shigella*, and *Campylobacter*.[119] Many of the patients with reactive arthritis with axial symptoms fulfill the new ASAS classification criteria, but there is no evidence that the infections that precede reactive arthritis development play a role in AS/axSpA that lacks typical clinical features of reactive arthritis.

Biomechanical Stress

Biomechanical stress may play a role in axSpA, and a study has shown that long-lasting AS patients with higher level of work-related physical activity during their working life had greater functional limitations.[120] The same group of investigators later reported that occupational activities, such as bending, twisting, and stretching, were associated with worse functional status and radiographic damage in patients having AS for ≥20 years. Exposure to whole-body vibration was associated only with more radiographic damage.[121] These findings provide support for the role of mechanical stress in the progression of AS, rather than its initiation. However, a mouse model for SpA demonstrated that mechanical strain may indeed trigger entheseal inflammation and lead to new bone formation.[122] Actually, trauma has been proposed to precipitate chronic inflammatory arthritis since the 1940s,[123] and even earlier than that. Many case series and/or case reports have suggested a link between trauma and inflammatory arthritis, including AS,[124] reactive arthritis,[125,126] and peripheral SpA.[127-129] It is possible that injury may not have been related to the disease process but was likely to have been brought to the patient's recall, possibly during the immobilization at the hospital.[124] A recent longitudinal matched cohort study reported that patients with psoriasis with a previous exposure to trauma have a higher risk of developing psoriatic arthritis than those without.[130]

Smoking

There is as yet no evidence for association of smoking with susceptibility to AS, but smoking and hypertension were found to be associated with incident AS.[131] Therefore, patients with AS, especially those who have a family history of this disease or carry HLA-B*27 gene, should be encouraged to stop smoking.

DISEASE PROGRESSION

Radiographic change in the SIJs and spine is considered to reflect the disease progression in axSpA. However, there is no evidence that worsening of radiographic changes in the SIJs has any impact on patients' functional status and mobility, whereas structural damage in the spine and disease activity are shown to be determinants of the functional status and spinal mobility in early axSpA.[132]

Several studies have evaluated the risk of progression from the nonradiographic to the radiographic stage of axSpA. Before the introduction of the ASAS classification criteria, such studies had included patients with undifferentiated SpA (uSpA), and a systematic review of patients with uSpA has reported rates of development of radiographic sacroiliitis of 22%, 29%, and 39%, after 5, 8, and 10 years, respectively.[133] Recent study cohorts that have included patients with nr-axSpA as defined by the ASAS criteria (DESIR and EMBARK cohorts) indicated ≤1.6% rate of progression from nr-axSpA to AS over a period of 2 years[134,135] as compared with 9% true progression rate (defined as progression rate minus regression rate) observed in the GESPIC cohort comprising patients with axSPA,[136] and 4-year data (from RAPID axSpA trial cohort) noted almost no progression.[137] Markedly different ranges of rates of progression of 5%–6%,[138–140] 17%–25%,[139,141] and 26%–69%[139,141] have been reported after 5, 10, and 15 years of disease duration, respectively. Notably, the French cohort[141] that showed a very high progression rate over 15 years is a multiplex SpA family cohort. Higher genetic load, younger age at onset, and considerably longer disease duration may have contributed to the markedly higher progression rate at 15 years in this cohort.

Risk factors for radiographic progression in the SIJs include elevated CRP levels at baseline,[136] positive MRI at baseline,[134,139,140] and a low-grade radiographic sacroiliitis at baseline and buttock pain during follow-up.[141] In the DESIR cohort, HLA-B*27 and smoking status were identified as predictors of progression at 2 years,[134] but not at 5 years.[140] However, in the 5-year progression study, the association of positive MRI with progression was stronger among HLA-B*27-positive patients.

Progression of structural damage in the spine is more prevalent in the AS subset of axSpA.[142] In the GESPIC cohort, which is an axSpA cohort as stated earlier, new syndesmophyte formation was observed in 3.2% of nr-axSpA and 11.3% of AS patients.[142] Baseline structural damage, elevated CRP, and smoking status were associated with radiographic progression in that study. Another study reported a higher progression rate at 31% and found the presence of syndesmophyte as the best predictor of radiographic progression.[143] A 12-year follow-up study of long-lasting AS patients noted at least one new syndesmophyte formation in about 30% of the patients over 2 years and 60% of the patients over the whole study period.[144] 25% of the patients developed no syndesmophyte, whereas another 25% showed high level of progression. HLA-B*27 in men and a baseline modified Stoke Ankylosing Spondylitis Spinal Score (mSASSS) ≥10 were associated with radiographic progression.

MORTALITY

It is well known that the first report indicating an excess mortality in AS dates back to the 1960s and that leukemias and cancers due to irradiation therapy used for the treatment of AS at those times were the main source of mortality.[145] However, it is not perhaps as well known that even the actual number of deaths due to causes unrelated to the form of treatment in that study was also higher than the expected number estimates from national mortality rates.[145] Since then, several studies have been published on this topic.[16,82,146–152] Although some of the early studies reported an increased mortality or decreased survival in AS patients,[146,148,149] a few others found no difference as compared with general population.[16,82,147] However, the results of more recent studies with generally larger sample sizes have been more consistent in indicating an excess mortality rate in AS.[150–152] The most recent study from Sweden, involving 8600 AS patients diagnosed at rheumatology or internal medicine outpatient clinics in Sweden, demonstrated a hazard ratio (HR) of 1.60 (95% CI:

1.44–1.77) for total mortality, as compared with the general population. Mortality was increased significantly in both male (HR: 1.53, 95% CI: 1.36–1.72) and female patients (HR: 1.83, 95% CI: 1.50–2.22). Standardized mortality ratios (SMRs) from previous studies ranged from 1.33 to 1.80,[146,149–151] but significance level was reached in the total patient population and among males,[146,149–151] but not in female patients.[146,150,151] Amyloidosis,[149] cardiovascular and circulatory diseases (CVD),[148,150,152] and infections[151] were the leading cause of death in these studies. Increased mortality risk was associated with diagnostic delay, increased inflammation, and low intake of nonsteroidal antiinflammatory drugs in the study from Norway[150] and with lower level of education, general comorbidities (diabetes, infections, cardiovascular, pulmonary, and malignant diseases) and previous hip joint replacement surgery in the study from Sweden.[152]

A large population-based cohort study from Ontario, Canada, focused on vascular mortality in AS patients, without evaluating all-cause mortality.[153] This study reported an adjusted HR of 1.36 (95% CI: 1.13–1.65), for cardiovascular and cerebrovascular mortality, as compared with matched non-AS controls. Increased mortality risk was significant for the male patients (HR: 1.46, 95% CI: 1.13–1.87), but not for the female patients (HR: 1.24, 95% CI: 0.92–1.67). Interestingly, vascular death risk was found to be negatively associated with exposure to NSAIDs in patients aged 65 years or older, although this may be due to channeling bias as elderly patients with CVD are less likely to be prescribed NSAIDs.

A recent US study evaluated cause of death among the 12,484 AS patients admitted to the hospital between 2007 and 2011.[154] Of the 267 AS patients who died during their hospitalization, 55% were coded with a diagnosis of CVD. However, when the data were analyzed based on the principal diagnoses coded for the patients, sepsis (14%), spinal cord injury (9%), vertebral fractures (9%), respiratory failure (6%), and pneumonia (6%) were the top diagnostic categories. Cervical spine fracture with spinal cord injury had the strongest association with inpatient mortality with an odds ratio of 13.4 (95% CI: 8.00–22.6), whereas CVD had an odds ratio of 1.3 (95% CI: 1.0–1.7). Notably, among the hospitalized AS patients, falling was the primary mechanism of cervical fractures.

*HLA-B*27* has been reported to be positively associated with an increased mortality after adjustment for SpA, among US veterans clinically selected for *HLA-B*27* testing.[155] However, *HLA-B*27* positivity in patients without a diagnosis of SpA did not significantly influence mortality, suggesting that increased mortality in SpA cases may account for the observed increased mortality rates in *HLA-B*27*-positive veterans. Therefore, as stated in an accompanying editorial, these results should be interpreted with caution.[156]

REFERENCES

1. Porta M. *A Dictionary of Epidemiology.* Oxford University Press; 2008.
2. Ahrens W, Krickeberg K, Pigeot I. An introduction to epidemiology. In: *Handbook of Epidemiology.* Springer; 2014:3–41.
3. van der Linden SJ, Cats A, Valkenburg HA, Khan MA. Evaluation of the diagnostic criteria for ankylosing spondylitis: a proposal for modification of the New York criteria. *Clin Res.* 1983;(31):734A.
4. van der Linden SJ, Cats A, Valkenburg HA, Khan MA. Evaluation of the diagnostic criteria for ankylosing spondylitis: a proposal for modification of the New York criteria. *Br J Rheumatol.* 1984;(23):148.
5. van der Linden S, Valkenburg HA, Cats A. Evaluation of diagnostic criteria for ankylosing spondylitis. A proposal for modification of the New York criteria. *Arthritis Rheum.* 1984;27(4):361–368.
6. Rudwaleit M, van der Heijde D, Landewe R, et al. The development of Assessment of SpondyloArthritis international Society classification criteria for axial spondyloarthritis (part II): validation and final selection. *Ann Rheum Dis.* 2009;68(6):777–783.
7. Khan MA, van der Linden SM, Kushner I, Valkenburg HA, Cats A. Spondylitic disease without radiologic evidence of sacroiliitis in relatives of HLA-B27 positive ankylosing spondylitis patients. *Arthritis Rheum.* 1985;28(1):40–43.
8. Rudwaleit M, van der Heijde D, Landewe R, et al. The Assessment of SpondyloArthritis International Society classification criteria for peripheral spondyloarthritis and for spondyloarthritis in general. *Ann Rheum Dis.* 2011;70(1):25–31.
9. Dean LE, Jones GT, Macdonald AG, Downham C, Sturrock RD, Macfarlane GJ. Global prevalence of ankylosing spondylitis. *Rheumatology.* 2014;53(4):650–657.
10. Mikkelsen WM, Dodge HJ, Duff IF, Kato H. Estimates of the prevalence of rheumatic diseases in the population of Tecumseh, Michigan, 1959–60. *J Chronic Dis.* 1967;20(6):351–369.
11. Solomon L, Beighton P, Valkenburg HA, Robin G, Soskolne CL. Rheumatic disorders in the South African Negro. Part I. Rheumatoid arthritis and ankylosing spondylitis. *S Afr Med J.* 1975;49(32):1292–1296.
12. Stolwijk C, van Onna M, Boonen A, van Tubergen A. Global prevalence of spondyloarthritis: a systematic review and meta-regression analysis. *Arthritis Care Res.* 2016;68(9):1320–1331.

13. Gofton JP, Bennett PH, Smythe HA, Decker JL. Sacroiliitis and ankylosing spondylitis in North American Indians. *Ann Rheum Dis.* 1972;31(6):474–481.

14. Gomor B, Gyodi E, Bakos L. Distribution of HLA B27 and ankylosing spondylitis in the Hungarian population. *J Rheumatol Suppl.* 1977;3:33–35.

15. Atkins C, Reuffel L, Roddy J, Platts M, Robinson H, Ward R. Rheumatic disease in the Nuu-Chah-Nulth native Indians of the Pacific northwest. *J Rheumatol.* 1988;15(4):684–690.

16. Carter ET, McKenna CH, Brian DD, Kurland LT. Epidemiology of ankylosing spondylitis in Rochester, Minnesota, 1935–1973. *Arthritis Rheum.* 1979;22(4):365–370.

17. Gran JT, Husby G, Hordvik M. Prevalence of ankylosing spondylitis in males and females in a young middle-aged population of Tromso, northern Norway. *Ann Rheum Dis.* 1985;44(6):359–367.

18. Lutalo SK. Chronic inflammatory rheumatic diseases in black Zimbabweans. *Ann Rheum Dis.* 1985;44(2):121–125.

19. Oen K, Postl B, Chalmers IM, et al. Rheumatic diseases in an Inuit population. *Arthritis Rheum.* 1986;29(1):65–74.

20. Boyer GS, Lanier AP, Templin DW. Prevalence rates of spondyloarthropathies, rheumatoid arthritis, and other rheumatic disorders in an Alaskan Inupiat Eskimo population. *J Rheumatol.* 1988;15(4):678–683.

21. Boyer GS, Lanier AP, Templin DW, Bulkow L. Spondyloarthropathy and rheumatoid arthritis in Alaskan Yupik Eskimos. *J Rheumatol.* 1990;17(4):489–496.

22. Boyer GS, Templin DW, Lanier AP. Rheumatic diseases in Alaskan Indians of the southeast coast: high prevalence of rheumatoid arthritis and systemic lupus erythematosus. *J Rheumatol.* 1991;18(10):1477–1484.

23. Boyer GS, Templin DW, Cornoni-Huntley JC, et al. Prevalence of spondyloarthropathies in Alaskan Eskimos. *J Rheumatol.* 1994;21(12):2292–2297.

24. Wigley RD, Zhang NZ, Zeng QY, et al. Rheumatic diseases in China: ILAR-China study comparing the prevalence of rheumatic symptoms in northern and southern rural populations. *J Rheumatol.* 1994;21(8):1484–1490.

25. Chou CT, Pei L, Chang DM, Lee CF, Schumacher HR, Liang MH. Prevalence of rheumatic diseases in Taiwan: a population study of urban, suburban, rural differences. *J Rheumatol.* 1994;21(2):302–306.

26. Benevolenskaya LI, Boyer GS, Erdesz S, et al. Spondylarthropathic diseases in indigenous circumpolar populations of Russia and Alaska. *Rev Rhum Engl Ed.* 1996;63(11):815–822.

27. Brown MA, Jepson A, Young A, Whittle HC, Greenwood BM, Wordsworth BP. Ankylosing spondylitis in West Africans—evidence for a non-HLA-B27 protective effect. *Ann Rheum Dis.* 1997;56(1):68–70.

28. Dans LF, Tankeh-Torres S, Amante CM, Penserga EG. The prevalence of rheumatic diseases in a Filipino urban population: a WHO-ILAR COPCORD study. World health organization. International league of associations for rheumatology. Community oriented programme for the control of the rheumatic diseases. *J Rheumatol.* 1997;24(9):1814–1819.

29. Kaipiainen-Seppanen O, Aho K, Heliovaara M. Incidence and prevalence of ankylosing spondylitis in Finland. *J Rheumatol.* 1997;24(3):496–499.

30. Braun J, Bollow M, Remlinger G, et al. Prevalence of spondylarthropathies in HLA-B27 positive and negative blood donors. *Arthritis Rheum.* 1998;41(1):58–67.

31. Akkoc N, Khan MA. Overestimation of the prevalence of ankylosing spondylitis in the Berlin study: comment on the article by Braun et al. *Arthritis Rheum.* 2005;52(12):4048–4049.

32. Hukuda S, Minami M, Saito T, et al. Spondyloarthropathies in Japan: nationwide questionnaire survey performed by the Japan Ankylosing Spondylitis Society. *J Rheumatol.* 2001;28(3):554–559.

33. Bruges-Armas J, Lima C, Peixoto MJ, et al. Prevalence of spondyloarthritis in Terceira, Azores: a population based study. *Ann Rheum Dis.* 2002;61(6):551–553.

34. Cardiel MH, Rojas-Serrano J. Community based study to estimate prevalence, burden of illness and help seeking behavior in rheumatic diseases in Mexico City. A COPCORD study. *Clin Exp Rheumatol.* 2002;20(5):617–624.

35. Dai SM, Han XH, Zhao DB, Shi YQ, Liu Y, Meng JM. Prevalence of rheumatic symptoms, rheumatoid arthritis, ankylosing spondylitis, and gout in Shanghai, China: a COPCORD study. *J Rheumatol.* 2003;30(10):2245–2251.

36. Minh Hoa TT, Darmawan J, Chen SL, Van Hung N, Thi Nhi C, Ngoc An T. Prevalence of the rheumatic diseases in urban Vietnam: a WHO-ILAR COPCORD study. *J Rheumatol.* 2003;30(10):2252–2256.

37. Alamanos Y, Papadopoulos NG, Voulgari PV, Karakatsanis A, Siozos C, Drosos AA. Epidemiology of ankylosing spondylitis in Northwest Greece, 1983–2002. *Rheumatology.* 2004;43(5):615–618.

38. Al-Awadhi AM, Olusi SO, Moussa M, et al. Musculoskeletal pain, disability and health-seeking behavior in adult Kuwaitis using a validated Arabic version of the WHO-ILAR COPCORD Core Questionnaire. *Clin Exp Rheumatol.* 2004;22(2):177–183.

39. Zeng QY, Chen R, Xiao ZY, et al. Low prevalence of knee and back pain in southeast China; the Shantou COPCORD study. *J Rheumatol.* 2004;31(12):2439–2443.

40. Bakland G, Nossent HC, Gran JT. Incidence and prevalence of ankylosing spondylitis in Northern Norway. *Arthritis Rheum.* 2005;53(6):850–855.

41. Haq SA, Darmawan J, Islam MN, et al. Prevalence of rheumatic diseases and associated outcomes in rural and urban communities in Bangladesh: a COPCORD study. *J Rheumatol.* 2005;32(2):348–353.

42. Saraux A, Guillemin F, Guggenbuhl P, et al. Prevalence of spondyloarthropathies in France: 2001. *Ann Rheum Dis.* 2005;64(10):1431–1435.

43. Trontzas P, Andrianakos A, Miyakis S, et al. Seronegative spondyloarthropathies in Greece: a population-based study of prevalence, clinical pattern, and management. The ESORDIG study. *Clin Rheumatol.* 2005;24(6):583–589.

44. De Angelis R, Salaffi F, Grassi W. Prevalence of spondyloarthropathies in an Italian population sample: a regional community-based study. *Scand J Rheumatol.* 2007;36(1):14–21.

45. Veerapen K, Wigley RD, Valkenburg H. Musculoskeletal pain in Malaysia: a COPCORD survey. *J Rheumatol.* 2007;34(1):207–213.

46. Davatchi F, Jamshidi AR, Banihashemi AT, et al. WHO-ILAR COPCORD study (stage 1, urban study) in Iran. *J Rheumatol.* 2008;35(7):1384.

47. Onen F, Akar S, Birlik M, et al. Prevalence of ankylosing spondylitis and related spondyloarthritides in an urban area of Izmir, Turkey. *J Rheumatol.* 2008;35(2):305–309.

48. Adomaviciute D, Pileckyte M, Baranauskaite A, Morvan J, Dadoniene J, Guillemin F. Prevalence survey of rheumatoid arthritis and spondyloarthropathy in Lithuania. *Scand J Rheumatol.* 2009;37(2):113–119.

49. Joshi VL, Chopra A. Is there an urban-rural divide? Population surveys of rheumatic musculoskeletal disorders in the Pune region of India using the COPCORD Bhigwan model. *J Rheumatol.* 2009;36(3):614–622.

50. Liao ZT, Pan YF, Huang JL, et al. An epidemiological survey of low back pain and axial spondyloarthritis in a Chinese Han population. *Scand J Rheumatol.* 2009;38(6):455–459.

51. Reyes-Llerena GA, Guibert-Toledano M, Penedo-Coello A, et al. Community-based study to estimate prevalence and burden of illness of rheumatic diseases in Cuba: a COPCORD study. *J Clin Rheumatol.* 2009;15(2):51–55.

52. Anagnostopoulos I, Zinzaras E, Alexiou I, et al. The prevalence of rheumatic diseases in central Greece: a population survey. *BMC Musculoskelet Disord.* 2010;11:98.

53. Eaton WW, Pedersen MG, Atladottir HO, Gregory PE, Rose NR, Mortensen PB. The prevalence of 30 ICD-10 autoimmune diseases in Denmark. *Immunol Res.* 2010;47(1–3):228–231.

54. Geirsson AJ, Eyjolfsdottir H, Bjornsdottir G, Kristjansson K, Gudbjornsson B. Prevalence and clinical characteristics of ankylosing spondylitis in Iceland - a nationwide study. *Clin Exp Rheumatol.* 2010;28(3):333–340.

55. Hanova P, Pavelka K, Holcatova I, Pikhart H. Incidence and prevalence of psoriatic arthritis, ankylosing spondylitis, and reactive arthritis in the first descriptive population-based study in the Czech Republic. *Scand J Rheumatol.* 2010;39(4):310–317.

56. Alvarez-Nemegyei J, Pelaez-Ballestas I, Sanin LH, Cardiel MH, Ramirez-Angulo A, Goycochea-Robles MV. Prevalence of musculoskeletal pain and rheumatic diseases in the southeastern region of Mexico. A COPCORD-based community survey. *J Rheumatol Suppl.* 2011;86:21–25.

57. Haglund E, Bremander AB, Petersson IF, et al. Prevalence of spondyloarthritis and its subtypes in southern Sweden. *Ann Rheum Dis.* 2011;70(6):943–948.

58. Karkucak M, Cakirbay H, Capkin E, et al. The prevalence of ankylosing spondylitis in the Eastern black sea region of Turkey. *Eur J Gen Med.* 2011;8(1):40–45.

59. Pelaez-Ballestas I, Sanin LH, Moreno-Montoya J, et al. Epidemiology of the rheumatic diseases in Mexico. A study of 5 regions based on the COPCORD methodology. *J Rheumatol Suppl.* 2011;86:3–8.

60. Rodriguez-Amado J, Pelaez-Ballestas I, Sanin LH, et al. Epidemiology of rheumatic diseases. A community-based study in urban and rural populations in the state of Nuevo Leon, Mexico. *J Rheumatol Suppl.* 2011;86:9–14.

61. Cakir N, Pamuk ON, Dervis E, et al. The prevalences of some rheumatic diseases in western Turkey: Havsa study. *Rheumatol Int.* 2012;32(4):895–908.

62. Reveille JD, Witter JP, Weisman MH. Prevalence of axial spondylarthritis in the United States: estimates from a cross-sectional survey. *Arthritis Care Res.* 2012;64(6):905–910.

63. Pelaez-Ballestas I, Navarro-Zarza JE, Julian B, et al. A community-based study on the prevalence of spondyloarthritis and inflammatory back pain in mexicans. *J Clin Rheumatol.* 2013;19(2):57–61.

64. Strand V, Rao SA, Shillington AC, Cifaldi MA, McGuire M, Ruderman EM. Prevalence of axial spondyloarthritis in United States rheumatology practices: assessment of SpondyloArthritis International Society criteria versus rheumatology expert clinical diagnosis. *Arthritis Care Res.* 2013;65(8):1299–1306.

65. Haroon NN, Paterson JM, Li P, Haroon N. Increasing proportion of female patients with ankylosing spondylitis: a population-based study of trends in the incidence and prevalence of AS. *BMJ Open.* 2014;4(12):e006634.

66. Kassimos DG, Vassilakos J, Magiorkinis G, Garyfallos A. Prevalence and clinical manifestations of ankylosing spondylitis in young Greek males. *Clin Rheumatol.* 2014;33(9):1303–1306.

67. Koko V, Ndrepepa A, Skenderaj S, Ploumis A, Backa T, Tafaj A. An epidemiological study on ankylosing spondylitis in southern Albania. *Mater Sociomed.* 2014;26(1):26–29.

68. Munoz-Ortego J, Vestergaard P, Rubio JB, et al. Ankylosing spondylitis is associated with an increased risk of vertebral and nonvertebral clinical fractures: a population-based cohort study. *J Bone Miner Res.* 2014;29(8):1770–1776.

69. van Hoeven L, Luime J, Han H, Vergouwe Y, Weel A. Identifying axial spondyloarthritis in Dutch primary care patients, ages 20-45 years, with chronic low back pain. *Arthritis Care Res.* 2014;66(3):446–453.

70. Costantino F, Talpin A, Said-Nahal R, et al. Prevalence of spondyloarthritis in reference to HLA-B27 in the French population: results of the GAZEL cohort. *Ann Rheum Dis.* 2015;74(4):689–693.

71. Exarchou S, Lindstrom U, Askling J, et al. The prevalence of clinically diagnosed ankylosing spondylitis and its clinical manifestations: a nationwide register study. *Arthritis Res Ther.* 2015;17:118.

72. Hamilton L, Macgregor A, Toms A, Warmington V, Pinch E, Gaffney K. The prevalence of axial spondyloarthritis in the UK: a cross-sectional cohort study. *BMC Musculoskelet Disord.* 2015;16:392.

73. Onen F, Solmaz D, Cetin P, et al. Prevalence of inflammatory back pain and axial spondyloarthritis among university employees in Izmir, Turkey. *J Rheumatol.* 2015;42(9):1647–1651.

74. Sliwczynski A, Raciborski F, Klak A, et al. Prevalence of ankylosing spondylitis in Poland and costs generated by AS patients in the public healthcare system. *Rheumatol Int.* 2015;35(8):1361–1367.

75. van Hoeven L, Vergouwe Y, de Buck PD, Luime JJ, Hazes JM, Weel AE. External validation of a referral rule for axial spondyloarthritis in primary care patients with chronic low back pain. *PloS One.* 2015;10(7): e0131963.

76. Curtis JR, Harrold LR, Asgari MM, et al. Diagnostic prevalence of ankylosing spondylitis using computerized health care data, 1996 to 2009: underrecognition in a US health care setting. *Perm J.* 2016;20(4):4–10.

77. Dean LE, Macfarlane GJ, Jones GT. Differences in the prevalence of ankylosing spondylitis in primary and secondary care: only one-third of patients are managed in rheumatology. *Rheumatology.* 2016;55(10):1820–1825.

78. Barnabe C, Jones CA, Bernatsky S, et al. Inflammatory arthritis prevalence and health services use in the first nations and non-first nations populations of Alberta, Canada. *Arthritis Care Res.* 2017;69(4):467–474.

79. Videm V, Thomas R, Brown MA, Hoff M. Self-reported diagnosis of rheumatoid arthritis or ankylosing spondylitis has low accuracy: data from the Nord-Trondelag health study. *J Rheumatol.* 2017;44(8):1134–1141.

80. Reveille JD, Weisman MH. The epidemiology of back pain, axial spondyloarthritis and HLA-B27 in the United States. *Am J Med Sci.* 2013;345(6):431–436.

81. Bohn R, Cooney M, Deodhar A, Curtis JR, Golembesky A. Incidence and prevalence of axial spondyloarthritis: methodologic challenges and gaps in the literature. *Clin Exp Rheumatol.* 2017.

82. Carbone LD, Cooper C, Michet CJ, Atkinson EJ, O'Fallon WM, Melton 3rd LJ. Ankylosing spondylitis in Rochester, Minnesota, 1935-1989. Is the epidemiology changing? *Arthritis Rheum.* 1992;35(12):1476–1482.

83. Kaipiainen-Seppanen O, Aho K. Incidence of chronic inflammatory joint diseases in Finland in 1995. *J Rheumatol.* 2000;27(1):94–100.

84. Savolainen E, Kaipiainen-Seppanen O, Kroger L, Luosujarvi R. Total incidence and distribution of inflammatory joint diseases in a defined population: results from the Kuopio 2000 arthritis survey. *J Rheumatol.* 2003;30(11):2460–2468.

85. Yamaguchi A, Tsuchiya N, Mitsui H, et al. Association of HLA-B39 with HLA-B27-negative ankylosing spondylitis and pauciarticular juvenile rheumatoid arthritis in Japanese patients. Evidence for a role of the peptide-anchoring B pocket. *Arthritis Rheum.* 1995;38(11):1672–1677.

86. Calin A, Elswood J, Rigg S, Skevington SM. Ankylosing spondylitis–an analytical review of 1500 patients: the changing pattern of disease. *J Rheumatol.* 1988;15(8):1234–1238.

87. Webers C, Essers I, Ramiro S, et al. Gender-attributable differences in outcome of ankylosing spondylitis: long-term results from the Outcome in Ankylosing Spondylitis International Study. *Rheumatology.* 2016;55(3): 419–428.

88. Rudwaleit M, Haibel H, Baraliakos X, et al. The early disease stage in axial spondylarthritis: results from the German Spondyloarthritis Inception Cohort. *Arthritis Rheum.* 2009;60(3):717–727.

89. Ciurea A, Scherer A, Weber U, et al. Age at symptom onset in ankylosing spondylitis: is there a gender difference? *Ann Rheum Dis.* 2014;73(10):1908–1910.

90. Collantes E, Zarco P, Munoz E, et al. Disease pattern of spondyloarthropathies in Spain: description of the first national registry (REGISPONSER) extended report. *Rheumatology.* 2007;46(8):1309–1315.

91. Benegas M, Munoz-Gomariz E, Font P, et al. Comparison of the clinical expression of patients with ankylosing spondylitis from Europe and Latin America. *J Rheumatol.* 2012;39(12):2315–2320.

92. Bodur H, Ataman S, Bugdayci DS, et al. Description of the registry of patients with ankylosing spondylitis in Turkey: TRASD-IP. *Rheumatol Int.* 2012;32(1):169–176.

93. Gensler LS, Ward MM, Reveille JD, Learch TJ, Weisman MH, Davis Jr JC. Clinical, radiographic and functional differences between juvenile-onset and adult-onset ankylosing spondylitis: results from the PSOAS cohort. *Ann Rheum Dis.* 2008;67(2):233–237.

94. Kim TJ, Kim TH. Clinical spectrum of ankylosing spondylitis in Korea. *Joint Bone Spine.* 2010;77(3):235–240.

95. Polley HF, Slocumb CH. Rheumatoid spondylitis: a study of 1,035 cases. *Ann Intern Med.* 1947;26(2):240–249.

96. Lee W, Reveille JD, Davis Jr JC, Learch TJ, Ward MM, Weisman MH. Are there gender differences in severity of ankylosing spondylitis? Results from the PSOAS cohort. *Ann Rheum Dis.* 2007;66(5):633–638.

97. Gladman DD, Rahman P, Cook RJ, et al. The spondyloarthritis research consortium of Canada registry for spondyloarthritis. *J Rheumatol.* 2011;38(7):1343–1348.

98. Baumberger H, Khan MA. SAT0417 Gradual progressive change to equal prevalence of ankylosing spondylitis among males and females in Switzerland: data from the swiss ankylosing spondylitis society (SVMB). *Ann Rheum Dis.* 2017;76(suppl 2):929.

99. Rusman T, van Vollenhoven RF, Horst-Bruisma vd. Gender differences in axial spondyloarthritis: women are not so lucky. *Curr Rheumatol Rep.* 2018;20(6):35. In press.

100. Dougados M, d'Agostino MA, Benessiano J, et al. The DESIR cohort: a 10-year follow-up of early inflammatory back pain in France: study design and baseline characteristics of the 708 recruited patients. *Joint Bone Spine revue du rhumatisme.* 2011;78(6):598–603.

101. Molto A, Paternotte S, van der Heijde D, Claudepierre P, Rudwaleit M, Dougados M. Evaluation of the validity of the different arms of the ASAS set of criteria for axial spondyloarthritis and description of the different imaging abnormalities suggestive of spondyloarthritis: data from the DESIR cohort. *Ann Rheum Dis.* 2015;74(4):746–751.

102. Poddubnyy D, Inman R, Sieper J, Akar S, Muñoz-Fernández S, Hojnik M. SAT0395 Similarities and differences between non-radiographic and radiographic axial spondyloarthritis in proof cohort. *Ann Rheum Dis.* 2017;76(suppl 2). 921–921.

103. van den Berg R, de Hooge M, van Gaalen F, Reijnierse M, Huizinga T, van der Heijde D. Percentage of patients with spondyloarthritis in patients referred because of chronic back pain and performance of classification criteria: experience from the Spondyloarthritis Caught Early (SPACE) cohort. *Rheumatology.* 2013;52(8):1492–1499.

104. Brewerton DA, Hart FD, Nicholls A, Caffrey M, James DC, Sturrock RD. Ankylosing spondylitis and HL-A 27. *Lancet.* 1973;1(7809):904–907.

105. Caffrey MF, James DC. Human lymphocyte antigen association in ankylosing spondylitis. *Nature.* 1973;242(5393):121.

106. Schlosstein L, Terasaki PI, Bluestone R, Pearson CM. High association of an HL-A antigen, W27, with ankylosing spondylitis. *N Engl J Med.* 1973;288(14):704–706.

107. Hersh AH, Stecher RM, Solomon WM, Wolpaw R, Hauser H. Heredity in ankylosing spondylitis; a study of fifty families. *Am J Hum Genet.* 1950;2(4):391–408.

108. Geirsson AJ, Kristjansson K, Gudbjornsson B. A strong familiality of ankylosing spondylitis through several generations. *Ann Rheum Dis.* 2010;69(7):1346–1348.

109. Calin A, Brophy S, Blake D. Impact of sex on inheritance of ankylosing spondylitis: a cohort study. *Lancet.* 1999;354(9191):1687–1690.

110. Miceli-Richard C, Said-Nahal R, Breban M. Impact of sex on inheritance of ankylosing spondylitis. *Lancet.* 2000;355(9209):1097–1098; author reply 1098.

111. Brophy S, Taylor G, Blake D, Calin A. The interrelationship between sex, susceptibility factors, and outcome in ankylosing spondylitis and its associated disorders including inflammatory bowel disease, psoriasis, and iritis. *J Rheumatol.* 2003;30(9):2054–2058.

112. Jimenez-Balderas FJ, Zonana-Nacach A, Sanchez ML, et al. Maternal age and family history are risk factors for ankylosing spondylitis. *J Rheumatol.* 2003;30(10):2182–2185.

113. Costello ME, Ciccia F, Willner D, et al. Brief report: intestinal dysbiosis in ankylosing spondylitis. *Arthritis Rheumatol.* 2015;67(3):686–691.

114. Breban M, Tap J, Leboime A, et al. Faecal microbiota study reveals specific dysbiosis in spondyloarthritis. *Ann Rheum Dis.* 2017;76(9):1614–1622.

115. Lozupone CA, Stombaugh JI, Gordon JI, Jansson JK, Knight R. Diversity, stability and resilience of the human gut microbiota. *Nature.* 2012;489(7415):220–230.

116. Montoya J, Matta NB, Suchon P, et al. Patients with ankylosing spondylitis have been breast fed less often than healthy controls: a case-control retrospective study. *Ann Rheum Dis.* 2016;75(5):879–882.

117. Lindstrom U, Exarchou S, Lie E, et al. Childhood hospitalisation with infections and later development of ankylosing spondylitis: a national case-control study. *Arthritis Res Ther.* 2016;18(1):240.

118. Kaarela K, Jantti JK, Kotaniemi KM. Similarity between chronic reactive arthritis and ankylosing spondylitis. A 32-35-year follow-up study. *Clin Exp Rheumatol.* 2009;27(2):325–328.

119. Braun J, Kingsley G, van der Heijde D, Sieper J. On the difficulties of establishing a consensus on the definition of and diagnostic investigations for reactive arthritis. Results and discussion of a questionnaire prepared for the 4th International Workshop on Reactive Arthritis, Berlin, Germany, July 3-6, 1999. *J Rheumatol.* 2000;27(9):2185–2192.

120. Ward MM, Weisman MH, Davis Jr JC, Reveille JD. Risk factors for functional limitations in patients with long-standing ankylosing spondylitis. *Arthritis Rheum.* 2005;53(5):710–717.

121. Ward MM, Reveille JD, Learch TJ, Davis Jr JC, Weisman MH. Occupational physical activities and long-term functional and radiographic outcomes in patients with ankylosing spondylitis. *Arthritis Rheum.* 2008;59(6):822–832.

122. Jacques P, Lambrecht S, Verheugen E, et al. Proof of concept: enthesitis and new bone formation in spondyloarthritis are driven by mechanical strain and stromal cells. *Ann Rheum Dis.* 2014;73(2):437–445.

123. Ryden E. Chronic polyarthritis and trauma. *Acta Med Scand.* 1943;114(4–5):442–469.

124. Jacoby RK, Newell RL, Hickling P. Ankylosing spondylitis and trauma: the medicolegal implications. A comparative study of patients with non-specific back pain. *Ann Rheum Dis.* 1985;44(5):307–311.

125. Wisnieski JJ. Trauma and Reiter's syndrome: development of 'reactive arthropathy' in two patients following musculoskeletal injury. *Ann Rheum Dis.* 1984;43(6):829–832.

126. Masson G, Thomas P, Bontoux D, Alcalay M. Influence of trauma on initiation of Reiter's syndrome and ankylosing spondylitis. *Ann Rheum Dis.* 1985;44(12):860–861.

127. Olivieri I, Gemignani G, Christou C, Pasero G. Trauma and seronegative spondyloarthropathy: report of two more cases of peripheral arthritis precipitated by physical injury. *Ann Rheum Dis.* 1989;48(6):520–521.

128. Olivieri I, Gherardi S, Bini C, Trippi D, Ciompi ML, Pasero G. Trauma and seronegative spondyloarthropathy: rapid joint destruction in peripheral arthritis triggered by physical injury. *Ann Rheum Dis.* 1988;47(1):73–76.

129. Olivieri I, Gemignani G, Christou C, Semeria R, Giustarini S, Pasero G. The triggering role of physical injury in the onset of peripheral arthritis in seronegative spondyloarthropathy. *Rheumatol Int.* 1991;10(6):251–253.

130. Thorarensen SM, Lu N, Ogdie A, Gelfand JM, Choi HK, Love TJ. Physical trauma recorded in primary care is associated with the onset of psoriatic arthritis among patients with psoriasis. *Ann Rheum Dis.* 2017;76(3):521–525.

131. Videm V, Cortes A, Thomas R, Brown MA. Current smoking is associated with incident ankylosing spondylitis – the HUNT population-based Norwegian health study. *J Rheumatol.* 2014;41(10):2041–2048.

132. Poddubnyy D, Listing J, Haibel H, Knuppel S, Rudwaleit M, Sieper J. Functional relevance of radiographic spinal progression in axial spondyloarthritis: results from the German SPondyloarthritis Inception Cohort. *Rheumatol (Oxf)*. 2018;57(4):703–711.

133. Xia Q, Fan D, Yang X, et al. Progression rate of ankylosing spondylitis in patients with undifferentiated spondyloarthritis: a systematic review and meta-analysis. *Med (Baltim)*. 2017;96(4):e5960.

134. Dougados M, Demattei C, van den Berg R, et al. Rate and predisposing factors for sacroiliac joint radiographic progression after a two-year follow-up period in recent-onset spondyloarthritis. *Arthritis Rheumatol*. 2016;68(8):1904–1913.

135. Dougados M, Maksymowych WP, Landewe RBM, et al. Evaluation of the change in structural radiographic sacroiliac joint damage after 2 years of etanercept therapy (EMBARK trial) in comparison to a contemporary control cohort (DESIR cohort) in recent onset axial spondyloarthritis. *Ann Rheum Dis*. 2018;77(2):221–227.

136. Poddubnyy D, Rudwaleit M, Haibel H, et al. Rates and predictors of radiographic sacroiliitis progression over 2 years in patients with axial spondyloarthritis. *Ann Rheum Dis*. 2011;70(8):1369–1374.

137. van der Heijde D, Baraliakos X, Hermann KA, et al. Limited radiographic progression and sustained reductions in MRI inflammation in patients with axial spondyloarthritis: 4-year imaging outcomes from the RAPID-axSpA phase III randomised trial. *Ann Rheum Dis*. 2018;77(5):699–705.

138. Sepriano A, Rudwaleit M, Sieper J, van den Berg R, Landewe R, van der Heijde D. Five-year follow-up of radiographic sacroiliitis: progression as well as improvement? *Ann Rheum Dis*. 2016;75(6):1262–1263.

139. Wang R, Gabriel SE, Ward MM. Progression of nonradiographic axial spondyloarthritis to ankylosing spondylitis: a population-based cohort study. *Arthritis Rheumatol*. 2016;68(6):1415–1421.

140. Dougados M, Sepriano A, Molto A, et al. Sacroiliac radiographic progression in recent onset axial spondyloarthritis: the 5-year data of the DESIR cohort. *Ann Rheum Dis*. 2017;76(11):1823–1828.

141. Costantino F, Zeboulon N, Said-Nahal R, Breban M. Radiographic sacroiliitis develops predictably over time in a cohort of familial spondyloarthritis followed longitudinally. *Rheumatology*. 2017;56(5):811–817.

142. Poddubnyy D, Haibel H, Listing J, et al. Baseline radiographic damage, elevated acute-phase reactant levels, and cigarette smoking status predict spinal radiographic progression in early axial spondylarthritis. *Arthritis Rheum*. 2012;64(5):1388–1398.

143. Baraliakos X, Listing J, Rudwaleit M, et al. Progression of radiographic damage in patients with ankylosing spondylitis: defining the central role of syndesmophytes. *Ann Rheum Dis*. 2007;66(7):910–915.

144. Ramiro S, Stolwijk C, van Tubergen A, et al. Evolution of radiographic damage in ankylosing spondylitis: a 12 year prospective follow-up of the OASIS study. *Ann Rheum Dis*. 2015;74(1):52–59.

145. Brown WM, Doll R. Mortality from cancer and other causes after radiotherapy for ankylosing spondylitis. *Br Med J*. 1965;2(5474):1327–1332.

146. Radford EP, Doll R, Smith PG. Mortality among patients with ankylosing spondylitis not given X-ray therapy. *N Engl J Med*. 1977;297(11):572–576.

147. Kaprove RE, Little AH, Graham DC, Rosen PS. Ankylosing spondylitis: survival in men with and without radiotherapy. *Arthritis Rheum*. 1980;23(1):57–61.

148. Khan MA, Khan MK, Kushner I. Survival among patients with ankylosing spondylitis: a life-table analysis. *J Rheumatol*. 1981;8(1):86–90.

149. Lehtinen K. Mortality and causes of death in 398 patients admitted to hospital with ankylosing spondylitis. *Ann Rheum Dis*. 1993;52(3):174–176.

150. Bakland G, Gran JT, Nossent JC. Increased mortality in ankylosing spondylitis is related to disease activity. *Ann Rheum Dis*. 2011;70(11):1921–1925.

151. Mok CC, Kwok CL, Ho LY, Chan PT, Yip SF. Life expectancy, standardized mortality ratios, and causes of death in six rheumatic diseases in Hong Kong, China. *Arthritis Rheum*. 2011;63(5):1182–1189.

152. Exarchou S, Lie E, Lindstrom U, et al. Mortality in ankylosing spondylitis: results from a nationwide population-based study. *Ann Rheum Dis*. 2016;75(8):1466–1472.

153. Haroon NN, Paterson JM, Li P, Inman RD, Haroon N. Patients with ankylosing spondylitis have increased cardiovascular and cerebrovascular mortality: a population-based study. *Ann Intern Med*. 2015;163(6):409–416.

154. Wysham KD, Murray SG, Hills N, Yelin E, Gensler LS. Cervical spinal fracture and other diagnoses associated with mortality in hospitalized ankylosing spondylitis patients. *Arthritis Care Res*. 2017;69(2):271–277.

155. Walsh JA, Zhou X, Clegg DO, Teng C, Cannon GW, Sauer B. Mortality in American veterans with the HLA-B27 gene. *J Rheumatol*. 2015;42(4):638–644.

156. Haroon N. Does a positive HLA-B27 test increase your risk of mortality? *J Rheumatol*. 2015;42(4):559–560.

Classification Criteria for Axial Spondyloarthritis

VICTORIA NAVARRO-COMPÁN, PHD, MD • ATUL DEODHAR, MD, MRCP

INTRODUCTION

The term "spondyloarthritis" (SpA) has been traditionally used to describe a group of rheumatic diseases that share common clinical, pathogenic, genetic, and radiographic characteristics. The most representative disease of this group is ankylosing spondylitis (AS), but other entities such as psoriatic arthritis, SpA associated with inflammatory bowel disease, reactive arthritis, and undifferentiated SpA are also included within this group. Nevertheless, this traditional concept of SpA is evolving. Currently, patients tend to be classified according to the area of predominant symptoms into two subgroups: (1) axial SpA (characterized by predominant involvement of the spine and/or sacroiliac joints) and (2) peripheral SpA (with peripheral arthritis, enthesitis, and/or dactylitis). Although this concept seems less specific, using this dichotomy may provide more relevant information in clinical practice than classification based on the different entities, because treatment efficacy in axial and peripheral manifestations has been shown to differ, whatever the disease entity.

In this regard, an early diagnosis in patients with SpA is becoming increasingly important because therapies can be even more effective if used in early stages of the disease. However, this aim is not easy to achieve. Similar to the majority of rheumatic diseases, the diseases included within SpA categorization differ in their presentations and natural course and lack a clinical, laboratory, or imaging biomarker beyond sacroiliitis to serve as a "gold standard" for diagnosis. As more effective treatment modalities become available, development of classification criteria has been an important focus of research in this field during the past decades.

DISTINCTION BETWEEN CLASSIFICATION CRITERIA AND DIAGNOSTIC CRITERIA

Diagnostic and classification criteria play central roles in clinical rheumatology, but unfortunately they are not always properly applied. Diagnostic and classification criteria are not interchangeable, and its misuse may lead to confusion. Therefore, it is essential to understand what are the differences between classification and diagnostic criteria.[1]

The mix-up between diagnosis and classification may partially proceed from the fact that the same clinical, laboratory, and imaging features are used both for diagnostic purposes and to classify patients with SpA. However, the way in which they are incorporated is different. Classification consists of applying common clinical characteristics to group homogenous patients together to decide about their possible inclusion in a clinical trial or observational study. By contrast, the objective of diagnostic criteria is to help in the diagnosis process of a patient individually. In making a diagnosis, the clinician has to exclude other diseases ("look-alikes") that may have similar clinical presentation(s). When making the diagnosis, the clinical value of any diagnostic test or criterion depends highly on the pretest probability or, in case of an individual patient, on the prevalence of the disease in the population. This contrasts with the classification criteria, which are to be applied only in patients who have been already previously diagnosed with the disease.[2] Therefore, whereas classification criteria must be highly specific and should not contain too many false positives, diagnostic criteria must be highly sensitive, which means that they may contain false positives and have low specificity. In this sense, classification criteria must therefore allow a categorical answer (yes/no) to the question of whether a patient fulfill these criteria or not, whereas diagnostic criteria should allow us to establish the degree of confidence in the diagnosis (very high, probable, or possible).[3]

In clinical practice, in the absence of diagnostic criteria, classification criteria are often used to assist in the diagnostic process of a disease. However, the fact of making a diagnosis only because the patient meets a set of classification criteria can lead to errors in the diagnosis, especially if this is done in a

Axial Spondyloarthritis. https://doi.org/10.1016/B978-0-323-56800-5.00004-7

population with a low pretest probability of the condition. The relevance of this will be discussed later in this chapter.

To date, there are no diagnostic criteria developed for any diseases within the SpA spectrum. Recently, fundamental concerns related to diagnostic criteria in rheumatology have been pointed out, and these concerns have led to the decision by the American College of Rheumatology (ACR) and the European League against Rheumatism to not endorse diagnostic criteria for rheumatic diseases anymore.[1] Therefore, it seems the development of diagnostic criteria for SpA will remain an unmet need.

DIAGNOSTIC ALGORITHM: UTILITY OF THE TYPICAL SPONDYLOARTHRITIS FEATURES

In 2006, a new algorithm was published for the early diagnosis of SpA with predominant axial manifestations, known as the Berlin algorithm.[4] When developing this algorithm, the positive and negative likelihood ratio of each one of the clinical, laboratory, and imaging manifestations of patients with axial SpA was taken into account. These typical manifestations included inflammatory back pain, enthesitis (heel pain), peripheral arthritis, dactylitis, anterior uveitis, psoriasis, inflammatory bowel disease, a positive family history of SpA, good response to nonsteroidal antiinflammatory drugs, elevated acute phase reactants, presence of HLA-B27, sacroiliitis on magnetic resonance imaging (MRI), and sacroiliitis on plain radiographs. The different values for sensitivity, specificity, positive likelihood

ratio, and negative likelihood ratio for each of the characteristics are shown in Fig. 4.1.

Based on this, the diagnostic probability of the disease can be estimated by multiplying the values of the positive likelihood ratios of the characteristics present in a certain patient. Nevertheless, when using this tool in individual cases, it is important to note that for the calculation of the diagnostic probability through this pyramid, a prevalence of the disease in patients with chronic low back pain of 5% is assumed, which may not be appropriate for all settings.

In 2013, a Dutch group proposed a modification of the Berlin diagnostic algorithm.[5] In the initial Berlin algorithm, the starting point was inflammatory back pain. However, a subsequent study in two international cohorts of patients with recent axial SpA showed that this feature may not be present in up to 30% of patients with axial SpA. Therefore, to avoid missing the diagnosis of these patients, the Assessment of SpondyloArthritis international Society (ASAS) group decided to accept and endorse the proposed modification to the diagnostic algorithm, in which the entry criterion is chronic low back pain, which may have "inflammatory" or "mechanical" characteristics. This algorithm is presented in Fig. 4.2.

EVOLUTION OF THE CLASSIFICATION CRITERIA FOR SPONDYLOARTHRITIS

The concept of SpA was proposed in 1974 to highlight the relationship between AS and the other entities that had previously been described as separate diseases

Manifestation	Sensitivity (%)	Specificity (%)	Positive likelihood ratio	Negative likelihood ratio
Inflammatory back pain	71-75	75-80	3.1	0.33
Positive family history for SpA	7-36	93-99	6.4	0.72
Good response to NSAIDs	61-67	80-85	5.1	0.27
Enthesitis (heel pain)	16-37	89-94	3.4	0.71
Peripheral arthritis	40-62	90-98	4.0	0.67
Dactylitis	12-24	96-98	4.5	0.85
Inflammatory bowel disease	5-8	97-99	4.0	0.97
Psoriasis	10-20	95-97	2.5	0.94
Anterior uveitis	10-22	97-99	7.3	0.80
HLA-B27 positive	83-96	90-96	9.0	0.11
Elevated Acute Phase Reactants	38-69	67-80	2.5	0.63
Sacroiliitis on MRI	60-85	90-97	20.0	0.41
Sacroiliitis on x-Ray	40	98	20.0	0.61

FIG. 4.1 Diagnostic utility of the typical manifestations of axial spondyloarthritis.

(e.g., psoriatic arthritis, reactive arthritis). However, the typical phenotype of AS with fusion of the sacroiliac joints and of the spine was found in some postmortem specimens as early as the 17th century, although it was not until 1960 when the first criteria to classify or diagnose patients with AS were formulated.[6]

The Rome criteria were the first criteria established for the classification of AS (1961). After the exclusion of chest pain (due to its low specificity) and uveitis (due to its low sensitivity), the New York classification criteria for AS emerged in 1966. Subsequently, as a consequence of the relevance of the inflammatory character of low back pain, the modified New York criteria for classifying AS were developed in 1984. According to these criteria, a patient can be classified as AS if he/she has at least one of the following clinical criteria (inflammatory back pain, limited mobility of the lumbar spine, or limitation of the chest expansion) plus a radiological criterion (bilateral grade 2 radiographic sacroiliitis or unilateral grade 3–4 radiographic sacroiliitis) (Fig. 4.3).

Until the past decade, these criteria have been the most used to classify patients with AS. However, to fulfill these criteria, patients are required to present a substantial degree of structural damage of the sacroiliac joints (i.e., radiographic sacroiliitis according to modified New York criteria), which usually appears only after several years of clinical symptoms and disease

onset. Therefore, the modified New York criteria are not appropriate to classify patients at early stages of the disease. In addition, these criteria include only axial symptoms, and patients presenting with peripheral symptoms would not be classified as suffering from AS.

Based on this, two sets of classification criteria for SpA were introduced almost at the same time. These criteria were the Amor criteria[7] and the European Spondyloarthropathy Study Group (ESSG) criteria.[8] Their development was very relevant for the field of SpA. Both criteria were refined not only with the objective of classifying patients with SpA but also to be able to cover a broader clinical spectrum of the disease by including a subgroup of undifferentiated SpA. To fulfill these criteria, the presence of structural damage was optional (but not obligatory) and therefore the identification of patients with SpA at the beginning of the disease was in principle feasible.

The Amor criteria were published in 1990 and consist of a list of clinical, genetic, and radiographic signs and do not require an entry criterion. The different clinical items in the criteria contribute 1 point, 2 points, or 3 points, and a total score of 6 or more classifies a patient as SpA. The Amor criteria included for the first time peripheral features and good response to nonsteroidal antiinflammatory drugs. As mentioned, radiographic sacroiliitis was not required to fulfill the criteria, but it had the highest score (3 points). Thus,

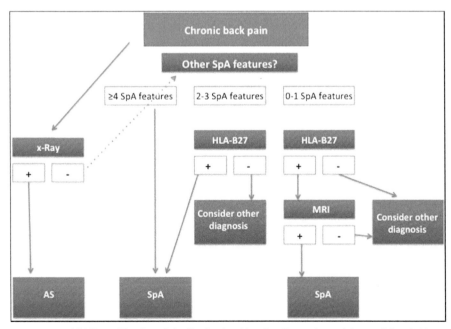

FIG. 4.2 ASAS modification of the Berlin algorithm for diagnosing axial spondyloarthritis.

Modified New York criteria for ankylosing spondylitis (1984)	
Clinical criteria	Low back pain and stiffness for more than 3 months that improves with exercise, but is not relieved by rest.
	Limitation of motion of the lumbar spine in the sagittal and frontal planes.
	Limitation of chest expansion relative to normal values correlated for age and sex.
Radiological criterion	Sacroiliitis grade >2 bilaterally or grade 3–4 unilaterally.

Definite AS if the radiological criterion is associated with at least one clinical criterion.

FIG. 4.3 Modified New York criteria for ankylosing spondylitis.

although classification of early disease was possible through the employment of these criteria, in practice, this was not really feasible (Fig. 4.4).

The ESSG criteria were proposed in 1991. These criteria were the predecessor of the criteria developed later because the entry criteria focused on the two predominant symptoms of SpA: (1) the presence of inflammatory lumbar pain and (2) the presence of (oligo) asymmetric peripheral arthritis. To fulfill the ESSG criteria, in addition to one of these two entry criteria, patients are required to have at least one of the following as a minor criterion: enthesitis, a positive family history, psoriasis, inflammatory bowel disease, urethritis/cervicitis/acute diarrhea within the previous month, buttock pain, and sacroiliitis (Fig. 4.5). The presence of radiographic sacroiliitis was just one of these minor criteria, which favored the identification of SpA at an early stage of the disease.

THE NEED FOR NEW CRITERIA

The need to develop new classification criteria for patients with SpA was felt once again in early 2000, mainly because of major advances in two related fields—the emergence of MRI to assess early inflammatory changes in the sacroiliac joints, and the advent of new and effective medication to treat AS.[2] Some other reasons included the limited sensitivity and specificity, as well as the inability of the existing classification criteria to identify early stages of axial SpA, and the necessity to separately identify axial and peripheral SpA.

Based on these reasons, the ASAS group decided to start an international study to develop a new set of validated classification criteria.

DEVELOPMENT AND VALIDATION OF THE ASAS (ASSESSMENT OF SPONDYLOARTHRITIS INTERNATIONAL SOCIETY) CRITERIA

To develop the new criteria, a three-step process was applied. First, 20 expert ASAS members developed candidate classification criteria for axial SpA using a paper patients scoring exercise and using items from existing criteria. In a second step, a prospective, international study with 25 participant centers including more than 600 patients with chronic back pain referred to rheumatologists for suspicion of axial SpA was carried out. Part of the cohort (40%) was used to refine the criteria, and the remainder (60%) was used to validate it. The external "gold" standard for evaluation of these criteria was the rheumatologist's expert opinion of the SpA diagnosis after incorporating lab and imaging data with clinical evaluation. Finally, the new classification criteria were formally voted upon at an ASAS annual meeting.[9]

The ASAS criteria were published in 2009 (for axial SpA) and 2011 (for peripheral SpA) classifying patients into two groups according to the predominant manifestations (axial or peripheral) of the disease.[9,10] The criteria for axial SpA and for peripheral SpA are detailed in Fig. 4.6. Overall, these criteria showed

A. Clinical Symptoms / History	Score
1. Pain at night	1
2. Assymmetrical oligoarthritis	2
3. Gluteal (buttock) pain (any)	1
or	
alternating gluteal pain	2
4. Sausage like digit or toe (dactylitis)	2
5. Enthesitis (heel)	2
6. Uveitis	2
7. Urethritis/Cervicitis within 1 month before onset of arthritis	1
8. Diarrheae within 1 month before onset of arthritis	1
9. Psoriasis, balanitis or inflammatory bowel disease	2
B. Radiographs	
10. Sacroiliitis (grade 2 bilaterally or grade 3 unilaterally)	3
C. Genetical background	
11. HLA-B27 positive or positive family history for AS, ReA, uveitis, psoriasis or IBD	2
D. Good response to NSAIDs	
12. Good response to NSAIDs in less than 48 h, or relapse of the pain in less 2 than 48 h if NSAIDs discontinued	2

FIG. 4.4 Amor classification criteria for spondyloarthritis. At least 6 points are necessary.

Inflammatory spinal pain	OR	Synovitys (asymmetric or predominantly in the lower limbs)
Plus at least one of the following:		
Positive family history		
Psoriasis		
Inflammatory bowel disease		
Urethritis, cervicitis or acute diarrhea within one month before arthritis		
Alternating buttock pain		
Enthesopaty		
Sacroiliitis		

FIG. 4.5 ESSG (European Spondyloarthropathy Study Group) classification criteria.

sensitivity of 80% and a specificity of 83% to classify patients with SpA.

The ASAS classification criteria for axial SpA were developed with an entry requirement of presence of low back pain for at least 3 months that has its onset before age 45 years. The criteria have two possible entry doors or "arms": the imaging arm (through the presence of sacroiliitis on radiography or MRI) and the clinical arm (through the presence of HLA-B27). To classify a patient as axial SpA, in addition to one

Axial Spondyloarthritis	Peripheral Spondyloarthritis
In patients with ≥ 3 months back pain and age at onset <45 years	In patients with peripheral symptoms ONLY
Sacroiliitis on imaging plus at least one SpA feature or **HLA-B27 plus at least two SpA features**	**Arthritis or enthesitis or dactylitis plus**
Inflammatory back pain	**At least one SpA feature**
Arthritis	Uveitis
Enthesitis (heel)	Psoriasis
Uveitis	Inflammatory bowel disease
Dactylitis	Preceding infection
Psoriasis	HLA-B27 positive
Inflammatory bowel disease	Sacroiliitis on imaging
Good response to NSAIDs	**OR**
Family history for SpA	**At least two SpA feature**
HLA-B27 positive	Arthritis
Elevated CRP	Enthesitis
	Dactylitis
	Inflammatory bowel disease
	Family history for SpA

FIG. 4.6 ASAS classification criteria for axial and peripheral spondyloarthritis.

of these entry criteria, the presence of at least one (or two, in case of the clinical arm) of the typical characteristics of SpA is required (Fig. 4.6). These characteristics include inflammatory back pain, inflammatory arthritis, enthesitis (heel preferred), uveitis, dactylitis, psoriasis, inflammatory bowel disease, good response to nonsteroidal antiinflammatory drugs, family history of SpA, presence of HLA-B27, and elevated CRP.

In the original study, the ASAS criteria for axial SpA showed an overall sensitivity of 83% and a specificity of 84%. The imaging arm showed excellent specificity (98%) but had low sensitivity (66%), whereas the clinical arm has reasonably good specificity (83%) but low sensitivity (57%). Recently, the predictive validity of the ASAS criteria for axial SpA after 4 years of follow-up was established using data from 22 centers participating in the original development study. In this study, the positive predictive value of the axial SpA criteria to forecast an expert's

diagnosis of axial SpA after more than 4 years was shown to be excellent, and the imaging arm and clinical arm had similar predictive validity and were complementary.[11] However, this study had its own limitations, as direct follow-up was limited to 35% of original patient participants (although information was collected on additional 25% by telephone interviews), and because the follow-up examination and diagnosis were established by the same expert, it was vulnerable to significant bias.

Recently, data from a metaanalysis including nine studies with more than 5500 patients have been published.[12] The results of this metaanalysis support the good performance of the ASAS SpA criteria as tested against the rheumatologist's diagnosis. The entire set of the ASAS SpA classification criteria yielded 73% sensitivity and 88% specificity. The corresponding values for the ASAS axial SpA classification criteria were 82% and 89%, respectively. On splitting the axial SpA criteria, both the imaging arm and the clinical arm showed a very low sensitivity (30% and 23%, respectively), but a very high specificity (97% and 94%, respectively). The ASAS peripheral SpA classification criteria had 63% sensitivity and 87% specificity.

The ASAS criteria are increasingly being used in clinical trials and are widely accepted. In the past, most clinical trials in the field of SpA were conducted in patients with AS with average disease duration of 5–10 years. The newer pharmaceutical trials are using the ASAS criteria, which allow inclusion of patients with early disease to assess the efficacy of new drugs in the full spectrum of the disease.

A NEW ENTITY: NON-RADIOGRAPHIC AXIAL SPONDYLOARTHRITIS

As a consequence of the development of the ASAS criteria for axial SpA, a new term was coined: "non-radiographic axial SpA" (nr-axSpA). These are the patients who have a clinical picture of AS but do not exhibit radiographic sacroiliitis. Initially, this concept was thought to represent "preradiographic" axial SpA, but in the past decade, it has been shown that not all patients with this entity develop radiographically defined sacroiliitis over time, and therefore this term was modified to "non-radiographic axial SpA." Moreover, several cohort studies examined the demographic and clinical features of patients with nr-axSpA in comparison with AS patients, concluding that both disorders represent different ends of the same disease spectrum. During recent years, many concerns have been raised around this clinical entity. These include diminished association with HLA-B27 and gender equality in prevalence compared with AS; however, some have argued that HLA-B27 and male sex may be risk factors for radiographic progression.[13,14] The response to TNF inhibitor treatment relative to placebo has a delta value of 16%–30% for nr-axSpA versus 31%–38% for AS patients.[15] Despite these differences, there is a general acceptance that nr-axSpA and AS belong to the same disease spectrum and that the current treatment strategies are similar for both.[16]

IS IT TIME FOR NEW CRITERIA?

Almost a decade after the ASAS classification criteria were developed, the question of whether or not these criteria should be revised is frequently raised in many forums.[17] Some concerns stem from the observations that the prevalence of HLA-B27 varied between 29% and 100% in patients of white European descent diagnosed as axial SpA in the original study (wide variations

in HLA-B27 prevalence were seen in centers from the same country). The specificity of "positive MRI diagnosis" has also been questioned, as patients with nonspecific back pain have demonstrated similar MRI findings in 20%–30% cases.[18,19] The apparent lack of specificity of the criteria reported in some studies might have been the result of erroneous use of these criteria for diagnostic purposes. In the approval process of two anti-TNF agents by the Food and Drug Administration, these critical points had been fundamental.

The debate regarding "is it time to renew the ASAS criteria for axial SpA?" is divided into two camps. Some experts have concerns regarding possible overdiagnosis of axial SpA by physicians erroneously using the ASAS criteria to diagnose the disease because of the lack of diagnostic criteria. In this sense, specific concerns are the lack of homogeneity between the clinical and imaging arms, which have performed differently in validation studies. The specificity of the clinical arm has been questioned. As an example, an HLA-B27 positive young female patient with fibromyalgia could be misclassified as axial SpA based on "soft" features such as positive family history and good response to nonsteroidal anti-inflammatory drugs. In this scenario, it has been argued that the subjective and objective features of SpA may not necessarily have the same importance, and hence all features in the ASAS criteria should not have the same weight. This group of experts has also expressed concerns regarding the specificity of the current MRI positivity definition, the circularity of arguments regarding the use of MRI in the diagnosis of axSpA, and the HLA-B27 prevalence in the original study as mentioned before. Accordingly, this group of experts defend the need to methodologically improve the development of the criteria including rigorous assessment of potential candidate criteria sets, discrete choice experiments to allow consideration of feature weights, and separate evaluation of the structural and inflammatory lesions to establish the MRI definition of sacroiliitis.[20] Opposing this view, other experts claim that classification criteria should not be used for diagnosis and that an expert rheumatologist should make the diagnosis based on full evaluation of all clinical, laboratory, and imaging information, but importantly by clinical reasoning that actively excludes other diagnoses.[21] In addition, based on the results of a recent study,[22] fibromyalgia patients rarely fulfill the ASAS classification criteria (in particular, its clinical arm), and therefore, the ASAS criteria perform well if correctly applied.[23] According to these experts, efforts should be allocated to educate rheumatologists worldwide to not use the axial SpA classification criteria for diagnosis and for treatment indication, and for interpreting MRI results in a "global" way. Extensive discussions and debates between these two groups have led to development of a research agenda to validate, and if need be modify, the existing ASAS classification criteria for axial SpA.

RESEARCH AGENDA TO FURTHER VALIDATE OR IMPROVE THE CURRENT CLASSIFICATION CRITERIA

The Spondyloarthritis Research and Treatment Network (SPARTAN) organization from North America and ASAS have joined forces to run the "Classification of Axial Spondyloarthritis Inception Cohort" (CLASSIC) study. The aim of this study is not to develop new criteria but to validate the ASAS axial SpA classification criteria in a worldwide study, which will run with appropriate sample size calculations for North America and the rest of the world. A minimum sensitivity and specificity have been established (75% and 90%, respectively). If this is achieved, the study will end and the ASAS classification criteria will be validated. However, if this is not achieved, further actions will be taken to improve the sensitivity and specificity of the ASAS criteria. These actions may include, but may not be restricted to, strengthening of the MRI positivity definition by including structural damage definition, weighting the SpA features, dividing the SpA features as "major" and "minor," etc.

Finally, we must remember the words by a senior rheumatologist from Mayo Clinic when discussing classification or diagnostic criteria for any disease. Dr. Gene Hunder wrote "The process of disease description needs to be dynamic, with additions or changes to criteria and definitions, as more is learned about these illnesses. We must keep in mind that classification criteria and diagnoses are not diseases. They are descriptors that change as new knowledge is acquired."[24]

CONFLICT OF INTEREST

Victoria Navarro and Atul Deodhar are members of ASAS, and Atul Deodhar is also a member and former chairman of SPARTAN.

REFERENCES

1. Landewe RB, van der Heijde DM. Why CAPS criteria are not diagnostic criteria? *Ann Rheum Dis.* 2017;76(4):e7.
2. Rudwaleit M, Khan MA, Sieper J. The challenge of diagnosis and classification in early ankylosing spondylitis: do we need new criteria? *Arthritis Rheum.* 2005;52(4):1000–1008.
3. Aggarwal R, Ringold S, Khanna D, et al. Distinctions between diagnostic and classification criteria? *Arthritis Care Res.* 2015;67(7):891–897.
4. Rudwaleit M, Feldtkeller E, Sieper J. Easy assessment of axial spondyloarthritis (early ankylosing spondylitis) at the bedside. *Ann Rheum Dis.* 2006;65(9):1251–1252.
5. van den Berg R, de Hooge M, Rudwaleit M, et al. ASAS modification of the Berlin algorithm for diagnosing axial spondyloarthritis: results from the SPondyloArthritis Caught Early (SPACE)-cohort and from the Assessment of SpondyloArthritis international Society (ASAS)-cohort. *Ann Rheum Dis.* 2013;72(10):1646–1653.
6. Taurog JD, Chhabra A, Colbert RA. Ankylosing spondylitis and axial spondyloarthritis. *N Engl J Med.* 2016;374(26):2563–2574.
7. Amor B, Dougados M, Listrat V, et al. Evaluation of the amor criteria for spondylarthropathies and European spondylarthropathy study group (ESSG). A cross-sectional analysis of 2,228 patients. *Ann Med Interne.* 1991;142(2):85–89.
8. Dougados M, van der Linden S, Juhlin R, et al. The European Spondylarthropathy Study Group preliminary criteria for the classification of spondylarthropathy. *Arthritis Rheum.* 1991;34(10):1218–1227.
9. Rudwaleit M, van der Heijde D, Landewe R, et al. The development of Assessment of SpondyloArthritis international Society classification criteria for axial spondyloarthritis (part II): validation and final selection. *Ann Rheum Dis.* 2009;68(6):777–783.
10. Rudwaleit M, van der Heijde D, Landewe R, et al. The Assessment of SpondyloArthritis International Society classification criteria for peripheral spondyloarthritis and for spondyloarthritis in general. *Ann Rheum Dis.* 2011;70(1):25–31.
11. Sepriano A, Landewe R, van der Heijde D, et al. Predictive validity of the ASAS classification criteria for axial and peripheral spondyloarthritis after follow-up in the ASAS cohort: a final analysis. *Ann Rheum Dis.* 2016;75(6):1034–1042.
12. Sepriano A, Rubio R, Ramiro S, Landewe R, van der Heijde D. Performance of the ASAS classification criteria for axial and peripheral spondyloarthritis: a systematic literature review and meta-analysis. *Ann Rheum Dis.* 2017;76(5):886–890.
13. Molto A, Paternotte S, van der Heijde D, Claudepierre P, Rudwaleit M, Dougados M. Evaluation of the validity of the different arms of the ASAS set of criteria for axial spondyloarthritis and description of the different imaging abnormalities suggestive of spondyloarthritis: data from the DESIR cohort. *Ann Rheum Dis.* 2015;74(4):746–751.
14. Navarro-Compan V, Machado PM. Spondyloarthropathies: sacroiliac joint radiographic progression - speed and determinants. *Nat Rev Rheumatol.* 2016;12(7):380–382.
15. Sepriano A, Regel A, van der Heijde D, et al. Efficacy and safety of biological and targeted-synthetic DMARDs: a systematic literature review informing the 2016 update of the ASAS/EULAR recommendations for the management of axial spondyloarthritis. *RMD Open.* 2017;3(1):e000396.

16. Slobodin G, Eshed I. Non-radiographic axial spondyloarthritis. *Isr Med Assoc J*. 2015;17(12):770–776.
17. Akkoc N, Khan MA. ASAS classification criteria for axial spondyloarthritis: time to modify. *Clin Rheumatol*. 2016;35(6):1415–1423.
18. Weber U, Ostergaard M, Lambert RG, et al. Candidate lesion-based criteria for defining a positive sacroiliac joint MRI in two cohorts of patients with axial spondyloarthritis. *Ann Rheum Dis*. 2015;74(11):1976–1982.
19. Arnbak B, Jensen TS, Egund N, et al. Prevalence of degenerative and spondyloarthritis-related magnetic resonance imaging findings in the spine and sacroiliac joints in patients with persistent low back pain. *Eur Radiol*. 2016;26(4):1191–1203.
20. Dubreuil M, Deodhar AA. Axial spondyloarthritis classification criteria: the debate continues. *Curr Opin Rheumatol*. 2017;29(4):317–322.
21. Deodhar A. Axial spondyloarthritis criteria and modified NY criteria: issues and controversies. *Clin Rheumatol*. 2014;33(6):741–747.
22. Baraliakos X, Regel A, Kiltz U, et al. Patients with fibromyalgia rarely fulfil classification criteria for axial spondyloarthritis. *Rheumatology*. 2017 (Epub ahead of print).
23. Rudwaleit M. Fibromyalgia is not axial spondyloarthritis: towards an appropriate use of the ASAS classification criteria for axial SpA. *Rheumatology*. 2017 (Epub ahead of print).
24. Hunder GG. The use and misuse of classification and diagnostic criteria for complex diseases. *Ann Intern Med*. 1998;129(5):417–418.

CHAPTER 5

Genetics of Axial Spondyloarthritis

MATTHEW A. BROWN, MBBS, MD, FRACP, FAHMS, FAA •
HUJI XU, MD, PHD • JOHN D. REVEILLE, MD

GENETIC EPIDEMIOLOGY

The strong tendency of AS to run in families was recognized long ago and shown to be greater even than for rheumatoid arthritis.[1] Pooled analyses of familial recurrence studies show that the likelihood of recurrence in monozygotic (MZ) twins was 63%, first-degree relatives 8.2%, second-degree relatives 1.0%, and third-degree relatives 0.7%. The recurrence rate in parent-child pairs (7.9%) was similar to the sibling recurrence risk (8.2%).[2] Modeling studies using these data demonstrate that AS is not a monogenic disease (i.e., caused by a single allelic variant, HLA-B27) but is likely at least oligogenic. Higher recurrence risk has been reported for spondyloarthropathy overall (10.6% parent-child, 13.9% sibling recurrence), perhaps because of the inclusion of diseases other than AS, such as undifferentiated spondyloarthritis, which are common in the community.[3]

Using the outstanding Icelandic genealogical resources, it was demonstrated that the recurrence risk ratios (likelihood of disease in relatives of a proband compared with likelihood in general population) were for first-degree relatives 94, second-degree relatives 25, and third-degree relatives 3.5. The study also demonstrated increased genetic sharing measured as the "kinship coefficient," the probability that two randomly selected alleles at an autosomal locus, one from each individual, are inherited from a common ancestor. The kinship coefficient for AS was 75 and for IBD 14.5, indicating far higher familiality for AS than IBD. The risk of Crohn disease or ulcerative colitis was significantly increased in families of AS cases, with first-degree risk ratios, respectively, of 3.7 and 2.9 for these conditions, providing the first genetic epidemiology evidence of the association of these conditions.

Twin studies have confirmed the high heritability of AS, suggesting that most of the high familiality is due to shared genetic rather than environmental factors. Two major twin studies, one in the British population[4] and one in Danish and Norwegian twins,[5] estimated the heritability of AS to be >90%. This estimate should be viewed with caution because of the relatively small number of twin pairs available for study and the possibility of ascertainment bias in a condition in which a high proportion of cases in the community are as yet undiagnosed.

Recently, methods have been developed to assess heritability using unrelated individuals. Using dense SNP data from genome-wide association studies, the extent of sharing of genetic factors captured by the SNP data between cases can be compared with healthy controls.[6] In diseases in which genetic variants captured by the SNP data play a role in disease risk, the cases share SNP alleles overall to a greater extent than controls. The level of "heritability" demonstrated by this approach depends on the heritability of the disease and whether that heritability is due to genetic variants either genotyped by or in linkage disequilibrium with the genotyped SNPs. A major advantage of this approach is that it is not biased by ascertainment. In the UK Biobank, heritability of AS was estimated at 69.1%, compared with 20.9% for Crohn disease, 15.9% for ulcerative colitis, and 16.3% for rheumatoid arthritis (http://www.nealelab.is/blog/2017/9/15/heritability-of-2000-traits-and-disorders-in-the-uk-biobank).

This approach can also be used to assess the extent of sharing of genetic factors between different diseases. Early studies showed association in AS of *KIF21B* and *STAT3* and confirmed the association of *IL23R* with AS, loci known to be associated with inflammatory bowel disease.[7] A systematic review of sharing of associated SNPs between different immune-mediated diseases showed that there was a high degree of sharing of loci between AS and IBD and that this was nearly all concordant (same SNP, same direction of association).[8] The extent of this sharing was then quantified in a study using the Illumina Immunochip, a SNP microarray targeting immunogenetic loci of interest.[9] This found that there was very strong genetic correlation (r_g) between AS and ulcerative colitis ($r_g = 0.47$) and Crohn disease ($r_g = 0.49$), and also moderate sharing with psoriasis ($r_g = 0.28$) and primary sclerosing cholangitis ($r_g = 0.33$).

Axial Spondyloarthritis. https://doi.org/10.1016/B978-0-323-56800-5.00005-9

In the same study, the extent to which this high heritability is due to HLA-B27 was estimated. The major histocompatibility complex (MHC, the region at which HLA-B27 is encoded) was found to contribute 20.44% of heritability, and the remaining 113 loci identified to that point contributed a further 7.38% of heritability.[9] This is similar to the previous estimates from twin[4] and linkage studies[10,11] and confirms the substantial non-MHC heritability involved in AS susceptibility.

Clinical manifestations of AS are also potentially heritable, and limited studies have been performed in twins and families to estimate the role of genetics in this area. Family studies found heritability of the Bath Ankylosing Spondylitis Disease Activity Index (BASDAI) of 0.49, Bath Ankylosing Spondylitis Index (BASFI) of 0.76, and age at symptom onset 0.33.[12,13] Radiographic severity as assessed using the Bath Ankylosing Spondylitis Radiology Index has also been reported to be heritable (h2 = 0.62).[14]

Major Histocompatibility Complex Genetics

Since the discovery of the association of HLA-B27 and AS in 1973 in the United Kingdom[15] and the United States,[16] this has persisted as the best example of a disease association with a hereditary marker. To date, over 174 protein allotypes of HLA-B27 have been described (Fig. 5.1) (https://www.ebi.ac.uk/cgi-bin/ipd/imgt/hla/get_allele.cgi?). *HLA-B*27:05* is the most common subtype, with a worldwide distribution, and is almost certainly the "ancestral" *HLA-B*27* allele, present in *Homo sapiens* before departing from Africa more than 80,000 years ago. In fact, sequence similarities of HLA-B27 have been observed in MHC class I alleles from chimpanzees in Africa.[17]

HLA-B*27:05 is likely to be an ancient specificity, probably the "parent" HLA-B27 allele, and other *HLA-B*27* subtypes are likely derived from it. The major and most frequently occurring "subtypes" of *HLA-B*27* include *B*27:02*, found primarily in those of European

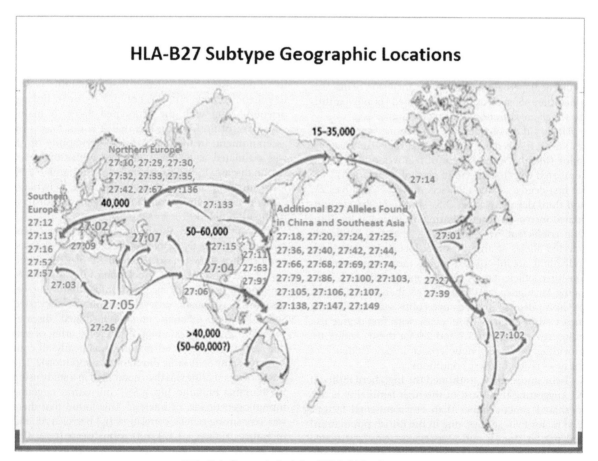

FIG. 5.1 Suggested origin of HLA-B27 subtypes.

27:05

SUBTYPES DIRECTLY DERIVED FROM B*27:05		
27:01 (NA)	27:92
27:03 (AF)	27:93
27:09 (SAR)	27:95
27:10 (EU)	27:96
27:13 (EU)	27:97
27:14 (EU,NA)	27:98
27:17	27:99
27:19	27:103
27:23	27:104
27:28	27:110
27:29 (SCA)	27:111
27:31	27:117
27:32 (EU)	27:118
27:34	27:121
27:35 (SCA)	27:122
27:37	27:123
27:38	27:124
27:39 (NA)	27:126
27:41	27:127
27:45	27:128
27:46	27:129
27:47	27:131
27:48	27:132
27:50	27:133 (CR)
27:51	27:135
27:52 (EU)	27:137
27:53	27:139
27:54	27:140
27:55	27:141
27:56	27:143
27:58	27:144
27:60	27:145
27:61	27:146
27:67 (EU)	27:148
27:70	27:150
27:71	27:151
27:72	27:152
27:73	27:155
27:74 (EA)	27:156
27:76	27:158
27:78	27:159
27:80	27:160
27:81	27:161
27;82	27:162
27:84	27:166
27:85	27:167
27:87	27:169
27:88	27:170
27:90	27:174

27:02 (EU)
N-77, I-80, A-81
27:30 (EU)
27:57 (TU)
27:62 (EU)
27:75
27:77
27:83
27:102 (SA)
27:116
27:119
27:134
27:157
27:163
27:171
27:172

27:04 (EA)
S-77, E-152
27:15 (EA)
27:25 (EA)
27:36 (EA)
27:63 (PH)
27:66 (EA)
27:68 (EA)
27:69 (EA)
27:79 (EA)
27:86 (EA)
27:100 (EA)
27:105 (EA)
27:108
27:109
27:112
27:113
27:114
27:115
27:120
27:147 (EA)
27:149 (EA)
27:165
27:173

27:06 (SEA, PH)
D-114, Y-116
27:21
27:91 (PH)
27:106 (EA)
27:107 (EA)
27:138 (EA)

27:07 (EU, EA, NA)
S-97, H-113, N-114, Y-116
27:11 (JA)
27:20 (EA)
27:24 (EA)
27:27 (NA)
27:43 (EA)
27:125
27:130
27:136 (EU)
27:153
27:164
27:168

27:08 (EU)
S-77, N-80, R 82, G-83
27:16 (EU)
27:26 (AF)
27:33 (EU)
27:40 (EA)
27:42 (EA)
27:44 (EA)
27:89

27:12 (EU)
79-T,80-N, 81 T
27:18 (EA)
27:153

or Mediterranean ancestry, *B*27:03*, found in West Africa, *B*27:04*, primarily seen in those of eastern Asian descent, and *B*27:06*, found in those of southeast Asian, Indonesian, and Philippine ancestry. *HLA-B*27:07* is likely a very ancient allele, diverging from *HLA-B*27:05* before extensive dispersal of *H. sapiens* from Africa ensued, as it has been found in cell lines of individuals from Wales, India, and Eastern Asia. *HLA-B*27:01* has been identified in individuals from North America, including Caucasians, Latinos, and Blacks, and may be of Native American (likely NaDene) origin. *HLA-B*27:08* has been seen in individuals from northern Europe, and *HLA-B*27:09* from natives of Sardinia (and rarely Italy perhaps reflecting migration from the former). One HLA-B27 subtype, *HLA-B*27:22*, was withdrawn, having resulted from a DNA sequencing error, and three subtypes, *B*27:59*, *B*27:64* and *B:27:65*, contain intraexonic deletions and are likely not expressed at the cell surface. Most of the "major" subtypes derived from *HLA-B*27:05* are associated with AS susceptibility or at least have been primarily described in patients with AS, although two subtypes, *HLA-B*27:06* and *B*27:09*, are not disease-associated.

The other alleles *of HLA-B*27* have arisen by single or few amino acid substitutions from *HLA-B*27:05* or from the major subtypes. For the most part, these alleles are rare and have been encountered in small numbers of individuals, largely from specific geographic locations, suggesting more recent evolution (Fig. 5.2).

Other HLA genes have also been implicated in addition to *HLA-B*27*. However, linkage disequilibrium (LD) with *HLA-B*27* has made it difficult to resolve whether they play an independent role themselves, which would provide additional clues to AS pathogenesis, and potentially serve as biomarkers of diagnosis. The most consistent association has been at *HLA-B60* (known at the DNA level as *B*40*).[18,19] The initial observation was made as far back as 1989 and has been extensively replicated in whites and in Asians,[20] although the odds ratios are much weaker than with *HLA-B27*. Nonetheless, the same gene:gene interaction has been observed between *HLA-B*40* and *ERAP1* (see below) as has been seen with *HLA-B*27*.[21]

Other *HLA-B* locus alleles have also been implicated, including *HLA-B*14* in West Africans with axial SpA.[22] A large study examining 7264 MHC SNPs in 9069 AS cases and 13,578 population controls of European descent using the Illumina Immunochip microarray and controlling for the effects of *HLA-B*27:02* and *B*27:05*, where HLA-alleles were determined by imputation, identified significantly increased frequencies of HLA-B*13:02, B*40:01, B*40:02, B*47:01, B*51:01, and

negative associations with *HLA-B*07:02* and *B*57:01*.[21] *HLA-B*7* has been shown in the Chinese population to be strongly protective against AS (heterozygote odds ratio 0.15).[23] *HLA-B*15* has been implicated in Colombian and Mexican patients with peripheral spondyloarthritis.[24,25] However, the relative risks that these genes carry for AS susceptibility are relatively small compared with *HLA-B27*, and their overall contribution to disease susceptibility is much less.

The HLA-A locus, specifically the allele *HLA-A*02:01*, was also found to be independently associated with AS in whites in the imputation study above.[21] In Koreans, association with *HLA-C*1502* was observed.[26]

Immediately centromeric to *HLA-B* in the MHC lies the major histocompatibility complex I polypeptide-related sequence A (*MICA*) locus, which encodes a membrane-bound protein acting as a ligand to stimulate an activating receptor, NKG2D, expressed on the surface of human NK cells, gd T cells, and CD8+ ab T cells. Given the role of membrane-bound MICA in acting as a signal during the early immune response against infection and its expression and its high expression in intestinal epithelium, it was natural to consider *MICA* as a candidate locus for AS. Early studies in small European descent and Asian cohorts suggest an association with AS (15–18),[27,28,29] but subsequently this was shown to be due to linkage disequilibrium (LD) with *HLA-B*27*.[30–32] Zhou et al. reported in a sequencing-based study of moderately large cohorts of US whites and Han Chinese an association of AS in whites with *MICA*007* and in Chinese with *MICA*007* and *019*,[33] but this could not be confirmed in a much larger study where the *MICA* alleles were determined by imputation.[34] Thus, any role that MICA genes might have in AS susceptibility remains to be demonstrated.

Given the known involvement of CD4+ T cells in SpA, it is not surprising that involvement with MHC class II alleles is likely relevant to disease pathogenesis. Associations with *HLA-DRB1*01* and *HLA-DRB1*04:04* have been reported in UK AS patients and from French spondyloarthritis families.[35,36] Similarly, the association with *HLA-DRB1*01:03*, which has been previously associated with inflammatory bowel disease[37] and axial enteropathic arthritis,[38] was seen by imputation in AS.[21] In the same study, *HLA-DRB1*15:01* and its linked allele *DQB1*06:02* were actually decreased in frequency[21] in patients with AS in general. Studies with acute anterior uveitis (AAU) in AS, compared with AS without AAU, have demonstrated unique associations with *HLA-DRB1*01:03*, *DQB1*05*, and with the *HLA-DRB5* locus, a gene which is only found on

HLA-DRB1*15- and DRB1*16-bearing HLA haplotypes, as well as with the class I allele HLA-B*08.[39] The HLA-DP locus, including both HLA-DPA1 and HLA-DPB1 genes, has also been implicated in older studies as well as more recently by imputation.[21,40,41]

Other genes in the MHC that have been studied include TNF-alpha1,[42] TAP1,[43] and LMP2,[40,44] although the level of association of these findings has not been definitive and the associations have not been confirmed.

Overall, the relative contribution of the MHC, the major region in AS susceptibility, is complex, with the overwhelming effect provided by HLA-B27 itself and minor additional risk (and likely some interactive effects) from other MHC genes.

NON–MAJOR HISTOCOMPATIBILITY COMPLEX GENETICS

Table 5.1 lists the current known loci associated with AS at genome-wide significance levels. These are derived from either genome-wide association studies (GWAS),[32,45,46] more targeted studies using SNP microarrays such as nonsynonymous SNP-targeted chips,[47] Immunochip[9,48,49] or Exomechip,[50] or candidate gene genotyping.[7,51] Although suggestive association

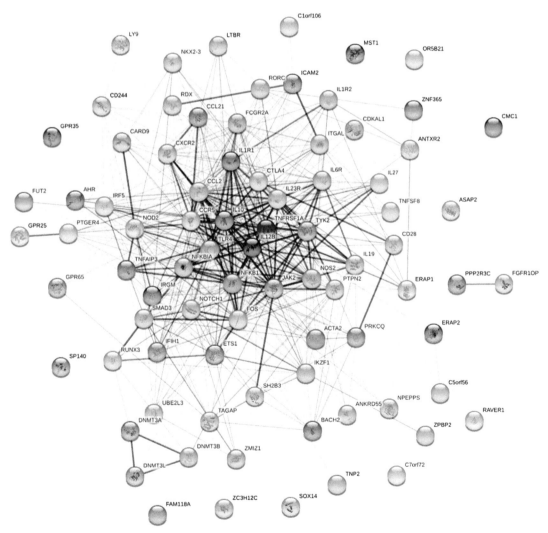

FIG. 5.2 Protein-protein interaction pathway analysis of AS-associated genes using the STRING database revealing key pathways involved in disease pathogenesis.

findings have been reported from family-based studies, as these are not as yet genetically definitive, they will not be discussed further here.[52] It is notable that only two non-MHC loci have been detected at genome-wide significance level first in candidate gene studies (*ANTXR2*[51] and *C1orf106/GPR25*[7]), and in both cases, the studies were informed by prior GWAS studies. This highlights the problems with many genetic studies that are either underpowered to achieve robust, genome-wide, significance levels, or which use study designs, which do not control for population stratification, or use genotyping methods that are not as robust as SNP microarrays; such studies have nearly all not proven robust nor provided definitive association findings.

The associations listed in Table 5.1 contribute ~7%–8% of the known genetic risk for AS.[9] In total, 115 non-MHC loci have been associated with AS either at genome-wide levels of significance ($P<5 \times 10^{-8}$) in an AS-specific analysis or in a set-based metaanalysis, with demonstration of an association of AS independently at that locus. Gene annotations have been given where there is a clear candidate gene on the basis of function and/or only one candidate gene at the locus. Note that for the most part, these annotations cannot be considered definite as few loci have been extensively studied in AS to ensure definitive statements can be made. Nonetheless, these annotations should be considered fairly robust. This represents a treasure trove of biologic information about the etiopathogenesis of AS, and potential therapeutic targets, which the functional genomics and immunology community need to focus on to better dissect and translate into clinical outcomes. The fact that common variant genomic findings have been demonstrated to be powerful predictors of

TABLE 5.1
Established Genetic Associations With AS (Either Genome-Wide Significance (GWS) ($P<5 \times 10^{-8}$) With Confirmation ($P<.05$) in Another Dataset or $P<5 \times 10^{-8}$ in Set-Based Metaanalysis (SMR) With $P<.05$ as an Individual Disease)

SNP	CHR	Position	Gene	A1	A2	OR	MAF	Significance
rs11249215	1	25297184	RUNX3	A	G	1.19	0.48	GWS
rs6600247	1	25305114	RUNX3	T	C	0.83	0.51	GWS
rs80174646	1	67708155	IL23R	T	G	0.60	0.066	GWS
rs10889676	1	67722567	IL23R	A	C	1.16	0.30	GWS
rs4129267	1	154426264	IL6R	T	C	0.85	0.39	GWS
rs12131796	1	200878727	C1orf106/GPR25	A	G	0.83	0.27	GWS
rs2666218	2	9402988	ASAP2	G	A	1.12	0.28	GWS
rs10865331	2	62551472	2p15 Intergenic	A	G	1.3	0.4	GWS
rs4851529	2	102647300	IL1R2	A	G	0.88	0.41	GWS
rs871656	2	102771282	IL1R1	A	T	0.87	0.19	GWS
rs11306716	2	204707771	CD28/CTLA4	I	D	1.14	0.48	GWS
rs3749171	2	241569692	GPR35	T	C	1.18	0.18	GWS
rs10510607	3	28286261	CMC1	T	C	0.87	0.17	GWS
rs6781808	3	137441372	SOX14	C	T	1.14	0.20	GWS
rs12504282	4	80927001	ANTXR2	C	T	0.88	0.43	GWS
rs3774937	4	103434253	NFKB1	C	T	1.120	0.33	GWS
rs11750385	5	10521668	Uncertain	G	T	1.11	0.37	GWS
rs469758	5	96121715	ERAP1	C	T	1.34	0.34	GWS
rs2549803	5	96174929	ERAP1	T	C	0.87	0.37	GWS
rs2910686	5	96252589	ERAP2	C	T	1.21	0.44	GWS

TABLE 5.1

Established Genetic Associations With AS (Either Genome-Wide Significance (GWS) ($P<5\times10^{-8}$) With Confirmation ($P<.05$) in Another Dataset or $P<5\times10^{-8}$ in Set-Based Metaanalysis (SMR) With $P<.05$ as an Individual Disease)—cont'd

SNP	CHR	Position	Gene	A1	A2	OR	MAF	Significance
rs6556416	5	158818745	IL12B	C	A	1.17	0.83	GWS
rs56167332	5	158827769	IL12B	A	C	1.13	0.34	GWS
rs2328530	6	20643727	CDKAL1	G	A	0.88	0.20	GWS
rs6908425	6	20728731	CDKAL1	C	T	1.2	0.78	GWS
rs67025039	6	167415404	FGFR1OP	I	D	1.21	0.48	GWS
rs1525735	7	17197571	AHR	C	T	1.17	0.45	GWS
rs1250573	10	81042475	ZMIZ1	A	G	0.89	0.31	GWS
rs1800682	10	90749963	ACTA2	G	A	0.89	0.46	GWS
rs10748781	10	101283330	NKX2-3	C	A	1.11	0.43	GWS
rs7115956	11	109956346	ZC3H12C/RDX	C	T	1.23	0.49	GWS
rs7933433	11	128194450	ETS1	T	G	1.12	0.34	GWS
rs1860545	12	6446777	TNFRSF1A	A	G	0.85	0.41	GWS
rs11616188	12	6502742	LTBR	A	G	1.11	0.42	GWS
rs11624293	14	88488821	GPR65	C	T	1.23	0.087	GWS
rs26528	16	28517709	IL27	C	T	1.17	0.46	GWS
rs34670647	16	30171017	Uncertain	D	I	1.23	0.48	GWS
rs9797244	17	26097131	NOS2	C	T	1.14	0.19	GWS
rs2779255	17	26137540	NOS2	C	T	1.11	0.38	GWS
rs12943464	17	45690351	NPEPPS	A	T	1.15	0.48	GWS
rs196941	17	62147192	ERN1/ICAM2	G	C	1.14	0.24	GWS
rs9977672	21	40463283	21q22 Intergenic	A	G	0.83	0.26	GWS
rs1569414	22	45727565	FAM118A	G	T	0.87	0.27	GWS
rs6426833	1	20171860	Uncertain	G	A	1.05	0.46	SBM
rs7517847	1	67681669	IL23R	G	T	0.93	0.43	SBM
rs183686347	1	67703442	IL23R	A	G	1.78	0.0019	SBM
rs4845604	1	151801680	RORC	A	G	1.08	0.15	SBM
rs4971079	1	155130391	Uncertain	A	G	1.076	0.46	SBM
rs1333062	1	160846284	LY9/CD244	T	G	0.91	0.32	SBM
rs10800314	1	161472789	FCGR2A	C	A	1.07	0.35	SBM
rs61802846	1	161473873	FCGR2A	C	A	1.11	0.13	SBM
rs3024493	1	206943968	IL10/IL19	A	C	1.10	0.16	SBM
rs12075255	1	206961628	IL10/IL19	A	G	0.93	0.15	SBM
rs13407913	2	25097644	Uncertain	G	A	1.06	0.43	SBM
rs201014116	2	25500905	DNMT3A	C	A	1.07	0.31	SBM
rs72871627	2	163136942	IFIH1	G	A	1.28	0.0099	SBM

Continued

TABLE 5.1
Established Genetic Associations With AS (Either Genome-Wide Significance (GWS) ($P<5\times10^{-8}$) With Confirmation ($P<.05$) in Another Dataset or $P<5\times10^{-8}$ in Set-Based Metaanalysis (SMR) With $P<.05$ as an Individual Disease)—cont'd

SNP	CHR	Position	Gene	A1	A2	OR	MAF	Significance
rs7426056	2	204612058	CD28/CTLA4	A	G	1.06	0.23	SBM
rs11676348	2	219010146	CXCR2	T	C	1.06	0.48	SBM
rs12694846	2	231148128	SP140	G	A	1.08	0.26	SBM
rs4676406	2	241579108	GPR35	G	T	0.94	0.48	SBM
rs1001007	3	46428658	CCR5	A	G	0.94	0.40	SBM
rs3197999	3	49721532	MST1	A	G	1.09	0.28	SBM
rs1992661	5	40414989	PTGER4	G	A	0.93	0.39	SBM
rs9687958	5	40496423	PTGER4	G	T	0.95	0.32	SBM
rs71624119	5	55440730	ANKRD55	A	G	0.94	0.24	SBM
rs17622517	5	131803537	C5orf56	C	T	1.15	0.084	SBM
rs11749391	5	150229066	IRGM	C	T	1.13	0.082	SBM
rs1267499	6	14715882	6p23 Intergenic	T	C	0.92	0.19	SBM
rs72928038	6	90976768	BACH2	A	G	1.08	0.17	SBM
rs582757	6	138197824	TNFAIP3	C	T	1.06	0.27	SBM
rs2451258	6	159506600	TAGAP	C	T	1.09	0.34	SBM
rs2301436	6	167437988	FGFR1OP	T	C	0.91	0.48	SBM
rs12718244	7	50175654	C7orf72	A	G	1.05	0.40	SBM
rs4917129	7	50323174	IKZF1	T	C	0.95	0.40	SBM
rs4728142	7	128573967	IRF5	A	G	1.07	0.44	SBM
rs10758669	9	4981602	JAK2	C	A	1.06	0.35	SBM
rs2812378	9	34710260	CCL21	G	A	1.09	0.33	SBM
rs726657	9	117696336	TNFSF8	T	C	0.92	0.42	SBM
rs4986790	9	120475302	TLR4	G	A	0.90	0.057	SBM
rs141992399	9	139259592	CARD9	G	C	0.48	0.0067	SBM
rs10870077	9	139263891	CARD9	G	C	1.09	0.43	SBM
rs3124998	9	139389432	NOTCH1	T	C	1.21	0.027	SBM
rs2236379	10	6527143	PRKCQ	A	G	1.07	0.25	SBM
rs10761648	10	64354262	ZNF365	T	C	1.09	0.17	SBM
rs7915475	10	64381668	ZNF365	G	A	0.93	0.32	SBM
rs11190133	10	101278725	NKX2-3	T	C	0.88	0.30	SBM
rs10750899	11	58284951	Uncertain	G	A	1.23	0.013	SBM
rs11236797	11	76299649	Uncertain	A	C	1.105	0.45	SBM
rs11221322	11	128346793	ETS1	C	T	1.14	0.162	SBM
rs11221332	11	128380974	ETS1	T	C	1.09	0.23	SBM
rs12369214	12	107198611	Uncertain	A	G	0.95	0.37	SBM

TABLE 5.1
Established Genetic Associations With AS (Either Genome-Wide Significance (GWS) ($P<5\times10^{-8}$) With Confirmation ($P<.05$) in Another Dataset or $P<5\times10^{-8}$ in Set-Based Metaanalysis (SMR) With $P<.05$ as an Individual Disease)—cont'd

SNP	CHR	Position	Gene	A1	A2	OR	MAF	Significance
rs3184504	12	111884608	SH2B3	T	C	0.92	0.49	SBM
rs8006884	14	35563211	Uncertain	C	T	1.10	0.35	SBM
rs2145623	14	35839236	NFKBIA	C	G	0.94	0.28	SBM
rs1569328	14	75741751	FOS	T	C	0.94	0.17	SBM
rs35874463	15	67457698	SMAD3	G	A	1.13	0.049	SBM
rs367569	16	11365500	TNP2	T	C	0.95	0.29	SBM
rs11574938	16	30485393	ITGAL	G	C	1.08	0.47	SBM
rs2066845	16	50756540	NOD2	C	G	0.78	0.015	SBM
rs72796367	16	50762771	NOD2	C	T	0.79	0.023	SBM
rs5743293	16	50763781	NOD2	I	D	0.82	0.024	SBM
rs9889296	17	32570547	CCL2/7/8/11	A	G	0.93	0.28	SBM
rs35736272	17	38032680	ZPBP2	C	T	1.07	0.46	SBM
rs1292035	17	57989557	Uncertain	A	G	1.10	0.19	SBM
rs12968719	18	12879466	PTPN2	A	G	1.12	0.12	SBM
rs74956615	19	10427721	RAVER1	A	T	0.81	0.049	SBM
rs35018800	19	10464843	TYK2	A	G	0.60	0.0088	SBM
rs12720356	19	10469975	TYK2	C	A	1.09	0.084	SBM
rs587259	19	34656406	LSM14	T	C	0.95	0.37	SBM
rs679574	19	49206108	FUT2	G	C	1.07	0.46	SBM
rs4243971	20	30849517	Uncertain	T	G	0.92	0.44	SBM
rs6058869	20	31348750	DNMT3B	T	C	1.09	0.40	SBM
rs2823288	21	16820888	21q21 Intergenic	A	G	1.06	0.29	SBM
rs4456788	21	45616324	ICOSLG/DNMT3L	G	A	1.08	0.39	SBM
rs2266961	22	21928597	UBE2L3	G	C	1.10	0.20	SBM
rs2143178	22	39660829	PDFGFB	C	T	0.90	0.17	SBM

CHR, chromosome; *MAF*, minor allele frequency in controls. Position is for human genome build 37. A1 and A2 are the two SNP alleles. OR and MAF are for the A1 allele.

likely success in drug development pipelines highlights the value of these data to therapeutic development.[53,54]

Cytokine Pathways

Pathway analysis (Fig. 5.2) using the STRING protein-protein interaction database shows that many of the genetic associations identified to date are involved in either the IL-23 pathway, TNF pathway, or related cytokines including IL-1, IL-6, IL-10, and IL-27.

IL-23 Pathway Genes

The first two genes associated with AS at genome-wide significance were *IL23R* and *ERAP1*. At roughly the same time that *IL23R* was found to be associated with AS, the same variants were also found to be associated with psoriasis[55,56] and inflammatory bowel disease.[57] Certainly for AS, and arguably for any rheumatic disease, this was the first definitive evidence that this pathway was involved in its pathogenesis and stimulated the development of new agents targeting this pathway as well as the repositioning of agents being trialed in other diseases to their use in these three conditions.

Fine-mapping studies of the *IL23R* locus show that there are multiple independent signals involved, with the largest such study finding four independent associations using conditional regression methods.[9] The two strongest of these associations are with the coding SNP rs11209026 (Arg381Gln), with the low frequency "A" allele affording protection from AS. This variant has been shown to lead to reduction in IL-23-induced IL-17A and IL-22 production and STAT3 phosphorylation,[58-61] as well as reduced circulating Th17 and Tc17 cell numbers.[60] The functional effect of other *IL23R* variants is not yet established, including the East Asian AS-associated variant rs76418789 (Gly149Arg).[62]

The relative strength of association of variants at this locus with different rheumatic diseases varies, and it is likely that this contributes to the difference in phenotype between diseases. For example, in Behcet disease, the association at this locus is primarily with SNPs, which lie in the intergenic region between *IL23R* and *IL12RB2*,[63] rather than those within *IL23R*, which are the most strongly associated with AS, psoriasis, and IBD. Studies of this region in AS suggest that the key SNP in the *IL23R-IL12RB2* intergenic region is rs11209032[32] and that the risk variants of this SNP lead to increased Th1 lymphocyte numbers,[64] in contrast to the effects of the *IL23R* variants such as rs11209026 discussed above, which primarily involve IL-17-producing cell types. Similar differences are also seen at many other loci associated with different diseases and likely lead to fine differences in expression in different tissues and in response to different stimuli.

Discordant associations are also observed, often involving SNPs associated with AS and classical autoimmune diseases.[8] For example, *IL27* SNPs are associated with AS[49] and IBD,[65] and the AS/IBD-protective variants are discordantly associated with type 1 diabetes.[66] IL-27 plays roles in balancing the relative activity of Th1 and Treg cells, and Th17 lymphocytes,[67] providing a likely explanation for the differential association of variants in this gene in diseases, which are driven by either of these lymphocyte subsets.

Since the discovery of these *IL23R* associations, multiple other genes in this pathway have been reported to be associated with AS. Polymorphisms of *IL12B*, encoding the IL-12p40 protein that forms half of the IL-23 and IL-12 heterodimers, are also associated with AS,[7] psoriasis,[56] and IBD.[68] However, polymorphisms of *IL23A*, which encodes IL-23p19 the other half of the IL-23 heterodimer, are associated with psoriasis[69] and

psoriatic arthritis,[70] but not to date with AS or inflammatory bowel disease. Although it is possible that with larger datasets, association between these genes and each of these genes may be demonstrated, it appears more likely that the genetic associations in these key IL-23 pathway cytokine genes are different between diseases, perhaps explaining some of the difference in response seen with inhibitors of different IL-23 pathway components.

IL-23R signals through JAK2 and STAT3. AS is associated with *JAK2*, suggesting that JAK inhibitors with effects on this tyrosine kinase may be effective for the disease. Recent trial data show beneficial effects of tofacitinib, a predominant JAK1 and JAK3 inhibitor with some effects on JAK2, in AS.[71] Although JAK2 inhibition would be expected to cause anemia through suppression of erythropoiesis, it will be interesting to see if future trials of JAK inhibitors with more JAK2 inhibition are more effective in AS, as the genetics would predict.

AS is also associated with *TYK2*, which is involved in downstream signaling from type I IFN, IL-12, and IL-23. The AS-protective primary *TYK2* SNP, rs34536443, has been shown to lead to reduced signaling in response to IFN, IL-12 and IL-23 and is not associated with increased risk of infectious diseases in biobank population data.[72] This supports Tyk2 as a potential therapeutic target for AS, among other diseases.

The IL-23 pathway is well known to interact with other cytokine pathways, and this likely explains the association of genes encoding multiple other cytokines and cytokine receptors with AS. These include *IL10*, which has immunoregulatory functions, and the *IL10* family member *IL19*, which has antiinflammatory effects, suppressing expression of IL-1, IL-6, and TNF.[73] IL-19 levels have been found to inversely correlate with disease activity in spondyloarthritis, although no difference in plasma IL-19 levels was found in axial or peripheral spondyloarthritis compared with healthy controls.[74] IL-19 production is upregulated by TLR4 and was shown to decrease production of CCL2 and IL-10. This is notable because *TLR4*, *CCL2*, and *IL10* are all AS-associated. This suggests this may be an important regulatory network in axial spondyloarthritis and a potential link between bacterial exposure and inflammation in AS.

AS is very responsive to inhibition of TNF and consistent with that is associated with the main TNF-receptor, *TNFR1*, and with other elements of the TNF pathway, including *NFKB1*, *NFKBIA*, and *TNFAIP3*. NFKβ is a transcription factor formed by dimerization of a range of proteins, often including NKFB (encoded by

NFKB1). NFKBIA inhibits NFKB1 activity, and *TNFAIP3* encodes A20, a ubiquitin-editing enzyme involved in suppressing NFKB activity.[75] Thus, the genetic findings also strongly implicate TNF and associated pathways in AS pathogenesis likely through NFKβ activation.

As noted with IL-23 pathway members, the genetic associations involved in this pathway show striking differences between diseases, which are likely to affect phenotype and treatment response. The AS-protective variant in *TNFR1* leads to loss of the transmembrane domain of the receptor and increased serum TNFR1, which downregulates TNF by acting as a soluble inhibitor, akin to the action of etanercept.[76] The same variant is also a risk factor for multiple sclerosis, consistent with the fact that TNF-inhibitor treatment can exacerbate or induce multiple sclerosis.[76]

Aminopeptidase Genes

The other major group of genes discovered in the first major SNP microarray genetic association study performed in AS was the M-aminopeptidases. Association was broadly seen across the chromosome 5q15 locus including with SNPs in the endoplasmic reticulum aminopeptidases *ERAP1* and *ERAP2*.[47,77] This association has been widely replicated with AS and with the broader axial spondyloarthritis disease grouping since then including in Asian populations[78,79] and major European ethnicities.[80-82] It is apparent that both *ERAP1* and *ERAP2* are AS-associated.

A key finding has been that the *ERAP1* genetic association is restricted to HLA-B27 positive cases[32] or HLA-B40-positive/HLA-B27-negative cases.[21] *ERAP1* is also associated with HLA-Cw6-positive psoriasis[83] and HLA-B51-positive Behcet disease.[84] *ERAP2* is associated with inflammatory bowel disease, where the major HLA associations are with HLA class II genes.[85] *ERAP1/2* is associated with the HLA-A29-associated immune-mediated disease birdshot retinopathy,[86] but as the disease is rare, dissection of the locus has not been achieved. The involvement of M1-aminopeptidases with AS has been further reinforced by the finding of the association of *NPEPPS* (puromycin-sensitive aminopeptidase) with AS.[49]

A key question in determining the functional mechanisms operating at this locus is which variants are involved. Haplotypic evolution studies suggested that a two-variant model most likely explains the ERAP1 association.[32] A Bayesian fine-mapping study determined the 99% credible interval for the ERAP1 associations was chr5: 96121151-96126308 (HG19 build).[87] The key SNP from conditional regression mapping, rs30187 (Lys528Arg), lies within this region,[32,49] along with 11

other variants. Two of these are coding and have minor allele frequency >1% (rs10050860) (Asn575Asp), and rs78649652 (Arg514Gly), which has low MAF (1.2%) and is therefore unlikely to be driving the association. Using recombinant ERAP1 protein, it has been shown that the protective rs30187 variant leads to reduced catalytic activity, whereas no effect was seen with rs10050860.[32]

It has been suggested that the association of *ERAP1* SNPs was driven by multiple SNPs operating in a haplotype.[88,89] However, in these studies, the direction of association of the key AS-associated variant rs30187 was the inverse of what has been reported in multiple international studies,[90] and a large-scale sequencing and imputation study has shown that many of the variants and haplotypes either do not exist or are much rarer in the population than previously reported.[91] Studies of the functional effects of haplotypes that do not exist, where whether the haplotype is involved in AS risk is unknown, or which involve variants not directly associated with AS, provide results the relevance of which to AS cannot be interpreted.[92,93]

Chromosome 5q15 variants also have marked effects on ERAP1/2 transcription.[94-96] Using RNA-seq, it was demonstrated that the second *ERAP1* haplotype tagged by rs10050860 is driven by effects on ERAP1 splicing leading to mRNA degradation, most likely due to rs7063 that lies within a splice junction site.[97] This finding defines the second ERAP1 haplotype and key functional variant and mechanism. The protective haplotype was associated with reduced translated ERAP1 protein, consistent with loss of function of ERAP1 being protective for AS.

At *ERAP2*, the AS-protective haplotype carries a synonymous SNP rs2248374, which has been shown to lead to skipping of an exon splice site, leading to premature termination of transcription and production of mRNA that is then subject to nonsense mediated decay, with no ERAP2 protein ultimately translated. This in turn leads to reduced MHC class I surface expression.[98] Other eQTL effects seen at ERAP2 also showed consistent direction of association, with AS-protective variants associated with reduced ERAP2 expression.[97]

NPEPPS, and ERAP1 and ERAP2 and are involved in peptide trimming in the cytosol and endoplasmic reticulum, respectively, before HLA class I presentation. ERAP1 operates as "molecular ruler," trimming peptides down to the optimal length for HLA class I presentation.[99] This process may lead either to the production of new antigens or to their destruction, possibly explaining how ERAP1 variants associated with protection from AS and psoriasis increase the risk of

Behcet disease. Marked effects of ERAP1 and ERAP2 variation on the peptidome presented by the different HLA class I alleles involved have been demonstrated, consistent with a mechanism of action through shaping the peptidome.[100–103] How this might lead to disease remains uncertain, with data to support effects on antigen presentation to T cells or KIR-bearing NK or CD8 T cells, on HLA class I folding and HLA-B27 homodimer formation (reviewed in Refs. 104,105). Whatever the downstream mechanism, the consistent finding with AS-associated protective variants at ERAP1 and ERAP2 that they are associated with loss of function supports efforts to target this system as a potential therapy for AS, psoriasis, and inflammatory bowel disease.

Epigenetics

Epigenetics is broadly distinguished from genetics through its influence on DNA function other than through change in the actual DNA sequence. This may involve addition of moieties directly to the DNA (for example, methyl groups), or alternately histone modification such as acetylation, with effects on chromatin structure and packing. Epigenetic effects are dynamic and responsive to environmental stimuli, whereas DNA, with the exception of random mutations, is stable in sequence during life. Epigenetic profiles also vary between cell types, whereas the sequence of DNA is the same in all cells in the one individual. Although genetic sequence is inherited through meiosis directly, thereby ensuring Mendelian inheritance of monogenic traits and diseases, epigenetic variation is less strictly inherited. Recent studies have estimated that the heritability of methylation in peripheral blood is ~20%,[106] although this varied between sites and was higher particularly at sites where the methylation is influenced by SNP variation.[107] Interestingly, from the perspective of a disease with a strong MHC association, a GWAS of cis-methylation effects found strong association between MHC SNPs and methylation at the locus, raising the possibility that methylation may be another mechanism by which MHC SNPs operate to influence HLA-associated disease risk.

DNA Methyl Transferase Associations

The demonstration of association of three different DNA methyltransferase genes with AS (*DNMT3A*, *DNMT3B*, and *DNMT3L*) indicates that methylation effects are involved in AS pathogenesis.[9] DNMT3 methyltransferases are involved in both de novo methylation and maintenance of inherited patterns of methylation.[108] DNMT3L is a factor that stimulates DNTM3-mediated methylation in poorly methylated sites by

anchoring the DNA methylation machinery onto chromatin. This attenuates the restrictions of the intrinsic DNMT3 flanking sequence preferences and thus promotes the formation of less restricted methylation patterns.[109] Further fine-mapping and functional studies are required to determine the effect of AS-associated genetic variants in and around these genes on their function.

Epigenetic Mapping

To date, only limited candidate gene methylation studies have been published in AS, with no adequately powered epigenome-wide association study reported (one study with five cases and five controls published[110]). Adequately powered studies with appropriate designs to control for covariates such as age, gender, medication effects, and smoking are clearly indicated in AS.

The increasing amount of publicly available information regarding epigenetic markers of gene activation facilitates functional genomic studies and enables hypothesis-free methods for identifying key cell and tissue types through which disease-associated genetic variants drive disease pathogenesis. This approach has been applied to AS genetic associations. The findings support the key role of cells of the immune system in driving AS pathogenesis, particularly CD4- and CD8-positive lymphocytes, but also T-regulatory cells, CD14-positive monocytes, and Th17 lymphocytes. Of particular interest, given the strong correlation between AS and IBD genetic associations, the study suggests involvement of multiple gastrointestinal mucosal tissues and cell types in the mechanism by which AS genetic associations lead to disease.[111]

Many of the genetic associations of AS involve transcription factors or regulators (*BACH2*, *EOMES*, *ETS1*, *IKZF1*, *NKX2-3*, *RUNX3*, *Tbx21*, *ZMIZ1*) or cytokines/cytokine receptor (discussed above), which are involved in lymphocyte activation/differentiation. AS-associated variants in these genes have been shown to have effects on CD8 lymphocytes (e.g., *RUNX3*[32,112]) as well as on innate lymphoid and NK cells (e.g., *Tbx21*[113]). Better epigenetic annotation data would be extremely valuable in these studies, enabling translation of the genetic findings. Although transcription factors themselves are not easily targeted therapeutically, understanding the disease processes they are involved in, genes whose transcription they regulate and cells and tissues whose properties and activities they affect will increase our understanding of the pathogenesis of AS and hopefully inform new therapy development.

GENETICS OF AXIAL SPONDYLOARTHRITIS IN EAST ASIANS

MHC Region

The prevalence of HLA-B27 positivity in the Chinese and Korean populations has been reported to be from 4% to 8% and from 2.3% to 7%, respectively,[114,115] which is lower than that in Caucasians but much higher than that in the Japanese population (1%).[116] To date, the most accurate tag SNP of *HLA-B27* is rs116488202 in both Europeans and Asians,[5] which is superior to the previously reported tag SNPS rs4349859 and rs13202464.[6] As in other ethnic groups, more than 80% of Chinese AS patients are *HLA-B27* positive with the primary subtype being *HLA-B*2704*, followed by *HLA-B*2705*.[7] The distribution of HLA-B27 subtypes reveals substantial demographic and geographic diversity. *HLA-B*2704* is a major subtype in Chinese individuals overall and particularly so in southern China, whereas *B*2705* is more common in northern Chinese.[8] It has been confirmed in both Taiwanese and mainland Chinese Han populations that *HLA-B*2704* is more commonly associated with AS than *HLA-B*2705*.[117,118] *HLA-B*2705* is the predominant subtype in Koreans.[119] *HLA-B*2706*, which is more prevalent in Malay descendants,[120–122] has a relatively weak association with AS compared with the *HLA-B*2704* subtype. *HLA-B*2706* has also been reported in Chinese Han descendants living in Taiwan.[123]

As has been demonstrated in Caucasians, the MHC associations of AS in East Asians is complex and not restricted to *HLA-B27*. Associations have been reported with *HLA-B60* and with MHC I chain-related gene A (*MICA*).[33,124] A recent case-control study in Korean additionally identified association with AS at *HLA-C*1502*.[18] Further dense SNP mapping of the locus may be of benefit to better define the MHC associations of the disease in Asian populations.

Non-MHC Loci

As discussed above, AS is strongly associated with variants in MHC region and HLA alleles, and multiple non-MHC genetic variants have been robustly associated with the disease. A large-scale multiethnic case-control association study performed with Illumina Immunochip microarray provided a new perspective on the similarities and differences in AS susceptibility between East Asian and Caucasians. A total of 13 loci had at least nominal levels of association in East Asians (Chinese, Koreans, Taiwanese), whereas 23 achieved genome-wide significance in white Europeans.[5] Because of the limited sample size of East Asian cohort in the Immunochip study, the power of the East Asian cohort was much inferior to that of the European cohort. However,

more than 40% of loci associated with AS in Europeans have been validated in East Asians (Fig. 5.3).These validated loci include *ERAP1*, *GPR35*, *HHAT*, *HLA-B*, *ICOSLG*, *IL23R*, *IL27*, *NOS2*, *NPEPPS*, *RUNX3*, *TBX21*, *TYK2*, *UBE2E3*, *UBE2L3*, *ZMIZ*1 and two intergenic regions (chromosomes 2p15 and 21q22).[125]

In addition, a GWAS study in Han Chinese identified two AS associated loci (*HAPLN1-EDIL3* and *ANO6*).[126] However, these findings have not been replicated in larger studies in either East Asians or Caucasians[125] and are thus likely false-positive findings.

Although in most cases, genetic associations were shared in both East Asians and Europeans, consistent with a common ancestral origin of the disease-associated SNPs, the associated variants are in some cases different. Taking interleukin-23 receptor (*IL23R*) gene, for example, the primarily associated variants indicated diversity between different Europe and Asia. rs11209026, a key nonsynonymous SNP in *IL23R* associated with AS in Caucasians, was not polymorphic in East Asians.[20] A low-frequency visitant in *IL23R*, rs76418789, has been reported to potentially attenuate the protective effects of *IL23R* against AS in Han Chinese.[62] The same SNP was also nominally associated with ankylosing spondylitis in Europeans. The minor allele frequency (MAF) of rs76418789 was about 3.7% in East Asians but only 0.34% in Europeans, and hence the association was not easily observed in Europeans. Among the other AS-associated loci defined in Europeans but not in East Asians, only the primary associated variant rs17765610 on *BACH2* presents a diverse frequency of over six times greater in Europeans than in East Asians (East Asians, 1.8%; Europeans, 11.8%).[5] These findings suggest that the differences in association findings between east Asians and Europeans are not due to differences in frequency of associated variants.

Prospects

The similarities and differences in the genetic features of AS between East Asia and other ethnic populations have demonstrated the utility of gene mapping in probing the genetic diversity among different ancestry groups. It is of great importance to confirm the associated loci in populations of different ancestries, which is a crucial indicator of the overall significance of defining the true disease-causing variant. The identification of genetic signatures in both the East Asian and European populations will provide additional details for unraveling the genetic basis of AS and other autoimmune diseases. Therefore, further transethnic genetic studies of multi-omics analyses, microbiota, and environmental factors are needed in expended cohorts.

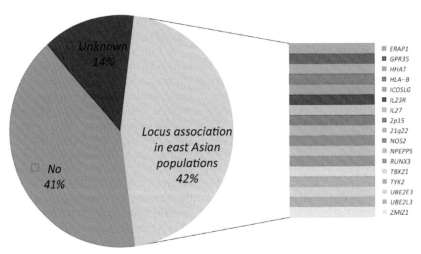

FIG. 5.3 Overlap of locus association in East Asian population in all genetic loci associated with AS. *No*, no association in East Asians reported, despite genome-wide significant associations in European descent populations. Association is defined as a concordant (same direction) association with *P* < .05 in the East Asian population.

The Future

We are still at a fairly early phase of AS genetic studies, with the largest GWAS in the disease having only 3023 cases in its discovery arm.[32] Although progress has been made through efficient use of targeted lower-cost SNP microarrays, much of the genome has not been studied in adequately powered studies. There is a strong linear correlation between sample size and number of loci identified in common heritable diseases.[127] At some point though, additional genetic discoveries do not add to biologic understanding as markers tend to fall either in the same genes or in closely related genes and thus contribute less. We are clearly well short of this point in AS.

Larger studies will also be required to assist in fine-mapping and rare variant studies. In a study involving 33,595 inflammatory bowel disease cases and 34,257 controls, researchers were able to define single causative variants at 18/94 loci studies with >95% certainty and at additional 27 loci with greater than 50% certainty.[128] This greatly simplifies the challenges of dissecting the functional mechanisms involved at each locus.

At this stage, no rare variant (minor allele frequency <1%) has been robustly associated with AS,

although rare variants within genes already identified by common variant studies have been reported.[49,62] The early suggestion that common disease heritability was largely caused by rare variants[129] has not panned out, and analyses have demonstrated that in common traits such as height where sufficiently large sample sizes have been studied, that rare variants play a small minority role.[6]

Nonetheless, there are a lot of potential values in identifying low frequency or rare variants of more major effect, as they indicate that the gene or pathway involved is likely to be less redundant and therefore has greater potential as a therapeutic target. Multi-case family studies tend simply to find high numbers of founders carrying major genes such as *HLA-B27* and have thus been relatively uninformative. Whole genome or even targeted sequencing is extremely expensive compared with SNP microarrays. The increasing power of imputation, which with modern SNP microarray data and large public reference panels can provide good coverage of variants down to a minor allele frequency of 0.5%, means that except for very rare variants, SNP microarrays remain the genotyping approach of choice for common diseases such as AS. There will not be sufficient cases for this approach to succeed. Therefore, large SNP microarray studies using imputation to investigate low frequency and rare variant associations are the most informative at this stage.

Large-scale studies will also enable development of genetic risk algorithms. Given the high heritability of AS, it should be possible to develop genetic risk algorithms, which are capable of accurate discrimination between cases and controls. This could be very helpful particularly in early or even preclinical settings, changing the practice of AS management toward early intervention approaches for which there is evidence that they are more effective. A genetic risk score for AS would also help in redefining nonradiographic disease, assisting in the validation of new classification criteria for early AS.

These studies will also be required to identify genetic associations of AS-associated features such as overall disease activity, radiographic progression, and the genetic factors involved in acute anterior uveitis and other AS-associated traits. Early studies of anterior uveitis have identified particularly the novel association of *CDKAL1* and increased association of *ERAP1* variants and HLA-B27 with AS complicated by eye disease,[39,130] but large cohorts will be required for study because of the high penetrance of uveitis in AS patients.

Another alternative to identify novel, including rare, variants is to study novel populations. To date, there has been no GWAS of AS in India, although the disease has similar prevalence there to other populations studied. There is also limited information available about AS genetics in Mediterranean countries. The findings of the only AS-GWAS in East Asians[126] unfortunately proved unreliable,[49] and thus more information is required about AS in China and Korea in particular.

We also would greatly benefit from a comprehensive set of transcriptional data on relevant cell and tissue types from AS cases, preferably with associated methylation and genomic and proteomic data. Whatever cell type people study, there will inevitably be criticism that "it is not the key cell type involved in AS" or that it is the wrong tissue, but pragmatically circulating immune cells are at least accessible and are moderately correlated in behavior to the immune cells in the gut and entheses.

The final main challenge is ensuring engagement between the genomics and other relevant communities required to translate these data, including the immunology and microbiology communities and

pharmaceutical industry. Successful translation of these fascinating discoveries depends on their involvement.

REFERENCES

1. de Blecourt J, Polman A, de Blecourt-Meindersma T. Hereditary factors in rheumatoid arthritis and ankylosing spondylitis. *Ann Rheum Dis.* 1961;20:215–223.
2. Brown MA, Laval SH, Brophy S, Calin A. Recurrence risk modelling of the genetic susceptibility to ankylosing spondylitis. *Ann Rheum Dis.* 2000;59(11):883–886.
3. Dernis E, Said-Nahal R, D'Agostino MA, Aegerter P, Dougados M, Breban M. Recurrence of spondylarthropathy among first-degree relatives of patients: a systematic cross-sectional study. *Ann Rheum Dis.* 2009;68(4):502–507.
4. Brown MA, Kennedy LG, MacGregor AJ, et al. Susceptibility to ankylosing spondylitis in twins: the role of genes, HLA, and the environment. *Arthritis Rheum.* 1997;40(10):1823–1828.
5. Pedersen OB, Svendsen AJ, Ejstrup L, Skytthe A, Harris JR, Junker P. Ankylosing spondylitis in Danish and Norwegian twins: occurrence and the relative importance of genetic vs. environmental effectors in disease causation. *Scand J Rheumatol.* 2008;37(2):120–126.
6. Yang J, Benyamin B, McEvoy BP, et al. Common SNPs explain a large proportion of the heritability for human height. *Nat Genet.* 2010;42(7):565–569.
7. Danoy P, Pryce K, Hadler J, et al. Association of variants at 1q32 and STAT3 with ankylosing spondylitis suggests genetic overlap with Crohn's disease. *PLoS Genet.* 2010;6(12):e1001195.
8. Parkes M, Cortes A, van Heel DA, Brown MA. Genetic insights into common pathways and complex relationships among immune-mediated diseases. *Nat Rev Genet.* 2013;14(9):661–673.
9. Ellinghaus D, Jostins L, Spain SL, et al. Analysis of five chronic inflammatory diseases identifies 27 new associations and highlights disease-specific patterns at shared loci. *Nat Genet.* 2016;48(5):510–518.
10. Brown MA, Pile KD, Kennedy LG, et al. A genome-wide screen for susceptibility loci in ankylosing spondylitis. *Arthritis Rheum.* 1998;41(4):588–595.
11. Laval SH, Timms A, Edwards S, et al. Whole-genome screening in ankylosing spondylitis: evidence of non-MHC genetic-susceptibility loci. *Am J Hum Genet.* 2001;68(4):918–926.
12. Brown MA, Brophy S, Bradbury L, et al. Identification of major loci controlling clinical manifestations of ankylosing spondylitis. *Arthritis Rheum.* 2003;48(8):2234–2239.
13. Hamersma J, Cardon LR, Bradbury L, et al. Is disease severity in ankylosing spondylitis genetically determined? *Arthritis Rheum.* 2001;44(6):1396–1400.
14. Brophy S, Hickey S, Menon A, et al. Concordance of disease severity among family members with ankylosing spondylitis? *J Rheumatol.* 2004;31(9):1775–1778.

15. Brewerton DA, Hart FD, Nicholls A, Caffrey M, James DC, Sturrock RD. Ankylosing spondylitis and HL-A 27. *Lancet*. 1973;1(7809):904–907.

16. Schlosstein L, Terasaki PI, Bluestone R, Pearson CM. High association of an HL-A antigen, W27, with ankylosing spondylitis. *N Engl J Med*. 1973;288(14):704–706.

17. Lawlor DA, Warren E, Taylor P, Parham P. Gorilla class I major histocompatibility complex alleles: comparison to human and chimpanzee class I. *J Exp Med*. 1991;174(6):1491–1509.

18. Robinson WP, van der Linden SM, Khan MA, et al. HLA-Bw60 increases susceptibility to ankylosing spondylitis in HLA-B27+ patients. *Arthritis Rheum*. 1989;32(9):1135–1141.

19. Brown MA, Pile KD, Kennedy LG, et al. HLA class I associations of ankylosing spondylitis in the white population in the United Kingdom. *Ann Rheum Dis*. 1996;55(4):268–270.

20. Wei JC, Tsai WC, Lin HS, Tsai CY, Chou CT. HLA-B60 and B61 are strongly associated with ankylosing spondylitis in HLA-B27-negative Taiwan Chinese patients. *Rheumatology*. 2004;43(7):839–842.

21. Cortes A, Pulit SL, Leo PJ, et al. Major histocompatibility complex associations of ankylosing spondylitis are complex and involve further epistasis with ERAP1. *Nat Commun*. 2015;6:7146.

22. Lopez-Larrea C, Mijiyawa M, Gonzalez S, et al. Association of ankylosing spondylitis with HLA-B*1403 in a West African population. *Arthritis Rheum*. 2002;46(11):2968–2971.

23. Yi L, Wang J, Guo X, et al. Profiling of HLA-B alleles for association studies with ankylosing spondylitis in the Chinese population. *Open Rheumatol J*. 2013;7:51–54.

24. Santos AM, Pena P, Avila M, et al. Association of human leukocyte A, B, and DR antigens in Colombian patients with diagnosis of spondyloarthritis. *Clin Rheumatol*. 2017;36(4):953–958.

25. Londono J, Santos AM, Pena P, et al. Analysis of HLA-B15 and HLA-B27 in spondyloarthritis with peripheral and axial clinical patterns. *BMJ Open*. 2015;5(11):e009092.

26. Kim K, Bang SY, Lee S, et al. An HLA-C amino-acid variant in addition to HLA-B*27 confers risk for ankylosing spondylitis in the Korean population. *Arthritis Res Ther*. 2015;17:342.

27. Amroun H, Djoudi H, Busson M, et al. Early-onset ankylosing spondylitis is associated with a functional MICA polymorphism. *Hum Immunol*. 2005;66(10):1057–1061.

28. Tsuchiya N, Shiota M, Moriyama S, et al. MICA allele typing of HLA-B27 positive Japanese patients with seronegative spondylarthropathies and healthy individuals: differential linkage disequilibrium with HLA-B27 subtypes. *Arthritis Rheum*. 1998;41(1):68–73.

29. Ricci-Vitiani L, Vacca A, Potolicchio I, et al. MICA gene triplet repeat polymorphism in patients with HLA-B27

30. Yabuki K, Ota M, Goto K, et al. Triplet repeat polymorphism in the MICA gene in HLA-B27 positive and negative caucasian patients with ankylosing spondylitis. *Hum Immunol*. 1999;60(1):83–86.

31. Martinez-Borra J, Gonzalez S, Lopez-Vazquez A, et al. HLA-B27 alone rather than B27-related class I haplotypes contributes to ankylosing spondylitis susceptibility. *Hum Immunol*. 2000;61(2):131–139.

32. Evans DM, Spencer CC, Pointon JJ, et al. Interaction between ERAP1 and HLA-B27 in ankylosing spondylitis implicates peptide handling in the mechanism for HLA-B27 in disease susceptibility. *Nat Genet*. 2011;43(8):761–767.

33. Zhou X, Wang J, Zou H, et al. MICA, a gene contributing strong susceptibility to ankylosing spondylitis. *Ann Rheum Dis*. 2014;73(8):1552–1557.

34. Cortes A, Gladman D, Raychaudhuri S, et al. Imputation-based analysis of MICA alleles in the susceptibility to ankylosing spondylitis. *Ann Rheum Dis*. 2018;77(11):1691–1692.

35. Said-Nahal R, Miceli-Richard C, Gautreau C, et al. The role of HLA genes in familial spondyloarthropathy: a comprehensive study of 70 multiplex families. *Ann Rheum Dis*. 2002;61(3):201–206.

36. Brown MA, Kennedy LG, Darke C, et al. The effect of HLA-DR genes on susceptibility to and severity of ankylosing spondylitis. *Arthritis Rheum*. 1998;41(3):460–465.

37. Goyette P, Boucher G, Mallon D, et al. High-density mapping of the MHC identifies a shared role for HLA-DRB1*01:03 in inflammatory bowel diseases and heterozygous advantage in ulcerative colitis. *Nat Genet*. 2015;47(2):172–179.

38. Orchard TR, Thiyagaraja S, Welsh KI, Wordsworth BP, Hill Gaston JS, Jewell DP. Clinical phenotype is related to HLA genotype in the peripheral arthropathies of inflammatory bowel disease. *Gastroenterology*. 2000;118(2):274–278.

39. Robinson PC, Claushuis TA, Cortes A, et al. Genetic dissection of acute anterior uveitis reveals similarities and differences in associations observed with ankylosing spondylitis. *Arthritis Rheumatol*. 2015;67(1):140–151.

40. Ploski R, Maksymowych W, Forre O. HLA-DR8 and susceptibility to acute anterior uveitis in ankylosing spondylitis: comment on the article by Monowarul Islam et al. *Arthritis Rheum*. 1996;39(2):351–352.

41. Diaz-Pena R, Aransay AM, Bruges-Armas J, et al. Fine mapping of a major histocompatibility complex in ankylosing spondylitis: association of the HLA-DPA1 and HLA-DPB1 regions. *Arthritis Rheum*. 2011;63(11):3305–3312.

42. Hohler T, Schaper T, Schneider PM, Meyer zum Buschenfelde KH, Marker-Hermann E. Association of different tumor necrosis factor alpha promoter allele frequencies with ankylosing spondylitis in HLA-B27 positive individuals. *Arthritis Rheum*. 1998;41(8):1489–1492.

43. Fraile A, Collado MD, Mataran L, Martin J, Nieto A. TAP1 and TAP2 polymorphism in Spanish patients with ankylosing spondylitis. *Exp Clin Immunogenet.* 2000;17(4):199–204.

44. Maksymowych WP, Wessler A, Schmitt-Egenolf M, et al. Polymorphism in an HLA linked proteasome gene influences phenotypic expression of disease in HLA-B27 positive individuals. *J Rheumatol.* 1994;21(4):665–669.

45. Reveille J, Sims A, Maksymowych W, et al. Genomewide association study in ankylosing spondylitis identifies major non-MHC genetic determinants of disease susceptibility. *Arthritis Rheum.* 2008;(suppl 1):S1186.

46. Australo-Anglo-American Spondyloarthritis C, Reveille JD, Sims AM, et al. Genome-wide association study of ankylosing spondylitis identifies non-MHC susceptibility loci. *Nat Genet.* 2010;42(2):123–127.

47. Burton PR, Clayton DG, Cardon LR, et al. Association scan of 14,500 nonsynonymous SNPs in four diseases identifies autoimmunity variants. *Nat Genet.* 2007;39(11):1329–1337.

48. Cortes A, Brown MA. Promise and pitfalls of the Immunochip. *Arthritis Res Ther.* 2011;13(1):101.

49. International Genetics of Ankylosing Spondylitis C, Cortes A, Hadler J, et al. Identification of multiple risk variants for ankylosing spondylitis through high-density genotyping of immune-related loci. *Nat Genet.* 2013;45(7):730–738.

50. Robinson PC, Leo PJ, Pointon JJ, et al. Exome-wide study of ankylosing spondylitis demonstrates additional shared genetic background with inflammatory bowel disease. *NPJ Genom Med.* 2016;1:16008.

51. Karaderi T, Keidel SM, Pointon JJ, et al. Ankylosing spondylitis is associated with the anthrax toxin receptor 2 gene (ANTXR2). *Ann Rheum Dis.* 2014;73(11):2054–2058.

52. O'Rielly DD, Uddin M, Codner D, et al. Private rare deletions in SEC16A and MAMDC4 may represent novel pathogenic variants in familial axial spondyloarthritis. *Ann Rheum Dis.* 2016;75(4):772–779.

53. Cook D, Brown D, Alexander R, et al. Lessons learned from the fate of AstraZeneca's drug pipeline: a five-dimensional framework. *Nat Rev Drug Discov.* 2014;13(6):419–431.

54. Nelson MR, Tipney H, Painter JL, et al. The support of human genetic evidence for approved drug indications. *Nat Genet.* 2015;47(8):856–860.

55. Cargill M, Schrodi SJ, Chang M, et al. A large-scale genetic association study confirms IL12B and leads to the identification of IL23R as psoriasis-risk genes. *Am J Hum Genet.* 2007;80(2):273–290.

56. Nair RP, Ruether A, Stuart PE, et al. Polymorphisms of the IL12B and IL23R genes are associated with psoriasis. *J Invest Dermatol.* 2008;128(7):1653–1661.

57. Duerr RH, Taylor KD, Brant SR, et al. A genome-wide association study identifies IL23R as an inflammatory bowel disease gene. *Science.* 2006;314(5804):1461–1463.

58. Di Meglio P, Villanova F, Napolitano L, et al. The IL23R A/Gln381 allele promotes IL-23 unresponsiveness in human memory T-helper 17 cells and impairs Th17 responses in psoriasis patients. *J Invest Dermatol.* 2013;133(10):2381–2389.

59. Di Meglio P, Di Cesare A, Laggner U, et al. The IL23R R381Q gene variant protects against immune-mediated diseases by impairing IL-23-induced Th17 effector response in humans. *PLoS One.* 2011;6(2):e17160.

60. Sarin R, Wu X, Abraham C. Inflammatory disease protective R381Q IL23 receptor polymorphism results in decreased primary CD4+ and CD8+ human T-cell functional responses. *Proc Natl Acad Sci USA.* 2011;108(23):9560–9565.

61. Pidasheva S, Trifari S, Phillips A, et al. Functional studies on the IBD susceptibility gene IL23R implicate reduced receptor function in the protective genetic variant R381Q. *PLoS One.* 2011;6(10):e25038.

62. Davidson SI, Jiang L, Cortes A, et al. Brief report: high-throughput sequencing of IL23R reveals a low-frequency, nonsynonymous single-nucleotide polymorphism that is associated with ankylosing spondylitis in a Han Chinese population. *Arthritis Rheum.* 2013;65(7):1747–1752.

63. Remmers EF, Cosan F, Kirino Y, et al. Genome-wide association study identifies variants in the MHC class I, IL10, and IL23R-IL12RB2 regions associated with Behcet's disease. *Nat Genet.* 2010;42(8):698–702.

64. Roberts AR, Vecellio M, Chen L, et al. An ankylosing spondylitis-associated genetic variant in the IL23R-IL12RB2 intergenic region modulates enhancer activity and is associated with increased Th1-cell differentiation. *Ann Rheum Dis.* 2016;75(12):2150–2156.

65. Wang K, Baldassano R, Zhang H, et al. Comparative genetic analysis of inflammatory bowel disease and type 1 diabetes implicates multiple loci with opposite effects. *Hum Mol Genet.* 2010;19(10):2059–2067.

66. Barrett JC, Clayton DG, Concannon P, et al. Genome-wide association study and meta-analysis find that over 40 loci affect risk of type 1 diabetes. *Nat Genet.* 2009;41(6):703–707.

67. Neufert C, Becker C, Wirtz S, et al. IL-27 controls the development of inducible regulatory T cells and Th17 cells via differential effects on STAT1. *Eur J Immunol.* 2007;37(7):1809–1816.

68. Fisher SA, Tremelling M, Anderson CA, et al. Genetic determinants of ulcerative colitis include the ECM1 locus and five loci implicated in Crohn's disease. *Nat Genet.* 2008;40(6):710–712.

69. Nair RP, Duffin KC, Helms C, et al. Genome-wide scan reveals association of psoriasis with IL-23 and NF-kappaB pathways. *Nat Genet.* 2009;41(2):199–204.

70. Bowes J, Orozco G, Flynn E, et al. Confirmation of TNIP1 and IL23A as susceptibility loci for psoriatic arthritis. *Ann Rheum Dis.* 2011;70(9):1641–1644.

71. van der Heijde D, Deodhar A, Wei JC, et al. Tofacitinib in patients with ankylosing spondylitis: a phase II, 16-

week, randomised, placebo-controlled, dose-ranging study. *Ann Rheum Dis.* 2017;76(8):1340–1347.

72. Diogo D, Bastarache L, Liao KP, et al. TYK2 protein-coding variants protect against rheumatoid arthritis and autoimmunity, with no evidence of major pleiotropic effects on non-autoimmune complex traits. *PLoS One.* 2015;10(4):e0122271.

73. Azuma YT, Matsuo Y, Kuwamura M, et al. Interleukin-19 protects mice from innate-mediated colonic inflammation. *Inflamm Bowel Dis.* 2010;16(6):1017–1028.

74. Kragstrup TW, Andersen T, Holm C, et al. Toll-like receptor 2 and 4 induced interleukin-19 dampens immune reactions and associates inversely with spondyloarthritis disease activity. *Clin Exp Immunol.* 2015;180(2):233–242.

75. Lee EG, Boone DL, Chai S, et al. Failure to regulate TNF-induced NF-kappaB and cell death responses in A20-deficient mice. *Science.* 2000;289(5488):2350–2354.

76. Gregory AP, Dendrou CA, Attfield KE, et al. TNF receptor 1 genetic risk mirrors outcome of anti-TNF therapy in multiple sclerosis. *Nature.* 2012;488(7412):508–511.

77. Tsui FW, Haroon N, Reveille JD, et al. Association of an ERAP1 ERAP2 haplotype with familial ankylosing spondylitis. *Ann Rheum Dis.* 2010;69(4):733–736.

78. Davidson SI, Wu X, Liu Y, et al. Association of ERAP1, but not IL23R, with ankylosing spondylitis in a Han Chinese population. *Arthritis Rheum.* 2009;60(11):3263–3268.

79. Li C, Lin Z, Xie Y, et al. ERAP1 is associated with ankylosing spondylitis in han Chinese. *J Rheumatol.* 2010;38(2):317–321.

80. Pimentel-Santos FM, Ligeiro D, Matos M, et al. Association of IL23R and ERAP1 genes with ankylosing spondylitis in a Portuguese population. *Clin Exp Rheumatol.* 2009;27(5):800–806.

81. Pazar B, Safrany E, Gergely P, Szanto S, Szekanecz Z, Poor G. Association of ARTS1 gene polymorphisms with ankylosing spondylitis in the Hungarian population: the rs27044 variant is associated with HLA-B*2705 subtype in Hungarian patients with ankylosing spondylitis. *J Rheumatol.* 2010;37(2):379–384.

82. Kadi A, Izac B, Said-Nahal R, et al. Investigating the genetic association between ERAP1 and spondyloarthritis. *Ann Rheum Dis.* 2013;72(4):608–613.

83. Strange A, Capon F, Spencer CC, et al. A genome-wide association study identifies new psoriasis susceptibility loci and an interaction between HLA-C and ERAP1. *Nat Genet.* 2010;42(11):985–990.

84. Kirino Y, Bertsias G, Ishigatsubo Y, et al. Genome-wide association analysis identifies new susceptibility loci for Behcet's disease and epistasis between HLA-B*51 and ERAP1. *Nat Genet.* 2013;45(2):202–207.

85. Franke A, McGovern DP, Barrett JC, et al. Genome-wide meta-analysis increases to 71 the number of confirmed Crohn's disease susceptibility loci. *Nat Genet.* 2010;42(12):1118–1125.

86. Kuiper JJ, Van Setten J, Ripke S, et al. A genome-wide association study identifies a functional ERAP2 haplotype associated with birdshot chorioretinopathy. *Hum Mol Genet.* 2014;23(22):6081–6087.

87. van de Bunt M, Cortes A, Consortium I, Brown MA, Morris AP, McCarthy MI. Evaluating the performance of fine-mapping strategies at common variant GWAS loci. *PLoS Genet.* 2015;11(9):e1005535.

88. Reeves E, Elliott T, Edwards CJ, James E. Both rare and common ERAP1 allotypes have distinct functionality defined by polymorphic context and are important in AS association. *Proc Natl Acad Sci USA.* 2017;114(9):E1575–E1576.

89. Reeves E, Edwards CJ, Elliott T, James E. Naturally occurring ERAP1 haplotypes encode functionally distinct alleles with fine substrate specificity. *J Immunol.* 2013;191(1):35–43.

90. Robinson PC, Brown MA. ERAP1 biology and assessment in Ankylosing Spondylitis. *Proc Natl Acad Sci USA.* 2015;112(15):E1816.

91. Roberts AR, Appleton LH, Cortes A, et al. ERAP1 association with ankylosing spondylitis is attributable to common genotypes rather than rare haplotype combinations. *Proc Natl Acad Sci USA.* 2017;114(3):558–561.

92. Rastall DPW, Alyaquob FS, O'Connell P, et al. Mice expressing human ERAP1 variants associated with ankylosing spondylitis have altered T-cell repertoires and NK cell functions, as well as increased in utero and perinatal mortality. *Int Immunol.* 2017;29(6):277–289.

93. Seregin SS, Rastall DP, Evnouchidou I, et al. Endoplasmic reticulum aminopeptidase-1 alleles associated with increased risk of ankylosing spondylitis reduce HLA-B27 mediated presentation of multiple antigens. *Autoimmunity.* 2013;46(8):497–508.

94. Dixon AL, Liang L, Moffatt MF, et al. A genome-wide association study of global gene expression. *Nat Genet.* 2007;39(10):1202–1207.

95. Harvey D, Pointon JJ, Evans DM, et al. Investigating the genetic association between ERAP1 and ankylosing spondylitis. *Hum Mol Genet.* 2009;18(21):4204–4212.

96. Costantino F, Talpin A, Evnouchidou I, et al. ERAP1 gene expression is influenced by nonsynonymous polymorphisms associated with predisposition to spondyloarthritis. *Arthritis Rheumatol.* 2015;67(6):1525–1534.

97. Hanson AL, Cuddihy T, Haynes K, et al. Genetic variants in ERAP1 and ERAP2 associated with immune-mediated diseases influence protein expression and the isoform profile. *Arthritis Rheumatol.* 2018;70(2):255–265.

98. Andres AM, Dennis MY, Kretzschmar WW, et al. Balancing selection maintains a form of ERAP2 that undergoes nonsense-mediated decay and affects antigen presentation. *PLoS Genetics.* 2010;6(10):e1001157.

99. Chang SC, Momburg F, Bhutani N, Goldberg AL. The ER aminopeptidase, ERAP1, trims precursors to lengths of MHC class I peptides by a "molecular ruler" mechanism. *Proc Natl Acad Sci USA.* 2005;102(47):17107–17112.

100. Alvarez-Navarro C, Martin-Esteban A, Barnea E, Admon A, Lopez de Castro JA. ERAP1 polymorphism relevant to inflammatory disease shapes the peptidome of the

birdshot chorioretinopathy-associated HLA-A*29:02 antigen. *Mol Cell Proteomics.* 2015;17(8):1564–1577.

101. Sanz-Bravo A, Campos J, Mazariegos MS, Lopez de Castro JA. Dominant role of the ERAP1 polymorphism R528K in shaping the HLA-B27 Peptidome through differential processing determined by multiple peptide residues. *Arthritis Rheumatol.* 2015;67(3):692–701.

102. Guasp P, Alvarez-Navarro C, Gomez-Molina P, et al. The peptidome of Behcet's disease-associated HLA-B*51:01 includes two subpeptidomes differentially shaped by endoplasmic reticulum aminopeptidase 1. *Arthritis Rheumatol.* 2016;68(2):505–515.

103. Martin-Esteban A, Sanz-Bravo A, Guasp P, Barnea E, Admon A, Lopez de Castro JA. Separate effects of the ankylosing spondylitis associated ERAP1 and ERAP2 aminopeptidases determine the influence of their combined phenotype on the HLA-B*27 peptidome. *J Autoimmun.* 2017;79:28–38.

104. Lopez de Castro JA, Alvarez-Navarro C, Brito A, Guasp P, Martin-Esteban A, Sanz-Bravo A. Molecular and pathogenic effects of endoplasmic reticulum aminopeptidases ERAP1 and ERAP2 in MHC-I-associated inflammatory disorders: towards a unifying view. *Mol Immunol.* 2016;77:193–204.

105. Kenna TJ, Robinson PC, Haroon N. Endoplasmic reticulum aminopeptidases in the pathogenesis of ankylosing spondylitis. *Rheumatology (Oxf).* 2015;54(9):1549–1556.

106. McRae AF, Powell JE, Henders AK, et al. Contribution of genetic variation to transgenerational inheritance of DNA methylation. *Genome Biol.* 2014;15(5):R73.

107. Shah S, McRae AF, Marioni RE, et al. Genetic and environmental exposures constrain epigenetic drift over the human life course. *Genome Res.* 2014;24(11):1725–1733.

108. Rhee I, Jair KW, Yen RW, et al. CpG methylation is maintained in human cancer cells lacking DNMT1. *Nature.* 2000;404(6781):1003–1007.

109. Wienholz BL, Kareta MS, Moarefi AH, Gordon CA, Ginno PA, Chedin F. DNMT3L modulates significant and distinct flanking sequence preference for DNA methylation by DNMT3A and DNMT3B in vivo. *PLoS Genet.* 2010;6(9):e1001106.

110. Hao J, Liu Y, Xu J, et al. Genome-wide DNA methylation profile analysis identifies differentially methylated loci associated with ankylosis spondylitis. *Arthritis Res Ther.* 2017;19(1):177.

111. Li Z, Haynes KH, Pennisi DJ, et al. Epigenetic and gene expression analysis of ankylosing spondylitis-associated loci implicate immune cells and the gut in the disease pathogenesis. *Gene Immun.* 2017;18(3):135–143.

112. Vecellio M, Roberts AR, Cohen CJ, et al. The genetic association of RUNX3 with ankylosing spondylitis can be explained by allele-specific effects on IRF4 recruitment that alter gene expression. *Ann Rheum Dis.* 2016;75(8):1534–1540.

113. MC L PK, ME C, et al. Enhanced expression of the transcription factor T-bet alters pro-inflammatory cytokine profile in ankylosing spondylitis. *Arthritis Rheumatol.* 2015;67(suppl 10):S2829.

114. Kim TJ, Kim TH. Clinical spectrum of ankylosing spondylitis in Korea. *Joint Bone Spine.* 2010;77(3):235–240.

115. Yang M, Xu M, Pan X, et al. Epidemiological comparison of clinical manifestations according to HLA-B*27 carrier status of Chinese ankylosing spondylitis patients. *Tissue Antigens.* 2013;82(5):338–343.

116. Feltkamp TE, Mardjuadi A, Huang F, Chou CT. Spondyloarthropathies in eastern Asia. *Curr Opin Rheumatol.* 2001;13(4):285–290.

117. Yang KL, Chen IH, Hsiao CK, et al. Polymorphism of HLA-B27 in Taiwanese Chinese. *Tissue Antigens.* 2004;63(5):476–479.

118. Liu Y, Jiang L, Cai Q, et al. Predominant association of HLA-B*2704 with ankylosing spondylitis in Chinese Han patients. *Tissue Antigens.* 2010;75(1):61–64.

119. Park SH, Kim J, Kim SG, Kim SK, Chung WT, Choe JY. Human leucocyte antigen-B27 subtypes in Korean patients with ankylosing spondylitis: higher B*2705 in the patient group. *Int J Rheum Dis.* 2009;12(1):34–38.

120. Gonzalez-Roces S, Alvarez MV, Gonzalez S, et al. HLA-B27 polymorphism and worldwide susceptibility to ankylosing spondylitis. *Tissue Antigens.* 1997;49(2):116–123.

121. Lopez-Larrea C, Sujirachato K, Mehra NK, et al. HLA-B27 subtypes in Asian patients with ankylosing spondylitis. Evidence for new associations. *Tissue Antigens.* 1995;45(3):169–176.

122. Ren EC, Koh WH, Sim D, Boey ML, Wee GB, Chan SH. Possible protective role of HLA-B*2706 for ankylosing spondylitis. *Tissue Antigens.* 1997;49(1):67–69.

123. Hou TY, Chen HC, Chen CH, Chang DM, Liu FC, Lai JH. Usefulness of human leucocyte antigen-B27 subtypes in predicting ankylosing spondylitis: Taiwan experience. *Intern Med J.* 2007;37(11):749–752.

124. Ho HH, Chen JY. Ankylosing spondylitis: Chinese perspective, clinical phenotypes, and associated extra-articular systemic features. *Curr Rheumatol Rep.* 2013;15(8):344.

125. Brown MA, Kenna T, Wordsworth BP. Genetics of ankylosing spondylitis--insights into pathogenesis. *Nat Rev Rheumatol.* 2016;12(2):81–91.

126. Lin Z, Bei JX, Shen M, et al. A genome-wide association study in Han Chinese identifies new susceptibility loci for ankylosing spondylitis. *Nat Genet.* 2011;44(1):73–77.

127. Visscher PM, Brown MA, McCarthy MI, Yang J. Five years of GWAS discovery. *Am J Hum Genet.* 2012;90(1):7–24.

128. Huang H, Fang M, Jostins L, et al. Fine-mapping inflammatory bowel disease loci to single-variant resolution. *Nature.* 2017;547(7662):173–178.

129. McCarthy MI, Abecasis GR, Cardon LR, et al. Genome-wide association studies for complex traits: consensus, uncertainty and challenges. *Nat Rev Genet.* 2008;9(5):356–369.

130. Robinson PC, Leo PJ, Pointon JJ, et al. The genetic associations of acute anterior uveitis and their overlap with the genetics of ankylosing spondylitis. *Genes Immun.* 2016;17(1):46–51.

CHAPTER 6

The Gut Microbiome and Ankylosing Spondylitis

PETER R. STERNES, PHD • MATTHEW A. BROWN, MBBS, MD, FRACP, FAHMS, FAA

There is strong evidence from a range of sources that ankylosing spondylitis (AS) occurs as a result of aberrant interactions between the gut microbiome and a genetically primed host-immune system.

EPIDEMIOLOGY

The high heritability of AS (>90%) indicates that the environmental trigger for the disease is likely ubiquitous.[1,2] This hypothesis is supported by the absence of common source outbreaks of the disease and the largely (with the exception of West Africa) similar global prevalence in relation to the major genetic risk factor, HLA-B27. Furthermore, although AS is rare in HLA-B27-positive West Africans living in West Africa,[3] the disease is seen in their descendants living in other environments such as the United States and the Azores, indicating that environmental factors operate to either protect from disease in West Africa or induce disease in other environments.

It has long been known that reactive arthritis, which in ~10% of cases leads to the development of AS and chronic reactive arthritis clinically indistinguishable from AS,[4] can be triggered by either gastrointestinal (Salmonella, Shigella, Campylobacter, Yersinia) or urogenital (Chlamydia) bacterial infections. The majority of AS cases do not evolve after a reactive arthritis like illness, however, suggesting that either the environmental triggers or host genetics are different.

AS AND INFLAMMATORY BOWEL DISEASE

Increased gut permeability has been demonstrated in both AS patients and their first-degree relatives compared with unrelated healthy controls,[5–8] consistent with the hypothesis that increased "leakiness" to gut microbes may drive inflammation in the disease. Crohn disease is closely related to AS with a similar prevalence and high heritability. The two commonly cooccur with an estimated ~5% of AS patients developing Crohn disease and 4%–10% of Crohn disease patients developing AS.[9,10]

Up to 70% of AS patients have evidence of terminal ileitis resembling Crohn disease, suggesting that gut inflammation is important in the disease.[11,12] Patients with AS also have a high prevalence of elevated fecal calprotectin, a marker of gut inflammation. Elevation of fecal calprotectin has been shown in AS patients to predict development of clinical IBD.[13] Furthermore, in capsule endoscopy studies, it correlates with the appearance of mucosal inflammation characteristic of Crohn disease in AS patients,[14] even in the absence of a clinical diagnosis of Crohn disease.

GENETICS

Strong cofamiliality,[15] and the extensive sharing of genetic factors between inflammatory bowel disease and AS[16,17] suggest that they have a shared etiopathogenesis. This is consistent with the hypothesis that increased "leakiness" of the gut, and potentially the capability of HLA-B27 to present relevant microbial antigens, may alter the gut microbial composition and increase gut mucosal microbial dissemination, and hence drive inflammation in the disease.[18,19] Furthermore, analysis of the 114 loci currently known to be associated with AS shows that these disproportionately affect gene expression or lie within epigenetic marks of gene activation in gastrointestinal cells and tissues.[20] Thus, the genetic associations of AS operate to a significant extent by effects on the gastrointestinal tract.

Considering individual loci, many are known to have major roles in bacterial sensing or immunity. For example, GPR65 variants that are AS- as well as IBD-associated lead to impaired clearance of intracellular bacteria through effects on lysozymal function.[21] The AS-associated variant in FUT2 determines "secretor status," the ability to secrete blood group antigens, which has marked effects on the gut microbiome.[22] *C1orf106* variants associated with both AS and IBD have recently been shown to regulate epithelial cell adherens function, thereby affecting intestinal epithelial cell barrier leading to increased "leakiness" to bacteria.[23] These and other examples provide strong hypothesis-free evidence that the gut is not simply affected as a bystander in AS but is directly involved in the development of the disease.

HISTOPATHOLOGY AND SEROLOGY

Reduced expression of the intestinal barrier protein zonulin and histopathologic evidence of gut wall invasion by bacteria in AS further support this hypothesis.[24] In this study, Ciccia and colleagues demonstrated increased serum lipopolysaccharide in AS patients and that the number of mucosal wall inflammatory cells correlated with the number of invading bacteria.

The same group also demonstrated increased expression of the genes encoding the antimicrobial peptides human alpha-defensin 5 (HD-5), phospholipase A2 (PLA2), and lysozyme in AS gut mucosal biopsies, to a similar extent to that seen in Crohn disease, providing further indirect support for bacterial driven gut inflammation being involved in AS pathogenesis.[25]

Multiple serologic studies have been performed investigating the role of yeast and bacterial species in AS. Extensive investigation of the proposed role of *Klebsiella* species in AS pathogenesis has not proven conclusive,[26] and it is notable that no support for the involvement of *Klebsiella* has been identified by sequencing-based studies described below. AS patients have elevated levels of ASCA (anti-*Saccharomyces cerevisiae*), anti-I2 (associated with anti-*Pseudomonas* activity), and anti-CBir1 (antiflagellin) antibodies.[27] The latter is of particular note given the known involvement of flagellated bacteria in driving Th17 lymphocyte development.[28,29] This raises the specific hypothesis that flagellated bacteria specifically may have a role in AS pathogenesis.

ANIMAL MODELS AND HUMAN STUDIES

Experimental evidence from mouse and rat models of spondyloarthritis provides further evidence that spondyloarthritis is driven by gut microbial factors. In the SKG mouse and *B27*-transgenic rat models of spondyloarthritis, animals grown in sterile conditions remain healthy and bacterial recolonization of the gut is sufficient to lead to arthritis.[30,31] Dysbiosis has been shown

to be an early feature of disease in *HLA-B27* transgenic rats, preceding the onset of clinical disease in the gut or joints.[32]

The first direct evidence of dysbiosis in human AS came from studies using 16S rRNA community profiling, which showed that AS cases have a discrete intestinal microbial signature in the terminal ileum compared with healthy controls ($P < .001$).[33] This was driven by higher abundance of five families of bacteria, *Lachnospiraceae* ($P = .001$), *Ruminococcaceae* ($P = .012$), *Rikenellaceae* ($P = .004$), *Porphyromonadaceae* ($P = .001$), and *Bacteroidaceae* ($P = .001$), and decreases in abundance of two families, *Veillonellaceae* ($P = .01$) and *Prevotellaceae* ($P = .004$).

Gut dysbiosis in AS has subsequently been confirmed by other studies.[34,35] Wen et al. used shotgun sequencing of stool samples from 97 Chinese AS cases and 114 healthy controls and reported significant dysbiosis in the AS cases.[34] Breban et al.[35] used 16S rRNA profiling of the stool microbiome to study 87 patients with axial spondyloarthritis (42 with AS), 69 healthy controls, and 28 rheumatoid arthritis patients and demonstrated intestinal dysbiosis in the spondyloarthritis patients. *HLA-B27*-positive but not *HLA-B27*-negative siblings were shown to have increased carriage of the *Micrococcaceae* family (including the species *Rothia mucilaginosa* within it), several *Blautia* and *Ruminococcus* species, and *Eggerthella lenta*, as well as reduced carriage of *Bifidobacterium* and *Odoribacter* species. Stoll and colleagues studied enthesitis-related arthritis, a form of pediatric arthritis, which includes juvenile AS among other conditions. They showed significant reductions in *Faecalibacterium prausnitzii* and the *Lachnospiraceae* family (12% vs. 7.0%, $P = .020$) and an increase in *Bifidobacterium* (1.8% vs. 0%, $P = .032$). The reduction in *F. prausnitzii* is of particular interest given its reduced carriage in IBD and antiinflammatory properties thought, at least partly, to relate to its capacity to produce butyrate.[36] Lastly, Tito et al.[37] in a study of 27 spondyloarthritis patients (i.e., not necessarily AS) and 15 healthy controls using 16S rRNA profiling did not report dysbiosis associated with overall disease status, relative to healthy controls. However, they did report the association of *Dialister* species carriage in ileal or colonic mucosal biopsies with disease activity assessed by self-reported questionnaire (the Bath AS Disease Activity Index). The differences observed between these studies may relate to analytical differences such as handling of covariates, disease definition, sample site studied, ethnicity and diet, and the different methods used to profile the microbiome, as discussed below.

MICROBIOME-TARGETED TREATMENTS AND AS

Although many patients with AS follow diets, there is a paucity of evidence about their efficacy in the disease, with no formal trials reported to date of dietary interventions in AS. Anecdotal reports have been published suggesting that low-starch diets, by influencing the carriage of *Klebsiella* species, may influence disease activity.[38] However, formal reports of low-starch dietary interventions have not been published, and as mentioned above, early evidence that *Klebsiella* species are involved in AS pathogenesis has not subsequently borne out.

Probiotics are supplements of live microorganisms that are thought to have health-beneficial effects. Prebiotics are chemicals that induce the growth or activity of microorganisms that similarly are thought to benefit health. A clinical trial of probiotic therapy in AS did not show improvement in disease activity[39] although whether the treatment actually influenced microbiome composition in those treated was not clear. An Internet-enabled study of probiotics similarly showed no difference in arthritis outcomes.[40] To date, there has been no reported trial of prebiotics and AS.

Limited studies of antibiotic therapy have been reported in AS. An open-label 12-week trial of the fluoroquinolone antibiotic, moxifloxacin, reported reductions in a range of patient self-reported outcomes, although mean changes in the objective measures ESR (17.3–16.2 mm/h) and CRP (8.2–7.6 mg/L) were very minor, suggesting a modest effect on inflammation.[41] No other antibiotic trials have been reported.

Finally, no clinical trial or case series of fecal transplant therapy has been reported in AS to date.

UNANSWERED QUESTIONS

Although these studies are consistent with a role for disordered interaction between the immune system and gut microbiome in driving AS, they do not prove that this relationship is causative. It is possible that these findings are due to AS itself, rather than driving the disease. Furthermore, although human studies aim to control for treatment effects or effects of microbiome covariates (such as cigarette smoking) to varying extents, control for these covariates has been incomplete. Although the mouse and rat studies provide additional support, they are animal models that imperfectly represent human disease and may not reflect the actual disease process in humans.

The studies performed to date have focused particularly on the potential role of bacteria, based on the prior model of reactive arthritis and supported by the animal model studies. However, no studies have yet been published, which report on viruses or fungi. The application of whole-genome sequencing, also known as "shotgun metagenomics," may prove to be informative in future studies.

Assuming that gut bacteria are key drivers of the pathogenesis of AS, the mechanism involved is also unclear. The bacteria may be driving proinflammatory cytokine production, such as IL-23, in the gut wall in AS patients, leading to distant inflammation. This mechanism is supported by the demonstration in mice that elevation of IL-23 levels using IL-23 expression-driving minigenes leads to the development of spondyloarthritis.[42] It is also feasible that bacterial translocation from the gut occurs to sites of inflammation in AS, driving chronic arthritis, or that other mechanisms involving interaction between the gut and host mucosal immune systems are involved.

Whether one or a limited number of bacteria are involved is also not clear. The modest overlap in findings from gut microbiome studies so far has not highlighted a single bacterial species shared by all or a high proportion of cases, suggesting that multiple individual bacteria can either trigger or drive the disease or that combinations of bacteria are involved. The known interactive relationship between counts of bacteria genera suggests that interaction is likely to be involved.[33] Further elucidation of the microbes involved in increasing and decreasing risk of AS would be very helpful in informing future microbiome-targeted therapies.

SEQUENCING-BASED METHODS OF PROFILING THE MICROBIOME

Early microbial studies were restricted to culture-based methods, which were hamstrung by the relatively large number of species, which resisted cultivation.[43–48] Although the capacity to culture these microbes has improved, the advent of next-generation high-throughput sequencing has given rise to molecular methods such as marker gene amplicon analysis (also known as "metabarcoding") and shotgun metagenomics both of which have delivered rapid access to the identification and functional genomic study of previously unculturable organisms.[49,50]

When conducting a sequence-based microbiome study, there are many methodological choices at disposal, the choice of which can introduce a variety of technical variations in the study. These variations can obfuscate the main hypothesis and/or render the study incomparable with others that have utilized a different methodology. Factors can include sampling method,[51] DNA extraction protocol,[52] amplification, purification and quantification methods,[53] sequencing parameters (such as depth, read length, and platform), and the choice of bioinformatic methodology.[54,55]

METABARCODING

By far the most commonly used strategy for microbiome profiling in AS cases is the use of 16S rRNA amplicon sequencing, or metabarcoding, of bacterial species.[56] The ubiquitous 16S rRNA gene is composed of nine hypervariable regions, which are flanked by more highly conserved regions of DNA suitable for primer binding[57] This allows for PCR amplification and sequencing of hypervariable regions of broad range of prokaryotes. The high degree of variation in these amplicons allows them to be used as barcodes to identify the relative proportion of microbes within a sample. The most commonly used regions are the V1–V3, V4, and V4–V5, each of which can achieve genus-level sequence resolution, with the choice of region depending on which subset of the microbial community is of most interest.[58,59]

Metabarcoding remains the default strategy for sequence-based bacterial analysis because of reasonably powerful taxonomic assignment, low resource requirements, the presence of numerous curated databases for sequence comparison and taxonomic assignment, and the ability to PCR amplify and sequence bacterial DNA without human DNA contamination. However, there are also several key limitations that researchers should be aware of before interpreting these data[60]:

1. The 16S rRNA gene has variable copy numbers, which can result in biased estimation of organism abundance.[61]
2. Universal PCR priming sites in some organisms lack conservation leading to differences in PCR amplification efficiency and lack specificity for certain bacterial groups.[62,63]
3. The taxonomic resolution is typically insufficient to provide species-level identification and may be biased toward certain well-characterized taxa.[64,65]
4. Many databases contain sequences with errors or incorrect taxonomic annotations.[66]

Although metabarcoding is a powerful tool for assessing the phylogenetic distribution of the microbiome, the functional genomic content may only be inferred by indirect means. The most commonly used tool, PICRUSt,[67] uses an extended ancestral state reconstruction algorithm to infer the unknown gene content from the nearest sequenced organism in the phylogeny.

However, if a sample contains a large proportion of poorly characterized taxa, which are distantly related, the resulting gene content predictions are prone to inaccuracy. Furthermore, most species have not undergone comprehensive characterization of their intraspecific genetic variation.

To circumvent the above issues and to gain a direct insight into the functional genomic content of the samples, researchers are increasingly opting for a whole-genome sequencing or shotgun metagenomics approach; however, in the case of AS, only one such study exists to date.[34]

SHOTGUN METAGENOMICS

This more resource-intensive alternative to metabarcoding is also known simply as "metagenomics." This methodology bypasses the gene-specific amplification of microbial barcode sequences and performs untargeted sequencing of all fragmented DNA. Shotgun sequencing avoids a lot of the limitations of metabarcoding and can be used to profile the taxonomic composition at a higher resolution, for example, to the species and strain taxonomic levels.[68–72]

Several different bioinformatic methods of taxonomic classification exist with most methods relying on microbial genomes present in RefSeq[73]; however, some methods such as MetaPhlAn2[69] utilize many draft genomes from the Human Microbiome Project[74–77] and thus are particularly useful for human microbiome studies.[78]

The added utility of shotgun metagenomics also comes from the ability to directly determine the functional potential of microbial communities using either an assembly-based or assembly-free approach. Assembly-based methods require a high-quality metagenome assembly for which the functional genomic content can be determined using adaptions of single-genome gene prediction and annotation tools. On the other hand, assembly-free methods rely on translated nucleotide searches against functionally characterized protein families such as KEGG[79] and UniProt.[80] Regardless of which method is used, their effectiveness is ultimately underpinned by the comprehensiveness and accuracy of the functional databases used.

Despite the advantages and extraanalysis potential of shotgun metagenomics, there are also some important aspects, which limit its adoption as the default sequencing strategy[81,82]:

1. It remains very expensive to sequence metagenome samples (typically 1–10 gigabases per sample), and the analysis of many samples often requires substantial computational resources.

2. Although human mucosal tissues are of considerable interest, sequencing these samples often results in a high proportion of human DNA relative to the amount of microbial DNA. Molecular methods may be applied to selectively enrich microbial DNA before sequencing.
3. The comprehensiveness of microbial genome databases for taxonomic profiling is limited and is biased toward model organisms, known pathogens, and easily cultivatable microbes. The development of customized databases that have been supplemented with additional and/or more comprehensively assembled genomes may be used to enhance the profiling accuracy for the microbial species of interest.[83] Alternatively, mapping of sequencing reads to a highly curated database of marker genes may enhance taxonomic profiling accuracy.
4. Similar to (3), databases for the functional profiling of samples are limited because most of the genes lack properly validated annotations. Improving this issue requires substantial amounts of resource-intensive and low-throughput gene-specific functional studies.[81]

SAMPLING SITE

The sampling site for microbiome studies is an important consideration in the study design. The gut microbiota consists of two separate populations, the luminal microbiota and the mucosa-associated microbiota.[84,85] These two broad populations of microbiota are distinct,[86–89] and the mucosa-associated microbiota are believed to directly affect epithelial and mucosal function to a greater degree than luminal bacteria.[90] However, most AS studies, as well as other larger-scale studies such as the NIH Human Microbiome Project,[74–77] have focused on the collection of stool samples. Although stool may be the most convenient sample, it may only capture information about luminal microbiota, which are more transient compared with adherent microbes. On the other hand, the collection of mucosal samples via biopsy is an invasive procedure and is associated with risks such as the risk of perforation; these factors make it less suitable for large-scale studies. The study of IgA-coated bacteria isolated from stool samples or the use of rectal swabs[91] may prove to be an informative compromise between these two modes of collection.

DATA ANALYSIS

Quantitative metagenomics data are highly dimensional and suffer from a specific set of challenges because of the compositional nature of the taxonomic and functional profiling.[92] Consequently, if a microbe was to increase in abundance, all other microbes within a sample will appear to decrease in abundance, thus violating the assumption of sample independence and potentially causing false correlations. Despite sophisticated approaches to statistical transformation, the analysis of compositional data may remain a partially intractable problem.[93]

Several unsupervised methods have been deployed to unveil patterns within the data such as clustering and correlation of samples, and visualizations. Supervised methods have also been utilized and include statistical methods such as multivariate analysis of variance (ANOVA/PERMANOVA) for direct hypothesis testing between different groups or machine-learning classifiers that train models to label groups of samples, such as random forest or support vector machines.[81,94] Supervised methods can also be utilized for the visualization of data, such as a sparse partial least squares discriminant analysis (sPLSDA).[95] These methods can be used to investigate the community composition holistically; however, an alternative, more reductive, and univariate approach can be used to statistically test for association between specific microbial features (i.e., a genus) and the metadatum of interest (i.e., AS status).

Obfuscating the analysis are sources of covariation introduced from human behaviors such as exercise, diet and dietary supplements, smoking, alcohol consumption, and hygiene upon the microbiome. Although the effect of these behaviors and other factors such as age, gender, BMI, ethnicity, pregnancy, and drug treatment upon the gut microbiome have been shown to have varying degrees of influence,[96] collection of these metadata from patients and incorporation in the relevant statistical models represent another aspect of microbiome studies worth careful consideration.

STUDY DESIGN

Although sources of covariation can be included in the statistical modeling, under certain circumstances, some sources of covariation, notably antibiotic use, have a strong enough effect as to exclude samples from the study.[97–100] The NIH Human Microbiome Project[74–77] has relatively stringent inclusion/exclusion selection criteria for their study; however, this degree of stringency may not be pragmatic, and other studies have applied less stringent criteria empirically.[101]

In addition to exclusion of outlying subjects, careful consideration should also be applied to the selection of control subjects in case/control studies. Datasets derived from TwinsUK[102] and the Human Microbiome

Project[74–77] can potentially be used as healthy control sets. However, observable differences may be attributed to technical artifacts or sources of covariation. For this reason, most studies will require a collection of their own controls and cannot rely on these "universal" healthy control groups.[103]

Another important consideration for AS microbiome studies is the recruitment of an adequate number of subjects to enable enough statistical power for a detectable effect within the gut microbiome. More comparative groups, fewer subjects, greater within-group dissimilarity, and lesser effect sizes result in increased type II errors and decreased statistical significance.[104,105] It can be difficult to predict the minimum required sample size for detectable effects of AS upon the microbiome. A pilot study may be necessary to estimate the effect size and thus the required sampling size for studies with differing configurations of experimental parameters and study design.

Finally, given the flexible nature of the microbiome within individuals, whether to resample individuals over time or to sample individuals just once is a valid question. Many studies report that the adult fecal microbiota remain consistent over time,[75,96,106–108] indicating that the gut microbiome may be stable enough for single time point sampling. However, in the case of rheumatoid arthritis, differences between early-onset and chronic cases have been observed, with a key species, *Prevotella copri*, showing enrichment in early-onset rheumatoid arthritis cases and depletion in chronic rheumatoid arthritis cases.[109,110] These findings indicate that longitudinal studies of AS may be revealing and important for accurately determining the key species implicated in disease.

REFERENCES

1. Brown MA, Kennedy LG, MacGregor AJ, et al. Susceptibility to ankylosing spondylitis in twins: the role of genes, HLA, and the environment. *Arthritis Rheum.* 1997;40(10):1823–1828.
2. Pedersen OB, Svendsen AJ, Ejstrup L, Skytthe A, Harris JR, Junker P. Ankylosing spondylitis in Danish and Norwegian twins: occurrence and the relative importance of genetic vs. environmental effectors in disease causation. *Scand J Rheumatol.* 2008;37(2):120–126.
3. Brown MA, Jepson A, Young A, Whittle HC, Greenwood BM, Wordsworth BP. Ankylosing spondylitis in West Africans--evidence for a non-HLA-B27 protective effect. *Ann Rheum Dis.* 1997;56(1):68–70.
4. Kaarela K, Jantti JK, Kotaniemi KM. Similarity between chronic reactive arthritis and ankylosing spondylitis. A 32-35-year follow-up study. *Clin Exp Rheumatol.* 2009;27(2):325–328.
5. Martinez-Gonzalez O, Cantero-Hinojosa J, Paule-Sastre P, Gomez-Magan JC, Salvatierra-Rios D. Intestinal permeability in patients with ankylosing spondyllitis and their healthy relatives. *Rheumatology.* 1994;33(7):644–647.
6. Mielants H, De Vos M, Goemaere S, et al. Intestinal mucosal permeability in inflammatory rheumatic diseases. II. Role of disease. *J Rheumatol.* 1991;18(3):394–400.
7. Morris AJ, Howden CW, Robertson C, et al. Increased intestinal permeability in ankylosing spondylitis--primary lesion or drug effect? *Gut.* 1991;32(12):1470–1472.
8. Vaile J, Meddings J, Yacyshyn B, R AS, Maksymowych W. Bowel permeability and CD45RO expression on circulating CD20+ B cells in patients with ankylosing spondylitis and their relatives. *J Rheumatol.* 1999;26(1):128–135.
9. Palm O, Moum B, Ongre A, Gran JT. Prevalence of ankylosing spondylitis and other spondyloarthropathies among patients with inflammatory bowel disease: a population study (the IBSEN study). *J Rheumatol.* 2002;29(3):511–515.
10. Orchard TR, Holt H, Bradbury L, et al. The prevalence, clinical features and association of HLA-B27 in sacroiliitis associated with established Crohn's disease. *Aliment Pharmacol Ther.* 2009;29(2):193–197.
11. Mielants H, Veys EM, Cuvelier C, De Vos M, Botelberghe L. HLA-B27 related arthritis and bowel inflammation. Part 2. Ileocolonoscopy and bowel histology in patients with HLA-B27 related arthritis. *J Rheumatol.* 1985;12(2):294–298.
12. Ciccia F, Accardo-Palumbo A, Alessandro R, et al. Interleukin-22 and interleukin-22-producing NKp44+ natural killer cells in subclinical gut inflammation in ankylosing spondylitis. *Arthritis Rheum.* 2012;64(6):1869–1878.
13. Klingberg E, Strid H, Stahl A, et al. A longitudinal study of fecal calprotectin and the development of inflammatory bowel disease in ankylosing spondylitis. *Arthritis Res Ther.* 2017;19(1):21.
14. Kopylov U, Starr M, Watts C, Dionne S, Girardin M, Seidman EG. Detection of Crohn disease in patients with spondyloarthropathy: the SpACE capsule study. *J Rheumatol.* 2018;45(4):498–505.
15. Thjodleifsson B, Geirsson AJ, Bjornsson S, Bjarnason I. A common genetic background for inflammatory bowel disease and ankylosing spondylitis: a genealogic study in Iceland. *Arthritis Rheum.* 2007;56(8):2633–2639.
16. Ellinghaus D, Jostins L, Spain SL, et al. Analysis of five chronic inflammatory diseases identifies 27 new associations and highlights disease-specific patterns at shared loci. *Nat Genet.* 2016;48(5):510–518.
17. Parkes M, Cortes A, van Heel DA, Brown MA. Genetic insights into common pathways and complex relationships among immune-mediated diseases. *Nat Rev Genet.* 2013;14(9):661–673.

18. Cua DJ, Sherlock JP. Autoimmunity's collateral damage: gut microbiota strikes 'back'. *Nat Med.* 2011;17(9):1055–1056.

19. Costello ME, Elewaut D, Kenna TJ, Brown MA. Microbes, the gut and ankylosing spondylitis. *Arthritis Res Ther.* 2013;15(3):214.

20. Li Z, Haynes KH, Pennisi DJ, et al. Epigenetic and gene expression analysis of ankylosing spondylitis-associated loci implicate immune cells and the gut in the disease pathogenesis. *Gene Immun.* 2017;18(3):135–143.

21. Lassen KG, McKenzie CI, Mari M, et al. Genetic coding variant in GPR65 alters lysosomal pH and links lysosomal dysfunction with colitis risk. *Immunity.* 2016;44(6):1392–1405.

22. Kolde R, Franzosa EA, Rahnavard G, et al. Host genetic variation and its microbiome interactions within the human microbiome project. *Genome Med.* 2018;10(1):6.

23. Mohanan V, Nakata T, Desch AN, et al. C1orf106 is a colitis risk gene that regulates stability of epithelial adherens junctions. *Science.* 2018;359(6380):1161–1166.

24. Ciccia F, Guggino G, Rizzo A, et al. Dysbiosis and zonulin upregulation alter gut epithelial and vascular barriers in patients with ankylosing spondylitis. *Ann Rheum Dis.* 2017;76(6):1123–1132.

25. Ciccia F, Bombardieri M, Rizzo A, et al. Over-expression of paneth cell-derived anti-microbial peptides in the gut of patients with ankylosing spondylitis and subclinical intestinal inflammation. *Rheumatology (Oxford).* 2010;49(11):2076–2083.

26. Stone MA, Payne U, Schentag C, Rahman P, Pacheco-Tena C, Inman RD. Comparative immune responses to candidate arthritogenic bacteria do not confirm a dominant role for Klebsiella pneumonia in the pathogenesis of familial ankylosing spondylitis. *Rheumatology.* 2004;43(2):148–155.

27. Mundwiler M, Mei L, Landers C, Reveille J, Targan S, Weisman M. Inflammatory bowel disease serologies in ankylosing spondylitis patients: a pilot study. *Arthritis Res Ther.* 2009;11(6):R177.

28. Atarashi K, Tanoue T, Ando M, et al. Th17 cell induction by adhesion of microbes to intestinal epithelial cells. *Cell.* 2015;163(2):367–380.

29. Ivanov II , Atarashi K, Manel N, et al. Induction of intestinal Th17 cells by segmented filamentous bacteria. *Cell.* 2009;139(3):485–498.

30. Taurog JD, Richardson JA, Croft JT, et al. The germfree state prevents development of gut and joint inflammatory disease in HLA-B27 transgenic rats. *J Exp Med.* 1994;180(6):2359–2364.

31. Ruutu M, Velasco J, Aguirre D, et al. The role of gut microflora and autoreactive CD4+T cells in the development of spondyloarthritis and inflammatory bowel disease in beta-glucan-treated SKG mice. *Arthritis Rheum.* 2011;63(suppl 10):S668.

32. Gill T, Asquith M, Brooks SR, Rosenbaum JT, Colbert RA. Effects of HLA-B27 on gut microbiota in experimental spondyloarthritis implicate an ecological model of dysbiosis. *Arthritis Rheumatol.* 2018;70(4):555–565.

33. Costello ME, Ciccia F, Willner D, et al. Brief report: intestinal dysbiosis in ankylosing spondylitis. *Arthritis Rheumatol.* 2015;67(3):686–691.

34. Wen C, Zheng Z, Shao T, et al. Quantitative metagenomics reveals unique gut microbiome biomarkers in ankylosing spondylitis. *Genome Biol.* 2017;18(1):142.

35. Breban M, Tap J, Leboime A, et al. Faecal microbiota study reveals specific dysbiosis in spondyloarthritis. *Ann Rheum Dis.* 2017;76(9):1614–1622.

36. Stoll ML, Kumar R, Morrow CD, et al. Altered microbiota associated with abnormal humoral immune responses to commensal organisms in enthesitis-related arthritis. *Arthritis Res Thera.* 2014;16(6):486.

37. Tito RY, Cypers H, Joossens M, et al. Brief report: dialister as a microbial marker of disease activity in spondyloarthritis. *Arthritis Rheumatol.* 2017;69(1):114–121.

38. Ebringer A, Wilson C. The use of a low starch diet in the treatment of patients suffering from ankylosing spondylitis. *Clin Rheumatol.* 1996;15(suppl 1):62–66.

39. Jenks K, Stebbings S, Burton J, Schultz M, Herbison P, Highton J. Probiotic therapy for the treatment of spondyloarthritis: a randomized controlled trial. *J Rheumatol.* 2010;37(10):2118–2125.

40. Brophy S, Burrows CL, Brooks C, Gravenor MB, Siebert S, Allen SJ. Internet-based randomised controlled trials for the evaluation of complementary and alternative medicines: probiotics in spondyloarthropathy. *BMC Musculoskelet Disord.* 2008;9:4.

41. Ogrendik M. Treatment of ankylosing spondylitis with moxifloxacin. *South Med J.* 2007;100(4):366–370.

42. Sherlock JP, Joyce-Shaikh B, Turner SP, et al. IL-23 induces spondyloarthropathy by acting on ROR-gammat+ CD3+CD4-CD8- entheseal resident T cells. *Nat Med.* 2012;18(7):1069–1076.

43. Rodríguez–Valera F. Environmental genomics, the big picture? *FEMS Microbiol Lett.* 2004;231(2):153–158.

44. Handelsman J. Metagenomics: application of genomics to uncultured microorganisms. *Microbiol Mol Biol Rev.* 2005;69(1):195.

45. Riesenfeld CS, Schloss PD, Handelsman J. Metagenomics: genomic analysis of microbial communities. *Annu Rev Genet.* 2004;38:525–552.

46. Streit WR, Schmitz RA. Metagenomics–the key to the uncultured microbes. *Curr Opin Microbiol.* 2004;7(5):492–498.

47. DeLong EF. Microbial population genomics and ecology. *Curr Opin Microbiol.* 2002;5(5):520–524.

48. Edwards RA, Rohwer F. Viral metagenomics. *Nat Rev Microbiol.* 2005;3(6):504.

49. Rappé MS, Giovannoni SJ. The uncultured microbial majority. *Annu Rev Microbiol.* 2003;57(1):369–394.

50. Hugenholtz P. Exploring prokaryotic diversity in the genomic era. *Genom Biol.* 2002;3(2):0001. reviews0003.

51. Bag S, Saha B, Mehta O, et al. An improved method for high quality metagenomics DNA extraction from human and environmental samples. *Sci Rep.* 2016;6:26775.

52. Salonen A, Nikkilä J, Jalanka-Tuovinen J, et al. Comparative analysis of fecal DNA extraction methods with phylogenetic microarray: effective recovery of bacterial and archaeal DNA using mechanical cell lysis. *J Microbiol Methods.* 2010;81(2):127–134.

53. Gihring TM, Green SJ, Schadt CW. Massively parallel rRNA gene sequencing exacerbates the potential for biased community diversity comparisons due to variable library sizes. *Environ Microbiol.* 2012;14(2):285–290.

54. Janda JM, Abbott SL. 16S rRNA gene sequencing for bacterial identification in the diagnostic laboratory: pluses, perils, and pitfalls. *J Clin Microbiol.* 2007;45(9):2761–2764.

55. Clooney AG, Fouhy F, Sleator RD, et al. Comparing apples and oranges?: next generation sequencing and its impact on microbiome analysis. *PLoS One.* 2016;11(2):e0148028.

56. Neefs J-M, Van de Peer Y, De Rijk P, Chapelle S, De Wachter R. Compilation of small ribosomal subunit RNA structures. *Nucleic Acids Res.* 1993;21(13):3025–3049.

57. Kumar PS, Brooker MR, Dowd SE, Camerlengo T. Target region selection is a critical determinant of community fingerprints generated by 16S pyrosequencing. *PLoS One.* 2011;6(6):e20956.

58. Caporaso JG, Kuczynski J, Stombaugh J, et al. QIIME allows analysis of high-throughput community sequencing data. *Nat Methods.* 2010;7(5):335.

59. Klindworth A, Pruesse E, Schweer T, et al. Evaluation of general 16S ribosomal RNA gene PCR primers for classical and next-generation sequencing-based diversity studies. *Nucleic Acids Res.* 2013;41(1):e1.

60. Tyler AD, Smith MI, Silverberg MS. Analyzing the human microbiome: a "how to" guide for physicians. *Am J Gastroenterol.* 2014;109(7):983.

61. Kembel SW, Wu M, Eisen JA, Green JL. Incorporating 16S gene copy number information improves estimates of microbial diversity and abundance. *PLoS Comput Biol.* 2012;8(10):e1002743.

62. Sim K, Cox MJ, Wopereis H, et al. Improved detection of bifidobacteria with optimised 16S rRNA-gene based pyrosequencing. *PLoS One.* 2012;7(3):e32543.

63. Schloss PD, Gevers D, Westcott SL. Reducing the effects of PCR amplification and sequencing artifacts on 16S rRNA-based studies. *PLoS One.* 2011;6(12):e27310.

64. Claesson MJ, Wang Q, O'sullivan O, et al. Comparison of two next-generation sequencing technologies for resolving highly complex microbiota composition using tandem variable 16S rRNA gene regions. *Nucleic Acids Res.* 2010;38(22):e200.

65. Kim M, Morrison M, Yu Z. Evaluation of different partial 16S rRNA gene sequence regions for phylogenetic analysis of microbiomes. *J Microbiol Methods.* 2011;84(1):81–87.

66. Ashelford KE, Chuzhanova NA, Fry JC, Jones AJ, Weightman AJ. At least 1 in 20 16S rRNA sequence records currently held in public repositories is estimated to contain substantial anomalies. *Appl Environ Microbiol.* 2005;71(12):7724–7736.

67. Langille MG, Zaneveld J, Caporaso JG, et al. Predictive functional profiling of microbial communities using 16S rRNA marker gene sequences. *Nat Biotechnol.* 2013;31(9):814.

68. Ercolini D. Exciting strain–level resolution studies of the food microbiome. *Microb Biotechnol.* 2017;10(1):54–56.

69. Truong DT, Franzosa EA, Tickle TL, et al. MetaPhlAn2 for enhanced metagenomic taxonomic profiling. *Nat Methods.* 2015;12(10):902.

70. Scholz M, Ward DV, Pasolli E, et al. Strain-level microbial epidemiology and population genomics from shotgun metagenomics. *Nat Methods.* 2016;13(5):435.

71. Eren AM, Esen ÖC, Quince C, et al. Anvi'o: an advanced analysis and visualization platform for omics data. *Peer J.* 2015;3:e1319.

72. Luo C, Knight R, Siljander H, Knip M, Xavier RJ, Gevers D. ConStrains identifies microbial strains in metagenomic datasets. *Nat Biotechnol.* 2015;33(10):1045.

73. Pruitt KD, Tatusova T, Maglott DR. NCBI reference sequences (RefSeq): a curated non-redundant sequence database of genomes, transcripts and proteins. *Nucleic Acids Res.* 2006;35(suppl 1):D61–D65.

74. Huttenhower C, Gevers D, Knight R, et al. Structure, function and diversity of the healthy human microbiome. *Nature.* 2012;486(7402):207.

75. Methé BA, Nelson KE, Pop M, et al. A framework for human microbiome research. *Nature.* 2012;486(7402):215.

76. Turnbaugh PJ, Ley RE, Hamady M, Fraser-Liggett CM, Knight R, Gordon JI. The human microbiome project. *Nature.* 2007;449(7164):804.

77. Lloyd-Price J, Mahurkar A, Rahnavard G, et al. Strains, functions and dynamics in the expanded human microbiome project. *Nature.* 2017;550(7674):61.

78. Peabody MA, Van Rossum T, Lo R, Brinkman FS. Evaluation of shotgun metagenomics sequence classification methods using in silico and in vitro simulated communities. *BMC Bioinformatics.* 2015;16(1):362.

79. Kanehisa M, Goto S, Sato Y, Kawashima M, Furumichi M, Tanabe M. Data, information, knowledge and principle: back to metabolism in KEGG. *Nucleic Acids Res.* 2013;42(D1):D199–D205.

80. Consortium U. Activities at the universal protein resource (UniProt). *Nucleic Acids Res.* 2013;42(D1):D191–D198.

81. Quince C, Walker AW, Simpson JT, Loman NJ, Segata N. Shotgun metagenomics, from sampling to analysis. *Nat Biotechnol.* 2017;35(9):833.

82. Sharpton TJ. An introduction to the analysis of shotgun metagenomic data. *Front Plant Sci.* 2014;5:209.

83. Sternes PR, Lee D, Kutyna DR, Borneman AR. A combined meta-barcoding and shotgun metagenomic analysis of spontaneous wine fermentation. *Giga Sci.* 2017;6(7):1–10.

84. Ringel Y, Maharshak N, Ringel-Kulka T, Wolber EA, Sartor RB, Carroll IM. High throughput sequencing reveals distinct microbial populations within the mucosal and luminal niches in healthy individuals. *Gut Microb.* 2015;6(3):173–181.

85. Sartor RB. Gut microbiota: optimal sampling of the intestinal microbiota for research. *Nat Rev Gastroenterol Hepatol.* 2015;12(5):253.

86. Stearns JC, Lynch MD, Senadheera DB, et al. Bacterial biogeography of the human digestive tract. *Sci Rep.* 2011;1:170.

87. Morgan XC, Tickle TL, Sokol H, et al. Dysfunction of the intestinal microbiome in inflammatory bowel disease and treatment. *Genom Biol.* 2012;13(9):R79.

88. Eckburg PB, Bik EM, Bernstein CN, et al. Diversity of the human intestinal microbial flora. *Science.* 2005;308(5728):1635–1638.

89. Yasuda K, Oh K, Ren B, et al. Biogeography of the intestinal mucosal and lumenal microbiome in the rhesus macaque. *Cell Host Microb.* 2015;17(3):385–391.

90. Nishino K, Nishida A, Inoue R, et al. Analysis of endoscopic brush samples identified mucosa-associated dysbiosis in inflammatory bowel disease. *J Gastroenterol.* 2018;53(1):95–106.

91. Jones RB, Zhu X, Moan E, et al. Inter-niche and inter-individual variation in gut microbial community assessment using stool, rectal swab, and mucosal samples. *Sci Rep.* 2018;8(1):4139.

92. Friedman J, Alm EJ. Inferring correlation networks from genomic survey data. *PLoS Comput Biol.* 2012;8(9):e1002687.

93. Tsilimigras MC, Fodor AA. Compositional data analysis of the microbiome: fundamentals, tools, and challenges. *Ann Epidemiol.* 2016;26(5):330–335.

94. Pasolli E, Truong DT, Malik F, Waldron L, Segata N. Machine learning meta-analysis of large metagenomic datasets: tools and biological insights. *PLoS Comput Biol.* 2016;12(7):e1004977.

95. Lê Cao K-A, Costello M-E, Lakis VA, et al. MixMC: a multivariate statistical framework to gain insight into microbial communities. *PLoS One.* 2016;11(8):e0160169.

96. Costello EK, Lauber CL, Hamady M, Fierer N, Gordon JI, Knight R. Bacterial community variation in human body habitats across space and time. *Science.* 2009;326(5960):1694–1697.

97. Ubeda C, Taur Y, Jenq RR, et al. Vancomycin-resistant enterococcus domination of intestinal microbiota is enabled by antibiotic treatment in mice and precedes bloodstream invasion in humans. *J Clin Investig.* 2010;120(12):4332–4341.

98. Dethlefsen L, Huse S, Sogin ML, Reiman DA. The pervasive effects of an antibiotic on the human gut microbiota, as revealed by deep 16Ss rRNA Sequencing. *PLoS Biol.* 2008;6(11):2383–2401.

99. Dethlefsen L, Relman DA. Incomplete recovery and individualized responses of the human distal gut microbiota to repeated antibiotic perturbation. *Proc Natl Acad Sci USA.* 2011;108(suppl 1):4554–4561.

100. Cho I, Yamanishi S, Cox L, et al. Antibiotics in early life alter the murine colonic microbiome and adiposity. *Nature.* 2012;488(7413):621.

101. Koren O, Goodrich JK, Cullender TC, et al. Host remodeling of the gut microbiome and metabolic changes during pregnancy. *Cell.* 2012;150(3):470–480.

102. Spector TD, Williams FM. The UK adult twin registry (TwinsUK). *Twin Res Hum Genet.* 2006;9(6):899–906.

103. Goodrich JK, Di Rienzi SC, Poole AC, et al. Conducting a microbiome study. *Cell.* 2014;158(2):250–262.

104. Zar JH. *Biostatistical Analysis.* Pearson Education India; 1999.

105. Kelly BJ, Gross R, Bittinger K, et al. Power and sample-size estimation for microbiome studies using pairwise distances and PERMANOVA. *Bioinformatics.* 2015;31(15):2461–2468.

106. Ley RE, Turnbaugh PJ, Klein S, Gordon JI. Microbial ecology: human gut microbes associated with obesity. *Nature.* 2006;444(7122):1022.

107. Turnbaugh PJ, Hamady M, Yatsunenko T, et al. A core gut microbiome in obese and lean twins. *Nature.* 2009;457(7228):480.

108. Wu GD, Chen J, Hoffmann C, et al. Linking long-term dietary patterns with gut microbial enterotypes. *Science.* 2011;334(6052):105–108.

109. Scher JU, Sczesnak A, Longman RS, et al. *Prevotella Copri and Enhanced Susceptibility to Arthritis* Google Patents. 2016.

110. Scher JU, Sczesnak A, Longman RS, et al. Expansion of intestinal *Prevotella copri* correlates with enhanced susceptibility to arthritis. *elife.* 2013;2.

CHAPTER 7

Pathogenesis of Ankylosing Spondylitis

FRANCESCO CICCIA, MD, PHD • ARCHITA SRINATH, BSC •
FANXING ZENG, PHD • NIGIL HAROON, MD, PHD, DM

INTRODUCTION

Axial spondyloarthritis (axSpA) is a spectrum of chronic inflammatory arthritis predominantly involving the joints of the spine that **encompasses ankylosing spondylitis (**AS) that requires presence of definite X-ray changes of sacroiliitis. Because most studies on the pathogenesis of axSpA are done in patients with AS, we will be using the term AS predominantly in this chapter. Although spine is the primary target of disease, systemic as well as organ-specific inflammation including peripheral arthritis, enthesitis, psoriasis, colitis, and iritis can also be seen. There is also an increased risk of cardiovascular and cerebrovascular morbidity and mortality.[1] In addition to inflammation, osteoproliferation manifesting as pathologic new bone formation and bony ankylosis of the spine are important features. This chapter is an overview of the pathogenesis of AS, and it starts with the role of HLA-B27, followed by an introduction to aminopeptidases and other players in antigen processing and presentation. The gut-joint axis is discussed in some detail and finally bone formation pathways are explored. Detailed discussion on the genetics of AS is discussed in Chapter 5 and bone pathophysiology in Chapter 6.

The cause of AS is unknown and the basic mechanisms underlying chronic inflammation remain undefined. However, the complex pathogenesis of AS is slowly unraveling as a result of greater interest in this field and the rapid advances in high-throughput technology.

Elevated serum TNF and TNF expression in the sacroiliac joints are reported in AS.[2,3] TNF blockers provide significant symptomatic improvement and reduce spinal inflammation as evident from MRI studies.[4] TNF transgenic mice with a 3′-modified human TNF gene have overexpression of TNF. These mice develop sacroiliitis like AS.[5] Two metaanalysis studies showed no association of AS with TNF promoter polymorphisms.[6,7] Genome-wide scans reported an association with *TNFRSF1A*.[8,9] The Th17 pathway is in the limelight now in AS pathogenesis and therapeutics. IL-17-positive cells are seen in the facet joints of AS patients in much higher numbers compared with osteoarthritis patients.[10] AS is associated with *IL1RN* and other IL1 gene cluster members,[11-14] and GWAS showed association of AS with *IL1RII*.[8]

HLA-B27 IN THE PATHOGENESIS OF AS

The initial clues to the genetic basis of AS pathogenesis came from family and twin studies.[15,16] Although *HLA-B27* is the strongest MHC-I associated with AS, several other MHC-I alleles have been implicated in AS pathogenesis including *HLA-A2, HLA-B13, HLA-B40, HLA-B47,* and *HLA-DRB1*0103*.[17-20] The gene *HLA-B27* is found in 75%–95% of patients with AS, compared with 4%–8% of controls.[21-24] However, only 2% of all HLA-B27+ individuals develop AS. Thus *HLA-B27* appears to be important but not sufficient to cause disease. In addition, how HLA-B27 mediates the AS pathogenesis is not fully understood.

There is no perfect animal model for AS. The *HLA-B27/human β2m* transgenic rats develop arthritis, spondylitis, psoriasis, colitis, and uveitis, typical features seen in human SpA.[25] The onset and frequency of disease in the animals depends on a high number of transgene copies and the line of rats.[26] HLA-B27 being an MHC-I molecule, we would expect an immunologic interaction with CD8 T cells, leading to immune activation and AS pathogenesis. Although T cells are required for the development of SpA-like manifestations in the B27 rat model, it appears to be CD4 rather than CD8 dependent.[27]

The *HLA-B27* subtype specificity seen in AS is another interesting angle to the story. AS is associated strongly with *HLA-B*27:04, HLA-B*27:05,* and *HLA-B*27:02,* whereas individuals with *HLA-B27:06* and *HLA-B*27:09* do not develop classic AS.[24] Differential effects on folding capacity as well as peptide binding have been reported with AS-associated subtypes

Axial Spondyloarthritis. https://doi.org/10.1016/B978-0-323-56800-5.00007-2

compared with those not associated with AS.[28,29] Immunodominance may be another factor that modifies HLA-B27 responses. It was recently reported that in the presence of HLA-B7, there is lower B27-peptide complex–mediated cytotoxic T-cell (CTL) responses.[30]

Despite the high prevalence of *HLA-B27* in AS and the investigations done over the past 45 years, we still do not have a definitive explanation of how *HLA-B27* leads to AS pathogenesis. Based on its known properties and functions, several hypotheses have been put forward to link *HLA-B27* with pathogenesis of AS.

Arthritogenic Peptide Hypothesis

The "arthritogenic peptide hypothesis" postulates that HLA-B27 in its classical role as an MHC-I molecule presents special peptides to CD8+ T cells resulting in an arthritogenic immune response. It is possible that a unique peptide seen in the target tissue is preferentially presented by HLA-B27 unlike other protective MHC class I molecules. As a peptide-presenting molecule, the peptide binding grove's specificity would decide which peptides can be accommodated, which eventually results in a T-cell cascade, thereby leading to joint inflammation.[31,32] These B27 triggered T cell immune responses can also lead to protection against infections, such as have been reported against HCV infection as well as preventing progression to AIDS.[33,34] Extensive peptide studies have been conducted with HLA-B27 in the context of AS, and several peptides cross-reactive with infectious agents have been identified.[35-38] In search of peptides that bind in higher numbers to AS-associated B27 subtypes compared with nonassociated subtypes, several putative peptides were discovered.[39,40] Despite all these efforts, an arthritogenic peptide that leads to disease in AS has not been identified yet.

Natural Killer Cells and NK Cell Receptors in AS

Killer immunoglobulin-like receptors (KIRs) are natural killer (NK) cell receptors that can bind intact HLA-B27 heterotrimers, free heavy chains as well as dimers. KIR3DL1-expressing NK cells are increased in AS patients compared with healthy controls.[41] HLA-B27 free heavy chains can form dimers by disulfide bond formation at Cys67, and these B27 dimers can be recognized by KIR3DLI, KIR3DL2 as well as leukocyte immunoglobulin-like receptor (LILRB2).[42]

Interestingly, NK cell receptor expressed on T cells may be an important mediator of AS pathogenesis. The primary source of IL-17 in patients with AS is CD4 T cells expressing KIR3DL2. KIR3DL2-expressing NK cells survive longer when bound to HLA-B27, and this could lead to sustained production of IL-17. Direct in vitro evidence of enhanced cytokine production by KIR3DL1 or KIR3DL2 activation is lacking. However, in an animal model HD5, a monoclonal antibody that binds to B27 dimers and blocks their interaction with KIR reduced IL-17 and TNF production by CD4 T cells.[43] The "licensing" hypothesis is of interest as well. NK cells can respond to stimuli only if they are "licensed" to do so by an initial encounter with MHC-I. Licensing occurs via inhibitory receptors such as KIR3DL1 and KIR3DL2, and their presence could be responsible for increased T cell activation.[44]

Unfolded Protein Response

HLA-B27, compared with other MHC-I molecules, lacks stability and has a propensity to misfold. The misfolded free heavy chains of HLA-B27 are not transported appropriately to the surface. They can accumulate in the ER leading to cell stress and unfolded protein response (UPR). UPR activation results in downstream effects with release of proinflammatory cytokines. One of the major cytokines released by ER stress is IL-23.[45] UPR activation is seen in HLA-B27 transgenic rats and is associated with the onset of disease.[46]

Three pathways are activated as a result of cell stress: inositol-requiring kinase 1 (IRE-1), PKR-like ER kinase (PERK), and activating transcription factor 6 (ATF6) pathways. Binding protein (BiP) binds and stabilizes mediators in the basal state, and there is no cell stress. However, with UPR and cell stress, BiP is released and high levels of BiP can be used as a marker of UPR activation. XBP1s, a transcription factor that activates several genes, is generated by IRE-1 activation and splicing of X-box-binding protein 1 (XBP-1) RNA. Although ATF6 induces transcription of several genes including BiP, PERK activation leads to increased expression of CCAAT/enhancer-binding protein-homologous protein (CHOP), another marker of UPR activation.

One of the major issues with the UPR hypothesis is the difficulty to demonstrate UPR activation in AS patients because of the difficulty in accessing tissue. Moreover, UPR is heavily regulated and a snapshot at any one point may not reflect the true picture. Target specificity of UPR is also possible with UPR being important in certain tissues, whereas it is not the major mechanism in others. Macrophages of AS patients from synovial fluid can show UPR activation.[47] UPR may not be evident if we test peripheral blood cells. Interestingly, BiP has been reported to be higher in

HLA-B27-negative control dendritic cells (DCs) than in HLA-B27-positive AS patient–derived DC.[48] Similarly, no significant increase in UPR in the gut, synovium, or blood of AS patients was reported.[49,50]

AUTOPHAGY IN AS

The term "autophagy" is derived from two terms "auto" or self and "phagy" or eating. The literal meaning of autophagy is eating one's self. Rather than this being a suicidal process, as it may seem, this process helps to increase cell survival. During autophagy, cytoplasmic components that are in the early stages of dying are compartmentalized and transported to lysosomes for degradation. Thus, organelles such as mitochondria that are dysfunctional are removed to increase cell survival and prevent accelerated apoptosis.

Macroautophagy, the most common type of autophagy, starts with the formation of an isolation membrane called "phagophore" that elongates and subsequently engulfs a small pocket of cytoplasm. This leads to the formation of the autophagosome that compartmentalizes the organelles. When the autophagosome fuses with a lysosome, an autolysosome is born and most cytosolic proteins are degraded here. In chaperone-mediated autophagy, chaperones mediate the direct transfer of proteins across lysosomal membranes. In microautophagy, there is direct uptake into the lysosome by an invagination of the lysosomal membrane. Autophagy has been found to play an important role in a vast array of body functions including immunity, developmental, physiology, and homeostatic functions. Abnormalities in autophagy have been linked to several diseases including IBD, cancer, neurodegenerative diseases, hyperlipidemias, and cardiomyopathies.

In Crohn disease (CD), an important associated disease of AS, there is an association with autophagy genes ATG16L1, IRGM, and LRRK2. Recently, it was reported that autophagy rather than UPR may be a key factor in AS and CD gut inflammation.[49] Unfolded MHC-I free heavy chains and autophagy markers were upregulated in the gut of AS and HLA-B27-positive CD patients along with an upregulation of IL-23 production from the lamina propria cells. There is no strong genetic association identified between AS and autophagy. However, autophagy can lead to modification of HLA-B27-mediated AS pathogenesis. Autophagy can result in decreased HLA-B27 free heavy chain accumulation decreasing UPR or it could be a means of TAP-independent antigen presentation bypassing the ER.[51] Thus, autophagy should be studied further in AS pathogenesis.

ENDOPLASMIC RETICULUM AMINOPEPTIDASES IN THE PATHOGENESIS OF AS

In genome-wide association studies (GWAS), endoplasmic reticulum aminopeptidase 1 (ERAP1) was found to be strongly associated with AS.[8,52,53] There was a strong suggestion of functional interaction of ERAP1 and HLA-B27 based on their known functions and also because the ERAP1-AS association was restricted to HLA-B27+ AS patients.[9] It was later identified that ERAP1 association may be restricted to both HLA-B27 and HLA-B40+ patients with AS.[54] Thus likely there is a functional interaction with certain MHC-I molecules with specific/shared properties. ERAP1-deficient mice have altered MHC-peptide repertoire.[55] A change in ERAP1 levels caused a significant change in the peptide-MHC repertoire.[56] Subsequently, a study on multiplex AS families reported the association of AS with a haplotype of ERAP1/ERAP2.[57] The association of ERAP1 and ERAP2 in AS has been validated in multiple populations and large cohorts.[8] Beyond ERAP1 and ERAP2, a third gene in the family of M1 aminopeptidases, puromycin-sensitive amino peptidase (NPEPPS) is also associated with AS, although much work has not been done to understand the key variants and its functional impact.

ERAP1 and ERAP2, as the name suggests, are aminopeptidases found in the ER. They are complementary in action, clipping peptides for antigen presentation on MHC-I and with some overlap of substrate peptides. Although ERAP1 is seen in both humans and mice, ERAP2 is seen only in humans. The ERAP1 nonsynonymous single nucleotide polymorphism (nsSNP) rs27044 leads to the Q730E variation in ERAP1 and affects MHC-I free heavy chain (FHC) expression in HLA-B27+ AS patients.[58,59] The Q730E variant is known to have decreased aminopeptidase activity.[60] Decreased ERAP1 function is considered to be protective in AS. Potential mechanisms by which decreased ERAP1 function is protective include reduced generation of arthritogenic peptides or decreased B27-KIR-mediated T/NK cell activation.

ERAP1 is also known to cause clipping of membrane-bound cytokine receptors, and an abnormal functioning ERAP1 could potentially lead to reduced clipping and less cytokine receptors in circulation. However, there is no evidence that this action plays a role in the pathogenesis of AS.[61]

SEC16A AND AS

Interestingly, one more gene in the antigen processing and presentation pathway was recently identified.

In a study involving exome sequencing of a multigenerational family, a rare 9-base pair in-frame mutation in exon 3 of *SEC16A* was found in *HLA-B27+* family members affected by AS.[62] All nine family members who had *HLA-B27* and the *SEC16A* deletion developed axSpA over a period of time although only seven had AxSpA at the time of initial publication. Sec16a is involved in the formation of coat protein complex II (COPII) that aids transport of molecules from the ER to the Golgi apparatus, which is essential for export of all molecules synthesized in the ER, including MHC-peptide complexes. It is likely that Sec16a variants affect trafficking of HLA-B27 to the cell surface altering immune responses. Further studies in this area are warranted.

GUT IN AS PATHOGENESIS

The intestinal epithelial barrier in combination with the gut-associated lymphoid tissue plays a fundamental role in controlling the equilibrium between tolerance and immunity to non–self-antigens.[63] Dysregulation of this huge immune organ, in genetically susceptible individuals, may lead to intestinal and extraintestinal autoimmune disorders such as type 1 diabetes, celiac disease, AS, and RA.[63] The gastrointestinal tract is colonized by many trillions of microbes that represent the intestinal microbiota.[64] The perturbation of this homeostasis results in the so-called dysbiosis that influences the susceptibility of the host to different immune-mediated diseases and disorders.[64]

SpA includes a group of heterogeneous inflammatory conditions sharing common etiopathogenic mechanisms and clinical manifestations supported by complex genetic predispositions.[65] The concept of gut inflammation in patients with SpA includes patients showing clinically evident intestinal inflammation, Crohn disease (CD), or ulcerative colitis (UC), and patients who despite the absence of signs and symptoms of intestinal inflammation display a subclinical gut inflammation that has been described in up to 60% of patients with SpA.[66] A growing body of evidence suggests that subclinical gut inflammation in SpA, apparently driven by intestinal dysbiosis, is not the consequence of the systemic inflammatory process but rather an important pathophysiologic event by driving the activation and expansion of cells of the innate immune system, which can migrate from the intestine to sites of active extraintestinal inflammation, thus actively participating in the pathogenesis of the disease.

Historically, two main types of gut inflammation have been described in SpA patients: acute inflammation, resembling a self-limiting bacterial enterocolitis, and chronic inflammation, displaying altered intestinal architecture with strong infiltration of mononuclear cells eventually aggregated in lymphoid follicles, resembling the ileo-colitis seen in CD.[66] This morphologic classification, however, does not provide adequate information on the natural history of subclinical gut inflammation in patients with SpA. It is unclear in fact whether these are different stages of the same pathologic process in a continuum that sees the possible transition from the absence of inflammation to acute inflammation and finally chronic inflammation or whether instead they are completely different and independent biologic processes. Although it is not possible to exclude that genetic factors may be responsible for these alterations, similar epithelial damages have been described as consequence of the response of epithelial cells to bacterial toxins.

Increasing evidence suggests that the intestinal microbiota may play a role in initiating and maintaining the intestinal inflammation in patients with SpA. HLA-B27 has a role in shaping the gut microbiome as demonstrated in Lewis rats transgenic for HLA-B27 and human β2-microglobulin (hβ2m). There are significant differences in the cecal microbiota of HLA-B27 transgenic rats compared with wild-type Lewis rats.[67] The role of gut microbiome in AS pathogenesis is also suggested by studies demonstrating, in patients and first-degree relatives, an increased intestinal permeability.[68] It was also reported that patients with AS were breastfed less often than healthy controls and their healthy siblings (57% vs. 72%), giving an OR for AS onset of 0.53, indicating that breastfeeding reduces familial prevalence of AS.[69] It seems conceivable that in AS, the interaction between common environmental agents and the intestinal immune system in genetically susceptible individuals may play a pivotal role in the pathogenesis of the disease. Different studies have demonstrated the occurrence of dysbiosis in the gut of AS patients giving, however, different results regarding the composition of the gut microbiome.[70-75] The studies, however, gave different results possibly due to the fact that they evaluated different things and with different methods making it difficult to draw unequivocal conclusions. It also remains to be considered that different populations may have different microbial composition in relation to different dietetic habits. In a recent study, the presence of invasive bacteria was, in particular, associated with specific histologic alterations characterized by the detachment of basal membrane from the lamina propria, leading to the formation of vacuoles inside the villi and hemorrhagic extravasation.[76] AS ileal bacteria seem to be able to induce the activation of the zonulin pathway and the profound reduced expression of tight junction proteins by epithelial cells.[76] It is unclear whether these alterations are the cause or the consequence of intestinal dysbiosis. However, alterations of tight junctions were also present in HLA-B27 TG rats and were restored after antibiotic treatments, suggesting that intestinal dysbiosis might be responsible for the impairment of the epithelial barrier.[76]

In addition to the histologic alterations, the intestine of SpA patients is characterized by the abnormal activation of the innate and adaptive immune system and specific immunologic signatures. Immunologically, an impaired Th1 cytokine profile has been observed in gut mucosal lymphocytes from patients with SpA[77] together with a strong and significant upregulation of IL-23p19 transcripts.[78] In AS patients, IL-23, however, is not associated with upregulation of IL-17 and the IL-17-inducing cytokines IL-6 and IL-1beta. The absence of a full Th17 response in AS patients despite the high levels of IL-23 might suggest the occurrence of protective mechanisms in the AS gut such as the presence of an active Treg cell response, mainly dominated by IL-10 production,[79] and the increased expression of IL-22 responsible for the expansion of goblet cells and increased mucin expression.[80]

The overexpression of IL-23 raises the question of which biologic mechanisms underpin such increased expression. As referred to before, autophagy is a mechanism of controlled digestion of damaged organelles within a cell. The expression of macroautophagy genes has been proved to be significantly upregulated in comparison with healthy subjects, and the increased autophagy gene expression was correlated with augmented IL-23p19 levels and autophagy modulation was able to modulate the production of IL-23.[49]

The presence of high levels of IL-23 in AS gut seems to suggest a biologically relevance of this cytokine in the modulation of intestinal immune responses in AS. IL-23 has been demonstrated to be able by itself in promoting intestinal inflammation independently of effects on T cells and by expanding and activating innate lymphoid cells (ILCs) type 3.[81,82] IL-23R+ innate lymphoid cells type 3, capable to induce colitis in an IL-22- and IL-17-dependent mechanisms, have been demonstrated to be expanded in the gut of AS patients.[83,84] Interestingly, type 3 ILCs were also found to be expanded in the peripheral blood, synovial fluid, and the bone marrow of patients with AS and to express the homing integrin α4β7. In addition, MAdCAM1, the α4β7 ligand, was found to be highly represented in the gut and in the inflamed BM of AS, suggesting that a recirculation

of ILC3 between the gut and the BM may occur. Altogether these results suggest a role for IL-23-sensitized gut-resident ILC3, capable of producing IL17 and IL22, migration to joints, and the development of AS.[84] However, the factors influencing the maintenance of ILC3 in an activated state in extraintestinal sites are not clear. Recently, CX3CR1+ mononuclear phagocytes (MNPs) have been demonstrated to produce high levels of IL-23 and TL1A, efficiently supporting IL-22 production from ILC3.[85] Proinflammatory CX3CR1+CD59+ monocytes have been recently demonstrated to be expanded in the gut of AS patients compared with CD patients and controls.[86] Interestingly, gut-derived CD14++CD16+CX3CR1+CD59+CCR9+IL-23+TL1A+ cells were also expanded in the peripheral blood, synovial tissues, and BM of AS patients. Considering their expression of CCR9, a marker of intestinal homing, these cells might be of gut origin. The pathogenetic relevance of the recirculation of gut-derived immune cells seems to be supported by the evidence that blocking the a4b7 signaling with the low-affinity anti-a4b7 antibody, natalizumab, is effective in ameliorating the symptoms and preventing the radiographic progression of AS patients.[87] Recent evidences, however, indicate that treatment of IBD patients with the more specific anti-a4b7 vedolizumab may result in the induction of or flare of arthritis and/or sacroiliitis even though larger cohort studies are needed to provide information on the prevalence, the evolution, and underlying mechanism.[88]

These evidences highlight the complex relationships between bacteria and the innate and adaptive immune reactions in AS. The resulting continuous immune stimulation might induce, in genetically predisposed subjects, the selection of aberrant clones of cells of the immune system that from the intestine recirculate into extraintestinal sites inducing inflammation. Modulation of intestinal immune responses in SpA could represent in the future a keystone in the treatment of SpA.

NEW BONE FORMATION IN AS

Along with inflammation, osteoproliferation is an equally important feature of AS pathology. New bone formation in the spine and peripheral joints in AS is thought to be a repair mechanism in response to inflammation and osteodestruction. Endochondral and intramembranous ossification have been proposed to be closely linked to pathogenic bone formation in AS.[89,90]

Endochondral bone formation starts with terminal differentiation of chondrocytes, invasion of osteoblast precursors into the chondrocyte matrix, and finally replacement of cartilage by bone. Intramembranous ossification is associated with direct transformation of mesenchymal stem cells into osteoprogenitor cells. Evidence suggests that in AS, early mesenchymal expansion can be induced before the resolution of inflammation. When inflammation decreases, excessive tissue formation and ectopic chondrocyte formation can be seen. If inflammation is not resolved early enough, the structural damage will initiate osteoproliferation independent of the status of the inflammation.[91] It is now proposed that early treatment can suppress radiographic progression through inhibition of inflammation and subsequent invasion of subchondral granulation tissue.[92-94]

The pathogenesis and mediators of osteoproliferation in AS are largely unknown. Based on animal, immunohistochemistry, and histopathologic studies, several pathways have been proposed as important players in AS pathogenesis. Their primary role in AS is difficult to study because of the difficulty in accessing tissue. The majority of evidence stems from animal studies.

BMP

Bone morphogenetic proteins (BMPs) are multifunctional regulators in bone formation that belong to the transforming growth factor β (TGFβ) superfamily. BMPs promote osteoblastic gene transcription and joint ankylosis by activating Smad signaling cascades and p38/extracellular signal-regulated kinases (ERK)–dependent mitogen-activated protein kinase (MAPK) pathway.[95]

Unique BMP activation profiles have been associated with different stages of the bone development and AS disease process. BMP2 was found to be involved in early stage of endochondral ossification when mesenchymal progenitor cells differentiate into chondrocytes, whereas BMP6 and BMP7 play later roles in the prehypertrophic and hypertrophic chondrocytes differentiation.[96]

Several lines of studies indicate that abnormal BMP signaling pathway could be pathogenic in AS. Serum levels of BMP2, BMP4, BMP6, and BMP7 have been shown to be upregulated in AS patients. In addition, serum levels of BMP2, BMP4, and BMP7 were higher in AS patients with spinal fusion compared with patients without fusion.[97,98] BMP pathways are negatively regulated by BMP antagonist, noggin, which specifically binds to BMP2, BMP4, BMP6, and BMP7 and prevents them from binding to their receptor. The imbalance between BMPs and noggin is associated with the pathologic osteogenesis in AS. In the spontaneous model of arthritis in DBA/1 mice, expression of BMP2, BMP4, and BMP7 was elevated at sites of enthesitis and the addition of noggin-ameliorated entheseal ankylosis.[96] Xie et al. reported that bone marrow–derived mesenchymal stem cells (MSCs) from AS patients exhibited greater osteogenic differentiation capacity than MSCs from healthy controls because of enhanced BMP2 and decreased noggin secretion.[99] In addition, BMP6 polymorphisms have also been found to be associated with radiologic severity in AS patients.[100]

Wnt Pathway and DKK-1

Wnt signaling pathway mediated by wingless proteins (Wnt) is implicated in bone formation in AS. The canonical Wnt/β-catenin pathway has been implicated in inhibition of osteoclastogenesis as well as osteoblast differentiation, proliferation, and survival.[101,102] Wnt pathway is tightly regulated by several antagonists including Dickkopf-1 (DKK-1), expressed by osteocytes and osteoblasts, and sclerostin, expressed by osteocytes.[103] DKK-1 and sclerostin block Wnt from binding to its low-density lipoprotein receptor–related protein-5/6 (LRP5/6) on mesenchymal cells, leading to β-catenin degradation and osteoblast apoptosis.[104] Evidence indicates that the balance between Wnt pathway and its antagonists is crucial in the bone remodeling in AS. Decreased levels of DKK-1 and sclerostin along with hyperactive Wnt pathway have been found in a mouse model of AS.[105] Blockade of DKK-1 has been shown to reverse bone erosion, increase bone mass, and induce sacroiliac joint fusion in animal models.[106,107]

Serum DKK-1 and sclerostin have been found to be significantly lower in AS patients compared with healthy controls.[108] It has also been reported that DKK-1 is dysfunctional in AS patients.[109] Thus, the excessive bone formation in AS may be associated with overactivation of Wnt signaling and decreased functional levels of Wnt antagonists.

Hedgehog Pathway

The third pathway that is implicated in pathogenic osteoblastogenesis and new bone formation in AS is Hedgehog pathway. Hedgehog (Hh) pathway is stimulated by three major ligands, Indian Hedgehog (Ihh), Sonic Hedgehog (Shh), and Desert Hedgehog (Dhh) with Ihh being the main ligand in the process of endochondral ossification.[110] Ihh is primarily produced by prehypertrophic and hypertrophic chondrocytes and regulates parathyroid hormone–related protein

(PTHrP) in a negative feedback loop. Ihh binds to Hh receptor patched-1 (Ptch-1) and releases the G protein–coupled receptor–like molecule smoothened (Smo), which leads to the activation of glioma-associated-oncogene-homologues (Gli) including Gli1, Gli2, and Gli3. In the absence of PTHrP, mice exhibited aberrant prehypertrophic and hypertrophic chondrocytes in articular cartilage as well as nasal/costal cartilage destruction by mineralizing cells.[111] Blockade of Smo in a serum transfer–induced arthritis mouse model (K/B × N) significantly reduced osteophyte formation.[112] In a mouse model, chondrocyte-specific chronic activation of Hh pathway caused excessive chondrocyte proliferation in the intervertebral discs, leading to defective endochondral ossification and severe spinal malformation.[113] Daoussis et al. reported that serum Ihh levels were increased in AS patients and decreased following TNAα blocker treatment.[114] Interestingly, in a German cohort, serum Ihh levels were reported to be higher in HLA-B27 carriers compared with HLA-B27-negative individuals independent if they were healthy or with SpA.[115]

Macrophage Migration Inhibitory Factor

Macrophage migration inhibitory factor (MIF) is a pleiotropic cytokine that plays pivotal roles in adaptive and innate immune responses. MIF is known to be produced by a wide variety of cell types and to stimulate TNF and IL-6 expression through the activation of CD74/CD44 receptor complex pathways.

High levels of MIF have been reported in many autoimmune diseases and were associated with high disease activities of AS and RA.[116–119] MIF levels have also been shown to be correlated with the clinical index of AS.[118]

A series of reports support a conflicting theory that MIF plays roles in both sides of the bone-remodeling process. MIF is involved in fracture healing process by enhancing the expression of matrix metalloproteinase (MMP)-13 in osteoblasts and chondrocytes.[120] Jacquin et al. reported that MIF-deficient mice had decreased levels of bone turnover markers and decreased trabecular bone volume (TBV) in the femurs and vertebrae compared with wild-type (WT) mice. In addition, MIF inhibited osteoclast formation in cultured bone marrow and macrophage.[121] Deletion of CD74 abolished the effect of MIF on osteoclastogenesis, suggesting that MIF signals through CD74 and extracellular signal–regulated kinase (ERK)/mitogen-activated protein

kinase (MAPK) signaling.[122] Moreover, MIF has been shown to induce osteoblast mineralization in vitro through ERK and canonical Wnt/β-catenin pathway.[119]

On the contrary, MIF has been shown to facilitate the homing of osteoclast precursors to peripheral osteolytic lesions.[123] At the cartilage endplate (CEP), the activation of the MIF-CD74-ERK cascade led to degenerated chondrocytes.[124] In a K/B × N serum transfer–induced arthritis mouse model, MIF KO reduced RANKL-induced phosphorylation of NF-kb-p64 and ERK1/2 and further reduced osteoclastogenesis.[125]

Thus, the complexity of MIF-mediated bone-remodeling pathways indicates that the effect of MIF may highly depend on the local bone microenvironment. The exact roles of MIF in bone homeostasis remain to be elucidated.

IL23/IL17 Axis and Bone Remodeling in AS

The discovery of IL23/IL17 pathway has been a landmark in our understanding of autoimmune disorders. This pathway is thought to play a critical role in the disease pathogenesis of ankylosing spondylitis. IL23 is mainly produced by antigen-presenting cells (APCs) and is needed for the stabilization and expansion of Th17 cells that in turn secrete IL17A, IL17F, IL22, and IL21.[126]

Polymorphisms in the IL23R are strongly associated with AS in GWAS.[9] IL23 levels are also elevated in AS patients' serum and PBMC cultures.[127,128] Mice models provide conflicting evidence for the positive or negative involvement of IL23 with osteoclastogenesis. IL23 can stimulate RANK expression in murine myeloid precursor cells, which leads to their differentiation into osteoclasts.[129] In contrast, another study showed that mice lacking IL23p19 had 30% lower bone mineral density and trabecular bone mass.[130] These murine T cells also produced GM-CSF in response to IL23, which can inhibit osteoclastogenesis.[130] In 2012, Sherlock et al. showed that IL23 acts on ROR-γt+ CD3+CD4−CD8− entheseal T cells that express IL23R. They showed that IL23 overexpression using minicircle technology was sufficient to induce enthesitis and new bone formation as seen in AS patients.[131] Systemic overexpression of IL23 showed mouse paw swelling in a dose-dependent manner. Furthermore, 6 days after IL23 minicircle injection, severe entheseal inflammation developed. 18 days after injection, expansion of periosteal osteoblasts was seen. Cartilage, osteoid, chondrocytes, and new bone formation were also found in the articular structures of the mouse. As expected, IL23 stimulated the production of IL17 and IL22 from these ROR-γt+

CD3+CD4–CD8– entheseal T cells. It was shown that IL17 and IL23 alone had no effects in osteoproliferation.[131] However, overexpression of IL22 using minicircle technology was able to mimic new bone formation seen after IL23 overexpression. In vitro experiments using an osteoblast cell line showed that IL22 was able to upregulate genes related to osteoblast differentiation including alkaline phosphatase, Wnt family members, and bone morphogenic proteins.[131] These data taken together suggest that IL23 may not have a direct effect on bone formation in AS but may take on a more indirect role through the upregulation of IL22.

An interesting 2017 study showed that drug-induced ER stress of bone-derived cells (BdCs) from AS patients produced more secreted levels and mRNA transcripts of IL-23 than the same cells (also ER stressed) from healthy controls.[132] ER-stressed AS cells also exhibited increased osteogenic activity. RUNX2 knockout, a key transcription factor in osteoblast differentiation stimulation, in these BdCs was able to inhibit the expression of IL23.[132] These data elucidate a role for ER stress in AS osteoblasts that can contribute to inflammatory processes through the secretion of IL-23. It provides yet another link between inflammation and bone remodeling.

IL17 is a proinflammatory cytokine that has been implicated in a variety of autoimmune disorders. There are six cytokines that belong to the IL17 family: IL17A-F. Of these, IL17A and IL17F share the closest sequence homology and have been studied the most. Most commonly studied is the IL17 produced by Th17 cells. However, innate immune cells such as mast cells, innate lymphoid cells 3 (ILC3s), NKT cells, CD8+ T cells, NK cells, neutrophils, and γδ T cells also contribute to IL17 levels in the body.[133] Like IL23, IL17 has also been implicated in taking on a role in bone remodeling.

In isolated human mesenchymal stem cells (hMSCs), IL17A synergized with TNF alpha to form bone matrix. The two cytokines together also inhibited RANKL and DKK-1 expression, which points toward the milieu favoring osteoblastogenesis versus osteoclastogenesis.[134] IL17A and IL17F isolated from activated Th17 cells exhibited strong osteogenic effects when exposed to hMSCs.[135] A 2015 study discusses the role of IL17 secreted by δγ T cells in osteogenesis. They found that after fracture, the δγ T cell infiltrate doubled and IL17A secretion from these cells were crucial to new bone formation.[136] However, in the 2012 study by Sherlock et al., IL17A minicircle injection did not mimic IL23-dependent entheseal inflammation and in vitro (osteoblast cell line) osteoblastogenesis like IL22.[131] Another study using neonatal rat calvaria osteoblast precursor cells found IL17A to have negative effects on osteoblastogenesis.[137] When cultured with IL17 for 14 days, expression of osteoblast differentiation genes such as ALP and osteocalcin was decreased.[137] It can be inferred from these data that IL17A may have a role in driving uncommitted MSCs to osteoblast lineage but may have little effect on matured osteoblast cells.

Prostaglandin E2 and Its Interaction With EP4 in Bone Remodeling and Inflammation in AS

Prostaglandin E2 (PGE2) is a lipid molecule that promotes hormone-like effects in the body. Derived from arachidonic acid in the cellular membrane, the production of PGE2 is dependent on the cyclooxygenase enzymes 1 and 2 (COX1/2). The COX-2 enzymes are the site of inhibition for nonsteroidal antiinflammatory drugs (NSAIDs), which are commonly used to manage the symptoms of AS. Produced by mostly chondrocytes and fibroblasts, PGE2 can interact with one of four rhodopsin-like 7-transmembrane-spanning G protein–coupled receptors (GPCRs), which are named EP1-4. SNPs in the EP4 variant have been associated with ankylosing spondylitis in genome-wide association studies (GWAS).[9] Once EP4 is activated by PGE2, cyclic AMP is upregulated via adenylyl cyclase stimulation. PGE2 also has a variety of effects in the body, including being involved in bone remodeling as well as inflammation.

Knockout mice for each of the four PGE2 receptors as well as agonists and antagonists have been developed. Infusing PGE2 onto the periosteal surface of wild-type and EP1-3 knockout mice caused extensive callus formation at the site of infusion. However, EP4 knockout mice showed little to no callus formation.[138] Fractures in EP4 knockout mice also healed slower than fractures in wild-type mice. Although young EP4 knockout mice exhibited no skeletal phenotypes, aged EP4 KO mice showed low bone mass and less trabecular network density.[139] Bone marrow (BM) cells harvested from wild-type mice cultured with PGE2 for 3 weeks showed mineralized nodules and increases in RUNX-2 expression in a dose-dependent manner. However, BM cells isolated from EP4 KO mice showed little mineralization and RUNX-2 expression in response to PGE2 or vehicle control.[138] EP4 agonists were also shown to cause bone formation in wild-type and EP1-3 KO mice but not in EP4 KO mice. EP1-3 agonists did not cause bone formation.[138] Taken together, these studies show that EP4 and PGE2 interaction is necessary for proper bone remodeling and bone formation processes to occur. This may have implications in the aberrant cycles of bone formation and erosion seen in AS patients and calls for further exploration.

PGE2/EP4 interaction has also been implicated in driving Th17 cell phenotype. EP4 is present on both antigen-presenting cells and Th17 cells themselves.[140] On APCs, PGE2/EP4 interaction was shown to increase IL23 production, which in turn promotes the expansion of Th17 cells. When present on Th17 cells, EP4/PGE2 interaction can further IL23-mediated Th17 expansion.[140] Naïve T cells treated with PGE2 were shown to upregulate IL23 and IL1 receptors.[141] PGE2 also upregulates IL17 production from Th17 cells in the presence of APCs.[140] In bone marrow–derived dendritic cells, PGE2 synergistically induced IL23a expression with CD40 signaling. This effect was mimicked by an EP4 agonist.[142] In AS patients, Th17 cells, IL23, and IL17 have been shown to be elevated. Studying PGE2/EP4 interactions may provide further insight into the pathways that enhance the IL23/IL17 axis in AS. Moreover, β-glucan has been shown to elevate PGE2 levels. When SKG mice were injected with β-glucan, they develop SpA, which may underlie a mechanism of action for PGE2/EP4 in AS.[143] Finally, many genes in the IL17/IL23 pathway including the receptor for IL23 have been associated with AS in GWAS. PTGER4 mRNA levels were also found to be increased in synovial samples from AS patients when compared with noninflammatory arthritis or healthy controls.[9] These data can be taken together to suggest an involvement of PGE2/EP4 interaction in the inflammatory pathways implicated in AS. This receptor-ligand interaction requires further exploration to elucidate molecular mechanisms in the context of AS pathogenesis.

CONCLUSION

We have made significant strides in our understanding of AS pathogenesis. Studies on functional genomics have resulted in novel pathways being implicated in the pathogenesis of AS. The recognition of type 3 immunity as an important player in AS pathogenesis led to the introduction of IL-17 inhibitors in treatment. The gut-joint axis is being explored in great depth, and understanding the contribution of our microbiome in health and disease should help us elucidate better the impact of the environment on AS pathogenesis. The effect of TH17 cells, prostaglandins, and novel cytokines such as MIF on bone homeostasis implies that they are potentially amenable to therapeutic intervention.

REFERENCES

1. Haroon NN, Paterson JM, Li P, Inman RD, Haroon N. Patients with ankylosing spondylitis have increased cardiovascular and cerebrovascular mortality: a population-based study. *Ann Intern Med.* 2015;163:409–416.
2. Gratacos J, Collado A, Filella X, et al. Serum cytokines (IL-6, TNF-alpha, IL-1 beta and IFN-gamma) in ankylosing spondylitis: a close correlation between serum IL-6 and disease activity and severity. *Br J Rheumatol.* 1994;33:927–931.
3. Braun J, Xiang J, Brandt J, et al. Treatment of spondyloarthropathies with antibodies against tumour necrosis factor alpha: first clinical and laboratory experiences. *Ann Rheum Dis.* 2000;59(suppl 1):i85–i89.
4. Maksymowych WP, Salonen D, Inman RD, Rahman P, Lambert RG, CANDLE Study Group. Low-dose infliximab (3 mg/kg) significantly reduces spinal inflammation on magnetic resonance imaging in patients with ankylosing spondylitis: a randomized placebo-controlled study. *J Rheumatol.* 2010;37:1728–1734.
5. Redlich K, Gortz B, Hayer S, et al. Overexpression of tumor necrosis factor causes bilateral sacroiliitis. *Arthritis Rheum.* 2004;50:1001–1005.
6. Lee YH, Song GG. Lack of association of TNF-alpha promoter polymorphisms with ankylosing spondylitis: a meta-analysis. *Rheumatology.* 2009;48:1359–1362.
7. Li B, Wang P, Li H. The association between TNF-alpha promoter polymorphisms and ankylosing spondylitis: a meta-analysis. *Clin Rheumatol.* 2010;29:983–990.
8. Australo-Anglo-American Spondyloarthritis Consortium (TASC), Reveille JD, Sims AM, et al. Genome-wide association study of ankylosing spondylitis identifies non-MHC susceptibility loci. *Nat Genet.* 2010;42:123–127.
9. The Australo-Anglo-American Spondyloarthritis Consortium (TASC), The Wellcome Trust Case Control Consortium 2 (WTCCC2), Evans DM, et al. Interaction between ERAP1 and HLA-B27 in ankylosing spondylitis implicates peptide handling in the mechanism for HLA-B27 in disease susceptibility. *Nat Genet.* 2011;43:761–767.
10. Appel H, Maier R, Wu P, et al. Analysis of IL-17(+) cells in facet joints of patients with spondyloarthritis suggests that the innate immune pathway might be of greater relevance than the Th17-mediated adaptive immune response. *Arthritis Res Ther.* 2011;13:R95.
11. McGarry F, Neilly J, Anderson N, Sturrock R, Field M. A polymorphism within the interleukin 1 receptor antagonist (IL-1Ra) gene is associated with ankylosing spondylitis. *Rheumatology.* 2001;40:1359–1364.
12. Maksymowych WP, Rahman P, Reeve JP, Gladman DD, Peddle L, Inman RD. Association of the IL1 gene cluster with susceptibility to ankylosing spondylitis: an analysis of three Canadian populations. *Arthritis Rheum.* 2006;54:974–985.
13. Kim TJ, Kim TH, Lee HJ, et al. Interleukin 1 polymorphisms in patients with ankylosing spondylitis in Korea. *J Rheumatol.* 2008;35:1603–1608.

14. Chou CT, Timms AE, Wei JC, Tsai WC, Wordsworth BP, Brown MA. Replication of association of IL1 gene complex members with ankylosing spondylitis in Taiwanese Chinese. *Ann Rheum Dis.* 2006;65:1106–1109.

15. Jarvinen P. Occurrence of ankylosing spondylitis in a nationwide series of twins. *Arthritis Rheum.* 1995;38: 381–383.

16. Pedersen OB, Svendsen AJ, Ejstrup L, Skytthe A, Harris JR, Junker P. Ankylosing spondylitis in Danish and Norwegian twins: occurrence and the relative importance of genetic vs. environmental effectors in disease causation. *Scand J Rheumatol.* 2008;37:120–126.

17. Robinson WP, van der Linden SM, Khan MA, et al. HLA-Bw60 increases susceptibility to ankylosing spondylitis in HLA-B27+ patients. *Arthritis Rheum.* 1989;32:1135–1141.

18. Brown MA, Pile KD, Kennedy LG, et al. HLA class I associations of ankylosing spondylitis in the white population in the United Kingdom. *Ann Rheum Dis.* 1996;55:268–270.

19. Khan MA, Kushner I, Braun WE. Association of HLA-A2 with uveitis in HLA-B27 positive patients with ankylosing spondylitis. *J Rheumatol.* 1981;8:295–298.

20. Ranganathan V, Gracey E, Brown MA, Inman RD, Haroon N. Pathogenesis of ankylosing spondylitis - recent advances and future directions. *Nat Rev Rheumatol.* 2017;13:359–367.

21. Brewerton DA, Hart FD, Nicholls A, Caffrey M, James DC, Sturrock RD. Ankylosing spondylitis and HL-A 27. *Lancet.* 1973;1:904–907.

22. Schlosstein L, Terasaki PI, Bluestone R, Pearson CM. High association of an HL-A antigen, W27, with ankylosing spondylitis. *N Engl J Med.* 1973;288:704–706.

23. Khan MA. HLA-B27 and its subtypes in world populations. *Curr Opin Rheumatol.* 1995;7:263–269.

24. Khan MA. An update on the genetic polymorphism of HLA-B*27 with 213 alleles encompassing 160 subtypes (and still counting). *Curr Rheumatol Rep.* 2017;19:9. 017-0640-1.

25. Hammer RE, Maika SD, Richardson JA, Tang JP, Taurog JD. Spontaneous inflammatory disease in transgenic rats expressing HLA-B27 and human beta 2m: an animal model of HLA-B27-associated human disorders. *Cell.* 1990;63:1099–1112.

26. Taurog JD, Maika SD, Simmons WA, Breban M, Hammer RE. Susceptibility to inflammatory disease in HLA-B27 transgenic rat lines correlates with the level of B27 expression. *J Immunol.* 1993;150:4168–4178.

27. May E, Dorris ML, Satumtira N, et al. CD8 alpha beta T cells are not essential to the pathogenesis of arthritis or colitis in HLA-B27 transgenic rats. *J Immunol.* 2003;170:1099–1105.

28. Loll B, Fabian H, Huser H, et al. Increased conformational flexibility of HLA-B*27 subtypes associated with ankylosing spondylitis. *Arthritis Rheumatol.* 2016;68:1172–1182.

29. Rana MK, Luthra-Guptasarma M. Multi-modal binding of a 'self' peptide by HLA-B*27:04 and B*27:05 allelic

30. Akram A, Inman RD. Co-expression of HLA-B7 and HLA-B27 alleles is associated with B7-restricted immunodominant responses following influenza infection. *Eur J Immunol.* 2013;43:3254–3267.

31. Tanigaki N, Fruci D, Vigneti E, et al. The peptide binding specificity of HLA-B27 subtypes. *Immunogenetics.* 1994;40:192–198.

32. Fiorillo MT, Meadows L, D'Amato M, et al. Susceptibility to ankylosing spondylitis correlates with the C-terminal residue of peptides presented by various HLA-B27 subtypes. *Eur J Immunol.* 1997;27:368–373.

33. Fitzmaurice K, Hurst J, Dring M, et al. Additive effects of HLA alleles and innate immune genes determine viral outcome in HCV infection. *Gut.* 2015;64:813–819.

34. Schneidewind A, Brockman MA, Yang R, et al. Escape from the dominant HLA-B27-restricted cytotoxic T-lymphocyte response in Gag is associated with a dramatic reduction in human immunodeficiency virus type 1 replication. *J Virol.* 2007;81:12382–12393.

35. Ben Dror L, Barnea E, Beer I, Mann M, Admon A. The HLA-B*2705 peptidome. *Arthritis Rheum.* 2010;62: 420–429.

36. Lopez de Castro JA. The HLA-B27 peptidome: building on the cornerstone. *Arthritis Rheum.* 2010;62:316–319.

37. Alvarez-Navarro C, Cragnolini JJ, Dos Santos HG, et al. Novel HLA-B27-restricted epitopes from *Chlamydia trachomatis* generated upon endogenous processing of bacterial proteins suggest a role of molecular mimicry in reactive arthritis. *J Biol Chem.* 2013;288:25810–25825.

38. Daser A, Urlaub H, Henklein P. HLA-B27 binding peptides derived from the 57 kD heat shock protein of *Chlamydia trachomatis*: novel insights into the peptide binding rules. *Mol Immunol.* 1994;31:331–336.

39. Schittenhelm RB, Sian TC, Wilmann PG, Dudek NL, Purcell AW. Revisiting the arthritogenic peptide theory: quantitative not qualitative changes in the peptide repertoire of HLA-B27 allotypes. *Arthritis Rheumatol.* 2015;67: 702–713.

40. Schittenhelm RB, Sivaneswaran S, Lim K, Sian TC, Croft NP, Purcell AW. Human Leukocyte antigen (HLA) B27 allotype-specific binding and candidate arthritogenic peptides revealed through heuristic clustering of data-independent acquisition mass spectrometry (DIA-MS) data. *Mol Cell Proteomics.* 2016;15:1867–1876.

41. Scrivo R, Morrone S, Spadaro A, Santoni A, Valesini G. Evaluation of degranulation and cytokine production in natural killer cells from spondyloarthritis patients at single-cell level. *Cytometry B Clin Cytom.* 2011;80:22–27.

42. Bowness P. Hla-B27. *Annu Rev Immunol.* 2015;33:29–48.

43. Marroquin Belaunzaran O, Kleber S, Schauer S, et al. HLA-B27-Homodimer-Specific antibody modulates the expansion of pro-inflammatory T-cells in HLA-B27 transgenic rats. *PLoS One.* 2015;10:e0130811.

44. Long EO, Kim HS, Liu D, Peterson ME, Rajagopalan S. Controlling natural killer cell responses: integration of signals for activation and inhibition. *Annu Rev Immunol.* 2013;31:227–258.

45. DeLay ML, Turner MJ, Klenk EI, Smith JA, Sowders DP, Colbert RA. HLA-B27 misfolding and the unfolded protein response augment interleukin-23 production and are associated with Th17 activation in transgenic rats. *Arthritis Rheum.* 2009;60:2633–2643.

46. Turner MJ, Sowders DP, DeLay ML, et al. HLA-B27 misfolding in transgenic rats is associated with activation of the unfolded protein response. *J Immunol.* 2005;175:2438–2448.

47. Gu J, Rihl M, Marker-Hermann E, et al. Clues to pathogenesis of spondyloarthropathy derived from synovial fluid mononuclear cell gene expression profiles. *J Rheumatol.* 2002;29:2159–2164.

48. Campbell EC, Fettke F, Bhat S, Morley KD, Powis SJ. Expression of MHC class I dimers and ERAP1 in an ankylosing spondylitis patient cohort. *Immunology.* 2011;133:379–385.

49. Ciccia F, Accardo-Palumbo A, Rizzo A, et al. Evidence that autophagy, but not the unfolded protein response, regulates the expression of IL-23 in the gut of patients with ankylosing spondylitis and subclinical gut inflammation. *Ann Rheum Dis.* 2014;73:1566–1574.

50. Neerinckx B, Carter S, Lories RJ. No evidence for a critical role of the unfolded protein response in synovium and blood of patients with ankylosing spondylitis. *Ann Rheum Dis.* 2014;73:629–630.

51. Ciccia FHN. Autophagy in the pathogenesis of ankylosing spondylitis. *Clin Rheumatol.* 2016;35:1433–1436.

52. Wellcome Trust Case Control Consortium, Australo-Anglo-American Spondylitis Consortium (TASC), Burton PR, et al. Association scan of 14,500 nonsynonymous SNPs in four diseases identifies autoimmunity variants. *Nat Genet.* 2007;39:1329–1337.

53. Haroon N, Inman RD. Endoplasmic reticulum aminopeptidases: biology and pathogenic potential. *Nat Rev Rheumatol.* 2010;6:461–467.

54. Cortes A, Pulit SL, Leo PJ, et al. Major histocompatibility complex associations of ankylosing spondylitis are complex and involve further epistasis with ERAP1. *Nat Commun.* 2015;6:7146.

55. Hammer GE, Gonzalez F, James E, Nolla H, Shastri N. In the absence of aminopeptidase ERAAP, MHC class I molecules present many unstable and highly immunogenic peptides. *Nat Immunol.* 2007;8:101–108.

56. Blanchard N, Shastri N. Coping with loss of perfection in the MHC class I peptide repertoire. *Curr Opin Immunol.* 2008;20:82–88.

57. Tsui FW, Haroon N, Reveille JD, et al. Association of an ERAP1 ERAP2 haplotype with familial ankylosing spondylitis. *Ann Rheum Dis.* 2010;69:733–736.

58. Haroon N, Tsui FW, Uchanska-Ziegler B, Ziegler A, Inman RD. Endoplasmic Reticulum Aminopeptidase 1 (ERAP1) exhibits functionally significant interaction with HLA B27 and relates to subtype specificity in ankylosing spondylitis. *Ann Rheum Dis.* 2012;71:589–595.

59. Chen L, Ridley A, Hammitzsch A, et al. Silencing or inhibition of endoplasmic reticulum aminopeptidase 1 (ERAP1) suppresses free heavy chain expression and Th17 responses in ankylosing spondylitis. *Ann Rheum Dis.* 2016;75:916–923.

60. Evnouchidou I, Kamal RP, Seregin SS, et al. Coding single nucleotide polymorphisms of endoplasmic reticulum aminopeptidase 1 can affect antigenic peptide generation in vitro by influencing basic enzymatic properties of the enzyme. *J Immunol.* 2011;186:1909–1913.

61. Haroon N, Tsui FW, Chiu B, Tsui HW, Inman RD. Serum cytokine receptors in ankylosing spondylitis: relationship to inflammatory markers and endoplasmic reticulum aminopeptidase polymorphisms. *J Rheumatol.* 2010;37:1907–1910.

62. O'Rielly DD, Uddin M, Codner D, et al. Private rare deletions in SEC16A and MAMDC4 may represent novel pathogenic variants in familial axial spondyloarthritis. *Ann Rheum Dis.* 2016;75:772–779.

63. Peterson LW, Artis D. Intestinal epithelial cells: regulators of barrier function and immune homeostasis. *Nat Rev Immunol.* 2014;14:141–153.

64. Knight R, Callewaert C, Marotz C, et al. The microbiome and human biology. *Annu Rev Genom Hum Genet.* 2017;18:65–86.

65. Taurog JD, Chhabra A, Colbert RA. Ankylosing spondylitis and axial spondyloarthritis. *N Engl J Med.* 2016;374:2563–2574.

66. Mielants H, Veys EM, Cuvelier C, de Vos M. Ileocolonoscopic findings in seronegative spondylarthropathies. *Br J Rheumatol.* 1988;27(suppl 2):95–105.

67. Lin P, Bach M, Asquith M, et al. HLA-B27 and human beta2-microglobulin affect the gut microbiota of transgenic rats. *PloS One.* 2014;9:e105684.

68. Martinez-Gonzalez O, Cantero-Hinojosa J, Paule-Sastre P, Gomez-Magan JC, Salvatierra-Rios D. Intestinal permeability in patients with ankylosing spondylitis and their healthy relatives. *Br J Rheumatol.* 1994;33:644–647.

69. Montoya J, Matta NB, Suchon P, et al. Patients with ankylosing spondylitis have been breast fed less often than healthy controls: a case-control retrospective study. *Ann Rheum Dis.* 2016;75:879–882.

70. Costello ME, Ciccia F, Willner D, et al. Brief report: intestinal dysbiosis in ankylosing spondylitis. *Arthritis Rheumatol.* 2015;67:686–691.

71. Tito RY, Cypers H, Joossens M, et al. Brief report: dialister as a microbial marker of disease activity in spondyloarthritis. *Arthritis Rheumatol.* 2017;69:114–121.

72. Breban M, Tap J, Leboime A, et al. Faecal microbiota study reveals specific dysbiosis in spondyloarthritis. *Ann Rheum Dis.* 2017;76:1614–1622.

73. Wen C, Zheng Z, Shao T, et al. Quantitative metagenomics reveals unique gut microbiome biomarkers in ankylosing spondylitis. *Genome Biol.* 2017;18:142. 017-1271-6.

74. Stoll ML, Kumar R, Morrow CD, et al. Altered microbiota associated with abnormal humoral immune responses to commensal organisms in enthesitis-related arthritis. *Arthritis Res Ther.* 2014;16:486. 014-0486-0.

75. Scher JU, Ubeda C, Artacho A, et al. Decreased bacterial diversity characterizes the altered gut microbiota in patients with psoriatic arthritis, resembling dysbiosis in inflammatory bowel disease. *Arthritis Rheumatol.* 2015;67:128–139.

76. Ciccia F, Guggino G, Rizzo A, et al. Dysbiosis and zonulin upregulation alter gut epithelial and vascular barriers in patients with ankylosing spondylitis. *Ann Rheum Dis.* 2017;76:1123–1132.

77. Van Damme N, De Vos M, Baeten D, et al. Flow cytometric analysis of gut mucosal lymphocytes supports an impaired Th1 cytokine profile in spondyloarthropathy. *Ann Rheum Dis.* 2001;60:495–499.

78. Ciccia F, Bombardieri M, Principato A, et al. Overexpression of interleukin-23, but not interleukin-17, as an immunologic signature of subclinical intestinal inflammation in ankylosing spondylitis. *Arthritis Rheum.* 2009;60:955–965.

79. Ciccia F, Accardo-Palumbo A, Giardina A, et al. Expansion of intestinal CD4+CD25(high) Treg cells in patients with ankylosing spondylitis: a putative role for interleukin-10 in preventing intestinal Th17 response. *Arthritis Rheum.* 2010;62:3625–3634.

80. Ciccia F, Accardo-Palumbo A, Alessandro R, et al. Interleukin-22 and interleukin-22-producing NKp44+ natural killer cells in subclinical gut inflammation in ankylosing spondylitis. *Arthritis Rheum.* 2012;64:1869–1878.

81. Hue S, Ahern P, Buonocore S, et al. Interleukin-23 drives innate and T cell-mediated intestinal inflammation. *J Exp Med.* 2006;203:2473–2483.

82. Eken A, Singh AK, Treuting PM, Oukka M. IL-23R+ innate lymphoid cells induce colitis via interleukin-22-dependent mechanism. *Mucosal Immunol.* 2014;7:143–154.

83. Mjosberg J, Spits H. Human innate lymphoid cells. *J Allergy Clin Immunol.* 2016;138:1265–1276.

84. Ciccia F, Guggino G, Rizzo A, et al. Type 3 innate lymphoid cells producing IL-17 and IL-22 are expanded in the gut, in the peripheral blood, synovial fluid and bone marrow of patients with ankylosing spondylitis. *Ann Rheum Dis.* 2015;74:1739–1747.

85. Longman RS, Diehl GE, Victorio DA, et al. CX(3)CR1(+) mononuclear phagocytes support colitis-associated innate lymphoid cell production of IL-22. *J Exp Med.* 2014;211:1571–1583.

86. Ciccia F, Guggino G, Zeng M, et al. Pro-inflammatory CX3CR1(+) CD59(+) TL1A(+) IL-23(+) monocytes are expanded in patients with Ankylosing Spondylitis and modulate ILC3 immune functions. *Arthritis Rheumatol.* 2018. https://doi.org/10.1002/art.40582.

87. Ciccia F, Rizzo A, Guggino G, Bignone R, Galia M, Triolo G. Clinical efficacy of alpha4 integrin block with natalizumab in ankylosing spondylitis. *Ann Rheum Dis.* 2016;75:2053–2054.

88. Varkas G, Thevissen K, De Brabanter G, et al. An induction or flare of arthritis and/or sacroiliitis by vedolizumab in inflammatory bowel disease: a case series. *Ann Rheum Dis.* 2017;76:878–881.

89. Wendling D, Claudepierre P. New bone formation in axial spondyloarthritis. *Joint Bone Spine.* 2013;80:454–458.

90. Lories RJ, Haroon N. Bone formation in axial spondyloarthritis. *Best Pract Res Clin Rheumatol.* 2014;28:765–777.

91. Tseng HW, Pitt ME, Glant TT, et al. Inflammation-driven bone formation in a mouse model of ankylosing spondylitis: sequential not parallel processes. *Arthritis Res Ther.* 2016;18:35. 015-0805-0.

92. Bleil J, Maier R, Hempfing A, Sieper J, Appel H, Syrbe U. Granulation tissue eroding the subchondral bone also promotes new bone formation in ankylosing spondylitis. *Arthritis Rheumatol.* 2016;68:2456–2465.

93. Haroon N, Inman RD, Learch TJ, et al. The impact of tumor necrosis factor alpha inhibitors on radiographic progression in ankylosing spondylitis. *Arthritis Rheum.* 2013;65:2645–2654.

94. Molnar C, Scherer A, Baraliakos X, et al. TNF blockers inhibit spinal radiographic progression in ankylosing spondylitis by reducing disease activity: results from the Swiss Clinical Quality Management cohort. *Ann Rheum Dis.* 2018;77:63–69.

95. Biver E, Hardouin P, Caverzasio J. The "bone morphogenic proteins" pathways in bone and joint diseases: translational perspectives from physiopathology to therapeutic targets. *Cytokine Growth Factor Rev.* 2013;24:69–81.

96. Lories RJ, Derese I, Luyten FP. Modulation of bone morphogenetic protein signaling inhibits the onset and progression of ankylosing enthesitis. *J Clin Invest.* 2005;115:1571–1579.

97. Chen HA, Chen CH, Lin YJ, et al. Association of bone morphogenetic proteins with spinal fusion in ankylosing spondylitis. *J Rheumatol.* 2010;37:2126–2132.

98. Liao HT, Lin YF, Tsai CY, Chou TC. Bone morphogenetic proteins and Dickkopf-1 in ankylosing spondylitis. *Scand J Rheumatol.* 2018;47:56–61.

99. Xie Z, Wang P, Li Y, et al. Imbalance between bone morphogenetic protein 2 and noggin induces abnormal osteogenic differentiation of mesenchymal stem cells in ankylosing spondylitis. *Arthritis Rheumatol.* 2016;68:430–440.

100. Joo YB, Bang SY, Kim TH, et al. Bone morphogenetic protein 6 polymorphisms are associated with radiographic progression in ankylosing spondylitis. *PloS One.* 2014;9:e104966.

101. Monroe DG, McGee-Lawrence ME, Oursler MJ, Westendorf JJ. Update on Wnt signaling in bone cell biology and bone disease. *Gene.* 2012;492:1–18.

102. Duan P, Bonewald LF. The role of the wnt/beta-catenin signaling pathway in formation and maintenance of bone and teeth. *Int J Biochem Cell Biol.* 2016;77:23–29.

103. Johnson ML, Harnish K, Nusse R, Van Hul W. LRP5 and Wnt signaling: a union made for bone. *J Bone Miner Res.* 2004;19:1749–1757.

104. Mao B, Wu W, Davidson G, et al. Kremen proteins are Dickkopf receptors that regulate Wnt/beta-catenin signaling. *Nature.* 2002;417:664–667.

105. Haynes KR, Pettit AR, Duan R, et al. Excessive bone formation in a mouse model of ankylosing spondylitis is associated with decreases in Wnt pathway inhibitors. *Arthritis Res Ther.* 2012;14:R253.

106. Uderhardt S, Diarra D, Katzenbeisser J, et al. Blockade of Dickkopf (DKK)-1 induces fusion of sacroiliac joints. *Ann Rheum Dis.* 2010;69:592–597.

107. Diarra D, Stolina M, Polzer K, et al. Dickkopf-1 is a master regulator of joint remodeling. *Nat Med.* 2007;13:156–163.

108. Klingberg E, Nurkkala M, Carlsten H, Forsblad-d'Elia H. Biomarkers of bone metabolism in ankylosing spondylitis in relation to osteoproliferation and osteoporosis. *J Rheumatol.* 2014;41:1349–1356.

109. Daoussis D, Liossis SN, Solomou EE, et al. Evidence that Dkk-1 is dysfunctional in ankylosing spondylitis. *Arthritis Rheum.* 2010;62:150–158.

110. Long F, Zhang XM, Karp S, Yang Y, McMahon AP. Genetic manipulation of hedgehog signaling in the endochondral skeleton reveals a direct role in the regulation of chondrocyte proliferation. *Development.* 2001;128:5099–5108.

111. Chen X, Macica CM, Nasiri A, Broadus AE. Regulation of articular chondrocyte proliferation and differentiation by indian hedgehog and parathyroid hormone-related protein in mice. *Arthritis Rheum.* 2008;58:3788–3797.

112. Ruiz-Heiland G, Horn A, Zerr P, et al. Blockade of the hedgehog pathway inhibits osteophyte formation in arthritis. *Ann Rheum Dis.* 2012;71:400–407.

113. Dittmann K, Wuelling M, Uhmann A, et al. Inactivation of patched1 in murine chondrocytes causes spinal fusion without inflammation. *Arthritis Rheumatol.* 2014;66:831–840.

114. Daoussis D, Filippopoulou A, Liossis SN, et al. Anti-TNFalpha treatment decreases the previously increased serum Indian Hedgehog levels in patients with ankylosing spondylitis and affects the expression of functional Hedgehog pathway target genes. *Semin Arthritis Rheum.* 2015;44:646–651.

115. Aschermann S, Englbrecht M, Bergua A, et al. Presence of HLA-B27 is associated with changes of serum levels of mediators of the Wnt and hedgehog pathway. *Joint Bone Spine.* 2016;83:43–46.

116. Morand EF, Leech M, Weedon H, Metz C, Bucala R, Smith MD. Macrophage migration inhibitory factor in rheumatoid arthritis: clinical correlations. *Rheumatology.* 2002;41:558–562.

117. Radstake TR, Sweep FC, Welsing P, et al. Correlation of rheumatoid arthritis severity with the genetic functional variants and circulating levels of macrophage migration inhibitory factor. *Arthritis Rheum.* 2005;52:3020–3029.

118. Kozaci LD, Sari I, Alacacioglu A, Akar S, Akkoc N. Evaluation of inflammation and oxidative stress in ankylosing spondylitis: a role for macrophage migration inhibitory factor. *Mod Rheumatol.* 2010;20:34–39.

119. Ranganathan V, Ciccia F, Zeng F, et al. Macrophage migration inhibitory factor induces inflammation and predicts spinal progression in ankylosing spondylitis. *Arthritis Rheumatol.* 2017;69:1796–1806.

120. Onodera S, Nishihira J, Yamazaki M, Ishibashi T, Minami A. Increased expression of macrophage migration inhibitory factor during fracture healing in rats. *Histochem Cell Biol.* 2004;121:209–217.

121. Jacquin C, Koczon-Jaremko B, Aguila HL, et al. Macrophage migration inhibitory factor inhibits osteoclastogenesis. *Bone.* 2009;45:640–649.

122. Mun SH, Won HY, Hernandez P, Aguila HL, Lee SK. Deletion of CD74, a putative MIF receptor, in mice enhances osteoclastogenesis and decreases bone mass. *J Bone Miner Res.* 2013;28:948–959.

123. Movila A, Ishii T, Albassam A, et al. Macrophage migration inhibitory factor (MIF) supports homing of osteoclast precursors to peripheral osteolytic lesions. *J Bone Miner Res.* 2016;31:1688–1700.

124. Xiong C, Huang Y, Kang H, Zhang T, Xu F, Cai X. Macrophage inhibition factor-mediated CD74 signal modulate inflammation and matrix metabolism in the degenerated cartilage endplate chondrocytes by activating extracellular signal regulated kinase 1/2. *Spine.* 2017;42:E61–E70.

125. Gu R, Santos LL, Ngo D, et al. Macrophage migration inhibitory factor is essential for osteoclastogenic mechanisms in vitro and in vivo mouse model of arthritis. *Cytokine.* 2015;72:135–145.

126. Razawy W, van Driel M, Lubberts E. The role of IL-23 receptor signaling in inflammation-mediated erosive autoimmune arthritis and bone remodeling. *Eur J Immunol.* 2018;48:220–229.

127. Wang X, Lin Z, Wei Q, Jiang Y, Gu J. Expression of IL-23 and IL-17 and effect of IL-23 on IL-17 production in ankylosing spondylitis. *Rheumatol Int.* 2009;29:1343–1347.

128. Ugur M, Baygutalp NK, Melikoglu MA, Baygutalp F, Altas EU, Seferoglu B. Elevated serum interleukin-23 levels in ankylosing spondylitis patients and the relationship with disease activity. *Nagoya J Med Sci.* 2015;77:621–627.

129. Chen L, Wei XQ, Evans B, Jiang W, Aeschlimann D. IL-23 promotes osteoclast formation by up-regulation of receptor activator of NF-kappaB (RANK) expression in myeloid precursor cells. *Eur J Immunol.* 2008;38:2845–2854.

130. Quinn JM, Sims NA, Saleh H, et al. IL-23 inhibits osteoclastogenesis indirectly through lymphocytes and is required for the maintenance of bone mass in mice. *J Immunol.* 2008;181:5720–5729.

131. Sherlock JP, Joyce-Shaikh B, Turner SP, et al. IL-23 induces spondyloarthropathy by acting on ROR-gammat+

CD3+CD4-CD8- entheseal resident T cells. *Nat Med.* 2012;18:1069–1076.

132. Jo S, Koo BS, Lee B, et al. A novel role for bone-derived cells in ankylosing spondylitis: focus on IL-23. *Biochem Biophys Res Commun.* 2017;491:787–793.

133. Lubberts E. The IL-23-IL-17 axis in inflammatory arthritis. *Nat Rev Rheumatol.* 2015;11:415–429.

134. Osta B, Lavocat F, Eljaafari A, Miossec P. Effects of Interleukin-17A on osteogenic differentiation of isolated human mesenchymal stem cells. *Front Immunol.* 2014;5:425.

135. Croes M, Oner FC, van Neerven D, et al. Proinflammatory T cells and IL-17 stimulate osteoblast differentiation. *Bone.* 2016;84:262–270.

136. Ono T, Okamoto K, Nakashima T, et al. IL-17-producing gammadelta T cells enhance bone regeneration. *Nat Commun.* 2016;7:10928.

137. Kim YG, Park JW, Lee JM, et al. IL-17 inhibits osteoblast differentiation and bone regeneration in rat. *Arch Oral Biol.* 2014;59:897–905.

138. Yoshida K, Oida H, Kobayashi T, et al. Stimulation of bone formation and prevention of bone loss by prostaglandin E EP4 receptor activation. *Proc Natl Acad Sci USA.* 2002;99:4580–4585.

139. Li M, Healy DR, Li Y, et al. Osteopenia and impaired fracture healing in aged EP4 receptor knockout mice. *Bone.* 2005;37:46–54.

140. Yao C, Sakata D, Esaki Y, et al. Prostaglandin E2-EP4 signaling promotes immune inflammation through Th1 cell differentiation and Th17 cell expansion. *Nat Med.* 2009;15:633–640.

141. Boniface K, Bak-Jensen KS, Li Y, et al. Prostaglandin E2 regulates Th17 cell differentiation and function through cyclic AMP and EP2/EP4 receptor signaling. *J Exp Med.* 2009;206:535–548.

142. Ma X, Aoki T, Narumiya S. Prostaglandin E2-EP4 signaling persistently amplifies CD40-mediated induction of IL-23 p19 expression through canonical and noncanonical NF-kappaB pathways. *Cell Mol Immunol.* 2016;13:240–250.

143. Gagliardi MC, Teloni R, Mariotti S, et al. Endogenous PGE2 promotes the induction of human Th17 responses by fungal ss-glucan. *J Leukoc Biol.* 2010;88:947–954.

CHAPTER 8

Bone Pathophysiology in Axial Spondyloarthritis

RIK LORIES, MD, PHD

INTRODUCTION

Back pain, progressive stiffness, and increasing disability are characteristic symptoms of axial spondyloarthritis (axSpA), a common chronic inflammatory skeletal disease. The clinical signs are related to the presence of inflammation and of eventual bony ankylosis or fusion of the spine and sacroiliac joints (Fig. 8.1). The disease definition of axial spondyloarthritis has been defined by ASAS (Assessment of SpondyloArthritis International Society),[1] and the entity includes two forms: radiographic and nonradiographic axSpA (nraxSpA). Radiographic axSpA is largely identical to the formerly defined disease ankylosing spondylitis (AS), which can be classified using the modified New York criteria.[2] AS is distinguished from nraxSpA by the presence as opposed to the absence of structural damage to the bone that can be detected on conventional radiography. AxSpA is the main form of spondyloarthritis (SpA), a disease concept that also includes psoriatic arthritis (PsA), inflammatory bowel disease (IBD)–related arthritis, reactive arthritis (ReA), juvenile onset SpA, and undifferentiated SpA forms.

Remarkably, changes to the bony skeleton in axSpA are not only limited to the characteristic new bone formation that is leading to ankylosis but also include bone loss.[3] This apparent paradox may help to understand the underlying mechanisms as discussed below. In addition, it has become clear that not only the ankylosis process but also the loss of bone has clinical impact.[3]

Active inflammation and structural damage both contribute to the burden of disease for patients with axSpA.[5] The introduction of nuclear magnetic resonance imaging (NMR) has allowed the visualization of inflammatory processes in the spine and identified osteitis, enthesitis, and synovitis as key presentations. Clinically, these will translate as pain, stiffness, and loss of function.[6,7] On the other hand, structural damage has a complex impact on the patient. The effects can be explained by direct and indirect mechanisms. New bone formation leads to ankylosis of adjacent vertebrae and is the hallmark feature when studying structural progression of the disease.[8] Ankylosis of a specific segment of the spine will have a direct impact on mobility. In addition, structural changes will also have a mechanical consequence, for instance, leading to increased load in segments of the spine adjacent to the ankylosed vertebral bodies. Therefore, clinical management of patients with axSpA needs to take these factors into account, and the importance of addressing biomechanical problems in addition to treating inflammation cannot be underestimated.[9,10]

Interestingly, bone loss can appear as systemic bone loss, in particular in the vertebral bodies, and thereby increase the risk of spinal fractures.[3] In addition, bone erosions can be recognized, in particular, in the sacroiliac joints but also at the endplates of the vertebrae.

Studying structural damage in axSpA is not an easy task: human tissues are not readily available, ankylosis is a relatively slow process, and animal models can only partially mimic the human disorder. These challenges are not limited to better understanding of the molecular and cellular mechanisms of disease but equally include the clinical assessment and the impact of therapeutic interventions. Effectively, such clinical studies require a long-term follow-up. A key question in this context is the relationship between inflammation and new bone formation and the impact of current advanced therapies such as inhibition of cytokines tumor necrosis factor (TNF) and interleukin-17 (IL17). As further discussed below, the initial impact of these interventions may have been smaller than anticipated, but emerging data clearly suggest that long-term benefits at group and individual level can be expected.[11,12]

Axial Spondyloarthritis. https://doi.org/10.1016/B978-0-323-56800-5.00008-4

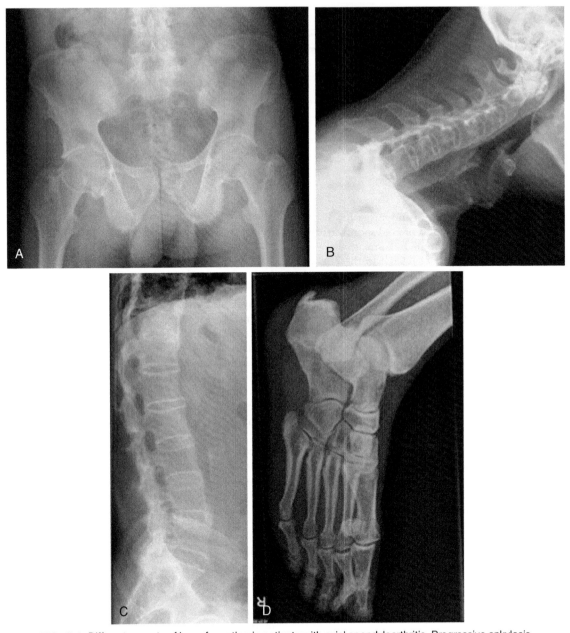

FIG. 8.1 Different aspects of bone formation in patients with axial spondyloarthritis. Progressive ankylosis of **(A)** the sacroiliac joints, **(B)** cervical spine, **(C)** lumbar spine. **(D)** An example of new bone formation at the Achilles' tendon insertion (enthesophytes). (Credit: reproduced from Lories RJ, Schett G. Pathophysiology of new bone formation and ankylosis in spondyloarthritis. *Rheum Dis Clin North Am*. 2012;38(3):555–567.)

CLINICAL IMPORTANCE OF BONE DISEASE IN AXSPA

Inflammation appears to be the main determinant of clinical symptoms in the initial phase of axSpA, whereas progression of ankylosis becomes more important as disease duration increases.[5] Therefore, assessment of the clinical and functional burden, and of the outcome of disease in these patients, should take into account both inflammation and structural damage to the spine. Mobility is negatively influenced by both spinal inflammation and the structural damage with its irreversible character, with a clear impact of both features on overall function.[5,13]

The emerging picture of these interactions remains complex. For instance, recent data suggest that in case of successful achievement of low disease activity after treatment with TNF inhibitors, overall functioning measured by scales such as the BASFI (Bath AS functional index) remained stable despite the presence of measurable disease progression. Additionally, fluctuation in clinical disease activity rather than structural disease progression predicted loss of function in this study.[14]

Although often overlooked by the striking visual and functional impact of ankylosis due to new bone formation, systemic bone loss also contributes to the burden of disease.[3] This systemic bone loss may evolve into clinically relevant osteoporosis and fractures. Different factors are likely contributing to this aspect of bone disease: the presence of proinflammatory cytokines that stimulate osteoclast differentiation and maturation, the lack of physical activity secondary to pain or limited spinal mobility, or malabsorption linked to the presence of inflammatory bowel disease.

The clinical impact of osteoporosis and associated factors in axSpA is important and may lead to severe complications, for example, when vertebral fractures in an ankylosed spine lead to acute neurologic complications.[15] Indeed, the combination of spinal ankylosis and trabecular bone loss secondary to inflammation puts the patients at risk for low-impact trauma fractures indicating that a systematic and in-depth clinical and imaging approach after low-impact trauma in axSpA patients should be part of the clinical care to avoid late-stage neurologic lesions due to fracture-associated instability of the spine. The risk for the occurrence of vertebral and nonvertebral fractures in patients with AS has been investigated in metaanalyses and clearly demonstrated a higher risk for vertebral, but not for hip, fractures.[3,16,17] Characteristics identified as major risk factors include male sex, disease duration, extent of structural damage on imaging, and low bone mineral density at hip and femoral neck.[17] These observations underline the importance of timely screening performed with dual-energy X-ray absorptiometry (DXA). Yet this is often difficult as BMD measurement of the spine in an anterior-posterior view can be inaccurate due to concurrent ankylosis.[3] DXA of the hip or lateral spine can be performed as an alternative, or the use of quantitative computed tomography can be considered when performance of DXA is not possible.[18]

THE MOLECULAR MECHANISMS UNDERLYING THE BONE FORMATION PROCESS

The ankylosis process in axSpA is an integral part of the disease and therefore pathologic but likely shares molecular mechanisms with physiologic bone forming processes as they occur during skeletal development and growth.[4] Therefore, important lessons can be learned from insights into these processes (Fig. 8.2). During development and growth, two distinct mechanisms can be recognized: endochondral bone formation (in which first a cartilage template is formed that is subsequently replaced by bone) and the direct differentiation of progenitor cells into bone formation, defined as membranous bone formation.[19] The former process establishes the shape of the bone and is continued in the growth plates. The latter is essential for cortical bone formation and growth. In addition, some bones of the skeleton, in particular, those of the skull, are entirely formed by membranous bone formation. During endochondral bone differentiation, progenitor cells first proliferate and form a cell condensation. Within that specific cell mass, cartilage differentiation is triggered. The chondrocytes proliferate and differentiate and ultimately become hypertrophic. The large hypertrophic chondrocytes produce a specific matrix that gets calcified, and these chondrocytes are replaced by osteoblasts differentiated from osteoprogenitor cells,[19] or they may transdifferentiate toward bone cells.[20]

After birth, skeletal homeostasis is maintained by the continuous renewal of bone in a process called bone remodeling that is based on the balanced activities of the bone-forming osteoblasts and the bone-resorbing osteoclasts.[4] Based on limited observations in human samples and on insights gained in mouse models, some zones with endochondral and membranous new bone formation can be recognized in axSpA.

Based on these similarities, it should not come as a surprise that molecular signaling pathways that drive ankylosis in axSpA include growth factors that are also playing a role in bone development, growth, and homeostasis, such as bone morphogenetic proteins (BMPs), Wnts, and Hedgehogs. In vitro, ex vivo, and animal model data provide strong support for this concept.[21]

Wnt

The Wnt signaling pathway plays an important role in skeletal development and growth.[22] Moreover, it is key regulator of the homeostatic bone remodeling throughout life. The balance between Wnts and some of their extracellular binding antagonists such

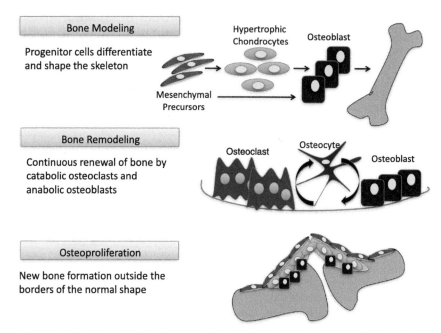

FIG. 8.2 Concepts of bone formation. Bone modeling is a developmental process that determines the shape and structure of the skeleton. In this well-orchestrated process, progenitors differentiate by endochondral or direct bone formation. Bone remodeling refers to the continuous renewal of the skeleton by bone-resorbing osteoclasts (multinucleated cells) and bone-forming osteoblasts. The osteocytes are mechanosensitive cells and orchestrate the bone remodeling cycle. Bone modeling in SpA is a disease-associated process, in which new bone formation is occurring outside the original borders of the skeleton. (Credit: reproduced from Lories RJ, Schett G. Pathophysiology of new bone formation and ankylosis in spondyloarthritis. *Rheum Dis Clin North Am.* 2012;38(3):555–567.)

as sclerostin is essential in the adaptation of bone toward mechanical loading. Wnt proteins make up a specific family of at least 15 secreted glycoproteins.[22] Complex interactions with different receptors can activate different signaling cascades, of which the beta-catenin-dependent canonical pathway is best studied.[22] The impact of Wnt signaling on new bone formation and ankylosis has been impressively demonstrated in a murine model that is characterized by the overexpression of TNF.[23] Systemic overexpression of human TNF leads to arthritis with prominent joint erosions and the complete absence of new bone formation, thus mimicking rheumatoid arthritis. However, administration of antibodies directed against Wnt antagonist Dickkopf-1 (DKK1) reverts this process. In the absence of any impact on inflammation, the structural damage phenotype is dramatically shifted from erosive disease toward ankylosing processes. Hence active Wnt signaling appears to stimulate the bone formation process.[23] First observed in the peripheral joints that are primarily affected in this

model, further investigation also identified inflammation and new bone formation in the sacroiliac joints.[24] Of particular interest from the clinical point of view, levels of Wnt antagonists such as DKK1 have been suggested as biomarkers for radiographic progression in patients with axSpA.[25]

Bone Morphogenetic Proteins

BMPs were originally identified as proteins isolated from the bone extracellular matrix that were capable of inducing new bone formation in vivo.[26] Thus, these potent growth factors were hypothesized to also play a role in the pathologic bone formation that characterizes axSpA. The first evidence that BMPs can play a role in the process of ankylosis was provided by studies in a mouse model of ankylosing enthesitis.[27] Upon grouped caging, male DBA/1 mice spontaneously develop peripheral arthritis of the toes of the hind-paws. Pathology analysis shows that the clinically apparent arthritis is caused by a short-lived phase of acute inflammation followed by extensive bone remodeling starting from the enthesis.[28] Distinct BMPs were identified in the progressive phase of the model, and overexpression of BMP-inhibitor noggin halted the pathologic bone-forming process in both preventive and therapeutic experiments.[27]

Translational evidence for the involvement of BMPs as well as for Wnts in axSpA patients unfortunately remains limited. Histologic analysis suggests that active BMP signaling is found in the entheses of patients with peripheral SpA and enthesophyte formation.[27] Bone marrow stromal cell–derived mesenchymal stem cells (MSCs) from patients with AS appear to have an enhanced potential for osteogenic differentiation in comparison with controls.[29] This effect was explained by an imbalance between the levels of BMP2 and its antagonist noggin.[29] Of note, AS patients have increased levels of autoantibodies directed against noggin,[30] a remarkable observation that could indicate that the excessive bone formation is influenced by blocking the activity of a BMP antagonist. Of note, single nucleotide polymorphisms in the BMP6 gene were demonstrated to be associated with the degree of radiographic severity in AS.[31]

Hedgehogs

The hedgehog signaling pathway is a key regulator of bone development and growth as it stimulates the important differentiation of the chondrocytes toward hypertrophic cells. This transition is essential to replace the transient cartilage by bone. This principle could also apply to the process of ankylosis in axSpA. Effectively, inhibition of hedgehog signaling reduced osteophyte formation in the postinflammatory phase of an antibody-driven serum transfer mouse model of arthritis.[32] The effect was obtained by administration of a small molecule antagonist to the pathway. The authors argue that this pathway could be of particular interest for patient management, as the transition toward hypertrophy allows for more specific targeting that modulates the BMP and Wnt cascades that may have broader effects.[32] If this assumption is correct, targeting hedgehog may trigger less safety concerns that targets BMP and Wnt signaling. However, these concepts have not been tested in a patient context and should therefore be treated with caution.

An important question that remains open with regard to all of the abovementioned pathways is the precise reason for their renewed activation in the context of axSpA. Obvious factors put forward include the presence of inflammation and the different involved cytokines, as well as biomechanical factors. The latter concept is based on the central role of the enthesis in

the disease process. Indeed, the insertions of tendons and ligaments are not only sites of important biomechanical stress but also the sites where the first signs of new bone formation are often seen, in particular in rodent models.

DISEASE MECHANISMS—THE RELATIONSHIP BETWEEN INFLAMMATION AND NEW BONE FORMATION

Biologic therapies using antibodies or soluble receptors against cytokines TNF and interleukin-17 (IL17) have dramatically altered the therapeutic approach toward management of patients with axSpA.[33] Their efficacy in controlling signs and symptoms of the disease and the enormous impact on the quality of life of the patients are unprecedented. Interestingly, strong data also support that control of inflammation using anti-TNF molecules strongly reduced osteoporotic bone loss in axSpA patients.[16] Similar effects are anticipated with targeting IL17 as this cytokine boosts osteoclast differentiation.[34] However, the impact of these strategies on progression of structural damage characterized by ankylosis is far more contested and has been subject of considerable debate.

Nonsteroidal Antiinflammatory Drugs

NSAIDs were the cornerstone of axSpA treatment before the introduction of biologicals and remain an obligatory first-line option.[35] Historical data suggested that NSAIDs may have an inhibitory effect on ankylosis based on the results of a retrospective analysis using the now obsolete drug.[36] More enthusiasm was generated with the introduction of the selective COX2 inhibitors, as a trial with celecoxib suggested that sustained rather than intermittent celecoxib use had a significant effect on structural disease progression.[37] However, recent data from the ENRADAS study in which the effect of diclofenac was assessed could not confirm this effect.[35] Decreased levels of prostaglandin E2 (PGE2), a molecule hypothesized to have a stimulatory effect on osteoblast activity, were hypothesized to mediate such an effect. The question whether a specific COX2 inhibitor would be different from a conventional NSAID has not been assessed in this context. The impact of these data on clinical practice is also controversial: sustained therapy with NSAIDs, COX2 specific or not, and its perceived effect on structural disease progression may not outmatch the eventual side effects of the drug, in particular with concerns about the cardiovascular safety of COX2 inhibitors in at-risk populations.

TNF

Recent data indicate that sustained inhibition of inflammation by TNF antagonists in patients with axSpA had a slow but significant effect on structural disease progression.[11,12] This observation is in line with the clear clinical effect of the drugs not only in terms of short-term signs and symptoms but also the overall impact on functionality of the patients. Nevertheless, this concept has not always been clear and does not necessarily entail that the proinflammatory cytokine TNF would be a direct driver of the ankylosing process. In contrast, the effects on pathology-associated bone loss, typically triggered by increased osteoclast activity, can be more easily attributed to a direct effect of TNF.[38]

The original follow-up cohort studies associated with the key clinical trials for different anti-TNF molecules did not observe a significant effect on new bone formation within a 2-year time window compared with a historical control cohort.[39–41] In addition, animal models had previously suggested that blocking TNF was insufficient to control the process of ankylosing enthesitis in mice,[42] thereby suggesting that inflammation and new bone formation may be linked, but also molecularly independent processes.[43] The new bone formation process is indeed strongly associated with the activation of growth factor cascades as highlighted above. Moreover, in TNF overexpression models, the striking phenotype is bone destruction and no signs of ankylosis in the joints are recognized.[23,44]

As a consequence, the TNF-brake hypothesis was introduced and suggested that TNF directly inhibits new bone formation by increasing the levels of Wnt inhibitor DKK-1.[45] However, the basis for this hypothesis could not be substantiated, as this view would eventually suggest that progressive ankylosis could be accelerated by achieving control of inflammation. Such an observation has not been made in any of the pivotal human studies.[46]

Recently emerging data provide evidence that over the long term, anti-TNF will have a measurable structural effect. Haroon et al. first suggested that this occurs in patients where treatment was started in the early disease phase or when the treatment is continued beyond a 4-year period.[11] These data were corroborated by a recent study by Maas et al.[12] who showed a deflection in the linear course of structural progression in the spine after 6 and 8 years of TNF inhibition. Based on these observations, we have proposed that active inflammation acts as an indirect trigger for ankylosis by triggering loss of bone and spinal instability as further discussed below.[47] However, some in vitro studies on human mesenchymal stem cells suggested that TNF can have both stimulating and inhibitory effects on differentiation toward osteoblasts. The in vitro settings are in the way of a clear concept, as the effects appear to be strongly dependent on concentration and type of growth factor used and on the specific cells under investigation.[38]

In conclusion, the promising long-term results increasingly support the concept that sustained inhibition of inflammation by TNF antagonists will extend its beneficial effects on signs, symptoms, and functionality toward inhibition of structural disease progression. The underlying mechanisms proposed are the inhibition of triggers for new bone formation, a feature that could occur at the tissue or the molecular level, and obviously also the prevention of disease development in previously unaffected places.

IL17

Targeting IL17 was recently welcomed as a new option to treat axSpA patients.[48] The concept of targeting IL17 is strongly supported by genetic data and animal models.[49] Like TNF, it is possible that IL17 or its inhibition has an effect on both aspects of bone involvement in axSpA. Effectively, IL17 can trigger the production of RANKL, an essential factor for osteoclast differentiation and maturation, and therefore appears to stimulate inflammation-associated bone loss.[50] Such effects not only may have local consequences on the development of bone erosions but can also play at a systemic level leading to osteoporosis. In an interesting study, overexpression of IL17 in the skin of mice resulted not only in a psoriasis-like skin rash but also in bone loss.[51] Additional evidence supports the view that IL17 may also negatively affect osteoblast activity, thereby again contributing to loss of bone.[51,52]

Obviously, structural disease progression data are eagerly anticipated for IL17 inhibitors. Animal model data have further sparked this interest. In the model of ankylosing enthesitis that spontaneously occurs in male DBA/1 mice, inhibition of IL17 may be effective in preventing ankylosis.[53] Two years' data for secukinumab, a monoclonal antibody directed against IL17A, and new bone formation have become available.[54] This initial evidence suggests a low rate of radiographic progression during this time window, but long-term data will be necessary to find any evidence of differences with the TNF inhibitors. Such comparison will require a high level of caution. Data from different studies cannot directly be compared, as setup and populations may differ and as the availability of anti-TNF drugs at the moment where studies with anti-IL17 have been performed may have influenced the selection of patients that are considered to participate in current clinical trials.

WHAT IS DRIVING THE ANKYLOSING PROCESS?—NOVEL CONCEPTS

Mechanical loading and associated biomechanical stress at the cell or tissue level may play an important role in diseases such as axSpA. The sacroiliac joints provide a good example of this concept. Despite their limited range of motion, these joints connect the axial with the lower appendicular skeleton, thereby translating biomechanical forces from the upper body to the legs.[47] Any disease process affecting the spine or the sacroiliac joints will likely at least be influenced by these loads and forces. At the tissue level, axSpA and other forms of SpA have been linked with enthesitis as primary disease manifestations. The enthesis is a transition tissue connecting ligaments, tendons, and capsules with bone. In daily life, it appears likely that repetitive movements and associated entheseal strain will result in varying degrees of microdamage. In genetically susceptible individuals, this microdamage may become one of the triggers for inflammation. Likewise, microdamage may be the driven force behind an excessive attempt to repair. Within this concept, the progressive process of new bone formation leading to ankylosis would become a pathologic repair response triggered by microdamage and inflammation (Fig. 8.3). The seminal discovery that the enthesis in mice is also populated by a low amount of innate lymphoid cell–like T cells[55] suggests that such immune cells could play a role in detecting microdamage and initiating a repair response, a process in which IL17 may play a role.[56] Recent data suggest that such cells may also be found in humans.[56]

This hypothesis is further supported by the observation that reduction of biomechanical loading in the hind-paws by tail suspension was able to inhibit severity of arthritis in a TNF overexpression-driven mouse model, in which the cytokine is enhanced in those sites that have a natural expression of this disease-driving cytokine.[44] However, in this model, no new bone formation is recognized most likely due to the continued high levels of TNF. Alternatively, in the repair phase of an anticollagen type II antibody–driven mouse model of arthritis where inflammation wanes over time, tail suspension was effective in reducing the late ankylosing process of the peripheral joints.

Consequentially, inflammation can indeed be recognized and confirmed as key trigger for the ankylosing process. Two different cascades of events may play a role. First, local microdamage may trigger tissue resident progenitor cells to form new bone, a process that appears to be constrained by persisting inflammation. However, much like what is seen in rodent models, shifts in the extent and intensity of inflammation may provide windows for ill-directed repair efforts. Secondly, and maybe more importantly, inflammation results in local and systemic bone loss, a phenomenon particularly important in the spine. Bone loss in the trabeculae of the vertebral bodies and in the subchondral zones of the sacroiliac joints may lead to osteoporosis and fractures and is therefore directly clinically relevant. Additionally, loss of bone will affect the biomechanical properties of the spine and the sacroiliac joints, triggering instability at the tissue level. In an effort to regain stability, bone-forming processes are likely activated. However, the continued presence of inflammation in the vertebral bodies may inhibit any of these efforts at this site. In contrast, stability may be increased by

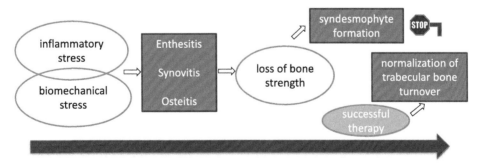

FIG. 8.3 Proposed sequence of events leading to ankylosis in axial spondyloarthritis. Inflammation at the enthesis, vertebral body, and synovium is triggered by inflammatory and biomechanical stress leading to bone loss. Reduced bone strength triggers a stabilizing anabolic effort resulting in syndesmophyte formation and progressive ankylosis. Successful treatment reduces inflammation and allows the bone metabolism to normalize, thereby taking away instability as driver of ankylosis. (Credit: reproduced from Neerinckx B, Lories RJ. Structural disease progression in axial spondyloarthritis: still a cause for concern? *Curr Rheumatol Rep*. 2017;19(3):14.)

the ankylosing process, compensatory stability for the spine but with a loss of normal mobility as the price to pay.[57]

CONCLUSION

AxSpA is characterized by inflammation and new bone formation, two different features that both can substantially contribute to the burden and impact of disease. New bone formation is an important feature of the disease, as it can lead to spinal or sacroiliac joint ankylosis, reduced mobility, and increased disability. Sometimes underestimated, partial ankylosis of the spine or the sacroiliac joints may fundamentally change the biomechanical properties of the axial skeleton and represent a trigger for mechanically induced pain. The direct or indirect role of inflammation in the onset and further progression of axSpA have been debated, and the full picture is not yet clear. Accumulating evidence does suggest that effective and sustained control of inflammation by specific interventions such as anti-TNF and anti-IL17 will have a positive long-term effect on structural damage including ankylosis.

CONFLICT OF INTEREST STATEMENT

Original research by the author is supported by FWO Vlaanderen and an "OT"-grant from KU Leuven. Leuven Research and Development, the technology transfer office of KU Leuven, has received speaker's and consultancy fees on behalf of R.L from Abbvie, Boehringer-Ingelheim, Celgene, Lilly, Janssen, Novartis, Merck, and Pfizer.

REFERENCES

1. Rudwaleit M, van der Heijde D, Landewe R, et al. The development of Assessment of SpondyloArthritis international Society classification criteria for axial spondyloarthritis (part II): validation and final selection. *Ann Rheum Dis.* 2009;68(6):777–783.
2. van der Linden S, Valkenburg HA, Cats A. Evaluation of diagnostic criteria for ankylosing spondylitis. A proposal for modification of the New York criteria. *Arthritis Rheum.* 1984;27(4):361–368.
3. Carter S, Lories RJ. Osteoporosis: a paradox in ankylosing spondylitis. *Curr Osteoporos Rep.* 2011;9(3):112–115.
4. Lories RJ, Schett G. Pathophysiology of new bone formation and ankylosis in spondyloarthritis. *Rheum Dis Clin N Am.* 2012;38(3):555–567.
5. Machado P, Landewe R, Braun J, Hermann KG, Baker D, van der Heijde D. Both structural damage and inflammation of the spine contribute to impairment of spinal mobility in patients with ankylosing spondylitis. *Ann Rheum Dis.* 2010;69(8):1465–1470.
6. Dougados M, Baeten D. Spondyloarthritis. *Lancet.* 2011;377(9783):2127–2137.
7. Lories RJ, Baeten DL. Differences in pathophysiology between rheumatoid arthritis and ankylosing spondylitis. *Clin Exp Rheumatol.* 2009;27(4 suppl 55):S10–S14.
8. Van Mechelen M, Gulino GR, de Vlam K, Lories R. Bone disease in axial spondyloarthritis. *Calcif Tissue Int.* 2018;102(5):547–558.
9. Vleeming A, Volkers AC, Snijders CJ, Stoeckart R. Relation between form and function in the sacroiliac joint. Part II: biomechanical aspects. *Spine.* 1990;15(2):133–136.
10. Vleeming A, Stoeckart R, Volkers AC, Snijders CJ. Relation between form and function in the sacroiliac joint. Part I: clinical anatomical aspects. *Spine.* 1990;15(2):130–132.
11. Haroon N, Inman RD, Learch TJ, et al. The impact of tumor necrosis factor alpha inhibitors on radiographic progression in ankylosing spondylitis. *Arthritis Rheum.* 2013;65(10):2645–2654.
12. Maas F, Arends S, Brouwer E, et al. Reduction in spinal radiographic progression in ankylosing spondylitis patients receiving prolonged treatment with TNF-alpha inhibitors. *Arthritis Care Res (Hoboken).* 2017;69(7):1011–1019.
13. Landewe R, Dougados M, Mielants H, van der Tempel H, van der Heijde D. Physical function in ankylosing spondylitis is independently determined by both disease activity and radiographic damage of the spine. *Ann Rheum Dis.* 2009;68(6):863–867.
14. Poddubnyy D, Fedorova A, Listing J, et al. Physical function and spinal mobility remain stable despite radiographic spinal progression in patients with ankylosing spondylitis treated with TNF-alpha inhibitors for up to 10 years. *J Rheumatol.* 2016;43(12):2142–2148.
15. Leone A, Marino M, Dell'Atti C, Zecchi V, Magarelli N, Colosimo C. Spinal fractures in patients with ankylosing spondylitis. *Rheumatol Int.* 2016;36(10):1335–1346.
16. Haroon NN, Sriganthan J, Al Ghanim N, Inman RD, Cheung AM. Effect of TNF-alpha inhibitor treatment on bone mineral density in patients with ankylosing spondylitis: a systematic review and meta-analysis. *Semin Arthritis Rheum.* 2014;44(2):155–161.
17. Pray C, Feroz NI, Haroon N. Bone mineral density and fracture risk in ankylosing spondylitis: a meta-analysis. *Calcif Tissue Int.* 2017;101(2):182–192.
18. Mandl P, Navarro-Compan V, Terslev L, et al. EULAR recommendations for the use of imaging in the diagnosis and management of spondyloarthritis in clinical practice. *Ann Rheum Dis.* 2015;74(7):1327–1339.
19. Lefebvre V, Bhattaram P. Vertebrate skeletogenesis. *Curr Top Dev Biol.* 2010;90:291–317.
20. Zhou X, von der Mark K, Henry S, Norton W, Adams H, de Crombrugghe B. Chondrocytes transdifferentiate into osteoblasts in endochondral bone during development, postnatal growth and fracture healing in mice. *PLoS Genet.* 2014;10(12):e1004820.
21. Gonzalez-Chavez SA, Quinonez-Flores CM, Pacheco-Tena C. Molecular mechanisms of bone formation in spondyloarthritis. *Joint Bone Spine.* 2016;83(4):394–400.

22. Nusse R, Clevers H. Wnt/beta-Catenin signaling, disease, and emerging therapeutic modalities. *Cell.* 2017;169(6):985–999.

23. Diarra D, Stolina M, Polzer K, et al. Dickkopf-1 is a master regulator of joint remodeling. *Nat Med.* 2007;13(2):156–163.

24. Uderhardt S, Diarra D, Katzenbeisser J, et al. Blockade of Dickkopf (DKK)-1 induces fusion of sacroiliac joints. *Ann Rheum Dis.* 2010;69(3):592–597.

25. Heiland GR, Appel H, Poddubnyy D, et al. High level of functional dickkopf-1 predicts protection from syndesmophyte formation in patients with ankylosing spondylitis. *Ann Rheum Dis.* 2012;71(4):572–574.

26. Urist MR. Bone: formation by autoinduction. *Science.* 1965;150(3698):893–899.

27. Lories RJ, Derese I, Luyten FP. Modulation of bone morphogenetic protein signaling inhibits the onset and progression of ankylosing enthesitis. *J Clin Investig.* 2005;115(6):1571–1579.

28. Lories RJ, Matthys P, de Vlam K, Derese I, Luyten FP. Ankylosing enthesitis, dactylitis, and onychoperiostitis in male DBA/1 mice: a model of psoriatic arthritis. *Ann Rheum Dis.* 2004;63(5):595–598.

29. Xie Z, Wang P, Li Y, et al. Imbalance between bone morphogenetic protein 2 and noggin induces abnormal osteogenic differentiation of mesenchymal stem cells in ankylosing spondylitis. *Arthritis Rheumatol.* 2016;68(2):430–440.

30. Tsui FW, Tsui HW, Las Heras F, Pritzker KP, Inman RD. Serum levels of novel noggin and sclerostin-immune complexes are elevated in ankylosing spondylitis. *Ann Rheum Dis.* 2014;73(10):1873–1879.

31. Joo YB, Bang SY, Kim TH, et al. Bone morphogenetic protein 6 polymorphisms are associated with radiographic progression in ankylosing spondylitis. *PLoS One.* 2014;9(8):e104966.

32. Ruiz-Heiland G, Horn A, Zerr P, et al. Blockade of the hedgehog pathway inhibits osteophyte formation in arthritis. *Ann Rheum Dis.* 2012;71(3):400–407.

33. Sieper J, Poddubnyy D. Axial spondyloarthritis. *Lancet.* 2017;390(10089):73–84.

34. Yago T, Nanke Y, Ichikawa N, et al. IL-17 induces osteoclastogenesis from human monocytes alone in the absence of osteoblasts, which is potently inhibited by anti-TNF-alpha antibody: a novel mechanism of osteoclastogenesis by IL-17. *J Cell Biochem.* 2009;108(4):947–955.

35. Sieper J, Listing J, Poddubnyy D, et al. Effect of continuous versus on-demand treatment of ankylosing spondylitis with diclofenac over 2 years on radiographic progression of the spine: results from a randomised multicentre trial (ENRADAS). *Ann Rheum Dis.* 2016;75(8):1438–1443.

36. Boersma JW. Retardation of ossification of the lumbar vertebral column in ankylosing spondylitis by means of phenylbutazone. *Scand J Rheumatol.* 1976;5(1):60–64.

37. Wanders A, Heijde Dv, Landewé R, et al. Nonsteroidal antiinflammatory drugs reduce radiographic progression in patients with ankylosing spondylitis: a randomized clinical trial. *Arthritis Rheum.* 2005;52(6):1756–1765.

38. Osta B, Benedetti G, Miossec P. Classical and paradoxical effects of TNF-alpha on bone homeostasis. *Front Immunol.* 2014;5:48.

39. van der Heijde D, Salonen D, Weissman BN, et al. Assessment of radiographic progression in the spines of patients with ankylosing spondylitis treated with adalimumab for up to 2 years. *Arthritis Res Ther.* 2009;11(4):R127.

40. van der Heijde D, Landewe R, Baraliakos X, et al. Radiographic findings following two years of infliximab therapy in patients with ankylosing spondylitis. *Arthritis Rheum.* 2008;58(10):3063–3070.

41. van der Heijde D, Landewe R, Einstein S, et al. Radiographic progression of ankylosing spondylitis after up to two years of treatment with etanercept. *Arthritis Rheum.* 2008;58(5):1324–1331.

42. Lories RJ, Derese I, de Bari C, Luyten FP. Evidence for uncoupling of inflammation and joint remodeling in a mouse model of spondylarthritis. *Arthritis Rheum.* 2007;56(2):489–497.

43. Lories RJ, Luyten FP, de Vlam K. Progress in spondylarthritis. Mechanisms of new bone formation in spondyloarthritis. *Arthritis Res Ther.* 2009;11(2):221.

44. Jacques P, Lambrecht S, Verheugen E, et al. Proof of concept: enthesitis and new bone formation in spondyloarthritis are driven by mechanical strain and stromal cells. *Ann Rheum Dis.* 2014;73(2):437–445.

45. Maksymowych WP, Chiowchanwisawakit P, Clare T, Pedersen SJ, Ostergaard M, Lambert RG. Inflammatory lesions of the spine on magnetic resonance imaging predict the development of new syndesmophytes in ankylosing spondylitis: evidence of a relationship between inflammation and new bone formation. *Arthritis Rheum.* 2009;60(1):93–102.

46. Baraliakos X, Haibel H, Listing J, Sieper J, Braun J. Continuous long-term anti-TNF therapy does not lead to an increase in the rate of new bone formation over 8 years in patients with ankylosing spondylitis. *Ann Rheum Dis.* 2014;73(4):710–715.

47. Van Mechelen M, Lories RJ. Microtrauma: no longer to be ignored in spondyloarthritis? *Curr Opin Rheumatol.* 2016;28(2):176–180.

48. Baeten D, Sieper J, Braun J, et al. Secukinumab, an Interleukin-17A inhibitor, in ankylosing spondylitis. *N Engl J Med.* 2015;373(26):2534–2548.

49. Cheung PP. Anti-IL17A in axial spondyloarthritis-where are we at? *Front Med (Lausanne).* 2017;4:1.

50. Croes M, Oner FC, van Neerven D, et al. Proinflammatory T cells and IL-17 stimulate osteoblast differentiation. *Bone.* 2016;84:262–270.

51. Uluckan O, Jimenez M, Karbach S, et al. Chronic skin inflammation leads to bone loss by IL-17-mediated inhibition of Wnt signaling in osteoblasts. *Sci Transl Med.* 2016;8(330):330ra337.

52. Uluckan O, Wagner EF. Role of IL-17A signalling in psoriasis and associated bone loss. *Clin Exp Rheumatol.* 2016;34(4 suppl 98):17–20.

53. Ebihara S, Date F, Dong Y, Ono M. Interleukin-17 is a critical target for the treatment of ankylosing enthesitis and psoriasis-like dermatitis in mice. *Autoimmunity.* 2015;48(4):259–266.

54. Braun J, Baraliakos X, Deodhar A, et al. Effect of secukinumab on clinical and radiographic outcomes in ankylosing spondylitis: 2-year results from the randomised phase III MEASURE 1 study. *Ann Rheum Dis.* 2017;76(6):1070–1077.

55. Sherlock JP, Joyce-Shaikh B, Turner SP, et al. IL-23 induces spondyloarthropathy by acting on ROR-gammat+ CD3+CD4-CD8- entheseal resident T cells. *Nat Med.* 2012;18(7):1069–1076.

56. Cuthbert RJ, Fragkakis EM, Dunsmuir R, et al. Human enthesis group 3 innate lymphoid cells. *Arthritis Rheumatol.* 2017;69(9):1816–1822.

57. Neerinckx B, Lories R. Mechanisms, impact and prevention of pathological bone regeneration in spondyloarthritis. *Curr Opin Rheumatol.* 2017;29(4):287–292.

58. Neerinckx B, Lories RJ. Structural disease progression in axial spondyloarthritis: still a cause for concern? *Curr Rheumatol Rep.* 2017;19(3):14.

CHAPTER 9

Clinical Assessment of Axial Spondyloarthritis

MARINA N. MAGREY, MD • UTA KILTZ, MD

INTRODUCTION

Spondyloarthritis (SpA) encompasses a group of complex diseases with highly varied manifestations (e.g., peripheral arthritis, spondylitis, enthesitis, dactylitis), resulting in highly variable patient experiences and impact on patient lives.[1-3] Patients with SpA may have predominant axial (axSpA) symptoms, and the major goal of management in these patients is to treat inflammation and to stop the structural damage, defined as new bone formation, resulting in complete or incomplete ankylosis of the spine. Because of the paucity of biomarkers for diagnosis, prognosis, disease activity, and predictive biomarkers of the response to biologic therapy in axSpA, a critical component of patient care includes a comprehensive assessment of disease activity, damage, and disability. Moreover, to reliably capture disease status and to measure treatment response, various assessment instruments have been developed.[4] There are two main types of outcome measures that are used clinically: "physician-reported outcomes" and "patient-reported outcomes."[5] Patient-reported outcomes (PROs) are pivotal in the assessment of global health, pain, stiffness, physical function, and decreased health-related quality of life (HRQoL). These outcome measures are quantifiable, reproducible, and easily measured in clinical practice. Based on treat-to-target recommendations in axSpA, the treatment target should be inactive disease/clinical remission and that low/minimal disease activity may be an alternative treatment target.[6] Hence, the emphasis is being placed not only on physician-reported outcomes but also on PROs to capture patient's experience of the disease and patient-perceived disability.[7] In this chapter, we will discuss various validated instruments that have been developed for clinical assessment of axSpA patients.

ASSESSMENT OF PATIENTS WITH AXIAL SPA

Assessment of disease status in axSpA encompasses measurement of pain, stiffness, fatigue, physical function, and HRQoL.[8] The various instruments used for assessment of patients with axSpA as shown in Table 9.1 were originally designed for use in patients with AS.

ASAS Core Set for Clinical Record Keeping

The Assessment of Spondyloarthritis Study Group (ASAS), a group of international experts in SpA, has established a core sets of variables to be measured in different settings as shown in Fig. 9.1 for assessment and monitoring of axSpA, including the ASAS cores set for clinical record keeping.[9,10] The core set includes the relevant domains, but specific instruments have been selected for each domain. The core set for clinical record keeping is shown in Table 9.2 and will be discussed in detail in this chapter.

ASSESSMENT OF DISEASE ACTIVITY IN AXIAL SPA

Bath Ankylosing Spondylitis Disease Activity Index

The evaluation of disease activity in axial SpA is complex and multifactorial with patients and physicians having a different perspective of the disease.[11] The Bath Ankylosing Spondylitis Disease Activity Index (BASDAI) is the traditional patient-reported outcome measure of disease activity in AS and is used routinely in clinical practice.[12] The questionnaire was initially created in Bath, England, and assesses the patient-reported severity of fatigue, spinal pain, peripheral joint pain, localized tenderness, quantity, and duration of morning stiffness using a 0–10 numeric rating scale (NRS) or 10-cm visual analog scale (VAS) with symptoms ranging from "none" to "very severe." The final BASDAI score is calculated by summing the first four questions and the average of the last two questions and dividing the result by 5. The score ranges from 0 (no disease activity) to 10 (very active disease). A cutoff of 4 is frequently used to define active disease, and a score of 4 or more is suggestive of high disease activity

Axial Spondyloarthritis. https://doi.org/10.1016/B978-0-323-56800-5.00009-6

warranting a change in therapy plan,[13,14] but this cut-off level does not have a firm justification. In addition, BASDAI scores did not correlate well with symptoms and clinical measurements of disease activity and/or MRI scores.[15,16]

TABLE 9.1
Showing Various Validated Instruments Developed for Clinical Assessment of Axial SpA

Measurement of Disease Activity	BASDAI, ASDAS, Enthesitis Index/Peripheral Joint Count, Acute Phase Reactants (ESR/CRP)
Measurement of physical function	BASFI, DFI, HAQ-S
Assessment of range of motion	BASMI
Disability/quality of life	ASASHI, ASQoL

ASASHI, ASAS Health Index; *ASDAS*, Ankylosing Spondylitis Disease Activity Index; *ASQoL*, Ankylosing Spondylitis Quality of Life; *BASDAI*, Bath Ankylosing Spondylitis Disease Activity Index; *BASFI*, Bath Ankylosing Spondylitis Functional Index; *BASMI*, Bath Ankylosing Spondylitis Metrology Index; *DFI*, Dougados Functional Index; *HAQ-S*, Health Assessment Questionnaire for the Spondyloarthropathies.

Given its ease in administration, interpretation, and a quick turnaround in results usually 0.5–2 min, the BASDAI has been successfully used not only in clinical practice but has been a gold standard for measuring disease activity in clinical trials. The tool is highly reliable with patients scoring similarly on consecutive days and highly sensitive to demonstrate an improvement in function as early as 3 weeks of physical therapy.[17] The minimum clinically important improvement (MCII) for BASDAI in patients with active disease (BASDAI> 4) has been identified to be 1.1 in one study.[18] However, fluctuations in reporting disease activity by using BASDAI have been seen and should be taken into account when treating a patient.[19] The ASAS group has described issues with the use of the traditional visual analog scale and instead now advocates for a switch to a numeric rating scale (NRS) as shown in Fig. 9.2. An important drawback of the BASDAI is that it is entirely patient-driven and many of the six items in the BASDAI are redundant (measuring the same construct), and they are not weighted.[20]

Ankylosing Spondylitis Disease Activity Score

To improve the objectivity of BASDAI, a highly discriminatory and validated instrument for assessing disease activity in SpA was developed in 2008 and was named

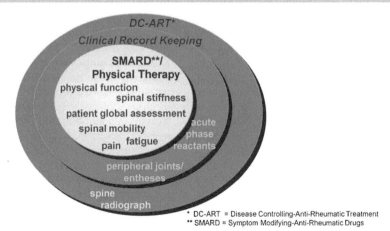

* DC-ART = Disease Controlling-Anti-Rheumatic Treatment
** SMARD = Symptom Modifying-Anti-Rheumatic Drugs

Adapted from van der Heijde D et al. J Rheumatol 1999;26:951-4 (with permission)
ASAS workshop Gent, Oct 2002

FIG. 9.1 Core domains for monitoring ankylosing spondylitis.

TABLE 9.2
ASAS Core Set for Clinical Record Keeping

Domain	Instrument
Physical function	*BASFI or DFI*
Pain	*VAS/NRS past week in spine, at night, due to AS and VAS/NRS past week, in spine due to AS*
Spinal mobility	Chest expansion and modified Schober and occiput-to-wall distance and lateral spinal flexion
Patient global assessment	*VAS/NRS past week*
Morning stiffness	*Duration of morning stiffness in spine past week*
Fatigue	*VAS/NRS past week*
Peripheral joints and entheses	A number of swollen joints (44 joint count) validated enthesitis indexes
Acute phase reactants	ESR

as the Ankylosing Spondylitis Disease Activity Score (ASDAS) and endorsed by ASAS.[21,22] The score includes patient-reported assessments of back pain (BASDAI question 2), duration of morning stiffness (BASDAI question 6), peripheral joint pain and/or swelling (BASDAI question 3), general well-being, and either the ESR (ASDAS-ESR) or the CRP (ASDAS-CRP) in a weighted manner. The ASDAS-CRP is recommended by ASAS, both for use in clinical practice and in clinical trials, but the ASDAS-ESR may be used as well. However, it should be clearly understood that these ASDAS versions with CRP or with ESR are not interchangeable. One version should be used consistently within patients or within a study. The ASDAS and aids for its calculation are available online at HYPERLINK "http://www.asas-group.org" and can also be calculated using an online calculator or an ASAP ASDAS App.

Various studies[23–25] have assessed the construct validity and responsiveness of the ASDAS and have found that its performance is better than patient-reported measures (including BASDAI) and acute-phase reactants, discriminating better between high and low disease activity status, and correlates well with changes in MRI inflammation scores at the sacroiliac joints or sacroiliac joints plus lumbar spine. The development and validation of ASDAS were based on conventional CRP values. It has been shown that when the

conventional CRP level is below the limit of detection or when the hsCRP level is <2 mg/L, the constant value of 2 mg/L should be used to calculate the ASDAS-CRP score.[26]

To define therapeutic goals and make treatment decisions objectively, one needs to understand various disease activity states and changes in them suggestive of response levels. It is particularly important to determine whether the treatment or the given intervention is working or not because the goal is to treat to the target. Cutoff values for disease activity states and improvement using the ASDAS have been developed. The same validated cutoff values apply to both the ASDAS-CRP and the ASDAS-ESR. The following cutoffs were initially selected with proven external validity and good performance: (1) ASDAS less than 1.3 to define inactive disease; (b) ASDAS greater or equal to 1.3 and less than 2.1 to define moderate disease activity; (3) ASDAS greater or equal to 2.1 and less than or equal to 3.5 to define high disease activity; (4) ASDAS greater than 3.5 to define very high disease activity. In the ASDAS cutoff validation study,[27] more patients achieved the inactive disease state compared with ASAS partial remission while retaining higher discriminatory capacity between treatment groups. Because ASDAS inactive disease is independent of structural damage, hence patients with the chronic deforming disease also easily achieve the score.

Recently the nomenclature of ASDAS was updated by ASAS. The "moderate disease activity" state is replaced by "low disease activity" state, better reflecting the opinion of patients and physicians about what ASDAS values ≥1.3 and <2.1 represent as shown in Fig. 9.3.[28] The reason for the change was based on the fact that the majority of patients in this ASDAS category have indeed mild disease activity, an observation that is in line with the external constructs that were used to derive the ASDAS cutoff of 2.1: patient and physician global assessments <3 using the 90% specificity criterion to determine the optimal cutoff.

The cutoffs selected for improvements were as follows:

1. .Change of 1.1 units for "clinically important improvement" (defined by using the patient's report of being "better" or "much better" since the start of treatment as an external criterion).
2. .Change of 2.0 units for "major improvement" (defined by using the patient's report of being "much better" since the start of treatment as an external criterion). Based on data-driven ASAS consensus process, the cutoff selected for "clinically important worsening" in axSpA is an increase in ASDAS of at least 0.9 points.[29]

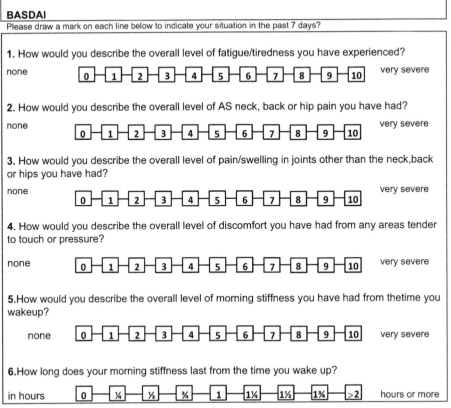

FIG. 9.2 BASDAI Numeric Rating Scale (questionnaire can be downloaded from www.asas-group.org).

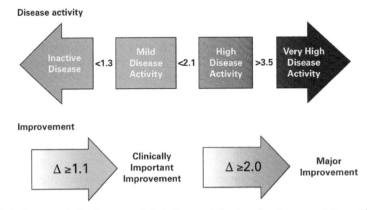

FIG. 9.3 Ankylosing spondylitis disease activity index—cutoff values for disease activity and improvement.

ASSESSING ENTHESITIS AND PERIPHERAL JOINTS IN AXSPA

Although axSpA predominantly affects axial skeleton, peripheral joint involvement and enthesitis are also important characteristics of the disease. Moreover, enthesitis in axSpA may define a subset of patients with the more severe disease. The first instrument for assessing enthesitis in axSpA is known as the Mander Enthesitis Index (MEI)[30] and includes 66 potential sites, graded for tenderness from 0 to 3 (0, no pain; 1, mild tenderness; 2,

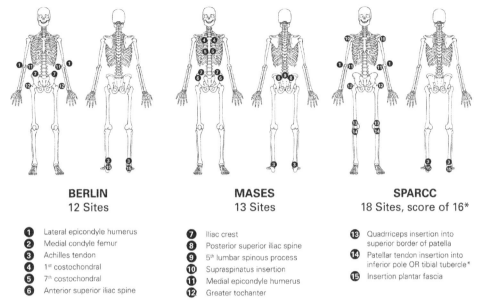

BERLIN	MASES	SPARCC
12 Sites	13 Sites	18 Sites, score of 16*

① Lateral epicondyle humerus
② Medial condyle femur
③ Achilles tendon
④ 1st costochondral
⑤ 7th costochondral
⑥ Anterior superior iliac spine

⑦ Iliac crest
⑧ Posterior superior iliac spine
⑨ 5th lumbar spinous process
⑩ Supraspinatus insertion
⑪ Medial epicondyle humerus
⑫ Greater tochanter

⑬ Quadrriceps insertion into superior border of patella
⑭ Patellar tendon insertion into inferior pole OR tibial tubercle*
⑮ Insertion plantar fascia

FIG. 9.4 Clinically feasible instruments to measure enthesitis in AxSpA. (Modified with permission from Mease PJ, et al. *J Rheumatol*. 2017;44(5). *All rights reserve*.)

moderate tenderness; or 3, tenderness severe enough to elicit a wince or withdrawal). These sites were identified from examination of patients with ankylosing spondylitis (AS) and subsequently validated in a similar group of AS patients. The MEI showed sensitivity to change in a large study of patients with ankylosing spondylitis,[31] but another study looking at the efficacy of infliximab in AS failed to demonstrate a change suggesting poor interobserver reliability and discrimination.[32] MEI has been found to be nonfeasible in clinical practice use because of time constraint.

Clinically feasible and validated instruments to measure entheseal inflammation have been developed as shown in Fig. 9.4. These include the Berlin Enthesitis Index (BEI),[33] the Maastricht AS Enthesitis Score (MASES),[34] and the San Francisco Index (SFI).[35] The SFI examines 17 sites with a scoring identical to the MEI. The MASES is easy to calculate and includes 13 sites as shown in Fig. 9.4. The BEI is similar to MASES and includes 12 sites. It did not perform better when tested in an AS study. Both the MASES and BEI are included in the ASAS core set for clinical evaluation.

Other validated enthesitis indices in axSpA include the Spondyloarthritis Research Consortium of Canada (SPARCC) Enthesitis Index, which was created using information from ultrasound and MRI studies.[36] The SPARCC score was developed using a full spectrum of SpA patients, but the feasibility and reproducibility were tested in a study using AS patients.[37] The study revealed that greater trochanter and supraspinatus entheses were the most frequently affected sites in these patients. The SPARCC Enthesitis Index has compared favorably with other instruments measuring enthesitis.[37] The Leeds Enthesitis Index (LEI) has been developed to measure entheseal inflammation in PsA and includes measurement of inflammation at six sites.[38] Both SPARCC and LEI are not included in the ASAS core sets as yet. ASAS does not recommend the use of enthesitis indices in daily clinical practice.

Peripheral joint involvement in axSpA is frequent and can be assessed using the 44-joint count. Presence of swelling is recorded, and the total score varies from 0 to 44.

SINGLE MEASURES FOR ASSESSING DISEASE ACTIVITY

Pain and Stiffness

Pain in axSpA is usually assessed by inquiring about the quantity of pain in the spine and how much of this pain is at night. The degree of both night pain and spinal pain during the day is measured by using either a VAS or an NRS. In general, the use of an NRS is preferred by patients and doctors. Morning stiffness in the spine is usually assessed for both aspects, duration and severity. Scores both for pain and morning stiffness (either on NRS or on VAS) range from 0 (none) to 10 (very severe). Pain and stiffness have a considerable influence on HRQoL in patients with AS. When assessing pain or stiffness, it is highly recommended to differentiate inflammatory from structural causes because of the impact on therapeutic options.

Fatigue

Patients with SpA are inquired about the overall level of fatigue as it has been described to be a major problem in patients with active AS, with up to 65% of the patients reporting this symptom.[39] The scores on the fatigue question of the BASDAI (question 1) have been shown to be significantly associated with scores on several dimensions of the quality of life instruments, suggesting that HRQoL is influenced by the degree of fatigue.[40] The degree of fatigue has also been assessed in controlled trials by using the Functional Assessment of Chronic Illness Therapy-Fatigue (FACIT-Fatigue) subscale, which is a 13-item composite score that uses a cross-cultural approach.[41]

Patient Global Assessment

The patient global assessment of disease activity is also very pertinent in axSpA as it gives the patient's perspective of his/her disease. It is usually assessed by the question: "How active was your spondyloarthritis in the last week?" and the answer is recorded on NRS or on a VAS with the score ranging from 0 (not active) to 10 (very active).[20] Treating physician can expect that a quarter of patient will report the global question discordant from the physician perspective.[42]

ASSESSMENT OF PHYSICAL FUNCTION

Monitoring of physical function in axSpA is a major outcome, as limited spinal mobility and decrease in function is a poor prognostic sign in these patients. Studies have shown that physical function in patients with axSpA is influenced not only by structural damage but also by disease activity (inflammation).[43-45] However, the function is also influenced by other factors including psychologic function and ability to cope with the disease.

Bath Ankylosing Spondylitis Functional Index

In 1994, a self-reported index using visual analog score was developed to define and monitor physical function in patients with AS.[46] The Bath Ankylosing Spondylitis Functional Index (BASFI) contains 10 questions related to activities of daily living, which are scored with a rating scale from 0 (no functional impairments) to 10 (maximal impairment). It contains eight items pertaining to everyday tasks and dependent on functional anatomy (bending, reaching, changing position, standing, turning, and climbing steps) and two items assessing the patients' ability to cope with everyday life. The mean of the individual scores is calculated to give the overall index score. It is available online at www.ASAS-group.org. The instrument is a reliable, valid, and feasible measure of physical function in patients with AS and takes less than 3 min to calculate. The minimum clinically important difference in BASFI from the patient's perspective has been reported as 7 mm or 17.5% with a sensitivity of 0.60 and specificity of 0.85, determined using receiver operating characteristic curve analyses.[47] However, the BASFI may not be sufficiently sensitive to detect subtle changes in functioning in patients without severe impairments.

Dougados Functional Index

It measures functional capacity of a person by assessing various activities of daily living; addressing aspects of dressing, bathing, standing, climbing stairs, bending, changing position, doing housework, coughing, and breathing deeply.[48] It uses a 3-point Likert response scale as follows: 0 = yes, with no difficulty; 1 = yes, but with difficulty; and 2 = impossible to do. Item scores are added to give a total functional index between 0 and 40. The DFI has been used in studies of disease outcome and in clinical trials and is considerably longer than BASFI questionnaire so not feasible for clinical practice.

Health Assessment Questionnaire for the Spondyloarthropathies

The Stanford Health Assessment Questionnaire Disability Index (HAQ-DI) was originally developed for the assessment of disability in patients with RA.[49] It focuses on two dimensions of health status, physical disability (eight categories), and pain. The eight categories review a total of 20 specific functions and evaluate patient's difficulty with activities of daily living over the past week. They include dressing and grooming, arising, eating, walking, hygiene, reaching, gripping, and errands and chores. It also identifies specific aids or devices utilized for assistance, as well as help needed from another person. The HAQ-DI was modified in 1990 for SpA (HAQ-S), incorporating additional five specific items pertaining to issues of physical functioning and impairment specific to patients with AS. These five items include neck function and static posture (driving a car, using a rear-vision mirror, carrying heavy groceries, sitting for long periods, and working at a desk). It is sensitive to change both in early disease and in advanced disease and is a good predictor of future disability and costs. HAQ-S has good face validity as the content is similar to the original HAQ-DI, which was tested in a group of 300 British AS patients[50,51] and also correlated well with it (Spearman's correlation coefficient 0.96). However, it only moderately correlated with other measures of physical functioning such as the DFI (r = 0.64).[52] It is routinely used for research purposes in axSpA but not in daily patient care. A study linking the BASFI, HAQ-S, and DFI questionnaires to the International Classification of Functioning, Disability, and Health (ICF) revealed a high level of concordance in terms of the domains of functioning and health.[53]

ASSESSMENT OF SPINAL MOBILITY

The Bath Ankylosing Spondylitis Metrology Index

To assess the spinal axial state (cervical, dorsal, lumbar, and hips) of individuals with axSpA and to characterize changes in the spinal mobility, a metrology index has been developed, the Bath Ankylosing Spondylitis Metrology Index (BASMI).[54] Five clinical measures that were found to be most reliable and clinically useful to reflect the axial status included: tragus-to-wall distance (TWD), cervical rotation, modified Schober test, lateral spinal flexion, and intermalleolar distance. In the original definition of the BASMI, each continuous assessment is converted into a nominal score of 0, 1, or 2, based on the conversion table shown in Table 9.3.

TABLE 9.3
The Bath Ankylosing Spondylitis Metrology Index (BASMI)

Measurement	LEVEL OF LIMITATION		
	0 = mild	1 = moderate	2 = severe
Tragus to wall	<15 cm	15–30 cm	>30 cm
Forward lumbar flexion	>4 cm	2–4 cm	<2 cm
Cervical rotation	>70°	20°–70°	<20°
Lateral spinal flexion	>10 cm	10–5 cm	<5 cm
Intermalleolar distance	>100 cm	70–100 cm	<70 cm

The sum of these scores is tabulated as whole numbers only, with a range from 0 to 10. To improve upon the BASMI where continuous measurements are converted into a nominal one, small changes in the assessments can be suppressed. A linear version of BASMI called BASMI-linear has been developed, in which the continuous scores are converted into a linear scale using five equations.[55] The BASMI-linear score is calculated by the mean of the five linear scores and ranges from 0 to 10. The BASMI-linear has shown to be more sensitive to change in clinical trials.

Although ASAS has adopted the BASMI as part of its core set for spinal mobility measurements in AS, it has also recommended using five different measures to assess mobility: chest expansion, modified Schober test, occiput-to-wall distance (OWD), cervical rotation, and lateral spinal flexion.[8,9] These measures are briefly described below; they are derived from the ASAS handbook and can be accessed from the ASAS website: www.ASAS-group.org.[20,56] Moreover, the pictures demonstrating examination techniques are well illustrated in the handbook.

Modified Schober Test

Lumbar spinal mobility is determined by placing a mark on the skin in the midline of the back at the level of posterior-superior iliac spine; a second mark is placed 10 cm above the midline with the patient erect and knees fully extended. The patient is then asked to maximally bend forward without bending the knees. The distance between the two marks on the back is measured and an increase in cm to the nearest 0.1 cm is recorded.

Lateral Lumbar Flexion

The patient stands as erect as possible, with the heels and back resting against the wall and knees fully extended and the arms fully hanging down by the sides. A mark is placed on the right thigh and another on the left thigh at the level of the patient's middle fingertip. The patient is then asked to bend sideward to the right as far as possible without rotating the back or bending the knees or lifting the heels, and a second mark is placed again at the level of the patient's middle fingertip. The distance between the two marks is measured in cm to the nearest 0.1 cm. The better of two tries is recorded. The same procedure is repeated on the left.

Occiput-to-Wall and Tragus-o-Wall Distance

The patient stands erect with the heels and back resting against the wall, and the chin held at the usual carrying level. The patient is asked to put maximal effort to touch the head against the wall. The distance between occiput and wall is measured in cm to the nearest 0.1 cm to calculate OWD. In the similar position, the distance between the tragus and the wall is measured twice in cm to the nearest 0.1 cm on the left and right side, averaging the best of the two sides.

Cervical Rotation

The patient is asked to sit straight in a chair with chin at the normal carrying level. The examiner places a goniometer at the top of the head in line with the nose and the patient is asked to rotate the neck maximally to the left, and the examiner follows with the goniometer. The angle between the first sagittal plane and the new plane after rotation is measured in degrees. The same procedure is followed for the right side. The final score for cervical rotation is calculated by averaging the best values for the two sides and recorded in degrees.

Intermalleolar Distance

It is measured with the patient lying with the legs separated as far apart as possible with the knees straight and the toes pointing upward. The distance between the medial malleoli is measured in cm. Alternatively, the intermalleolar distance is measured with the patient standing erect.

Chest Expansion

The patient is asked to rest his/her hands on or behind the head. The difference between maximal inspiration and expiration is measured at the fourth intercostal level anteriorly (or below the breast in females) in cm to the nearest 0.1 cm.

FUNCTIONING AND HEALTH STATUS, INCLUDING QUALITY OF LIFE (ASQoL, ASAS HI)

To assess the overall impact of chronic diseases, one needs to take into consideration the physical, mental, emotional, and social functioning of an individual in addition to traditionally defined outcome measures. Studies have shown that the impact of AS on employment and work disability is considerable,[57-59] and the various validated questionnaires to assess the quality of life in SpA are as follows:

Ankylosing Spondylitis Quality of Life Questionnaire (ASQoL): Health-related quality of life (HRQOL) questionnaire is a useful indicator of overall health status, as it captures information on the physical and mental health of individuals and quality of life.[59] ASQoL is an 18-item questionnaire, which is the most widely used instrument in SpA trials.[60-62] The 18 items that are being addressed are related to the impact of the disease on sleep, mood, motivation, coping, activities of daily living, independence, relationships, and social life. Each statement on the ASQoL is given a score of "1" or "0." A score of "1" is given where the item is affirmed, indicating adverse QoL. The items can be summed up to give a total score ranging from 0 to 18, with a lower score reflecting a higher HRQoL. Cases with more than three missing responses (i.e., more than 20%) cannot be allocated a total score. For cases with between one and three missing responses, the total score is calculated as follows: $T = 18x/18 - m$, where T is the total score, x is the total score for the items affirmed, and m is the number of missing items. The instrument has good reliability, sensitivity and responsiveness to change, and the construct validity with BASFI = 0.72.[63]

The ASAS Health Index

ASAS has developed the ASAS Health Index (ASAS HI), shown in Fig. 9.5, to adequately assess global functioning, including limitations in activities or social participation of patients with established axSpA. This questionnaire is based on the comprehensive ICF Core Set for axSpA.[64] It is a linear composite measure and contains 17 items (dichotomous response option: "I agree" and "I do not agree"), which cover most of the ICF core set.[65] The items address aspects of pain, emotional functions, sleep, sexual functions, mobility, self-care, and participation in the community life. The items can be summed up to give a total score ranging from 0 to 17, with a lower score indicating a better and a higher score indicating an inferior health status. Validity has been confirmed in a large international trial involving more than 20 countries. The ASAS HI has been translated so far into 517 languages.[66] It is important to emphasize that the ASAS HI is a health index and not an HRQoL instrument. Health is thereby operationalized through the ICF concept of functioning.

ASSESSING AND MONITORING TREATMENT

To measure response to therapy, ASAS has developed response criteria based on four domains: patient global, pain, function (assessed by BASFI), and inflammation (mean of BASDAI questions 5 and 6).[67] The first two response criteria (ASAS 20 and ASAS 40) are shown in Table 9.4. This table also lists the ASAS partial remission criteria that require a value not above 2 units (on a scale 0 to 10 scale) in each of the four domains.

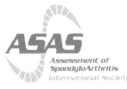

ASAS Health Index

Date: _____

Name: _____

Please answer all statements by placing one check mark per statement to indicate which response best applies to you **at this moment in time** taking into account your rheumatic disease (the term "rheumatic disease" contains all forms of spondyloarthritis including ankylosing spondylitis) .

1. Pain sometimes disrupts my normal activities.

    ☐ I agree

    ☐ I do not agree

2. I find it hard to stand for long.

    ☐ I agree

    ☐ I do not agree

3. I have problems running.

    ☐ I agree

    ☐ I do not agree

4. I have problems using toilet facilities.

    ☐ I agree

    ☐ I do not agree

5. I am often exhausted.

    ☐ I agree

    ☐ I do not agree

6. I am less motivated to do anything that requires physical effort.

    ☐ I agree

    ☐ I do not agree

7. I have lost interest in sex.

    ☐ I agree

    ☐ I do not agree

    ☐ Not applicable, I do not want to answer

8. I have difficulty operating the pedals in my car.

    ☐ I agree

    ☐ I do not agree

    ☐ Not applicable, I cannot / do not drive

www.ASAS-group.org

Developed by Assessment of SpondyloArthritis International Society (ASAS)

FIG. 9.5 ASAS Health Index.

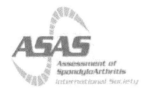

ASAS Health Index

9. I am finding it hard to make contact with people.

    ☐ I agree

    ☐ I do not agree

10. I am not able to walk outdoors on flat ground.

    ☐ I agree

    ☐ I do not agree

11. I find it hard to concentrate.

    ☐ I agree

    ☐ I do not agree

12. I am restricted in traveling because of my mobility.

    ☐ I agree

    ☐ I do not agree

13. I often get frustrated.

    ☐ I agree

    ☐ I do not agree

14. I find it difficult to wash my hair.

    ☐ I agree

    ☐ I do not agree

15. I have experienced financial changes because of my rheumatic disease.

    ☐ I agree

    ☐ I do not agree

16. I sleep badly at night.

    ☐ I agree

    ☐ I do not agree

17. I cannot overcome my difficulties.

    ☐ I agree

    ☐ I do not agree

Thank you for answering this questionnaire.

Developed by Assessment of SpondyloArthritis International Society (ASAS)

FIG. 9.5, cont'd

TABLE 9.4
ASAS Response and Remission Criteria

ASAS 20 response criteria	Improvement of >20% and >1 unit in at least three of four domains on a scale of 10
	No worsening of >20% and >1 unit in remaining domain on a scale of 10
ASAS 40 response criteria	Improvement of >40% and >2 unit in at least three domains on a scale of 10
	No worsening at all in remaining domain in at least three of the following four domains
ASAS partial remission	A value not above 2 units in each of the domains on a scale of 10

ASAS 5/6 Improvement Criteria

ASAS 5/6 response includes two additional domains (CRP and spinal mobility) in addition to the above-mentioned four domains.[68] To meet an ASAS 5/6 improvement, there should be an improvement of at least 20% in at least five of these six domains. It indicates a state of partial remission with very low disease activity, which is the goal of biologic therapy in axSpA.

BASDAI 50 Response

Based on ASAS consensus statement, response to TNF-α inhibitors is defined by improvement of at least 50% in the BASDAI score or an absolute change of 2 units (on a 0 to 10 scale) after 3 months of treatment with TNF-α inhibitors, together with an expert opinion compatible with improvement.[69]

CONCLUSION

Even though the standard of assessment has significantly improved in patients with axSpA, evaluation of the disease status is still challenging because of phenotypic heterogeneity of the disease that involves multidimensional assessment. ASAS has developed feasible core sets and new instruments (e.g., ASDAS and ASAS-HI) that have helped to create better understanding of all aspects of axSpA. The main clinical features in patients with axSpA are pain, stiffness, and fatigue, which are patient-reported complaints and can be easily assessed using the PROs to quantify the current disease state, to follow the disease progression and to measure the effect of any medical intervention.

REFERENCES

1. Taurog JD, Chhabra A, Colbert RA. Ankylosing spondylitis and axial spondyloarthritis. *N Engl J Med.* 2016;374:2563–2574.
2. Khan MA. Ankylosing spondylitis and related spondyloarthropathies: the dramatic advances in the past decade. *Rheumatology.* 2011;50:637–639.
3. Dougados M, Baeten D. Spondyloarthritis. *Lancet.* 2011;377:2127–2137.
4. Zochling J. Measures of symptoms and disease status in ankylosing spondylitis: ankylosing spondylitis disease activity score (ASDAS), ankylosing spondylitis quality of life scale (ASQoL), bath ankylosing spondylitis disease activity index (BASDAI), bath ankylosing spondylitis functional index (BASFI), bath ankylosing spondylitis global score (BAS-G), bath ankylosing spondylitis metrology index (BASMI), Dougados functional index (DFI), and health assessment questionnaire for the spondylarthropathies (HAQ-S). *Arthritis Care Res.* 2011;63(suppl 11):S47–S58.
5. Streiner DL, Norman GR. *Health Measurement Scales: A Practical Guide to Their Development and Use.* 4th ed. Oxford University Press; 2008. ISBN:978-0-19-923188.
6. Smolen JS, Schöls M, Braun J, et al. Treating axial spondyloarthritis and peripheral spondyloarthritis, especially psoriatic arthritis, to target: 2017 update of recommendations by an international task force. *Ann Rheum Dis.* 2018;77:3–17.
7. Nhan DT, Caplan L. Patient-reported outcomes in axial spondyloarthritis. *Rheum Dis Clin N Am.* 2016;42:285–299.
8. Sengupta R, Stone MA. The assessment of ankylosing spondylitis in clinical practice. *Nat Clin Pract Rheumatol.* 2007;3:496–503.
9. van der Heijde D, Calin A, Dougados M, Khan MA, van der Linden S, Bellamy N. Selection of instruments in the core set for DC-ART, SMARD, physical therapy, and clinical record keeping in ankylosing spondylitis. Progress report of the ASAS Working Group. *J Rheumatol.* 1999;26:951–954.
10. van der Heijde D, van der Linden S, Dougados M, Bellamy N, Russell AS, Edmonds J. Ankylosing spondylitis: plenary discussion and results of voting on selection of domains and some specific instruments. *J Rheumatol.* 1999;26:1003–1005.
11. Spoorenberg A, van Tubergen A, Landewé R, et al. Measuring disease activity in ankylosing spondylitis: patient and physician have different perspectives. *Rheumatology.* 2005;44:789–795.
12. Garrett S, Jenkinson T, Kennedy LG, et al. A new approach to defining disease status in ankylosing spondylitis: the bath ankylosing spondylitis disease activity index. *J Rheumatol.* 1994;21:2286–2291.
13. Braun J, Davis J, Dougados M, et al. First update of the international ASAS consensus statement for the use of anti-TNF agents in patients with ankylosing spondylitis. *Ann Rheum Dis.* 2006;65:316–320.

14. Zochling J, van der Heijde D, Burgos-Vargas R, et al. 'Assessment in AS' international working group; European League against Rheumatism. ASAS/EULAR recommendations for the management of ankylosing spondylitis. *Ann Rheum Dis.* 2006;65:442–452.

15. Machedo P, Landewé RB, Braun J, et al. MRI inflammation and its relation with measures of clinical disease activity and different treatment responses in patients with ankylosing spondylitis treated with a tumour necrosis factor inhibitor. *Ann Rheum Dis.* 2012;71:2002–2005.

16. Kiltz U, Baraliakos X, Karakostas P, et al. The degree of spinal inflammation is similar in patients with axial spondyloarthritis who report high or low levels of disease activity: a cohort study. *Ann Rheum Dis.* 2012;71:1207–1211.

17. Van Tubergen A, Landewe R, van der Heijde D, et al. Combined spa-exercise therapy is effective in patients with ankylosing spondylitis: a randomized controlled trial. *Arthritis Rheum.* 2001;45:430–438.

18. Kviatkovsky MJ, Ramiro S, Landewé R, et al. The minimum clinically important improvement and patient-acceptable symptom state in the BASDAI and BASFI for patients with ankylosing spondylitis. *J Rheumatol.* 2016;43:1680–1686.

19. Essers I, Boonen A, Busch M, et al. Fluctuations in patient reported disease activity, pain and global being in patients with ankylosing spondylitis. *Rheumatology.* 2016;55:2014–2022.

20. Landewé R, van Tubergen A. Clinical tools to assess and monitor spondyloarthritis. *Curr Rheumatol Rep.* 2015;17:47.

21. Lukas C, Landewe R, Sieper J, et al. Development of an ASAS-endorsed disease activity score (ASDAS) in patients with ankylosing spondylitis. *Ann Rheum Dis.* 2009;68:18–24.

22. van der Heijde D, Lie E, Kvien TK, et al. Assessment of SpondyloArthritis international Society (ASAS). ASDAS, a highly discriminatory ASAS endorsed disease activity score in patients with ankylosing spondylitis. *Ann Rheum Dis.* 2009;68:1811–1818.

23. Pedersen SJ, Sorensen IJ, Hermann KG, et al. Responsiveness of the Ankylosing Spondylitis Disease Activity Score (ASDAS) and clinical and MRI measures of disease activity in a 1-year follow-up study of patients with axial spondyloarthritis treated with tumour necrosis factor alpha inhibitors. *Ann Rheum Dis.* 2010;69:1065–1071.

24. Nas K, Yildirim K, Cevik R, et al. Discrimination ability of ASDAS estimating disease activity status in patients with ankylosing spondylitis. *Int J Rheum Dis.* 2010;13:240–245.

25. Aydin SZ, Can M, Atagunduz P, et al. Active disease requiring TNF-alpha antagonist therapy can be well discriminated with different ASDAS sets: a prospective, follow-up of disease activity assessment in ankylosing spondylitis. *Clin Exp Rheumatol.* 2010;28:752–755.

26. Machado P, Navarro-Compán V, Landewé R, van Gaalen FA, Roux C, van der Heijde D. Calculating the ankylosing spondylitis disease activity score if the conventional c-reactive protein level is below the limit of detection or if high-sensitivity c-reactive protein is used: an analysis in the DESIR cohort. *Arthritis Rheumatol.* 2015;67:408–413.

27. Machado P, Landewe R, Lie E, et al. Ankylosing Spondylitis Disease Activity Score (ASDAS): defining cut-off values for disease activity states and improvement scores. *Ann Rheum Dis.* 2011;70:47–53.

28. Machado PM, Landewé R, Heijde DV, Assessment of SpondyloArthritis International Society (ASAS). Ankylosing Spondylitis Disease Activity Score (ASDAS): 2018 update of the nomenclature for disease activity states. *Ann Rheum Dis.* 2018:pii: annrheumdis-2018-213184.https://doi.org/10.1136/annrheumdis-2018-213184.

29. Molto A, Gossec L, Meghnathi B, Landewé RBM, et al. ASAS-FLARE study group.An Assessment in SpondyloArthritis International Society (ASAS)-endorsed definition of clinically important worsening in axial spondyloarthritis based on ASDAS. *Ann Rheum Dis.* 2018;77:124–127.

30. Mander M, Simpson JM, McLellan A, Walker D, Goodacre JA, Dick WC. Studies with an enthesis index as a method of clinical assessment in ankylosing spondylitis. *Ann Rheum Dis.* 1987;46(3):197–202.

31. Auleley GR1, Benbouazza K, Spoorenberg A, et al. Evaluation of the smallest detectable difference in outcome or process variables in ankylosing spondylitis. *Arthritis Rheum.* 2002;47:582–587.

32. van der Heijde D1, Dijkmans B, Geusens P, et al. Efficacy and safety of infliximab in patients with ankylosing spondylitis: results of a randomized, placebo-controlled trial (ASSERT). *Arthritis Rheum.* 2005;52:582–591.

33. Braun J, Brandt J, Listing J, et al. Treatment of active ankylosing spondylitis with infliximab: a randomised controlled multicentre trial. *Lancet.* 2002;359(9313):1187–1193.

34. Heuft-Dorenbosch L, Spoorenberg A, van Tubergen A, et al. Assessment of enthesitis in ankylosing spondylitis. *Ann Rheum Dis.* 2003;62:127–132.

35. Clegg DO, Reda DJ, Weisman MH, et al. Comparison of sulfasalazine and placebo in the treatment of ankylosing spondylitis. A department of veterans affairs cooperative study. *Arthritis Rheum.* 1996;39:2004–12.

36. Gladman DD, Inman RD, Cook RJ, et al. International spondyloarthritis interobserver reliability exercise—the INSPIRE study: II. Assessment of peripheral joints, enthesitis, and dactylitis. *J Rheumatol.* 2007;34:1740–1745.

37. Maksymowych WP, Mallon C, Morrow S, et al. Development and validation of the spondyloarthritis research Consortium of Canada (SPARCC) enthesitis index. *Ann Rheum Dis.* 2009;68:948–953.

38. Healy PJ, Helliwell PS. Measuring clinical enthesitis in psoriatic arthritis: assessment of existing measures and development of an instrument specific to psoriatic arthritis. *Arthritis Rheum.* 2008;59:686–691.

39. Jones SD, Koh WH, Steiner A, Garrett SL, Calin A. Fatigue in ankylosing spondylitis: its prevalence and relationship to disease activity, sleep, and other factors. *J Rheumatol.* 1996;23:487–490.

40. van Tubergen A, Coenen J, Landewé R, et al. Assessment of fatigue in patients with ankylosing spondylitis: a psychometric analysis. *Arthritis Rheum.* 2002;47:8–16.

41. Revicki DA, Rentz AM, Luo MP, Wong RL. Psychometric characteristics of the short form 36 health survey and functional assessment of chronic illness Therapy-Fatigue subscale for patients with ankylosing spondylitis. *Health Qual Life Outcomes*. 2011;9:36.

42. Desthieux C1, Molto A2, Granger B3, Saraux A4, Fautrel B1, Gossec L1. Patient-physician discordance in global assessment in early spondyloarthritis and its change over time: the DESIR cohort. *Ann Rheum Dis*. 2016;75:1661–1666.

43. Machado P, Landewé R, Braun J, et al. A stratified model for health outcomes in ankylosing spondylitis. *Ann Rheum Dis*. 2011;70:1758–1764.

44. Machado P, Landewé R, Braun J, Hermann KG, Baker D, van der Heijde D. Both structural damage and inflammation of the spine contribute to impairment of spinal mobility in patients with ankylosing spondylitis. *Ann Rheum Dis*. 2010;69:1465–1470.

45. Landewé R, Dougados M, Mielants H, van der Tempel H, van der Heijde D. Physical function in ankylosing spondylitis is independently determined by both disease activity and radiographic damage of the spine. *Ann Rheum Dis*. 2009;68:863–867.

46. Calin A, Garrett S, Whitelock H, et al. A new approach to defining functional ability in ankylosing spondylitis: the development of the Bath Ankylosing Spondylitis Functional Index. *J Rheumatol*. 1994;21(12):2281–2285.

47. Pavy S, Brophy S, Calin A. Establishment of the minimum clinically important difference for the bath ankylosing spondylitis indices: a prospective study. *J Rheumatol*. 2005;32:80–85.

48. Dougados M, Gueguen A, Nakache JP, Nguyen M, Mery C, Amor B. Evaluation of a functional index and an articular index in ankylosing spondylitis. *J Rheumatol*. 1988;15:302–307.

49. Fries JF, Spitz P, Kraines RG, Holman HR. Measurement of patient outcome in arthritis. *Arthritis Rheum*. 1980;23:137–145.

50. Daltroy LH, Larson MG, Roberts NW, Liang MH. A modification of the health assessment questionnaire for the spondyloarthropathies. *J Rheumatol*. 1990;17:946–950.

51. Moncur C. Ankylosing spondylitis measures. *Arthritis Care Res*. 2003;49(suppl):S197–S209.

52. Ward MM, Kuzis S. Validity and sensitivity to change of spondylitis specific measures of functional disability. *J Rheumatol*. 1999;26:121–127.

53. Sigl T, Cieza A, van der Heijde D, Stucki G. ICF based comparison of disease specific instruments measuring physical functional ability in ankylosing spondylitis. *Ann Rheum Dis*. 2005;64:1576–1581.

54. Jenkinson TR, Mallorie PA, Whitelock HC, Kennedy LG, Garrett SL, Calin A. Defining spinal mobility in ankylosing spondylitis (AS). The bath AS metrology index. *J Rheumatol*. 1994;21:1694–1698.

55. van der Heijde D, Landewé R, Feldtkeller E. Proposal of a linear definition of the bath ankylosing spondylitis metrology index (BASMI) and comparison with the 2-step and 10-step definitions. *Ann Rheum Dis*. 2008;67(4):489–493.

56. Khan MA. *Ankylosing Spondylitis—Axial Spondyloarthritis*. 1st ed. 2016. 978-1-943236-08-4.

57. Dagfinrud H, Kjeken I, Mowinckel P, Hagen KB, Kvien TK. Impact of functional impairment in ankylosing spondylitis: impairment, activity limitation, and participation restrictions. *J Rheumatol*. 2005;32(3):516–523.

58. Boonen A, Chorus A, Miedema H, van der Heijde D, van der Tempel H, van der Linden S. Employment, work disability, and work days lost in patients with ankylosing spondylitis: a cross sectional study of Dutch patients. *Ann Rheum Dis*. 2001;60:353–358.

59. Revicki DA, Kleinman L, Cella D. A history of health-related quality of life outcomes in psychiatry. *Dialogues Clin Neurosci*. 2014;16:127–135.

60. Doward LC, Spoorenberg A, Cook SA, et al. Development of the ASQoL: a quality of life instrument specific to ankylosing spondylitis. *Ann Rheum Dis*. 2003;62:20–26.

61. Doward LC, McKenna SP, Meads DM, et al. Translation and validation of non-English versions of the ankylosing spondylitis quality of life (ASQOL) questionnaire. *Health Qual Life Outcomes*. 2007;5:7.

62. Ward MM. Health-related quality of life in ankylosing spondylitis: a survey of 175 patients. *Arthritis Care Res*. 1999;12(4):247–255.

63. Haywood KL, Garratt M, Jordan K, Dziedzic K, Dawes PT. Disease specific, patient-assessed measures of health outcome in ankylosing spondylitis: reliability, validity and responsiveness. *Rheumatology*. 2002;41:1295–1302.

64. Kiltz U, van der Heijde D, Boonen A, et al. Development of a health index in patients with ankylosing spondylitis (ASAS HI): final result of a global initiative based on the ICF guided by ASAS. *Ann Rheum Dis*. 2015;74:830–835.

65. Boonen A, Braun J, van der Horst Bruinsma IE, et al. ASAS/WHO ICF Core Sets for ankylosing spondylitis (AS): how to classify the impact of AS on functioning and health. *Ann Rheum Dis*. 2010;69:102–107.

66. Kiltz U. Measuring impairments of functioning and health in patients with axial spondyloarthritis by using the ASAS Health Index and the Environmental Item Set: translation and cross-cultural adaptation into 15 languages. *RMD Open*. 2016(2).

67. Anderson JJ, Baron G, van der Heijde D, Felson DT, Dougados M. Ankylosing spondylitis assessment group preliminary definition of short-term improvement in ankylosing spondylitis. *Arthritis Rheum*. 2001;44:1876–1886.

68. Brandt J, Listing J, Sieper J, Rudwaleit M, van der Heijde D, Braun J. Development and preselection of criteria for short term improvement after anti-TNF alpha treatment in ankylosing spondylitis. *Ann Rheum Dis*. 2004;63:1438–1444.

69. Braun J, Davis J, Dougados M, et al. First update of the international ASAS consensus statement for the use of anti-TNF agents in patients with ankylosing spondylitis. *Ann Rheum Dis*. 2006;65:316–320.

CHAPTER 10

Imaging in Axial Spondyloarthritis

WALTER P. MAKSYMOWYCH, MD, FRCP(C), MRCP(UK), FACP • ROBERT GEORGE WILLIAM LAMBERT, MB BCH,FRCR, FRCPC

Axial Spondyloarthritis (axSpA) comprises a group of inflammatory disorders that primarily affect the sacroiliac (SI) joints and structures of the spine and are characterized by the association with the HLA B27 gene. Imaging of the SI joints is an indispensable component of the diagnostic assessment of patients presenting with back pain and suspected axSpA, and with the advent of magnetic resonance imaging (MRI), more detailed assessment is now possible because active inflammation within soft tissues and bone, and not merely the structural damage that is a consequence of inflammation, can be visualized. This also allows the basic scientist to examine immunologic events in early disease, whereas the clinical researcher has additional objective measures to document inflammatory as well as structural lesions in the evaluation of therapeutic interventions and prognostic indicators. Four principal methods are currently used to evaluate the SI joints and spine of patients with axSpA: plain radiography, computed tomography (CT), scintigraphy, and MRI. Evaluation using sonography is primarily used to assess peripheral joints and entheses. In this chapter, we describe how each imaging modality can be used to assist the clinician in formulating diagnostic and therapeutic decisions and how imaging can be used as an outcome assessment tool for the basic and clinical researcher.

PLAIN RADIOGRAPHY

Plain radiography of the SI joints is still the cornerstone of diagnostic evaluation and classification of SpA. Abnormalities are limited to cancellous and/or cortical bone and include focal or diffuse sclerosis, erosion, and ankylosis. The earliest abnormality is visible as a loss of distinctness of the subchondral bone of the lower one-third of the iliac bone and is classically depicted as the serrated postage stamp (Fig. 10.1). This probably reflects early inflammation in the subchondral bone marrow of the cartilaginous portion of the joint with granulation tissue eroding through the overlying cartilage. As inflammation becomes more

extensive, the erosion becomes more obvious and may then affect the entire cortical bone of both joint surfaces in the joint, leading to apparent widening of the radiographic joint space. New bone formation and remodeling then leads to the appearance of progressive sclerosis and ankylosis across the joint space as subsequent features of disease.

DIAGNOSTIC EVALUATION USING RADIOGRAPHY

The increasing use of MRI in early axSpA has demonstrated the degree to which radiography lacks sensitivity for early diagnosis. A major reason for this is the complex anatomy of the joint so that the joint cavity is curved and obliquely orientated. The cartilaginous portion in the anteroinferior portion of the joint, which is the region primarily affected in early disease, is located laterally, whereas the posterior ligamentary portion is located medially. This, together with overlying bowel gas and soft tissue, creates difficulty in the interpretation of early subchondral changes using the conventional AP view, which permits only two-dimensional visualization of the joint with all structures and pathologic features superimposed. Erosion is therefore not reliably detected in early axSpA because it is either not in profile or is obscured by other structures.[1] Extensive training and assessment by more experienced readers does not enhance reliability of detection in early disease.

A variety of radiographic methodologies have been used in clinical practice for many years in the hope that these might enhance assessment of the SI joints (Fig. 10.2). These include oblique views of individual SI joints, which are taken at 25–30 degrees of patient rotation and are aimed at viewing the joints in profile by superimposing the anterior and posterior joint margins. A Ferguson view is commonly used to depict the SI joints in a more focused manner. The patient is in the same position as for the AP pelvis, but the tube is angled 30–35 degrees cranial and is centered to the midportion of the pelvis so that in the radiograph

Axial Spondyloarthritis. https://doi.org/10.1016/B978-0-323-56800-5.00010-2

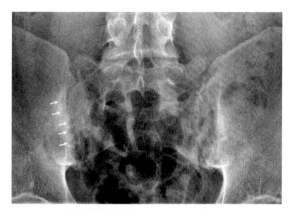

FIG. 10.1 A dedicated radiograph of the SI joints (Ferguson view) in a 39 year old man with bilateral grade 3 sacroiliitis shows erosion of subchondral bone with surrounding sclerosis. The smaller erosions in the upper half of the cartilage compartment of the right ilium (arrows) are projected free of overlying bowel gas and are easier to see. Focal subchondral erosions may create a serrated edge to the articular surface similar to a postage stamp. Larger erosion in the lower right SI joint is hard to distinguish from overlying bowel gas. On the left side, definite sclerosis is present with widening of the joint space due to ill-defined more confluent erosion, though visualization of erosion is challenging in the presence of overlying stool in the colon.

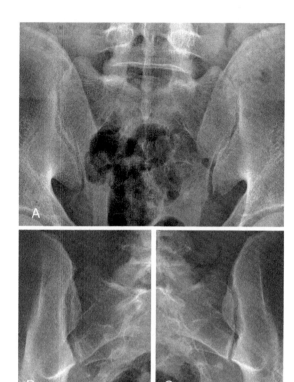

FIG. 10.2 Dedicated radiographs of SI joints in a normal subject. These may include an anterior-posterior (AP) view with 25– 30 degrees cranial angulation (Ferguson view (A)) and/or oblique views with 25– 30 degrees of patient rotation (B, C). The tilted orientation of the SI joint and its complex undulating contour may make it difficult to interpret SI joint radiographs and the standard pelvic projection may be supplemented by dedicated views of the SI joints. However, there is little evidence that the oblique projections provide significant additional information. Oblique views tend to obscure the lower one- third of the SI joints (although not in the case illustrated), which is the critical area for evaluation of early disease. Because of the significant additional radiation exposure, it is recommended that oblique views should not be performed.

the symphysis pubis does not obscure the SI joints. Despite the frequent use of these additional views, they do not enhance diagnostic accuracy when this methodology has been compared with CT evaluation.[2] Individual views have comparable diagnostic accuracy, and obtaining additional views when findings are equivocal on a single view only enhances diagnostic accuracy about 10%–15%. Consequently, only a single view is necessary, and additional views will only increase radiation exposure without enhancing diagnostic evaluation. If a pelvic radiograph is reported as equivocal for SpA and the clinical presentation is suspicious for axSpA, MRI of the pelvis is a more useful option than additional radiography (vide infra). Several prospective studies have also demonstrated that it is not worthwhile repeating pelvic radiography within 5 years, especially if the patient is symptomatic and unresponsive to conservative therapies, because only 10%–15% develop radiographic sacroiliitis after 5 years of follow-up.[3] Moreover, evidence of inflammation in the SI joints on MRI predicts the development of radiographic sacroiliitis.[4] Where important treatment decisions are to be made in early axSpA, MRI evaluation of the SI joints now represents best practice for diagnostic evaluation.

CLASSIFICATION OF AXIAL SPA USING RADIOGRAPHY
AxSpA has until recently been classified largely on the basis of radiographic findings of unequivocal

sacroiliitis as described in the modified New York (mNY) criteria.[5] Radiographic changes are graded according to the severity of abnormalities in the SI joints. At least bilateral grade 2, defined by small localized areas with erosion or sclerosis without alteration in joint width, or unilateral grade 3, defined by one or more of definite erosions, sclerosis, widening, or narrowing, must be present for classification of disease as being ankylosing spondylitis (AS). Prospective studies of patients presenting with clinical features of axSpA but short symptom duration of 3 years or less have shown that only about 15% would meet the mNY criteria.[3,6]

RADIOGRAPHY OF THE SACROILIAC JOINT IN JUVENILE SPA

Onset of axSpA before the age of 16 years is termed juvenile spondyloarthritis (JSpA). Up to 20% of patients with axSpA may have juvenile onset of disease. SI joint radiography in children is usually performed with a single AP projection to minimize radiation exposure. Interpretation of radiographic findings in a child is different from adults because the bone surface is normally irregular, and the radiographic joint space appears much wider because the cartilage is composed of both the articular surface and the centers of growth for the ilium and sacral ala. Consequently, reliable detection of erosion is challenging (Fig. 10.3) and, as in adults, clinical suspicion of axSpA with equivocal findings on radiography should prompt MRI evaluation. Erosion is more specific than sclerosis, and SI joint ankylosis is quite rare in children.

DIFFERENTIAL DIAGNOSIS OF RADIOGRAPHIC SACROILIITIS

Degenerative changes may be seen in 23.8% of primary care patients with back pain, particularly women, and SI joint findings may include sclerosis, subchondral cyst formation, joint space narrowing, osteophytes, and gas in the joint space.[7] The contour of the subchondral bone remains smooth and well defined, and radiographic evidence of erosion is rarely seen in SI joint osteoarthritis. In septic arthritis, there is typically unilateral erosion of subchondral bone and joint space widening. Reactive sclerosis is also frequently seen in subacute or chronic infection, but it is seldom pronounced. Osteitis condensans ilii (OCI) is most often a postpartum condition in which the iliac side of the SI joints becomes densely sclerotic in a characteristic

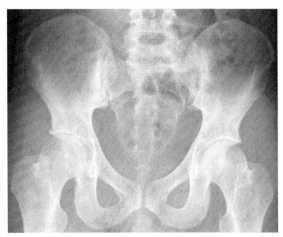

FIG. 10.3 AP radiograph of the pelvis in a young adult male shows mild subchondral sclerosis that is definitely present in the right ilium. However, erosion is hard to see and its presence is questionable. On the left side, no definite abnormality is seen with overlying colon interfering with interpretation. The radiograph does not meet modified New York criteria for sacroiliitis and if this is suspected clinically, then MRI or low-dose CT of the SI joints is recommended for further evaluation (see Fig. 4).

triangular distribution, being narrowest at the top and widest at the bottom of the SI joint. There may be some irregularity of the joint surfaces, but definite erosion is rarely seen on radiography. Other arthropathies and systemic disorders can affect the SI joints, however, they do not start in the SI joints and the clinical context will usually direct radiographic interpretation.

PLAIN RADIOGRAPHY OF THE SPINE

Plain radiography can show a variety of features in the spine, the earliest feature being the loss of the cortex at the corner of the vertebral body giving the appearance of erosion. Bone remodeling and new bone formation lead to the radiographic appearance of squaring and sclerosis at the vertebral corner. Further new bone formation extending vertically from the vertebral corner across the disc space to the adjacent vertebral corner in the form of an syndesmophyte may ultimately lead to complete ankylosis. This occurs not only at the vertebral rim but also in the interior of the disc. Spondylodiscitis is radiographically evident as disruption and loss of the vertebral endplate. Facet joint abnormalities consist of erosions, loss of joint space, and ankylosis, features that are not readily visible in the thoracic spine because of overlapping structures. They are visible on lateral radiographs of the cervical spine, whereas in the lumbar spine, oblique views may be required. The pace of radiographic progression in terms of new bone formation as detected by syndesmophytes, and ankylosis is variable but only about 20% of patients show progression over 2 years and until recently no treatment was available that could ameliorate this progression.[8] Consequently, there has been little interest in assessment of radiographic progression in either the SI joints or the spine, especially in routine practice. However, the introduction of highly effective antiinflammatory agents targeting cytokines involved in the pathogenesis of axSpA has rekindled interest in this area.

QUANTITATIVE ASSESSMENT OF PLAIN RADIOGRAPHIC CHANGE IN THE SI JOINTS AND SPINE

In the SI joints, the mNY criteria 0–4 grading scheme for radiographic sacroiliitis per SI joint has been used to develop a semiquantitative scale of severity ranging from 0–8.[9] When used in prospective studies, however, change in this severity score has been observed in both directions, that is, both worsening and improvement, which likely reflects some degree of measurement error.[10] Consequently, progression has been defined by calculating the net percentage of patients with progression defined as the number of patients with worsening minus the number of patients with improvement divided by the total study population.[3] This method has been used in a posthoc comparison of radiographic progression in the SI joints in clinical trial patients receiving tumor necrosis factor inhibitor (TNFi) versus those on conservative therapy over 2 years.[11]

The primary method used to assess radiographic progression in the spine is the modified Stoke Ankylosing Spondylitis Spine Score (mSASSS), which assesses sclerosis, erosion, squaring, syndesmophytes, and ankylosis at anterior vertebral corners of the cervical and lumbar spine on lateral radiographs. For an individual vertebral corner, the presence of ankylosis is scored 3, a syndesmophyte is scored 2, and the remaining abnormalities each receive a score of 1. The total scoring range is 0–72. At least 2 years' follow-up is required before change can be reliably detected, and over this time frame, about 40% of patients demonstrate radiographic progression.[12] Consequently, this method is still too insensitive for

use in routine practice and is not a suitable endpoint in placebo-controlled trials of disease-modifying therapies.

COMPUTED TOMOGRAPHY

CT of the SI joint is easier to interpret than plain radiography because of the absence of overlapping structures and sensitivity for detection of erosion and ankylosis is much better. The performance of plain radiography and CT of the SI joints was compared over a 2-year period in 910 patients with back pain.[13] Sacroiliitis was reported over twice as frequently with CT (25%) as with plain radiography (11%), and 41% of plain radiographic reports provided a false answer. A similar comparison was conducted in a French cohort of 489 patients with suspected SpA. Definite sacroiliitis was determined on plain radiographs in 6 (3.5%) patients and on CT scans in 32 (18.5%) patients.[14] Similar to plain radiography, CT primarily detects abnormalities in cancellous and cortical bone and therefore cannot directly assess inflammatory tissue or postinflammatory changes such as fat metaplasia that can be observed on MRI. However, direct comparison of diagnostic sensitivity and specificity performance of CT versus MRI in consecutive patients presenting with suspected early axSpA is lacking.

The primary limitation of pelvic CT is higher radiation dose, although improvements in CT technology and reconstruction software have increasingly allowed reduction of radiation dose to the level of plain radiography while maintaining diagnostic accuracy.[15,16] Annual background radiation has been estimated at 2.6 millisieverts (mSv).[17] A recent study estimated effective radiation dose from pelvic plain radiography and low-radiation CT that has been used in the assessment of renal colic: mean dose from SI joint radiographs was 0.15 mSv (range 0.07–1.38 mSv), mean dose from a single pelvic radiograph was 0.09 mSv (range 0.04–0.37 mSv), and mean dose from low-dose CT of the SI joints was 0.42 mSv (range 0.14–0.83 mSv).[16] Low-dose CT of the SI joint could be consistently performed with less than 1 mSv effective dose placing it in the same category of "minimal risk" (0.1–1 mSv) as SI joint radiography.[18] All CT studies were also deemed to be of diagnostic quality for global assessment of the SI joints (Fig. 10.4). In addition, CT scans can be more tightly collimated than radiography and so radiation exposure to the gonads with low-dose CT will actually be less than with radiography in all males and some females as the gonads will be further from the primary beam. This is highly relevant in a young adult population,

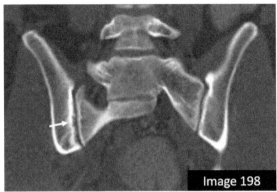 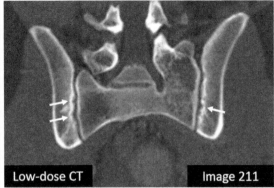

FIG. 10.4 Low-dose CT (LD-CT) performed for suspected ureteric calculus confirms the presence of sacroiliitis in a young adult male (same patient as Fig. 3). 1.5mm thick coronal images were reconstructed at 1mm increments. Small subchondral erosions (arrows) in the right ilium were seen on many of the images. However definite erosion of the left ilium was only seen on a single coronal slice (image 211). LD-CT provides excellent visualization of structural damage in the SI joints regardless of the orientation of the articular surface, and without superimposition of bony structures and overlying bowel. SI joint LD-CT can be consistently performed with radiation exposure of less than 1mSv which is in the same exposure range as radiography for the SI joints with oblique views, and with less radiation exposure than radiographs in some larger patients.[16]

as many subjects are likely to be of reproductive age. Although this methodology appears promising as a potential replacement for plain radiography of the SI joints, the use of CT in routine practice remains limited to the diagnostic evaluation of IBP where plain radiography shows normal SI joints and access to MRI is limited.

QUANTITATIVE ASSESSMENT OF RADIOGRAPHIC CHANGES ON CT

Plain radiographic assessment of radiographic changes in the spine is unreliable and omits the thoracic spine as well as posterior vertebral corners. CT of the spine is more sensitive, but radiation dosing for conventional CT is unacceptably high. A CT scan of the lumbar spine has an approximate dose of 8 millisieverts (mSv). A lower-dose CT protocol of the entire spine has been reported where the radiation dose has been estimated at 4 mSv.[19] This new method enabled the assessment of syndesmophytes and ankylosis along the entire perimeter of the vertebral endplates on either side of all the intervertebral disc spaces with enhanced image resolution. New bone growth was identified in five times as many patients when measured by low-dose CT than when measured by conventional radiography, with two-thirds of this new bone found in the thoracic spine.[20] In this method (the CT Syndesmophyte Score), new bone growth is scored by evaluating for the presence of syndesmophytes and

ankylosis, a score of 1 being assigned for a small syndesmophyte, which does not extend vertically beyond the midpoint of the intervertebral disc space, a score of 2 being assigned when it extends beyond the midpoint of the intervertebral disc space, and a score of 3 being assigned to each vertebral corner of an intervertebral disc space in the presence of complete bridging ankylosis.

ISOTOPIC IMAGING

Scintigraphy relies on abnormal uptake of radiotracer in areas of increased bone turnover and is more sensitive than plain radiography for detection of sacroiliitis, but the complex shape of the joint makes interpretation of planar images difficult. Inflammatory lesions in bone marrow are not directly visualized, and the scintigraphic activity reflects the impact of inflammation on bone turnover. Erosion, reparative lesions such as fat metaplasia, and ankylosis are not detected. Quantitative scanning of the SI joints has been evaluated as a diagnostic tool, although cutoffs that reliably distinguish patients from controls have proved difficult to establish. Sensitivity has ranged from 29% to 40%, whereas specificity was usually less than 80%. A recent systematic review concluded that isotopic imaging of the SI joints had low diagnostic utility for evaluation of IBP.[21] Consequently, use of this technique is decreasing in favor of MRI and will likely decrease further with the introduction of low-dose CT.

MAGNETIC RESONANCE IMAGING

A major advance in the field has been the development of MRI, which is superior to plain radiography and CT through its ability to visualize soft-tissue inflammation and inflammatory lesions within bone in three dimensions without interference from overlying structures. The objective evidence of inflammation provided by MRI is often not readily available on clinical evaluation because disease is often confined to the axial joints and laboratory markers of inflammation are positive in only 40%–50% of patients. Reliable quantitation of MRI inflammatory and structural abnormalities in the SI joints is now possible and is now increasingly being used to identity new therapeutic compounds in early phases of development, in registration trials of new agents, and for clinical research. In recent years, there has been greater understanding of the spectrum of acute and structural MRI features in the SI joints of patients with axSpA, appropriate indications for the use of MRI in diagnostic evaluation, the prognostic role of MRI, and its capacity to predict treatment response.

TECHNICAL CONSIDERATIONS

T1-weighted spin echo (T1W SE) images detect the signal from fat, which appears bright, whereas bone appears dark. T2-weighted (T2W) MRI sequences detect the signal from water, as may be observed in cysts, inflammatory infiltrates, and highly vascularized tissues such as tumors. Fluid is very bright on T2W MRI, whereas fat is variable and bone is black. However, the signal from water related to inflammation in the bone marrow will not be detected by T2W MRI because it will be obscured by the signal from marrow fat. Consequently, suppression of the signal from fat is necessary in MRI sequences used for detection of axSpA. These include short tau inversion recovery (STIR) and T2 fat-saturated (T2 fat-sat or T2FS) sequences where inflammatory lesions are characteristically present in subchondral bone and adjacent to entheses.

An alternative approach to the detection of inflammation is using a T1W sequence that is fat suppressed with assessment of contrast enhancement after intravenous administration of gadolinium (Gd). Gd accumulates at sites of increased vascularity and capillary permeability, where it alters the magnetic properties of surrounding soft tissues. This process can be followed over time, where both the rate and degree of Gd enhancement provide information on the severity of inflammation by quantifying the intensity (peak), the maximal rate (slope), and the time-to-peak enhancement of contrast.

NORMAL APPEARANCE OF THE SACROILIAC JOINT AND SPINE

For the SI joints, consecutive images 3 mm in thickness are obtained in the semicoronal orientation along the long axis of the sacral bone, which allows visualization of the cartilaginous portion of the joint, which is situated convex anteroinferiorly (Fig. 10.5). Axial sections, which are oriented perpendicular to semicoronal sections, may facilitate assessment of structural lesions, and allow superior evaluation of ligamentous structures in the posterosuperior portion of the joint (Fig. 10.6). Bone marrow fat in the iliac and sacral bones appears bright on a T1W SE sequence, whereas subchondral bone lining the joint cavity is dark (Fig. 10.5). When evaluating the joint from anterior to posterior slices, there is a transitional slice defined as the first slice in the cartilaginous portion that has a visible portion of the ligamentous joint. This appears bright because of the presence of fat surrounding the ligaments (Fig. 10.5). Further posteriorly, in the ligamentous compartment, there is both bright signal, indicating fat, and dark signal, indicating ligaments between iliac and sacral bones. On T2W fat-suppressed images assessed from anterior to posterior, bright signal is detected from presacral veins on anterior coronal slices through the joint (Fig. 10.5). Cortical bone and ligament appears dark on both sequences. Further posteriorly, bright signal can be seen in the spinal canal, reflecting cerebrospinal fluid. An initial study for diagnostic evaluation should consist of both a semicoronal T1W SE and either a STIR or T2FS sequence because they provide crucial complementary information. One sequence in the semiaxial plane, most often STIR or T2FS, may also contribute additional information.

The spine is imaged in the sagittal plane with consecutive slices of 3 mm thickness that extend laterally to depict the lateral spinal structures, including the costovertebral and costotransverse joints (Fig. 10.7). Imaging for evaluation of axSpA is conducted in two halves, cervicothoracic from C2 to T10 and thoracolumbar from T8 to S1. Often these images are reconstructed to show the entire spine in a single image. Dark cortical bone of the vertebral bodies and bright signal from fat in the bone marrow is readily visible on the T1W SE sequence. Bright signal from water in the cerebrospinal fluid is readily visible on an STIR/T2FS sequence in central sagittal slices. The vertebral pedicles, facet processes, head

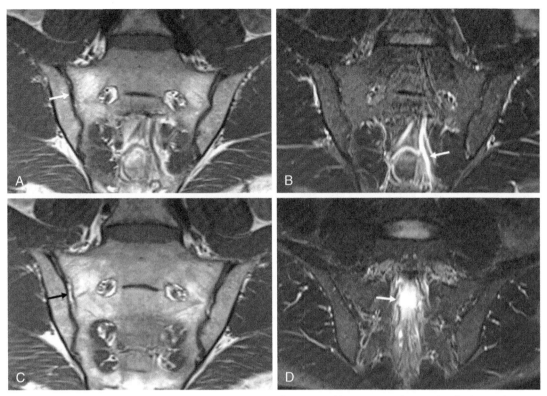

FIG. 10.5 MRI of SI joints in a healthy young subject. Semicoronal images are orientated to the long axis of the sacrum and T1W spin echo images (A - anterior slice, C - transitional slice) and STIR images (B - anterior slice, D - posterior slice) are most often acquired. On T1, bone marrow is brighter than muscle because of the higher fat content in bone marrow. The cortical bone appears as a thin dark line marking the joint outline (A – arrow). On STIR, fat signal is suppressed, bone marrow appears darker, and fluid signal is very bright as seen in presacral veins (B - arrow) and cerebrospinal fluid (D - arrow). The SI joints extend further anteriorly than sacral vertebral bodies, so anterior parts of the cartilage compartment are visualized on anterior slices (A), along with presacral soft tissues. The transitional slice (C) represents the start of the ligamentous compartment. The transitional slice is best identified on T1 when fat is seen in the centre of the joint (C - arrow) representing fat surrounding SI ligaments. Note that on any water-sensitive sequence, small blood vessels are frequently observed as small circular or curvilinear foci of bright signal adjacent to the perimeter of the joint or parallel to ligaments and should not be mistaken for bone marrow or soft tissue inflammation.

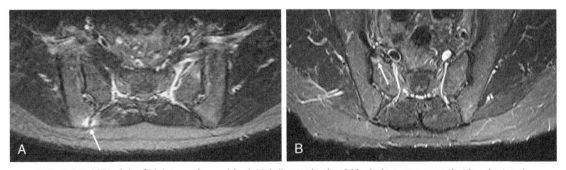

FIG. 10.6 MRI of the SI joints performed for initial diagnosis should include a sequence that is orientated perpendicular to the semicoronal sequences and axial or semiaxial STIR is often performed. This sequence may provide additional information and/or a second perspective of more subtle findings. Semiaxial STIR images in two different patients show: inflammatory enthesopathy at the right posteroinferior iliac spine (A – arrow) in a patient with subtle sacroiliitis due to SpA; and a small focus of bone marrow edema (BME) at the anterior border of the right sacral ala (B – arrow) with a typical configuration and location for biomechanical changes in a patient with sacroiliac osteoarthritis.

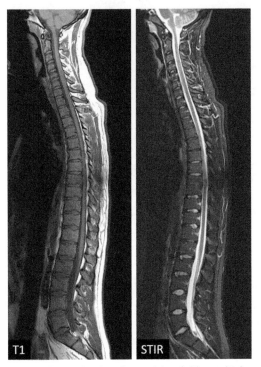

FIG. 10.7 For evaluation of spondyloarthritis, sagittal MRI of the entire spine can easily be acquired in under 10 minutes using large fields of view in two stations extending from C1 to T10, and from T8 to S3, composed into single whole spine images. Typically T1 and STIR are performed at 3mm thickness and extend further laterally than conventional spine MRI so as to include all the costovertebral and costotransverse joints. Good fat suppression is essential for detection of inflammation, and high resolution is required to interpret small lesions. STIR is usually performed in preference to T2 spin echo with fat saturation because of more consistent fat suppression over large fields of view with STIR.

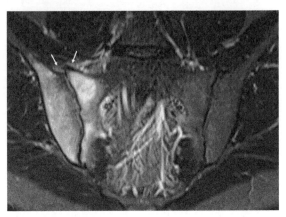

FIG. 10.8 STIR MRI of the SI joints in a 25 year old male demonstrates florid BME throughout the subchondral bone of the right SI joint. It is important to note that such extensive BME on one side of an SI joint due to SpA should always be associated with significant abnormality (BME or structural damage) on the other side of the same joint. Capsulitis is clearly present at the cranial border of the cartilage compartment (arrows) but there is no other soft-tissue inflammation.

of the adjacent rib, and transverse processes are all visible on lateral slices (Fig. 10.7). Routine imaging of the spine is not recommended for diagnostic purposes (vide infra).

EARLY MRI FEATURES OF SPONDYLOARTHRITIS

These are usually first seen as inflammatory lesions in the SI joints on T2W and/or contrast-enhanced MRI and include capsulitis, synovitis, and subchondral bone marrow inflammation[22,23] (Fig. 10.8). Dynamic MRI with Gd enhancement was used in the earliest studies to enhance the sensitivity of MRI in the detection of early sacroiliitis.[24] These included patients clinically characterized as having inflammatory low back pain but normal radiographs. Contrast MRI revealed enhancement of the joint capsule, synovium, and subchondral bone marrow, especially in the posterocaudal portion of the joint where the capsule attaches to bone. Subsequent studies using fat suppression techniques have similarly noted subchondral bone marrow edema (BME) as a consistent component of the early pathology of sacroiliitis. Direct CT-guided biopsy of the SI joints has also demonstrated significant correlations between the degree of Gd enhancement on MRI of the SI joints and the histopathologic grade of inflammation.[25]

As the BME lesion evolves, there is erosion of the subchondral bony plate, which may be observed soon after disease onset. Erosions develop adjacent to the joint space and are visible as loss of subarticular bone with decreased fat signal on T1W SE images, reflecting loss of marrow matrix adjacent to eroded bone (Fig. 10.9). Erosion may evolve from a focal defect in cortical bone to confluence of multiple erosions, resulting in extended erosion along the entire vertical height of the iliac cortical bone, leading to the appearance of pseudowidening of the joint space. There will be increased signal on fat-suppressed sequences at the site of erosion when inflammation is still active. When inflammation resolves, new tissue with high signal intensity

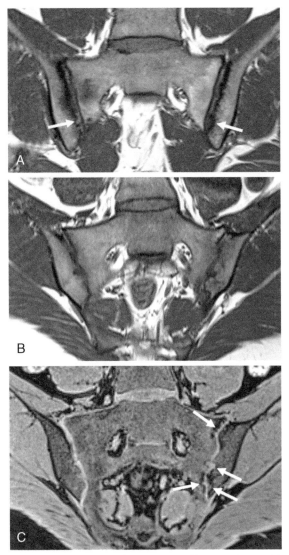

FIG. 10.9 T1 weighted images of the SI joints in two different patients illustrate the variable appearances of erosion in early sacroiliitis. In both cases, the normal subchondral cortex of the ilium is destroyed and the normal bone marrow signal at the site of erosion is diminished. In a 28 year old male patient (A) numerous tiny erosions in both joints are more prominent inferiorly (arrows) rendered more visible by adjacent reactive sclerosis that exaggerates the contrast at the surface of the bone. In a 16 year old with juvenile spondyloarthritis (B, C), the interpretation of the conventional T1 weighted spin echo sequence (B) is very challenging in part because the normal bone marrow in children is more erythropoietic with less fat content and often there is less sclerosis and less fat metaplasia in reaction to the erosion in juveniles. So while there is clear loss of definition of the subchondral cortices, the tissue contrast related to erosion is less apparent. In this situation, high resolution 3D imaging may be very useful such as with 3D VIBE with fat saturation (C). In this 1mm thick T1 weighted VIBE image, numerous tiny subchondral erosions (arrows) are clearly seen, more prominently on the left side. With high resolution 3D MRI sequences, erosion may be seen with similar conspicuity to high resolution CT (see Fig. 4)

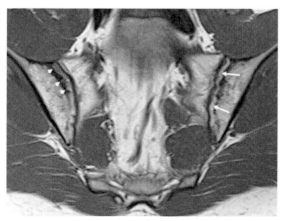

FIG. 10.10 Structural damage in sacroiliitis may have highly variable MRI appearances, especially after treatment. On this T1-weighted image in a young male patient, the right ilium shows subchondral sclerosis with erosion (arrowheads). On the left side, a well-defined serpiginous line of bright signal (arrows) parallels the distorted joint space on the articular side of iliac subchondral sclerosis. This is the typical appearance of backfill, which represents tissue metaplasia containing lipid-laden macrophages, filling the space created by erosion of subchondral bone and occurring as a repair process when inflammation subsides. Backfill may occur spontaneously or after biologic therapy.

appears on the T1W sequence in the erosion cavity and has been termed backfill (Fig. 10.10). Similarly, when subchondral BME resolves, new tissue with high signal intensity appears in the subchondral bone marrow and has been termed fat metaplasia. These appearances on the T1W SE sequence may be seen early after disease onset and reflect accumulation of fatty acids. Moreover, prospective assessment of MRI scans has confirmed this sequence of events.[26] The histopathologic counterpart to this reparative lesion is unknown but could reflect any type of tissue with extracellular and/or intracellular accumulation of fatty acids as in fibroblasts, macrophages, or adipocytes. A prospective analysis of patients followed over 2 years has shown that development of fat metaplasia on MRI is independently predictive of the development of ankylosis.[26] Fat metaplasia therefore appears to be an inherent characteristic of the tissue response following resolution of inflammation in the axial skeleton in SpA and supports the hypothesis that resolution of inflammation progresses to a stage of ankylosis through this key intermediary tissue.

Spinal abnormalities may also be observed on MRI soon after disease onset and are characterized by the presence of BME at vertebral corners and adjacent to the vertebral endplate (Fig. 10.11). Less frequently,

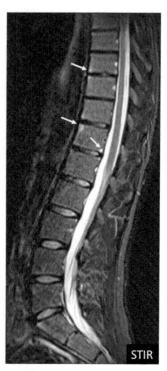

FIG. 10.11 Multiple corner inflammatory lesions (CIL) are seen on STIR (arrows) in a 34 year old man. These BME lesions are small with nonspecific shape but there is no evidence of significant disc degeneration and spine curvature is normal. They are clustered around the thoracolumbar junction between T9 and T12, and the appearances are highly suspicious for active inflammation due to SpA, if the clinical context is appropriate. (Also see T1W image performed at the same time in Fig. 13 and previous MRI in Fig. 14).

BME may be observed in lateral slices in the vertebral body, the pedicle, and the adjacent head of rib where it reflects costovertebral inflammation (Fig. 10.12). Fat metaplasia may then develop following resolution of inflammation at the same locations presumably reflecting the same processes that occur in the SI joints (Fig. 10.13). Prospective analysis has shown that fat metaplasia at vertebral corners is independently predictive of new bone formation observed on radiography as a syndesmophyte.[27]

MRI FEATURES IN ESTABLISHED SPONDYLOARTHRITIS

As disease progresses, there may be additional sites of inflammation such as the facet joints, which appears as BME in the facet processes, and costotransverse joints, which appears as BME in the transverse

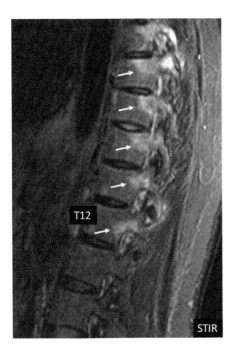

FIG. 10.12 Sagittal STIR MRI shows multiple foci of BME in the posterolateral aspects of the thoracic vertebral bodies (arrows). The shape, location and distribution of these lesions is typical of costovertebral joint inflammation. The BME lesions may be contiguous with but are not arising from the annulus fibrosus or vertebral endplate. At T7 and T8, the vertebral body BME is contiguous with facet joint inflammation via the pedicles but note that at T11 and T12, the BME lesions develop in an arc around the mid aspect of the posterior vertebral body and inferior pedicle with no contact with either endplate or facet joint. These lower lesions can only occur as a result of costovertebral joint inflammation and are pathognomonic for spondyloarthritis.

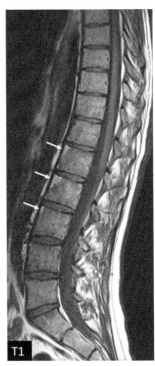

FIG. 10.13 Vertebral body corner lesions in spondylitis may have characteristic features. The corner fat lesions seen anteriorly in the lumbar spine (arrows) are longer in height than horizontal width. This is characteristic of SpA, and this shape is seldom seen with degeneration. There is no evidence of significant disc degeneration (see also STIR in Fig. 11 performed at the same time), and the size, shape, location and distribution of these corner fat lesions are typical for spondylitis. (Previous MRI scan on this 34-year-old man is illustrated in Fig. 14).

processes (Fig. 10.14). Inflammation may affect sacroiliac and spinal ligaments at their site of attachment to bone. More advanced structural changes include the development of bone sclerosis, characterized by low signal intensity on both T1W and T2W sequences, which is most readily observed in the SI joints. In the spine, erosive changes may affect vertebral corners and vertebral endplates, which are visible on T1W SE scans as full-thickness loss of the dark appearance of cortical bone at its anticipated location and loss of the normal bright appearance of adjacent bone marrow (Fig. 10.15). Ankylosis in the SI joints is evident as bone marrow signal on T1W sequences extending between the sacral and iliac bone marrow, with full-thickness loss of the dark appearance of the iliac and sacral cortical bone (Fig. 10.16). Intervertebral ankylosis may be observed both at the periphery and between

vertebral endplates in the interior of the intervertebral disc space (Fig. 10.17). Facet joint ankylosis is also observed as continuity of bone marrow signal across the joint space, which is no longer visible on T1W SE scans.

DIAGNOSTIC EVALUATION USING MRI

There has been relatively limited study of the sensitivity and specificity of MRI abnormalities for diagnosis in patients with early SpA, especially in unselected patients presenting with chronic back pain that may resemble SpA clinically. The gold standard for diagnosis requires unequivocal radiographic sacroiliitis, which means that assessment of diagnostic performance must be prospective to allow time for unequivocal radiographic abnormalities to develop. Consequently, it has

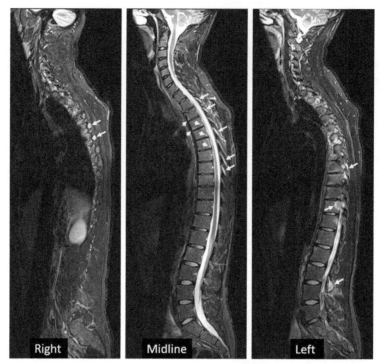

FIG. 10.14 In this 32-year-old man with early spondyloarthritis, multiple foci of bone marrow edema are scattered through the spine in a typical distribution for SpA: laterally in upper thoracic transverse processes (right - arrows); anterior and posterior corner inflammatory lesions (CIL) (midline - arrowheads) and spinous processes (midline - arrows); and facet and costovertebral joints (left - arrows).

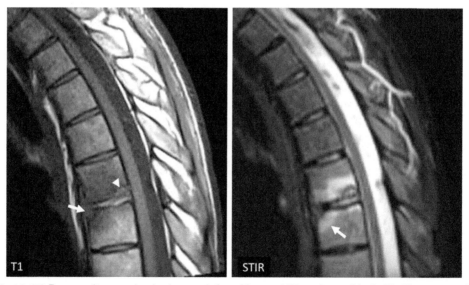

FIG. 10.15 Bone erosion may develop in association with spondylitis and spondylodiscitis. The corners of the vertebral body may be eroded in spondylitis and this is seen most often on T1W images anteriorly near the midline as full thickness loss of the dark appearance of cortical bone at its anticipated location and loss of the normal bright appearance of adjacent bone marrow (T1 - arrow). In this 29 year old man with known SpA, the anterior corner erosion has a thin sclerotic border that is better seen in T1W images, and surrounding BME (STIR - arrow). Findings of spondylodiscitis in SpA commonly include erosion, as seen here in the posterior aspect of the T7 vertebral endplate (T1 - arrowhead), with surrounding sclerosis and BME. Fat metaplasia in adjacent bone is also commonly seen in more chronic cases but soft tissue changes are minimal or absent. At the individual level, spondylodiscitis due to SpA may be hard to distinguish from other causes of discitis but it very rarely occurs in the absence of other more specific findings of SpA in the spine and SI joints.

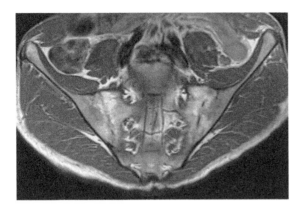

FIG. 10.16 In advanced disease, ankylosis is common in the SI joints and is seen on T1W sequences as bone marrow signal extending between the sacral and iliac bones with full-thickness loss of the dark appearance of the iliac and sacral subchondral cortices. The original joint line may be completely obliterated although thin linear remnants of the original joint may be visible.

been more feasible to conduct cross-sectional rather than prospective studies. One study compared scans from patients with scans from age- and sex-matched healthy controls and back conditions resembling SpA. Diagnostic utility of MRI was high for patients who had AS (sensitivity 0.90, specificity 0.97, positive likelihood ratio [LR] 44.6) as well as for patients diagnosed clinically as axSpA but without definite radiographic sacroiliitis (sensitivity 0.51, specificity 0.97, positive LR 26.0).[28]

A second study assessed MRI scans from two independent inception cohorts of consecutive patients aged ≤50 years presenting to a rheumatologist with back pain of undetermined etiology.[29] One cohort comprised patients with back pain of short symptom duration referred by primary care physicians to a rheumatologist for further evaluation of clinically suspected SpA. The second cohort comprised patients who presented with acute anterior uveitis and were referred for assessment of SpA if they indicated past or present back pain for at least 3 months. Sensitivity and specificity of MRI for nonradiographic axSpA,

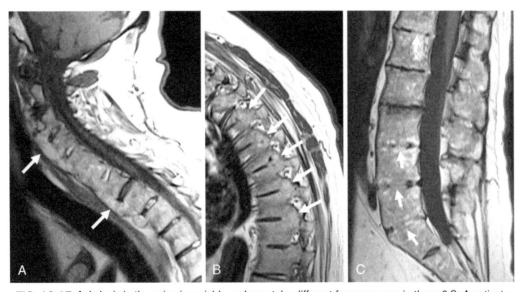

FIG. 10.17 Ankylosis in the spine is variable and may take different forms as seen in these 3 SpA patients aged over 60. Very thin linear syndesmophytes may not be visible on MRI at all and MRI is not sensitive for ankylosis unless bone marrow forms as part of the new bone formation. In a patient with psoriatic spondyloarthritis (A), exuberant anterior ossification (arrows) resembles DISH but the SpA has also caused complete ankylosis of one of the mid cervical discs with obliteration of the vertebral endplates which does not occur in degenerative ankylosis. In a patient with classical ankylosing spondylitis (B), the thoracic vertebrae are ankylosed laterally across the costovertbral joints (arrows) with relative preservation of the disc outline anteriorly. This pattern of ankylosis is pathognomonic for SpA. In the third patient with SpA (C), ankylosis has developed through the interior of the discs with bone marrow signal continuous between the vertebral bodies across the destroyed endplates (arrows).

defined according to rheumatologist expert opinion, compared with nonspecific back pain was 74%/44% and 95%/83%, for the first and second cohorts, respectively. A study of patients suspected of having SpA but without radiographic sacroiliitis that combined MRI and histopathologic assessment of SI joints after needle biopsy showed that specificity of MRI for sacroiliitis was 100%, whereas sensitivity was only 38%, using immunohistologic evidence of inflammation as the gold standard.[30] This study was conducted over a decade ago, and MRI technology has evolved considerably since then.

An expert task force of EULAR concluded, on the basis of 13 studies that evaluated the diagnostic utility of MRI, that assessment of the SI joints should be conducted if the diagnosis of axSpA cannot be established based on clinical features and conventional radiography, and axSpA is still suspected.[31] MRI of the SI joints is most useful diagnostically in those patients with a clinical suspicion of IBP who are HLA-B27-positive, have a normal or equivocal radiograph of the SI joints, have an insufficient symptomatic response to NSAIDs, and are considered candidates for more intensive therapy. Contrast-enhanced MRI is not recommended for routine use because its diagnostic performance is not superior to fat-suppressed sequences, but cost and inconvenience to patients are substantially greater. MRI of the spine in addition to the SI joints is not recommended for routine diagnostic practice because the incremental increase in diagnostic sensitivity is only 10%–15%.[32] It may be useful where SI joint features are equivocal for axSpA.

CLASSIFICATION OF SPONDYLOARTHRITIS USING MRI

The enhanced performance of MRI over radiography for detection of early SpA has led to its inclusion as a criterion for categorizing patients as having axSpA in the new ASAS classification criteria.[33] A positive MRI for the purposes of classification has been reported according to consensus opinion of rheumatologist and radiologist experts in the field.[34] This definition is based on the clear presence of BME/osteitis in subchondral bone on a fat-suppressed or contrast-enhanced sequence. The definition is met when there are at least two lesions on a single semicoronal slice or when a single lesion is present on two consecutive slices. It is important that this definition is not applied for diagnostic purposes. Controlled studies demonstrate BME meeting this

definition in the SI joints of up to 30% of mechanical back pain patients and healthy controls.[28,29] False-positive BME may be observed in the anterior sacrum and in the posteroinferior iliac bone because of signal from blood vessels located in close proximity to the joint at these locations.

Structural lesions in the SI joints on T1W MRI, especially erosions, may contribute to the decision by the observer that inflammatory lesions are genuinely due to SpA.[35] In one study where low-dose CT of the SI joints was used as the standard of reference, T1W MRI showed markedly better sensitivity with significantly more correct imaging findings compared with plain radiography for erosions.[15]

Fat metaplasia in the SI joints has also been evaluated for classification and diagnostic utility. In particular, fat metaplasia on T1W MRI adjacent to subchondral bone that has a distinct border and displays a homogeneous increase in T1W signal has high specificity for axSpA but by itself has low diagnostic utility because there are often other MRI features of SpA, such as erosions and BME. Appropriate evaluation of an MRI scan of the SI joints for both diagnosis and classification of axSpA should always include simultaneous assessment of T1W and fat-suppressed sequences because each sequence provides complementary information.

Several reports aimed at validating a definition of a positive spine MRI for classification of axSpA on the basis of the number of vertebral corners with BME and/or fat metaplasia have concluded that imaging of the spine does not materially contribute to MRI of the SI joints for purposes of either diagnosis or classification. However, inflammation in the costovertebral and costotransverse joints is highly specific for axSpA, particularly when it affects more than one vertebral unit.

MRI IN JUVENILE SPONDYLOARTHRITIS

The principles of MRI evaluation in children are similar to those in adults although MRI of the immature skeleton does confer some additional challenges (Fig. 10.18). Enthesitis and hip disease are more frequent than in adults. So the routine SI joint MRI protocol should be adjusted with expansion of the field of view and/or the number of slices in one of the acquisition planes so as to include the hips and entheses. Spinal MRI is not warranted for routine assessment because of the very low frequency of spinal abnormalities.

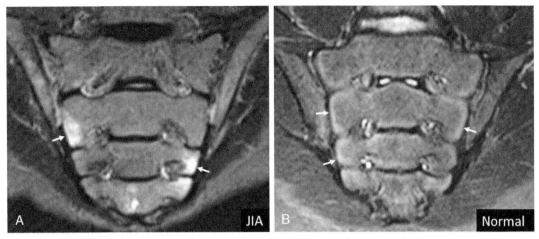

FIG. 10.18 In children, age-related normal variation should not be misinterpreted as bone marrow edema (BME) on coronal STIR MRI of the SI joints. Patchy sacral BME (A – arrows) is typical for active inflammation in a 12-year-old boy with known juvenile idiopathic arthritis. Normal periphyseal "flaring" (B - arrows) is present in a 7-year-old boy with a thin high signal rim in sacral subchondral bone, somewhat asymmetrical in intensity due to scan inhomogeneity.

The normal axial skeleton in children has a higher proportion of erythropoietic bone marrow and less fat content than in adults. Bone marrow therefore appears brighter on STIR or T2FS, making BME harder to detect than in adults. In addition, vascularity at sites of bone growth creates the appearance of a "subchondral flare" of brighter signal on STIR or T2FS in the subchondral bone. As in adults, there is little advantage to the use of contrast-enhanced MRI over STIR or T2FSA. Postinflammatory fat metaplasia in subchondral bone has much higher specificity than in adults because fatty replacement of normal marrow is not a feature of the juvenile axial skeleton. Erosion may be more difficult to discern because the normal bone-cartilage interface is very irregular in younger children. Subchondral sclerosis is one of the most frequent findings, but the density of the normal subchondral bone is variable so the diagnostic utility of this observation is limited.

DIFFERENTIAL DIAGNOSIS OF SPONDYLOARTHRITIS LESIONS ON MRI

Degenerative changes in the SI joints are frequent, even in the age group that develops axSpA. Small foci of sclerosis and/or BME without erosion are common, but significant fat metaplasia is seldom observed. Osteophytes may be evident at the periphery of the joint. The findings may sometimes be hard to distinguish from osteitis condensans ilii (OCI), and both of these conditions may cause broad areas of diffuse or dense sclerosis in subchondral bone, predominantly on the iliac side (Fig. 10.19). Mild BME may be seen, usually as a thin rim of BME surrounding the sclerotic bone. In the spine, degenerative disc disease and tears of the annulus fibrosus may present with BME adjacent to the vertebral endplate and at the vertebral corner. In more advanced disease, there is loss of disc height, irregularity of the vertebral endplates, and fat metaplasia along the vertebral endplates and at vertebral corners once BME has resolved (Fig. 10.20). Scheuermann's disease may be difficult to distinguish from the spondylodiscitis secondary to axSpA. It is characterized by irregularity of the vertebral endplate and loss of disc height as the disc herniates into the vertebral body.

Septic arthritis in the SI joints typically presents as a unilateral sacroiliitis and in the spine as spondylodiscitis at a single location. Inflammation is much more widespread on MRI and does not respect anatomical boundaries. It may extend far from the joint into adjacent soft tissues and result in abscess formation (Fig. 10.21). Destruction of joint surface and subchondral bone may be extensive. In the spine, prominent BME affecting an entire vertebral body with extension of inflammation into adjacent soft tissues may be observed in chronic recurrent multifocal osteomyelitis (Fig. 10.22). In contrast to

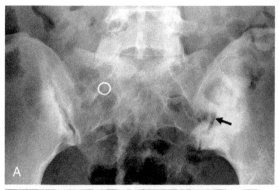

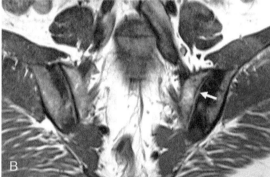

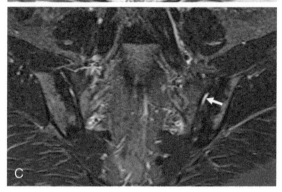

FIG. 10.19 Pelvic radiograph (A) and T1W (B) and STIR (C) MR images in a 35 year old female demonstrate typical findings of osteitis condensans ilii (OCI). Dense subchondral sclerosis is present on the iliac side of both SI joints, worse on the left side. There is no erosion with the smooth contour of the articular surface of the left ilium clearly seen on all the images (arrows). The STIR sequence also reveals a smooth linear focus of joint fluid that emphasizes the lack of erosion and the degenerative nature of the condition. Similar findings are often present to a much lesser extent on the sacral side. Although BME and fat metaplasia may be seen on MRI, these findings are usually minimal.

bacterial spondylodiscitis, the disc is usually not involved, there may be intervertebral ankylosis as well as erosive changes, and the degree of extension into soft tissues is less than that observed in septic discitis.

BME that is confined to a single bone in the SI joints is a common feature of stress fractures, which may be seen in overuse injuries and in osteoporotic patients with insufficiency fractures (Fig. 10.23). Fat metaplasia and joint erosion are not evident. A similar appearance of BME confined to a single bone may be observed with infiltrative and neoplastic lesions such as lymphoma. Prominent BME may be seen in the SI joint in female patients immediately postpartum and usually settles with conservative management.

Diffuse idiopathic skeletal hyperostosis (DISH) is characterized by bulky paravertebral ankylosis but may resemble the new bone spurs and ankylosis of axSpA, which can vary tremendously in appearance. Unlike axSpA, intradiscal and facet joint ankylosis are not a feature of this disease and abnormalities of the SI joints are confined to degenerative changes. However, capsular ossification of the SI and facet joints may simulate ankylosis although CT reveals that the ankylosis is confined to the periphery of the joint.

QUANTITATIVE ASSESSMENTS OF LESIONS OBSERVED ON MRI

Quantitative assessment of inflammatory and structural lesions is increasingly being used to assess the therapeutic potential of new agents in clinical trials of axSpA and as endpoints for assessment of prognostic tools. The primary method used for quantifying disease activity and structural lesions in the SI joints on MRI is the Spondyloarthritis Research Consortium of Canada (SPARCC) score. It is based on the assessment of consecutive semicoronal images that depict the cartilaginous portion of the SI joint and the subdivision of each SI joint into quadrants. In the inflammation scoring module, BME on STIR or T2FS scans is scored dichotomously as present/absent in each quadrant with additional weighting for intensity and depth (Fig. 10.24).[36] This method has been shown to be highly discriminatory in placebo-controlled clinical trials of both AS and nr-axSpA.[37] A similar approach is used to quantify fat metaplasia and erosion, whereas backfill and ankylosis are scored in SI joint halves rather than quadrants.[38] The SPARCC SIJ structural score has

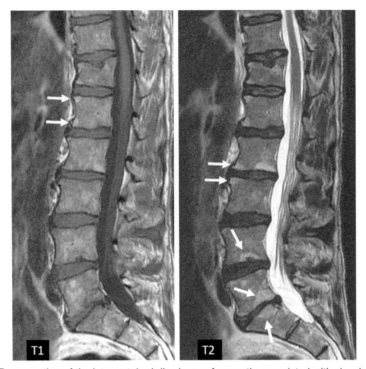

FIG. 10.20 Degeneration of the intervertebral disc is very frequently associated with signal changes in bone marrow, so called Modic changes. The location and signal intensity of the degenerative bone marrow lesions are often very similar to SpA lesions but distinguishing features may be identified. Degenerative corner lesions are usually associated with osteophytes, annular tears and/or nucleus pulposus degeneration. Modic changes related to the vertebral endplate are invariably associated with evidence of degeneration of the nucleus pulposus such as loss of disc height and signal intensity. In this 54 year old man with spondylosis, Modic type II fatty corner lesions are seen anteriorly in the L1 vertebral body (T1 - arrows) with anterior osteophytes and disc degeneration. The T2 image is not fat suppressed with both fluid and fat appearing bright so both Modic type I BME lesions and Modic type II fat lesions have bright signal. Multiple BME lesions are best seen at the vertebral anterior corners adjacent to the L2/3 intervertebral disc and at the endplates of L4, L5 and S1 (T2 – arrows).

also been shown to be discriminatory for treatment group differences in structural lesions in a 12-week placebo-controlled trial of a TNFi in patients with nonradiographic axSpA.[39] Pediatric versions of these two scoring methods have also been developed and validated.

Two primary methods have been used to quantify inflammation in the spine on MRI. Each is based on the assessment of a discovertebral unit, the region between two horizontal lines drawn through the middle of adjacent vertebrae. The Berlin method estimates the percent volume of this region affected by BME, whereas the SPARCC method divides this region into quadrants and scores BME dichotomously as present/absent in each quadrant on three consecutive sagittal slices with additional weighting for intensity and depth.

Online training modules for assessment of MRI lesions in the SI joints and BME in the spine have been developed (available at http://www.carearthritis.com/ MRI_scoring_modules.php).

FUTURE DIRECTIONS

Plain radiography of the SI joints for diagnosis of axSpA will increasingly be replaced by low-radiation CT and MRI of the SI joints as the imaging modalities of choice, particularly as therapeutic advances emphasize the need for early diagnosis and appropriate treatment intervention. There will be increased focus on new imaging

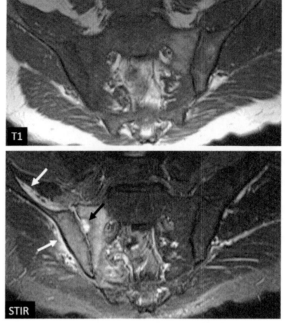

FIG. 10.21 Septic arthritis of the SI joint is usually unilateral and easily distinguished from inflammatory sacroiliitis. In this 43 year old man, extensive BME throughout the right ilium and sacrum is typical for septic arthritis and does not respect anatomical boundaries being associated with periosteal soft tissue inflammation (white arrows) that extends a long way from the joint. A solitary focus of bone destruction represents an intraosseous abscess (black arrow) and is large by comparison to SpA erosions. The left joint is normal and there is no fat metaplasia or other feature of SpA present.

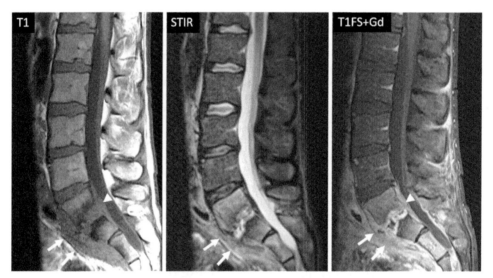

FIG. 10.22 Infectious discitis almost always involves the vertebral endplates with adjacent osteomyelitis and paravertebral inflammation. In a 43 year old man with infectious discitis, the T1W image demonstrates complete destruction of the outline of the vertebral endplates at L5/S1 with sclerosis of the non-eroded bone. Prominent paravertebral soft tissue inflammation anteriorly on all sequences (arrows) is consistent with inflammatory phlegmon demonstrating diffuse contrast enhancement on the T1W sequence with fat saturation following injection of intravenous gadolinium (T1FS+Gd). Posterior epidural inflammatory mass is better appreciated on T1 and T1FS+Gd (arrowheads). BME / osteitis is clearly present throughout the L5 and sacral vertebral bodies on both STIR and T1FS+Gd. While MRI of the spine for SpA can be completed with only T1W and STIR sequences, contrast enhanced sequences are often very important for identification or elucidation of infectious processes in the spine.

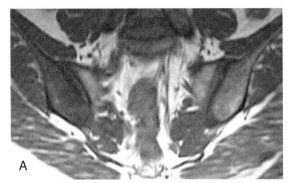

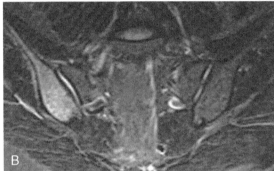

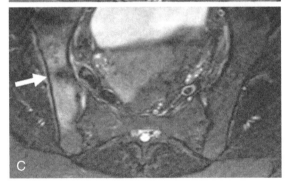

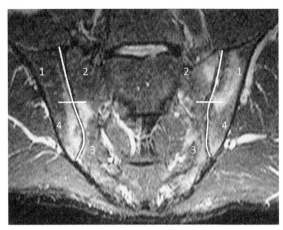

FIG. 10.24 The most common method used for quantifying disease activity and structural lesions in the SI joints on MRI is the Spondyloarthritis Research Consortium of Canada (SPARCC) score. The reader selects the 6 consecutive semicoronal images in the cartilaginous portion of the SI joint that demonstrate the most inflammation. Inflammation is only scored in the subchondral bone of the cartilaginous compartment. For each slice, each joint is divided into 4 sectors representing upper and lower iliac and sacral quadrants. BME on STIR or T2FS images (or osteitis on contrast enhanced images) are scored dichotomously as present/absent with an additional score of 1 for each joint if the BME has depth ≥ 1cm and an additional score of 1 for each joint if BME has intense signal ≥ CSF or well-visualized bright presacral veins. The maximum score for each slice is 12, and in the case illustrated, the score would be 11 with all quadrants positive for BME except the upper right sacrum, and with both joints positive for BME depth and intensity.

FIG. 10.23 A 37 year old HLA-B27 positive female with known uveitis presented with persistent right low back / buttock pain. MRI of the SI joints, performed for suspected sacroiliitis, demonstrates diffuse BME of the right ilium manifest as diminished bone marrow signal on coronal T1W image (A) and increased bone marrow signal on coronal STIR (B) and axial STIR (C). There is no evidence of erosion, fat metaplasia, enthesopathy or soft tissue abnormality and the left SI joint is normal. The articular surfaces are very smooth with thin well defined joint effusions seen in the joint spaces on STIR. The axial image (C) also demonstrates a think linear focus of bone sclerosis perpendicular to the medial iliac cortex immediately anterior to the right SI joint (arrow). The appearances are typical for an insufficiency type stress fracture of the ilium in the greater sciatic notch.

methodologies that are more sensitive to change in disease progression than plain radiography so that disease-modifying therapies can be more readily assessed in clinical trials. These will include low-radiation CT of the spine and MRI "bone-specific" sequences that use ultrashort echo time (UTE) and incorporate fat and adjacent soft-tissue suppression to directly image lamellar bone and produce images of cortical bone that are more similar in quality to that currently available by CT.

REFERENCES

1. van den Berg R, Lenczner G, Feydy A, et al. Agreement between clinical practice and trained central reading in reading of sacroiliac joints on plain pelvic radiographs. Results from the DESIR cohort. *Arthritis Rheumatol.* 2014;66:2403–2411.
2. Battistone MJ, Manaster BJ, Reda DJ, Clegg DO. Radiographic diagnosis of sacroiliitis-are sacroiliac views really better? *J Rheumatol.* 1998;25:2395–2401.

3. Dougados M, Sepriano A, Molto A, et al. Sacroiliac radiographic progression in recent onset axial spondyloarthritis: the 5-year data of the DESIR cohort. *Ann Rheum Dis.* 2017;76(11):1823–1828.

4. Bennett AN, McGonagle D, O'Connor P, et al. Severity of baseline magnetic resonance imaging-evident sacroiliitis and HLA-B27 status in early inflammatory back pain predict radiographically evident ankylosing spondylitis at eight years. *Arthritis Rheum.* 2008;58:3413–3418.

5. Van der Linden SM, Valkenburg HA, Cats A. Evaluation of diagnostic criteria for ankylosing spondylitis: a proposal for modification of the New York criteria. *Arthritis Rheum.* 1984;27:361–368.

6. van den Berg R, de Hooge M, van Gaalen F, Reijnierse M, Huizinga T, van der Heijde D. Percentage of patients with spondyloarthritis in patients referred because of chronic back pain and performance of classification criteria: experience from the Spondyloarthritis Caught Early (SPACE) cohort. *Rheumatology.* 2013;52:1492–1499.

7. O'Shea FD, Boyle E, Salonen DC, et al. Inflammatory and degenerative sacroiliac joint disease in a primary back pain cohort. *Arthritis Care Res.* 2010;62:447–454.

8. van der Heijde D, Salonen D, Weissman BN, et al. Assessment of radiographic progression in the spines of patients with ankylosing spondylitis treated with adalimumab for up to 2 years. *Arthritis Res Ther.* 2009;11:R127.

9. Poddubnyy D, Rudwaleit M, Haibel H, et al. Rates and predictors of radiographic sacroiliitis progression over 2 years in patients with axial spondyloarthritis. *Ann Rheum Dis.* 2011;70:1369–1374.

10. Sepriano A, Rudwaleit M, Sieper J, van den Berg R, Landewé R, van der Heijde D. Five-year follow-up of radiographic sacroiliitis: progression as well as improvement? *Ann Rheum Dis.* 2016;75(6):1262–1263.

11. Dougados M, Maksymowych WP, Landewé RBM, et al. Evaluation of the change in structural radiographic sacroiliac joint damage after 2 years of etanercept therapy (EMBARK trial) in comparison to a contemporary control cohort (DESIR cohort) in recent onset axial spondyloarthritis. *Ann Rheum Dis.* 2018;77(2):221–227.

12. Wanders AJ, Landewe RB, Spoorenberg A, et al. What is the most appropriate radiologic scoring method for ankylosing spondylitis? A comparison of the available methods based on the Outcome Measures in Rheumatology Clinical Trials filter. *Arthritis Rheum.* 2004;50:2622–2632.

13. Geijer M, Gothlin GG, Gothlin JH. The clinical utility of computed tomography compared to conventional radiography in diagnosing sacroiliitis. A retrospective study on 910 patients and literature review. *J Rheumatol.* 2007;34:1561–1565.

14. Devauchelle-Pensec V, D'Agostino MA, Marion J, et al. Computed tomography scanning facilitates the diagnosis of sacroiliitis in patients with suspected spondylarthritis: results of a prospective multicenter French cohort study. *Arthritis Rheum.* 2012;64:1412–1419.

15. Diekhoff T, Hermann KA, Greese J, et al. Comparison of MRI with radiography for detecting structural lesions of the sacroiliac joint using CT as standard of reference: results from the SIMACT study. Online First *Ann Rheum Dis.* March 10, 2017.

16. Chalal BS, Kwan ALC, Dhillon SS, et al. Radiation exposure to the sacroiliac joint from low-dose computed tomography compared to radiography. *AJR Am J Roentgenol.* 2018;211(5):1058–1062.

17. Mettler Jr FA, et al. Effective doses in radiology and diagnostic nuclear medicine. *Radiology.* 2008;248:254–263.

18. Martin CJ. Effective dose: how should it be applied to medical exposures? *Br J Radiol.* 2007;80:639–647.

19. De Bruin F, de Koning A, van den Berg R, et al. Development of the CT Syndesmophyte Score (CTSS) in patients with ankylosing spondylitis: data from the SIAS cohort. *Ann Rheum Dis.* 2018;77(3):371–377.

20. De Koning A, de Bruin F, van den Berg R, et al. Low-dose CT detects more progression of bone formation in comparison to conventional radiography in patients with ankylosing spondylitis: results from the SIAS cohort. *Ann Rheum Dis.* 2018;77(2):293–299.

21. Song IH, Carrasco-Fernandez J, Rudwaleit M, Sieper J. The diagnostic value of scintigraphy in assessing sacroiliitis in ankylosing spondylitis: a systematic literature search. *Ann Rheum Dis.* 2008;67:1535–1540.

22. Muche B, Bollow M, Francois RJ, Sieper J, Hamm B, Braun J. Anatomic structures involved in early- and late-stage sacroiliitis in spondylarthritis. *Arthritis Rheum.* 2003;48:1374–1384.

23. Puhakka KB, Jurik AG, Schiottz-Christensen B, et al. Magnetic resonance imaging of sacroiliitis in early seronegative spondylarthropathy. Abnormalities correlated to clinical and laboratory findings. *Rheumatol.* 2004;43:234–237.

24. Braun J, Bollow M, Eggens U, Konig H, Distler A, Sieper J. Use of dynamic magnetic resonance imaging with fast imaging in the detection of early and advanced sacroiliitis in spondyloarthropathy patients. *Arthritis Rheum.* 1994;37:1039–1045.

25. Bollow M, Fischer T, Reisshauer H, et al. Quantitative analyses of sacroiliac biopsies in spondylarthropathies: T cells and macrophages predominate in early and active sacroiliitis—cellularity correlates with the degree of enhancement detected by magnetic resonance imaging. *Ann Rheum Dis.* 2000;59:135–140.

26. Maksymowych WP, Wichuk S, Chiowchanwisawakit P, Lambert RG, Pedersen SJ. Fat metaplasia and backfill are key intermediaries in the development of sacroiliac joint ankylosis in patients with ankylosing spondylitis. *Arthritis Rheumatol.* 2014;66:2958–2967.

27. Chiowchanwisawakit P, Lambert RGW, Conner-Spady B, Maksymowych WP. Focal fat lesions at vertebral corners on magnetic resonance imaging predict the development of new syndesmophytes in ankylosing spondylitis. *Arthritis Rheum.* 2011;63:2215–2225.

28. Weber U, Lambert RG, Østergaard M, Hodler J, Pedersen SJ, Maksymowych WP. The diagnostic utility of magnetic resonance imaging in spondylarthritis: an international multicenter evaluation of one hundred eighty-seven subjects. *Arthritis Rheum.* 2010;62:3048–3058.

29. Weber U, Østergaard M, Lambert RGW, et al. Candidate lesion-based criteria for defining a positive sacroiliac joint MRI in two cohorts of patients with axial spondyloarthritis. online June *Ann Rheum Dis.* 2014;12.

30. Gong Y, Zheng N, Chen SB, et al. Ten years' experience with needle biopsy in the early diagnosis of sacroiliitis. *Arthritis Rheum.* 2012;64:1399–1406.

31. Mandl P, Navarro-Compán V, Terslev L, et al. EULAR recommendations for the use of imaging in the diagnosis and management of spondyloarthritis in clinical practice. *Ann Rheum Dis.* 2015;74(7):1327–1339.

32. Weber U, Zubler V, Zhao Z, et al. Does spinal MRI add incremental diagnostic value to MRI of the sacroiliac joints alone in non-radiographic axial spondyloarthritis? *Ann Rheum Dis.* 2015;74:985–992.

33. Rudwaleit M, van der Heijde D, Landewe R, et al. The development of Assessment of SpondyloArthritis international Society (ASAS) classification criteria for axial spondyloarthritis (Part II): validation and final selection. *Ann Rheum Dis.* 2009;68:777–783.

34. Rudwaleit M, Jurik AG, Hermann KGA, et al. Defining active sacroiliitis on magnetic resonance imaging (MRI) for classification of axial spondyloarthritis: a consensual approach by the ASAS/OMERACT MRI Group. *Ann Rheum Dis.* 2009;68:1520–1527.

35. Lambert RG, Bakker PA, van der Heijde D, et al. Defining active sacroiliitis on MRI for classification of axial spondyloarthritis: update by the ASAS MRI working group. *Ann Rheum Dis.* 2016;75:1958–1963.

36. Maksymowych WP, Inman RD, Salonen D, et al. Spondyloarthritis research Consortium of Canada magnetic resonance imaging index for assessment of sacroiliac joint inflammation in ankylosing spondylitis. *Arthritis Rheum.* 2005;53:703–709.

37. Lambert RGW, Salonen D, Rahman P, et al. Adalimumab significantly reduces both spinal and sacroiliac joint inflammation in patients with ankylosing spondylitis. *Arthritis Rheum.* 2007;56:4005–4014.

38. Maksymowych WP, Wichuk S, Chiowchanwisawakit P, Lambert RG, Pedersen SJ. Development and preliminary validation of the spondyloarthritis research consortium of Canada magnetic resonance imaging sacroiliac joint structural score. *J Rheumatol.* 2015;42:79–86.

39. Maksymowych WP, Wichuk S, Dougados M, et al. Modification of structural lesions on MRI of the sacroiliac joints by etanercept in the EMBARK trial: a 12-week randomised placebo-controlled trial in patients with non-radiographic axial spondyloarthritis. *Ann Rheum Dis.* 2018;77(1):78–84.

FURTHER READING

1. Maksymowych WP. Imaging in axial spondyloarthritis: evaluation of inflammatory and structural changes. *Rheum Dis Clin N Am.* 2016;42:645–662.

CHAPTER 11

Extraarticular Manifestations: Uveitis, Colitis, Psoriasis

SONAM KIWALKAR, MBBS • JAMES T. ROSENBAUM, MD, PHD • SERGIO SCHWARTZMAN, MD • JAN PETER DUTZ, MD, FRCPC • FILIP VAN DEN BOSCH, MD, PHD

INTRODUCTION

Extraarticular manifestations (EAMs) associated with axial spondyloarthritis (axSpA) include diseases or conditions involving the skin, eye, gastrointestinal, and cardiorespiratory systems. EAMs such as psoriasis, inflammatory bowel disease, and uveitis have well-established associations in observational studies, whereas the association between cardiovascular disease and ankylosing spondylitis (AS) is less validated. An epidemiologic study of 847 patients in Belgium with AS found that 42% had one or more EAMs, including acute anterior uveitis present in 27%, IBD in 10%, and psoriasis in 11%.[1] This illustrates the relatively high frequency of EAMs in axSpA patients. We will be focusing on acute anterior uveitis (AAU), inflammatory bowel disease (IBD), and psoriasis in this chapter.

EAMs in axSpA have gleaned increasing interest over the past few years for several reasons. It has been recognized that the presence of AAU, psoriasis, and IBD in patients with inflammatory back pain may help to make a diagnosis in patients with spondyloarthritis (SpA). This is underscored by the inclusion of EAMs in different criteria sets, which aim to classify SpA, such as the Amor criteria, the European Spondyloarthropathy Study Group (ESSG) criteria,[2,3] as well as the more recent Assessment of SpondyloArthritis International Society (ASAS) classification criteria for axial and peripheral SpA.[4,5] Secondly, EAMs tend to influence management choices. EAMs pose complex treatment decision questions that need to cross boundaries between specialties, thus mandating a multidisciplinary approach.[6] Different approved therapies for SpA may have greater impact on individual EAMs. Because of the chronicity of axSpA and its development in early adulthood, axSpA affects not only physical function and quality of life but also the ability to work and the use of health resources.[7] Consequently there is a burden to both patient and society. EAMs associated with AS contribute to this burden. For example, two patients with the same degree of back pain and radiographic findings will not share the same quality of life if one of them also has uveitis. EAMs can serve as a marker of severity of AS. In a longitudinal study, patients with AS and uveitis had a significant decline in Bath Ankylosing Spondylitis Functional Index (BASFI) scores compared with patients without uveitis.[8] Furthermore, patients with AS who also had psoriasis or IBD had a greater disease activity and lower physical function compared with those who did not have these comorbid conditions. Radiographic progression was worse for those with iritis and AS compared with those with AS alone.[9] Moreover, a recent study has investigated the economic burden of uveitis in French and German AS patients and found a substantially higher cost associated with the development of AAU among patients with AS.[10]

This chapter focuses on delineating the epidemiology, clinical characteristics, pathogenesis, and treatment challenges that rheumatologists face when dealing with EAMs.

EPIDEMIOLOGY OF EXTRAARTICULAR MANIFESTATIONS

Prevalence of EAMs

Although many studies report on the occurrence of EAMs, the prevalence of reported EAMs varies substantially based on the characteristics of cohorts and study design. To summarize and evaluate the published estimates for the prevalence of EAMs among patients with AS, Stolwijk et al. published a systematic review and metaanalysis. The pooled prevalence for acute anterior uveitis (AAU) was 25.8%.[11] The prevalence of AAU was associated with an increased duration of axSpA. It increased from 17.4% in studies including patients with a mean disease duration <10 year, to 38.5% in those studies with a mean disease duration

>20 years. In a supporting study that followed more than 1500 patients with AS there was a progressive increase of self-reported AAU with increased disease duration of AS. More than 50% of AS patients had AAU if they were followed for more than 40 years.[12] In studies where AAU was self-reported, there was higher prevalence compared with studies which required a diagnosis made by an ophthalmologist. The prevalence also varied according to geographical regions. Estimates were highest from North America (35.2%) and lowest in populations from Asia (21.4%) and Latin America (20.1%). The pooled prevalence of psoriasis was 9.3%, and for IBD it was 6.8%. Like AAU, the prevalence of psoriasis and IBD differed by geographical areas. The highest prevalence of psoriasis was from studies in Europe (10.9%) and the lowest was in Asia (3.2%). The highest prevalence of IBD was seen in Latin America (9.6%) and the lowest was seen in Asia (2.9%). It is well known that AAU is more prevalent in HLA-B27-positive patients compared with HLA-B27-negative patients.[12a,12b] Interestingly, in the meta-analysis published by Stolwijk et al.,[11] it was suggested that most differences between the geographical areas remained significant even after controlling for HLA-B27 in the multiregression analysis. This suggests that other environmental or epigenetic factors could play a role.

Prevalence of EAMs in AS Versus nr-axSpA

The early studies published on EAMs included patients with AS classified according to the modified New York criteria.[13] It was not until 2009, when ASAS classification criteria were developed to identify patients with early disease including nonradiographic axSpA (nr-axSpA) that this new group of patients was recognized. A meta-analysis published in 2016[14] was done with the objective to assess the prevalence of EAMs in AS and nr-axSpA. Table 11.1 depicts the results.

Conclusions from this study were as follows:
1. EAMs significantly contribute to the burden of both AS and nr-axSpA.
2. Uveitis has been reported to be more prevalent in AS than nr-AxSpA,[14] and it was hypothesized that the longer duration of disease in AS patients compared with nr-axSpA could account for the higher prevalence. However, a cross-sectional study published in 2009, which analyzed 462 patients (266 nr-axSpA and 236 AS) who were participants in the German SpA inception cohort, the prevalence of uveitis was not different between groups.[15] Because the prevalence of uveitis is high in both AS and nr-axSpA, ASAS recommends a combination

TABLE 11.1

Prevalence of Extraarticular Manifestations in Ankylosing Spondylitis and Nonradiographic axSpA

Features	Ankylosing Spondylitis	Non-Radiographic Axial Spondyloarthritis
Uveitis	23%	15.9%
Inflammatory bowel disease	4.1%	6.4%
Psoriasis	10.2%	10.9%
Symptom duration (years)	1.2–17.7	1.0–12.1

of AAU, HLA-B27 positivity, and inflammatory back pain to be sufficient to classify a patient with axSpA.[4,15]

Prevalence of EAMs in Pre- and Post-Biologic Eras

To compare the prevalence of EAMs in the pre- and post-anti-tumor necrosis factor (TNFi) periods, Varkas et al.[16] compared two large databases: a pre-TNF Belgian cohort (ASPECT) to a post-anti-TNF BelGian Inflammatory Arthritis and spoNdylitis cohorT (Be-GIANT). The results are shown in Table 11.2.

This study again suggests the EAMs seemed to increase with disease duration in both pre- and post-TNF periods and may be linked to longer cumulative exposure to the inflammation. Interestingly in this cohort, the frequency of uveitis and psoriasis does not seem to be diminished by the use of a TNFi.

Cumulative Incidence of EAMs

Previous studies have shown that prevalence of EAMs such as AAU, IBD, and psoriasis is increased in axSpA patients compared with the general population. Thus, it would be interesting to identify characteristics of patients who have an increased propensity to develop EAMs. Results from a 12-year OASIS cohort[17] tried to answer this question. When followed longitudinally for 12 years, patients who developed new IBD had a higher baseline Bath Ankylosing Spondylitis Disease Activity Index (BASDAI) and more spinal pain. None of the baseline characteristics contributed to the development of acute anterior uveitis or psoriasis in the study.

To determine the risk of acquiring an extraarticular manifestation during the course of the disease in

TABLE 11.2
Prevalence of EAMs

Features	ASPECT (N=847) COHORT		(BE-) GIANT (N=215) COHORT	
Disease Duration	Less than 10 years	More than 20 years	Less than 10 years	More than 10 years
EAMs free	70%	39%	71.5%	55.1%
Uveitis	15%	34%	11.1%	30.4%
Psoriasis	9%	6%	10.4%	8.7%
IBD	4%	11%	5.5%	1.4%

TABLE 11.3
Cumulative Incidence at Diagnosis and 20 Years Later

		AAU		IBD		PSORIASIS	
		axSpA pts	Controls	axSpA pts	Controls	axSpA pts	Controls
Cumulative incidence	At diagnosis	11.9%	0.5%	4.0%	0.6%	4.7%	2.6%
	After 20 years	24.5%	0.6%	7.5%	0.8%	10.1%	5.0%

patients with AS compared with the general population, Stolwijk et al. calculated cumulative incidence at diagnosis and 20 years after.[18] The findings are summarized in Table 11.3:

The cumulative incidence for AAU doubled after 20 years, which was significantly faster than controls. On the other hand, the cumulative incidence of psoriasis and IBD increased gradually over 20 years, with a slope comparable with controls.

Depending on the specific type of EAM, there may be different variables impacting on risk.

UVEITIS

Definition and Classification

Uveitis is defined as inflammation of the uvea, which corresponds to the middle layer of the eye. It consists of the iris and ciliary body forming the anterior uvea, and the choroid defining the posterior uvea. Intermediate uveitis refers to inflammatory cells in the vitreous humor, which fills the chamber posterior to the lens in the eye. It is useful to classify uveitis according to anatomy and clinical course (Fig. 11.1).

Acute Anterior Uveitis in axSpA

Large epidemiology studies have confirmed that anterior uveitis accounts for 81%–85% of all cases of uveitis.[19,20] Furthermore, HLA-B27 is associated in about 50% of instances of acute anterior uveitis (AAU).[21] HLA-B27-associated uveitis is typically anterior and

self-limited; the onset is usually sudden; and the inflammation is usually managed with just topical corticosteroids and topical cyclopentolate to dilate the pupil.[21] Because of the association of HLA-B27 with axSpA, it is not surprising that uveitis occurring in axSpA patients is predominantly anterior. In a study from a referral center in Paris, 175 HLA-B27-positive anterior uveitis patients were seen over a duration of 5 years.[22] On rheumatologic evaluation 77% had extraocular involvement and 46% had definite AS by the New York criteria. Demographic and clinical characteristics of uveitis and extraocular manifestations were noted. Patients with and without extraocular manifestations were compared. The study suggests the following:[22]

1. Rheumatologic symptoms preceded the first attack of uveitis in most cases (>80% cases).
2. The onset of extraocular symptoms occurrs at a younger age (26.4 ± 11.1 years), compared with the first attack of uveitis (34.0 ± 14.1 years).
3. Patients with SpA who were HLA-B27-positive had a greater number of recurrent attacks.

Similar findings were also suggested in a Chinese study.[23] Muñoz-Fernández et al. evaluated patients who have idiopathic recurrent HLA-B27-positive AAU (without a diagnosis of SpA). It was noted that a high percentage of these patients had enthesitis or an incomplete form of SpA.[24] A large multicentric, observational, prospective study, SENTINEL, published in 2016 investigated the prevalence of SpA in 798 patients with anterior uveitis. Patients were characterized as to HLA B27

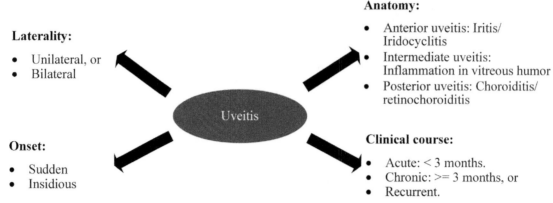

Laterality:

- Unilateral, or
- Bilateral

Onset:

- Sudden
- Insidious

Anatomy:

- Anterior uveitis: Iritis/ Iridocyclitis
- Intermediate uveitis: Inflammation in vitreous humor
- Posterior uveitis: Choroiditis/ retinochoroiditis

Clinical course:

- Acute: < 3 months.
- Chronic: >= 3 months, or
- Recurrent.

Uveitis

FIG. 11.1 Classification of uveitis.

status. 50.2% who presented with anterior uveitis were found to have axSpA. This percentage rose to 69.8% if patients were HLA-B27-positive.[25]

How often is acute anterior uveitis, the clinical manifestation that leads to a diagnosis of AS? Rosenbaum published a study in 1989, which included 236 consecutive patients with uveitis who were evaluated by a rheumatologist, of whom 13% had SpA. It was interesting to note that two-thirds of these patients were not known to have SpA before the eye inflammation. Similar results were seen in a study by Pato et al. who collected demographic data from 514 patients who were referred to the uveitis clinic. About one-fourth of the patients (22.7%) had some form of SpA, half of whom were diagnosed only after the first episode of uveitis. The undiagnosed SpA patients had shorter clinical evolution and less radiographic damage than those with known SpA.[26] Another study evaluated 394 patients with uveitis, of whom 18% had some form of SpA. Of these, less than half were undiagnosed, and uveitis was the first manifestation.[27] In summary then, AAU may be the first clinical manifestation of SpA. This suggests that the collaboration between ophthalmologists and rheumatologists greatly aids the diagnosis and treatment of such patients. To facilitate this process, a novel evidence-based algorithm called Dublin Uveitis Evaluation Tool (DUET) was proposed to guide ophthalmologists to refer AAU cases to rheumatology.

The DUET was published as a simple-to-follow, stepwise approach to effectively recognize SpA among patients with uveitis. First, the patient is thoroughly assessed through standardized clinical history, examination, and laboratory workup. If they do not carry a prior diagnosis of SpA, they are then queried as to whether they have had chronic (>3 months) back pain with onset of symptoms before the age of 45 years.

They are also screened for other joint pain and swelling. If they fulfill any of the above criteria, an HLA-B27 test is ordered. If positive, they are then referred to a rheumatologist. If negative, the patient would be then assessed for psoriasis. If psoriasis is evident on history or physical exam, the patient is also referred to a rheumatologist. This algorithm (96% sensitivity and 97% specificity) was created for appropriate and timely referral from ophthalmologists for the rapid diagnosis of SpA.[28]

Uveitis is reported to be the most common EAM in SpA.[29] The prevalence of uveitis among patients with SpA has been evaluated in several studies and is proposed to be roughly 10%–40%.[29-36] A metaanalysis of approximately 30,000 patients published in 2008 revealed that the prevalence of uveitis was 32.7% when these patients were followed for a mean duration of 17.7 years.[37] If the disease was diagnosed for less than 5 years, the prevalence of uveitis was 12.3%, whereas it rose to 42.8% if the follow-up was for 20–25 years. The prevalence of uveitis was higher in patients who were HLA-B27-positive. The authors also suggested that uveitis was acute in 88.7%, anterior in 90.5%, and unilateral in 87.3%. Recurrence occurred in 50.6%, whereas reduction of visual acuity was observed in 8.3%.

Uveitis seen in association with AS is foreshadowed by eye discomfort during a prodromal phase. This is followed by an acute onset of eye redness, pain, photophobia, and miosis. Visual acuity is generally preserved and, if diminished, is usually caused by cystoid macular edema. Pain is secondary to ciliary spasm due to anterior chamber inflammation. It can radiate all around the distribution of the first branch of the trigeminal nerve and the periorbital area. Complications associated with this type of uveitis consist mainly of hypopyon and posterior synechiae (pupil is adherent to lens). Although flares tend to be severe, appropriate treatment tends to resolve it in less than 3–4 months. Despite the recurrent nature of uveitis attacks, <5% developed visual impairment, and <2% developed legal blindness.[38] Another study confirmed that the prognosis in such patients was good, but among those who lost visual acuity, glaucoma or glaucoma surgery was frequently the cause.[17] On the other hand, uveitis seen in psoriatic arthritis or inflammatory bowel disease is sometimes insidious in onset, anterior or intermediate in location, bilateral, chronic, and more common in females.[39] See Table 11.4 for differences.

Possible Links between Uveitis and Ankylosing Spondylitis

The similarities and differences in the pathogenesis of uveitis and arthritis remain a subject of discussion and research. In 1973, Brewerton et al. established human leucocyte antigen (HLA)-B27 as a possible link between SpA and uveitis.[40] HLA-B27 transgenic rats and control nontransgenic rats were infected with *Salmonella* or *Yersinia*. After 7 days of infection, they developed AAU, which resembled human AAU. However, the expression of HLA-B27 did not appear to influence the incidence or severity of uveitis, suggesting that it is not the only contributing factor.[41] Another study in 1995 suggested that LMP2 and HLA-DR8 genes may influence the relative risk for AAU in patients with AS.[42] Robinson et al. in 2015 used high-density genotyping to investigate the genetic associations of AAU in patients. They compared 1711 patients with AAU (with or without AS) with 2339 with AS and no history of uveitis.[12] A summary of the results is depicted in Fig. 11.2: the authors concluded

that many genes predispose to both spondylitis and uveitis, but a few genes were identified that specifically predispose to uveitis.

The explanation for coexistence of uveitis and inflammatory arthritis is not well understood. There are a number of animal models that may provide some insight. Whereas most animal models do not display this coexistence, the SKG mouse model showed that after systemic injection with curdlan, arthritis, and unilateral uveitis coexisted, along with enthesitis, dactylitis, plantar fasciitis, vertebral inflammation, and ileitis.[43] Kezic et al. suggested that uveitis can coexist with arthritis in BALB/C mice when they are immunized with aggrecan. Administering IL-17 neutralizing antibodies in the murine model prevented arthritis and uveitis. This suggests a shared link in pathogenesis.[44] However, deletion of IFN (interferon) γ ameliorates arthritis but worsens uveitis. This suggests that the eye and arthritis inflammation pathways may diverge after a common

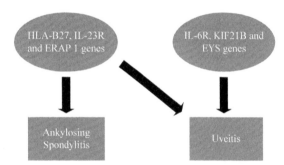

FIG. 11.2 Summary of results from high-density genotyping.[12]

TABLE 11.4
Patterns of Uveitis Associated With AS, PsA, and IBD

Features	UVEITIS	
	Ankylosing Spondylitis(AS)	**Psoriatic arthritis(PsA) and IBD Associated Arthritis**
Onset	Sudden	Insidious
Course of disease	Acute or Recurrent	Sometimes chronic
Anatomy	Anterior	Anterior or intermediate
LATERALITY		
Unilateral	52%	19%
Flip flop[a]	42%	19%
Bilateral	6%	63%
Gender	Males > Females	Females > males

[a]Flip flop: both eyes become involved, but not simultaneously.

point.[45] Arthritis and uveitis also coexist in the rat model of adjuvant arthritis, which is induced by the systemic injection of killed mycobacteria in mineral oil.[46]

Since the first suggestion that a common link exists between the pathogenesis of AAU and SpA, a great amount of research has been done. However, there still remain a lot of knowledge gaps, and the precise mechanism remains unclear.

Treatment

For simplicity, management of anterior uveitis can be broken down into two parts: the first section will be about management of acute flares, whereas the second will be a guide to prevent recurrences.

1. **Stepwise approach to treat acute anterior uveitis:**
   Therapy of axSpA-associated AAU consists of a short course of corticosteroids administered either topically, periocularly, or systemically. Patients usually respond well to topical corticosteroids. Periocular corticosteroid injection is useful when there is a lack of compliance with topical treatment, no improvement after initial topical treatment, flare-ups, or tendency to a chronic course after tapering-off of topical treatment. Oral corticosteroids may be required in cases of recalcitrant inflammation—although this approach may be restricted because of intolerance or side effects. A small percentage of patients have frequent recurrences, which may warrant prophylactic therapy to reduce disease occurrence (Fig. 11.3).

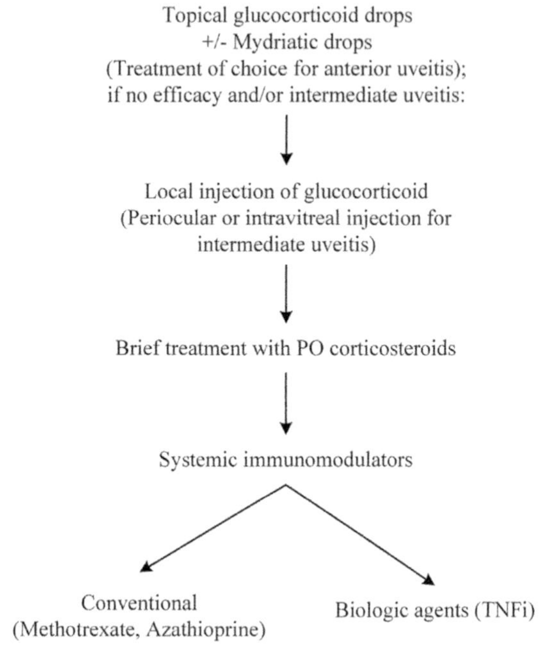

   Difluprednate can sometimes replace regional injection of corticosteroids to treat intermediate uveitis. It is a corticosteroid preparation with good distribution to the vitreous humor.

2. **Guide to prevent recurrences:**
   NSAIDs are frequently used to treat axSpA. Fiorelli et al. suggested that NSAIDs could reduce recurrence of uveitis.[47] 59 patients (of whom one-third were HLA-B27-positive) with recurrent uveitis were followed for a year before and after beginning NSAIDs. The number of relapses before treatment was 2.84 flares/year and that declined to 0.53 flares/year while on NSAIDs, showing a benefit. However, the data are retrospective and may possibly suffer from "regression to the mean" and so the role of NSAIDs in preventing attacks has not been shown definitively.[48] Anti-TNF antibody plus NSAIDs reduces the risk of uveitis to a greater extent than NSAIDs alone in AS patients with a history of uveitis.[48a] There are some positive data suggesting methotrexate prevents recurrence risk of anterior uveitis.[11,48b] Methotrexate and sulphasalazine reduced the uveitis relapse rate

Topical glucocorticoid drops
+/- Mydriatic drops
(Treatment of choice for anterior uveitis);
if no efficacy and/or intermediate uveitis:

↓

Local injection of glucocorticoid
(Periocular or intravitreal injection for intermediate uveitis)

↓

Brief treatment with PO corticosteroids

↓

Systemic immunomodulators

Conventional (Methotrexate, Azathioprine)   Biologic agents (TNFi)

FIG. 11.3 Simplified step-up approach use to treat acute noninfectious uveitis. Conventional treatment can also include use of mycophenolate, although methotrexate is most effective among them.

in HLA-B27-positive AAU patients, with methotrexate showing a beneficial effect on AAU-related macular edema.[48b] As discussed in the pathogenesis section, studies demonstrating subclinical intestinal inflammation and the role of gram-negative bacteria in patients with AAU have led to the hypothesis that sulfasalazine might prevent or improve eye disease. In a small retrospective analysis of 22 patients, Dougados suggested sulfasalazine was associated with prevention of recurrent attacks of SpA-associated uveitis.[49] Another study included patients who had at least two recurrent acute attacks of uveitis in the last year. 22 such patients were included, of which 10 patients were randomized to receive oral sulfasalazine and 12 patients were randomized to no treatment. Patients randomized to sulfasalazine had decreased number of uveitis recurrences compared with the placebo group.[50] Although sulfasalazine can be used to prevent uveitis, it may benefit only peripheral not axial manifestations in SpA.[51]

Based on data from 13 randomized clinical trials, it seems that the efficacy of all TNF inhibitors is comparable for axial and peripheral rheumatologic symptoms in axSpA. Despite the fact that it was not the primary aim to evaluate the efficacy of TNFi with regard to EAMs, a metaanalysis published by Braun et al., showed that infliximab decreased flares of AAU in patients with AS. Frequency of flares in the placebo arm was 15.6 per 100 patient-years, whereas frequency of flares in the infliximab arm was 3.4 per 100 patient-years. In the same trial, frequency of flares for patients on etanercept was 7.9 per 100 patient-years.[52] The difference between the incidence of acute uveitis flares between placebo and all TNF inhibitors was significant. Although the strength was stronger for infliximab ($P = 0.005$) than etanercept ($P = 0.05$). The difference in efficacy between infliximab and etanercept did not reach statistical significance ($P = 0.08$). To further evaluate the efficacy of etanercept in preventing uveitis relapse, Lie et al. in a Swedish registry compared the effects of adalimumab, etanercept, and infliximab on anterior uveitis occurrences in AS patients. 1365 patients with AS were included.[53] Compared with pretreatment rates, a reduction in rates of uveitis was observed for adalimumab and infliximab. There was an increase in rates of uveitis for etanercept.

In a subsequent study to evaluate the effect of adalimumab on the frequency of anterior uveitis, 1250 patients with active AS were evaluated.[54] They were enrolled in a multinational, open-labeled, uncontrolled study. Uveitis flares before and during adalimumab treatment were compared. As shown in the figure below, during adalimumab treatment, the rate of uveitis was reduced by 51% in all patients and by 58% in patients with a history of uveitis (Fig. 11.4).

Other anti TNF agents have been studied. A study done in 2016 compared incidence of uveitis flares in axSpA patients who were treated with certolizumab versus placebo. The rate of uveitis flares was lower in certolizumab (3.0 per 100 patient–years) than in placebo (10.3 per 100 patient–years)[55] A smaller trial demonstrated efficacy of golimumab in patients with recurrent uveitis who had AS.[56] Until more evidence is available, it can be concluded that TNFi (predominantly adalimumab and infliximab) seems to be more effective in lowering the recurrence rate of uveitis compared with etanercept.

There are some reports about etanercept causing de novo uveitis. A French nationwide study collected de novo onset of uveitis cases in patients on TNFi with rheumatologic diseases.[57] 31 cases were recorded, of which 19 occurred in AS. After normalizing for estimated number of patients treated with each medication, etanercept was associated with a greater number of uveitis cases than adalimumab and infliximab ($P < 0.01$). After excluding patients with underlying rheumatologic conditions, etanercept was again found to be statistically more likely to be associated with uveitis. Data from case series and reports show an additional 121 cases of new onset uveitis and also disclosed etanercept as the most common TNFi associated with uveitis. Further evidence emerges from the fact that uveitis, which can sometimes be bilateral, resolved on stopping the treatment, and in some cases, it recurred after a rechallenge.[58,58a,58b] Some patients benefited from switching to other TNFi.[58]

It is fair to say that etanercept has a greater propensity than monoclonal antibodies to cause de novo uveitis.[57,58,58a,58b] However, these findings do not support the use of infliximab or adalimumab over etanercept; rather, if a patient develops uveitis

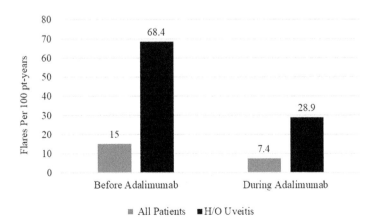

FIG. 11.4 Anterior uveitis flares before and during treatment with adalimumab.

TABLE 11.5
Available Treatment Modalities for axSpA and Uveitis in a Nutshell

Treatment Modalities	Axial Spondyloarthritis	Uveitis
Nonsteroidal antiinflammatory drugs (NSAIDs)	+	*
Sulfasalazine	Benefit for peripheral arthritis only	**
Monoclonal antibodies (adalimumab, infliximab)	+	+
Soluble receptor antibodies (etanercept)	+	−
Secukinumab (IL-17 inhibitor)	+	?

*Some evidence to suggest that use prevents attacks; no consistent benefit for active uveitis
**Strong evidence that use reduces frequency of attacks; no benefit for active uveitis

TABLE 11.6
Differences in Type I and Type II Peripheral Arthritis Seen in IBD

Type I Arthritis	Type II Arthritis
Pauciarticular	Polyarticular
Self-limited <10 weeks	Persistent for months to years
Parallels with intestinal activity	Independent of intestinal activity
Strongly associated with other EIMs	Weakly associated with other EIMs

EIMs, Extraintestinal Manifestations, e.g., Erythema Nodosum, Pyoderma Gangrenosum, and uveitis.

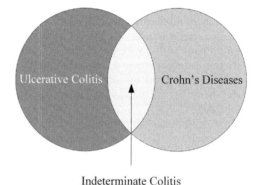

FIG. 11.5 Spectrum of IBD

during etanercept therapy, especially if the uveitis is severe or bilateral, then a change to infliximab or other monoclonal anti-TNF antibodies may be warranted.[59] Under such circumstances, uveitis is considered a paradoxical effect of TNF inhibitors that rheumatologists and ophthalmologists need to recognize.

Secukinumab has been studied in four randomized controlled trials for various forms of uveitis other than AAU. Three of these four studies failed to meet the primary efficacy endpoint.[60]

3. **Treat to target and the impact of uveitis**
Treat-to-target guidelines for SpA were published in 2018.[61] These guidelines conclude that the activity of uveitis should not be included in defining the activity of SpA. This recommendation makes sense because uveitis might be active independently of the spinal and joint disease and uveitis might respond to medication which is ineffective for the joints or vice versa. On the other hand, patients who experience uveitis often indicate that it has a marked effect on quality of life. (Table 11.5).

INFLAMMATORY BOWEL DISEASE
Definition and Classification
The spectrum of IBD includes ulcerative colitis, Crohn disease, and indeterminate colitis. It is characterized by chronic inflammation of the gut (Table 11.6; Fig. 11.5).

Approximately 10% of patients with IBD develop arthritis. It is the most common extraintestinal manifestation (EIM) of IBD.[62] Locomotor complications of IBD can be classified into peripheral and axial syndromes (Fig. 11.6).

To understand the natural history of arthritis in IBD patients, a large study was conducted about two decades ago in the United Kingdom.[63] Orchard et al. published the following results (Table 11.7).

It is interesting to note that, although type I peripheral arthritis is commonly associated with bowel relapses, it is certainly not the rule. Furthermore, in contrast to rheumatoid arthritis, IBD-associated peripheral arthritis is nonerosive or nondeforming.[64]

The chance of patients with SpA developing clinically apparent IBD is 5%–10%.[65] The following are some of the diagnostic clues that a rheumatologist should seek to diagnose IBD in axSpA patients:

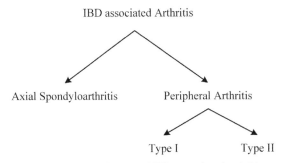

FIG. 11.6 Classification of IBD-associated arthritis.

TABLE 11.7
Prevalence of Peripheral Arthritis in IBD

INFLAMMATORY BOWEL DISEASE		Type I Arthritis	Type II Arthritis
Ulcerative colitis (n=976)	Prevalence	3.6%	2.5%
	Associated with intestinal activity	83%	29%
Crohn disease	Prevalence	6.0%	4.0%
	Associated with intestinal activity	76%	42%

1. Chronic diarrhea, chronic abdominal pain, rectal bleeding, weight loss, or persistent fever.
2. History or evidence of perianal fistula/abscess and anemia.
3. Family history of IBD.

Possible Links Between IBD and Ankylosing Spondylitis

For a long time, it has been recognized that about 60% of patients with SpA show microscopic inflammatory gut lesions, a fraction of which (10%) evolve into IBD. This evolution of gut histology was portrayed in a seminal paper in 1988 by Mielants et al.[66] Ileocolonoscopy was performed on 217 patients with SpA (except those with known inflammatory bowel disease). At baseline, 32% had normal gut histology, 23% had acute microscopic changes, and 45% had chronic microscopic changes. A few years later, 123 of those had the same procedure repeated.[67] 6% of patients with SpA without manifestations of overt IBD on initial examination developed IBD. Of these, seven had chronic gut inflammation and one had acute gut inflammation. All had active spondylitis on initial and subsequent visits. Accordingly, the authors suggested that persistently high articular disease activity, and inflammatory gut lesions at first ileocolonoscopy were risk factors to develop IBD. Of the 123 patients, 49

patients were sequentially rescoped.[62] Patients who had articular remission had normalization of endoscopic appearance and gut histology. On the other hand, those who had persistent articular complaints were associated with persistent gut inflammation and reappearance of gut inflammation during articular flare-ups. This confirms an association of inflammation of the bowel and the articular manifestations of SpA.

Similar results were documented even in the post-TNFi era. About 50% of the study population in 2012 had microscopic bowel inflammation. Compared with those who had a normal bowel biopsy, axSpA patients with microscopic bowel involvement were males, had a higher BASDAI, and were younger. Microscopic bowel inflammation was shown to be associated with a severe articular disease phenotype and extensive bone marrow edema of the sacroiliac joints.[68,69] These data solidify the link between mucosal inflammation and axSpA.

Another indication that a pathophysiologic connection exists between AS and IBD was suggested in a study by de Vries in 2010.[70] 55% of subjects with AS without overt IBD had a positive test for at least one of the following: perinuclear antineutrophil cytoplasmic antibody (ANCA), antibodies to the cell wall mannan of *Saccharomyces cerevisiae* (ASCA), or antibodies to porin protein C of *Escherichia coli* (OmpC). These serologic markers are often used to support a diagnosis of IBD, thus strengthening a common path of pathogenesis (Fig. 11.7).

It has been postulated that the progression of subclinical inflammation to overt IBD in axSpA patients is a cascade of events. This cascade represents an entire gamut—from prehistologic immune changes, to premacroscopic changes, to early preclinical changes, and finally to overt inflammatory bowel disease, which in turn is dictated by genetic or environmental factors. Further identification of biomarkers that are associated with progression toward overt IBD in patients with axSpA would open new routes in pathophysiology as well as early intervention (Fig. 11.8).

This brings us to the next question—is there an association between the presence of microscopic bowel inflammation and response to anti-TNF therapy? A prospective observational cohort trial proposed that the time to initiation of TNF inhibitor was sooner for patients with microscopic bowel inflammation, compared with those with normal biopsy findings.[71] Moreover, 10 of 11 patients with microscopic bowel inflammation showed clinically important Ankylosing Spondylitis Disease Activity Score (ASDAS) improvement, whereas this was only the case for 6/13 (46.2%) patients with normal bowel histology ($P<.05$). Even though associated with a more severe phenotype, it is reassuring that patients with microscopic bowel inflammation are responsive to treatment.

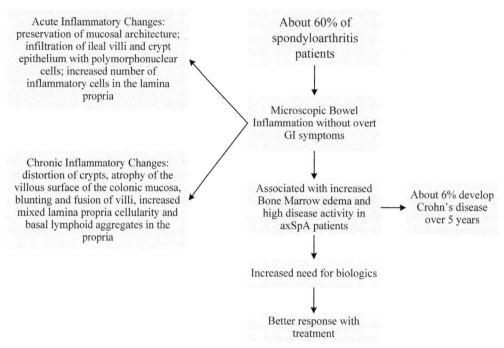

FIG. 11.7 Link between gut inflammation and spondyloarthritis.

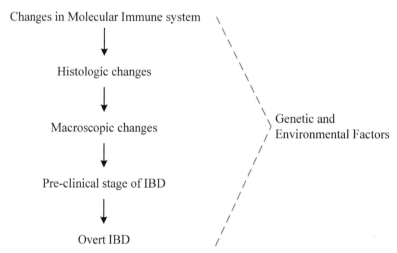

FIG. 11.8 Bowel of patients with axSpA and the immune cascade.

Presence of microscopic bowel inflammation on ileocolonoscopy in patients with axSpA thus seems to be a promising strategy to stratify patients to understand their prognosis. This should be weighed against the invasive procedure risk and cost associated with ileocolonoscopy. Calprotectin is a cytosolic protein expressed by phagocytic myeloid cells that is released at the site of inflammation. It activates the innate immune system via Toll-like receptors. Results from a study by Cypers et al.[72] suggested that a combination of serum and fecal calprotectin measurements in addition to C-reactive protein (C-RP) may be useful in identifying patients with axSpA at higher risk of subclinical bowel inflammation. Such patients might benefit from closer follow-up. Hence, markers like these could play a role in overall patient stratification. Nonetheless, larger studies are needed to provide more insight.

Subclinical or clinical inflammation of the gut in AS is of particular interest as this may provide a valuable clue for unscrambling the pathogenesis of the disease. A recent study[73] showed distinct microbial colonization in the terminal ileum for a small number of patients with AS using healthy individuals as controls. There was an increase in certain microbes—Lachnospiraceae, Ruminococcaceae, and Prevotellaceae, in AS patients. Interestingly, these bacterial species are also observed in a colitis model in mice.[74] Another study evaluated the microbiome of IBD patients with or without peripheral SpA. IBD patients with peripheral SpA revealed a selective enrichment in IgA-coated *E. coli* that was not present in patients without SpA. This strain of *E. coli* was similar to an adherent invasive *E. coli*, which has shown to induce Th17 helper cells. Furthermore, colonization of IL-10-deficient mice with SpA-derived E. coli led to a severe colitis and inflammatory arthritis. These data suggest that the gut microbiome can be a link between mucosal and systemic inflammation.[75]

A number of studies support increased intestinal permeability in AS patients, which is identical to IBD populations.[76] Understanding the complexity and dynamic nature of gut microbiology and its role in inflammatory disorders including SpA and IBD is a work in progress. Grasping this better may provide a window of opportunity to identify a common link between these diseases. This may open new avenues for antibiotic treatment, diet, probiotics, and even fecal transplant as future management options.

Treatment

The Italian Expert Panel[77] on the management of patients with coexisting SpA and IBD breaks down management of the coexisting conditions into two sets of recommendations: one set with active axSpA and the other with active IBD (Figs. 11.9 and 11.10):

1. **Patients with axSpA and active IBD:**

   The overall goal of active IBD therapy is to achieve corticosteroid-free clinical remission, mucosal healing, and decrease long-term complications requiring hospitalization and surgery. Nonsteroidal antiinflammatory drugs (NSAIDs) form the backbone of treatment of AS, as they reduce radiographic progression of the disease. Treatment with NSAIDs poses a challenge when trying to comanage a patient with AS and IBD. Evidence from case reports suggests that treatment with conventional NSAIDs is associated with intestinal relapses in patients with active IBD. Evans et al.[78] showed that NSAIDs are associated with increased admissions to the hospital because of flares or new onset of colitis. Contrary to earlier studies, a recent retrospective evaluation of the effect of NSAID therapy in IBD failed to reveal any correlation between NSAID use and active IBD.[79] These results were subsequently confirmed by a larger study of 629 IBD patients, which showed low-dose NSAID was not associated with an increased disease activity of IBD.[80] However, long-term and high dose of NSAIDs are often required to treat axSpA, which still remains problematic. Thus, given the available evidence, in daily practice, AS patients should be assessed thoroughly by taking a detailed history for symptoms, suggestive of IBD, and if present, they should refrain from NSAIDs or use them cautiously.

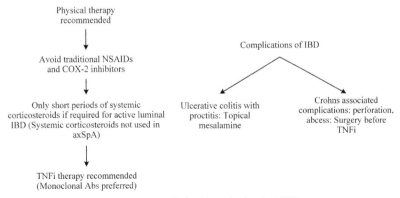

FIG. 11.9 axSpA with active luminal IBD.

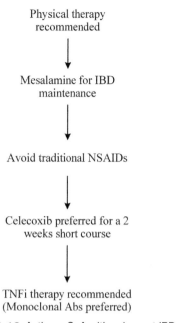

Physical therapy
recommended

↓

Mesalamine for IBD
maintenance

↓

Avoid traditional NSAIDs

↓

Celecoxib preferred for a 2
weeks short course

↓

TNFi therapy recommended
(Monoclonal Abs preferred)

FIG. 11.10 Active axSpA with quiescent IBD.

Short bursts of systemic corticosteroids can be used for moderate to severe flares of IBD, although it is definitely not the standard of care for treatment of axSpA.[81] Sulfasalazine can be used for IBD, but benefits only peripheral not axial manifestations in SpA.[51] Neither immunomodulators—methotrexate, nor azathioprine are effective for axSpA.[82,83] Thus the choice of therapy boils down to monoclonal TNFi.

Obstructive symptoms, intestinal perforation, or abscess requires surgical management that would precede any medical management for treatment of both intestinal and musculoskeletal symptoms. After surgery and complete resolution of the complication, TNFi should be restarted to prevent postoperative recurrences.[47,84] Management of perianal Crohn disease requires a dual strategy–surgical and medical. Surgery is required for septic complications, seton placement, and fistulectomy, whereas medical management requires antibiotics and TNFi as they are efficacious in inducing and maintaining healing of fistulas.[49,85,86]

2. Patients with active axSpA and quiescent IBD:
axSpA is managed in a step ladder fashion with physical therapy being one of the building blocks. Generally, NSAIDs are to be avoided in patients with IBD. An article published in 2005 shed light on the safety of celecoxib (selective COX 2 inhibitor) in patients with ulcerative colitis who were in

remission.[87] It was a 2-week short-term randomized controlled trial to evaluate risk of relapse or flare of IBD in patients using celecoxib compared with placebo. Relapse rate was comparable in both groups, and thus the 2015 ACR/SSA/SPARTAN guidelines conditionally recommend celecoxib over other NSAIDs for short courses owing to less potential harm. Thus, if required, celecoxib could be used for a short duration of time in patients with quiescent IBD. The treatment of choice for axSpA would be TNFi (monoclonal Abs). In quiescent IBD patients, mesalamine should be continued considering its efficacy in maintenance of remission and its possible preventive effect of colorectal cancer.[88,89]

To study the incidence of IBD in patients with AS treated with anti-TNF agents, Braun et al.[90] analyzed nine trials. Data were available for 1130 patients. Based on the results, infliximab was a preferred agent in patients with AS and IBD. After results of 2006 ATLAS trial[91] were available, the metaanalysis was updated to find the true incidence of flares or new onset of IBD in AS patients with infliximab, etanercept, and adalimumab. Rate of IBD flares (per 100 patient-years) for infliximab group was 0.2, etanercept was 2.2, and placebo was 1.3. Initially, adalimumab flare rate was 2.3, which decreased to 0.63 after tallying results from ATLAS trial. Thus, based on these results, both adalimumab and infliximab were associated with significant reduction in IBD flare rates compared with etanercept ($P < .01$).

Moreover, subcutaneous etanercept is not effective for treatment of patients with moderate to severe Crohn disease. It showed no greater benefit over placebo.[92] The mechanism underlying the differential efficacy of etanercept and infliximab in IBD is not entirely clear, but a number of possibilities are postulated. Please refer to Conclusions section for additional details. Furthermore, in a case series, three patients, who were treated with etanercept for AS, developed new onset of Crohn disease. One of the three patients was rechallenged with the etanercept and had a flare of Crohn disease, although he was on azathioprine.[93] The de novo flare of IBD is a thought-provoking hypothesis, and any causative role of etanercept remains unproven at this stage.

Secukinumab (IL-17 inhibitor) has proven to be effective in axSpA but not in IBD. Moreover, there have been reports of either new colitis onset or worsening with secukinumab. To understand whether secukinumab is really a culprit, pooled data were analyzed for 3430, 974, and 571 patients using secukinumab for psoriasis, PsA, and AS, respectively. The exposure-adjusted incidence rates for Crohn disease were 0.11, 0.07, and

0.77 per 1000 patient-years in psoriasis, PsA, and AS trials, respectively. The exposure-adjusted incidence rates for ulcerative colitis were 0.15, 0.14, and 0.29 per 1000 patient-years in psoriasis, PsA, and AS trials, respectively. Crohn disease has been reported at a rate of 0.25 cases per 100 patient-years among patients with psoriasis, 0.06 cases per 100 patient-years in PsA, and 0.7 cases per 100 patient-years in AS patients, who were treated only with placebo in these trials. The study suggested that overall there was no increase in incidence of IBD with secukinumab.[94] However, we do recommend avoiding secukinumab in patients with axSpA who have prominent bowel symptoms, even if a diagnosis of inflammatory bowel disease has not been definitively established.

The migration of inflammatory T cells into the gut mediates inflammation that characterizes IBD. These T cells with their surface expressed α4 β7 integrins bind to adhesion molecules (mucosal addressin cell adhesion molecule 1 = MAdCAM 1) present on endothelial cells in the gut. Please refer to Fig. 11.11. This interaction allows movement of T cells from the blood stream into the gut. Blocking this interaction prevents the downstream inflammatory cascade. Vedolizumab (VDZ) is a gut-specific humanized IgG1 monoclonal antibody to α4 β7 integrin that blocks its interaction with MAdCAM-1 and thus suppresses gut inflammation.[95,96]

Rubin et al. performed a posthoc analysis of the Gemini II study to investigate the effect of VDZ on extraintestinal manifestations. The data did not show a benefit of VDZ over placebo for arthritis in IBD patients. Furthermore, incidence of arthralgia was similar in VDZ and placebo group. This suggests that VDZ neither causes arthralgia as a side effect nor does it seem to have benefits on IBD associated arthritis.[97] Because of this neutral nature of VDZ on joints, a case report suggested a combination therapy of VDZ and etanercept (no efficacy in IBD) could be used to comanage active bowel disease in SpA. Granting no infections were observed in the patient, larger studies are needed to investigate this combination therapy further.[98]

Interestingly, a case series suggested that VDZ may cause de novo or exacerbate arthritis or sacroiliitis.[99] It is known that VDZ specifically blocks the interaction of integrins and adhesion molecules at the level of the gut. They postulate this could increase activated T cells drifting away from the gut to the joints.[100] This theory is supported by the fact that α4β7 integrins are expressed in inflamed joints.[101,102] The patients in this case series were HLA-B27 negative, had no family history of SpA, and had a dissociation of gut and joint response, further making an argument in support of de novo arthritis and sacroiliitis caused by VDZ. Because of the disparate data, larger cohort studies are needed to provide information

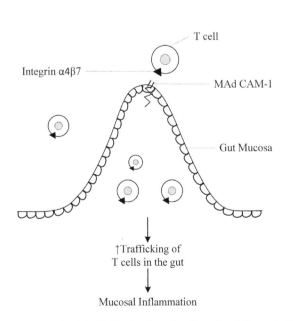 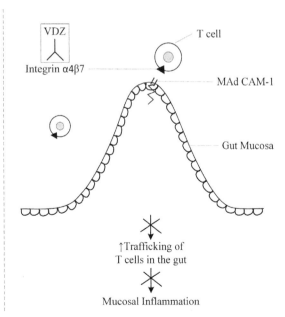

FIG. 11.11 Mechanism of action of vedolizumab (*MAd CAM-1*, mucosal addressin cell adhesion molecule-1; *VDZ*, vedolizumab).

on the prevalence, evolution, and mechanism of VDZ in IBD patients associated with arthritis.

Ustekinumab binds to p40 subunit of IL-12 and IL-23 and blocks further activation of Th1 cells (producing interferon-γ) and Th-17 cells (producing IL-17). Please refer to Fig. 11.12 for details. It induces response and remission in patients with moderately to severely active Crohn's disease that is refractory to either TNFi or conventional therapy.[104] Ustekinumab showed promising results for AS in a phase-II trial published in 2014.[103] Subsequently, three phase-III placebo controlled trials were undertaken. These subsequent trials failed to demonstrate efficacy in axSpA.[159] The first trial had 346 TNFi naïve patients with radiographic axSpA who had an inadequate response or intolerance to NSAIDs. ASAS40 response rates at week 24 were not significantly different among participants given ustekinumab 45mg (31.0%), ustekinumab 90mg (28.15%), or placebo (28.4%). Because primary and secondary endpoints were not met in this trial, the other two trials were terminated early. Since the two trials were discontinued, not all participants could reach the stipulated 24-week duration of the studies. Hence the efficacy analysis in the two trials were limited. In addition, a randomized controlled trial testing risankizumab, a monoclonal antibody that blocks IL-23 without affecting IL-12, also failed to show efficacy in the treatment of ankylosing spondylitis.[161] Thus,

IL-23 does not appear to be an effective target to treat joint disease associated with ankylosing spondylitis.

Although secukinumab works only for AS and vedolizumab and ustekinumab treat the gut, tofacitinib can be used in both – AS and IBD (Table 11.8).

Tofacitinib broadly inhibits janus kinases family (JAK 1, 2, and 3). In IBD patients, the dominant benefit is likely via JAK 1 inhibition, which then downregulates IL-6 and interferon-γ. Previous clinical trials have shown its utility in induction and maintenance of remission of moderate to severe ulcerative colitis.[105,106] Tofacitinib has also shown efficacy in AS patients in a randomized controlled trial, which demonstrated greater clinical efficacy than placebo in reducing signs and symptoms.[107]

PSORIASIS
Definition and Disease Burden

Like AS, psoriasis is a major histocompatibility class I (MHC-I)–associated, immune-mediated disorder. It is characterized by keratinocyte proliferation, which results in erythematous, scaly patches, and plaques on the trunk, extremities, scalp, or face as well as nail deformities. Psoriasis affects 2%–3% of the world population. It is not merely a cosmetic problem. Up to 55% of people with psoriasis face depression.[108] The disease is highly stigmatized because of the visible nature of the

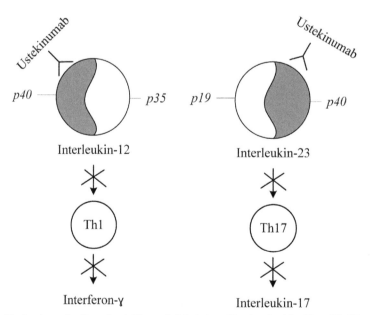

FIG. 11.12 Mechanism of action of ustekinumab (binds to p40 subunit of IL-12 and IL-23, preventing binding with NK or T cell surface receptors, inhibiting IL-12 signaling and further activation of Th1 cells to produce interferon gamma as well as IL-23 signaling and further activation of Th17 cells to produce IL-17).

TABLE 11.8
Available Treatment Modalities for axSpA and IBD in a Nutshell

Treatment Modalities	Axial Spondyloarthritis	IBD
Nonsteroidal antiinflammatory drugs (NSAIDs)	+	–
Sulfasalazine	Benefit for peripheral arthritis only	+
Monoclonal antibodies (adalimumab, infliximab)	+	+
Soluble receptor antibodies (etanercept)	+	–
Secukinumab (IL-17 inhibitor)	+	–
Ustekinumab (IL-12/23 inhibitor)	–	+
Vedolizumab (integrin inhibitor)	–	+
Tofacitinib (JAK inhibitor)	+ (limited data)	+

lesions.[109] Effective treatment of psoriasis is important as the disease reduces physical function, psychologic function, and quality of life.[110]

About 30% of patients with psoriasis have psoriatic arthritis, which is characterized by chronic inflammation of the peripheral joints, entheses, and the spine.[111] Occurrence of psoriasis is seen in approximately 5%–10% of patients with AS. Such patients tend to exhibit more peripheral joint involvement.[112] Association of axSpA with psoriasis was clearly found to produce a worse disease course than either primary AS or AS associated with IBD.[113] This warrants effective treatment of psoriasis in patients with axSpA.

Treatment

In case of scaling skin lesions, or nail changes, it is recommended that the patient be referred to a dermatologist. Skin manifestations of psoriasis respond to local corticosteroids or treatment with Psoralen plus Ultra-Violet A (PUVA) or Ultraviolet B (UVB) light.[65] NSAIDs do not play a role in treatment of skin or nail psoriasis. Evidence for sulfasalazine playing a role in the treatment of skin or nail psoriasis is scarce.[114] Methotrexate is proven to be effective in daily practice for treating skin and peripheral arthritis, despite a paucity of data from randomized controlled trials to support this.[115] However, none of the above medications benefits axial symptoms in axSpA.

On the other hand, TNFi, such as infliximab, etanercept, adalimumab, and golimumab, are efficacious for psoriasis as well as the axial manifestations of axSpA.[115] Interleukin-17 is an inflammatory cytokine secreted by Th 17 cells after induction by interleukin-23. Of the three interleukin-17 inhibitors available, secukinumab has been approved for the treatment of AS.[116] It has also shown significantly higher Psoriasis Area and Severity

Index (PASI 75) scores for skin psoriasis compared with placebo.[117] Several newer medications have been used to treat AS as well as psoriasis.

One such drug is apremilast. It is an oral phosphodiesterase 4 inhibitor used for the treatment of moderate to severe plaque psoriasis.[118–121] Phosphodiesterase 4 inhibition reduces production of multiple cytokines involved in the pathogenesis of psoriasis. It has shown some benefits in a randomized trial involving 38 patients with symptomatic AS.[122] There were trends suggesting greater improvement with apremilast, compared with placebo, but these differences did not achieve statistical significance. Larger trials of greater duration would be required to determine whether this medication will be of benefit to patients with AS.

Tofacitinib (small molecule JAK inhibitor) has also shown efficacy in AS and psoriasis patients. A randomized controlled trial demonstrated greater clinical efficacy with tofacitinib compared with placebo in reducing signs and symptoms of AS over a 12-week period.[107] It has also demonstrated efficacy for moderate to severe plaque psoriasis.[123–127]

Another drug that should be mentioned in this discussion is ustekinumab. Ustekinumab binds to p40 subunit of IL-12 and IL-23 and blocks further activation of Th1 cells (producing interferon-γ) and Th-17 cells (producing IL-17). Please refer to Fig. 11.12 for details. Prior study showed efficacy of blocking IL-12/23 axis in mouse models of psoriasis.[128] PHOENIX 1 and 2 are two randomized controlled trials that showed efficacy of ustekinumab in patients with severe plaque psoriasis.[129,130] Ustekinumab showed promising results for AS in a phase-II trial published in 2014.[103] Subsequently, three phase-III placebo controlled trials were undertaken, which failed to demonstrate efficacy in axSpA.[159] An editorial published in March 2018 speculated some reasons for this failure including different biologic mechanisms operating in the spine and the periphery, resulting in differential responses to IL-23 inhibition at these sites.[160]

There are emerging data that blocking IL-23 is more beneficial than combined blockade of IL-12/IL-23 in pathogenesis of psoriasis.[131] Guselkumab (selective IL-23 inhibitor) prevents the activation of only Th17 cells, sparing the Th1 cells and allowing IL-12-mediated interferon-γ release. This preferential effect is hypothesized to increase its safety profile. Refer to Fig. 11.13 for details. It has shown to be efficacious in clinical trials for patients with moderate to severe plaque-type psoriasis.[132–134] Preliminary data support the use in PsA and value for SpA is yet to be determined.[135]

In summary, tofacitinib (although not FDA approved for AS) may be used to treat patients with axSpA and concomitant psoriasis, if they do not respond to TNFi or secukinumab (Table 11.9).

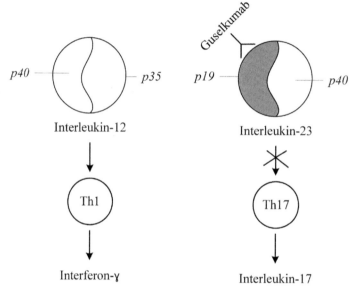

FIG. 11.13 Mechanism of action of guselkumab (binds to p19 subunit of IL-23, preventing binding with NK or T cell surface receptors, inhibiting IL-23 signaling and further activation of Th17 cells to produce IL-17 while causing no downstream effect via Th1 pathway).

TABLE 11.9
Available Treatment Modalities for axSpA and IBD in a Nutshell

Treatment Modalities	Axial Spondyloarthritis	Psoriasis
Nonsteroidal antiinflammatory drugs (NSAIDs)	+	−
Sulfasalazine	Benefit for peripheral arthritis only	−
Monoclonal antibodies (adalimumab, infliximab)	+	+
Soluble receptor antibodies (etanercept)	+	+
Secukinumab (IL-17 inhibitor)	+	+
Ustekinumab (IL-12/23 inhibitor)	−	+
Guselkumab (IL-23 inhibitor)	−	+
Tofacitinib (JAK inhibitor)	+ (limited data)	+
Apremilast (PDE-4 inhibitor)	−	+

Paradoxical Psoriasis

Treatment of any rheumatologic condition using TNFi agents could result in almost 1.5%–5% of patients developing paradoxical psoriasis.[136] Such eruptions are well documented in literature.[137–141] This paradoxical phenomenon is equally seen in males and females, and across all TNFi alike—suggesting it to be a class effect. The usual latency period of development is between 10 and 31 months. It occurs in 72% patients with no prior medical or family history of psoriasis. Multiple studies have shown that the skin morphology could be psoriasiform, plaque, palmoplantar pustular, or guttate.[137–141]

Nestle and Gilliet suggested injury or infection stimulates plasmacytic dendritic cells to produce interferon (INF)-α, which in turn produces psoriatic lesions.[142] It is hypothesized that TNFi unchecks INF-α causing its overproduction, which leads to psoriasis.[143,144] This has been supported by Gilliet who showed that elevated INF-α levels worsened psoriasis.[143,144] Mild to moderate skin lesions are treated with topical corticosteroids, vitamin D, UV light, methotrexate, or cyclosporine. In some severe cases, it requires switching to a different class of drugs such as interleukin-17 inhibitors.

Further studies are, however, needed to determine the exact mechanism of this phenomenon. It may help elucidate the pathogenetic link between psoriasis and axSpA.

POSTULATED REASONS FOR DIFFERENTIAL EFFICACY OF ETANERCEPT AND MONOCLONAL ANTIBODIES

Tumor necrosis factor inhibitors (TNFi) such as infliximab, adalimumab, golimumab, certolizumab, or etanercept have shown a significant improvement in both signs and symptoms of axSpA, as well as improvement in functional status and quality of life.[145–148] However, as discussed in Treatment and Paradoxical Psoriasis sections, etanercept has a poor therapeutic effect when managing patients with uveitis or IBD. To understand this, it is imperative to understand the structure and efficacy of the available TNFi agents along with their similarities and differences.

TNFi such as infliximab and adalimumab are monoclonal antibodies. Infliximab is a chimeric monoclonal antibody, whereas adalimumab is a humanized monoclonal antibody. They bind to both soluble and transmembrane forms of TNF molecules, i.e., monomers and trimers—to form stable complexes. Infliximab does not dissociate from the bound TNF molecules in radiolabeled assays.[149] In contrast, etanercept is a rigid p75 TNF receptor/Fc fusion protein. It binds only to the trimer form of TNF molecules. Radiolabeled binding assays have found that TNF-etanercept complexes are relatively

unstable.[149] TNF molecules that dissociate as a result of this unsteadiness have been found to be bioactive and could continue the inflammatory cascade.

Infliximab and adalimumab induce complement-dependent cytotoxicity—much more potently than etanercept.[150–154] Consequently, it is difficult for etanercept to make in vitro membrane attack complexes.

Metalloproteinases cleave TNFi at the hinge region. Infliximab and adalimumab are cleaved into Fc and Fab domains, whereas etanercept is cleaved into Fc and TNF-R2 (See Fig. 11.14). Free Fab domains can still antagonize TNF molecules, but TNF-R2 from etanercept loses this neutralization capability. Inflamed tissues have upregulated metalloproteinases, which could be another reason for the differential efficacy of etanercept in IBD and uveitis.[155]

Etanercept (unlike infliximab and adalimumab) binds and neutralizes lymphotoxin (LTα3 and LT α2β1). None of the TNFi can neutralize LT α1β2.[156] The latter has a regulatory role in intestinal inflammation. Further studies are required to understand the roll of lymphotoxin in treatment of IBD.[157]

Other possible explanations for the difference may be conceived as resulting either because of differences in their ability to[157]:

1. achieve serum concentration (pharmacokinetics),
2. therapeutic concentration in inflammatory microenvironments (tissue penetration), and
3. bind to TNFα molecules and induce treatment effects (mechanistic).

After reviewing the molecular biology of TNFi in this section and the differential effects of etanercept and monoclonal TNFi in clinical trials (refer to Sections Treatment and Paradoxical Psoriasis), an important question arises—how has this information affected real-life clinical practice? A cross-sectional study was published in 2012. It was designed to investigate the relationship between uveitis and parameters such as demographics, quality of life, medication use, and joint involvement in patients with SpA. Multivariate analysis showed that history of uveitis was positively associated with current use of infliximab and negatively associated with the current use of etanercept. It was the first study to suggest that the limited ability of etanercept to control uveitis appeared to impact prescribing practices.[158]

CONCLUSIONS

Population-based estimates of EAMs (AAU, IBD, and psoriasis) have shown a strong association between EAMs and AS in patients, as compared with the general population. Undoubtedly, they have a major impact on

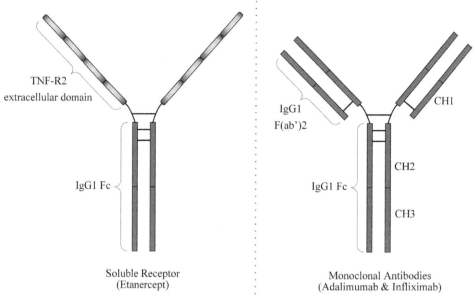

TNF-R2
extracellular domain

IgG1 Fc

Soluble Receptor
(Etanercept)

IgG1
F(ab')2

CH1

CH2

IgG1 Fc

CH3

Monoclonal Antibodies
(Adalimumab & Infliximab)

FIG. 11.14 Structural differences between soluble receptors and monoclonal antibodies.

TABLE 11.10
Available Treatment Modalities for axSpA and Extraarticular Manifestations in a Nutshell

Treatment Modalities	As	IBD	Psoriasis	Uveitis
Nonsteroidal antiinflammatory drugs (NSAIDs)	+	–	–	*
Sulfasalazine	Benefit for peripheral arthritis only	+	–	**
Monoclonal TNFi (adalimumab, infliximab)	+	+	+	+
Soluble receptor TNFi (etanercept)	+	–	+	–
Secukinumab (IL-17i)	+	–	+	–
Ustekinumab (IL-12/23i)	–	+	+	–
Guselkumab (IL-23i)	–	–	+	?
Vedolizumab (integrin inhibitor)	–	+	–	–
Tofacitinib (JAK inhibitor)	+ (limited data)	+	+	–
Apremilast (PDE-4 inhibitor)	–	–	+	–

*Some evidence to suggest that use prevents attacks; no consistent benefit for active uveitis
**Strong evidence that use reduces frequency of attacks; no benefit for active uveitis

the management of axSpA. They often require a multispecialty approach. Moreover, their presence increases the disease burden on individual patients, as well as society.

Recognizing its multifaceted nature, the American College of Rheumatology (ACR) and ASAS-EULAR guidelines state that the treatment of axSpA should be tailored according to the current levels of symptoms—be it axial spondylitis, peripheral arthritis, or extraarticular manifestations. As seen in the previous sections, it seems that the efficacy of all TNF inhibitors is comparable for managing axial and peripheral rheumatologic symptoms in axSpA. However, the presence of EAMs provides a basis to pick and choose between the best of the available options. Table 11.10 shows an overview of treatment of EAMs and axSpA:

There are still knowledge gaps in this field: we may not be aware of all comorbidities associated with AS. As newer therapeutic options and technologies evolve, life expectancy would improve, and more comorbidities may come to surface. We may not fully understand the mechanisms that account for these comorbidities. Finally, we still have to understand the differential effects of therapeutic options on AS and EAMs. For example, etanercept works on the inflammation of sacroiliac joint but not for uveitis. Another example is where NSAIDs are effective as the first-line therapy for AS but do not treat inflammation in the colon.

REFERENCES

1. Vander Cruyssen B, Ribbens C, Boonen A, et al. The epidemiology of ankylosing spondylitis and the commencement of anti-TNF therapy in daily rheumatology practice. *Ann Rheum Dis.* 2007;66(8):1072–1077. https://doi.org/10.1136/ard.2006.064543&.
2. Dougados M, Van Der LS, Juhlin R, et al. The European spondylarthropathy study group preliminary criteria for the classification of spondylarthropathy. *Arthritis Rheum.* 1991;34(10):1218–1227. https://doi.org/10.1002/art.1780341003.
3. Amor B, Dougados M, Mijiyawa M. Criteria of the classification of spondylarthropathies. *Rev Rhum Mal Osteoartic.* 1990;57(2):85–89. http://www.ncbi.nlm.nih.gov/pubmed/2181618.
4. Rudwaleit M, Van Der Heijde D, Landewé R, et al. The development of Assessment of spondyloArthritis international society classification criteria for axial spondyloarthritis (part II): validation and final selection. *Ann Rheum Dis.* 2009;68(6):777–783. https://doi.org/10.1136/ard.2009.108233.
5. Rudwaleit M, Van Der Heijde D, Landewé R, et al. The Assessment of SpondyloArthritis international Society classification criteria for peripheral spondyloarthritis and for spondyloarthritis in general. *Ann Rheum Dis.* 2011;70(1):25–31. https://doi.org/10.1136/ard.2010.133645.
6. Braun J, Van Den Berg R, Baraliakos X, et al. 2010 update of the ASAS/EULAR recommendations for the management of ankylosing spondylitis. *Ann Rheum Dis.* 2011;70(6):896–904. https://doi.org/10.1136/ard.2011.151027.
7. Braun J, Sieper J. Therapy of ankylosing spondylitis and other spondyloarthritides: established medical treatment, anti-TNF-alpha therapy and other novel approaches. *Arthritis Res.* 2002;4(5):307–321. https://doi.org/10.1186/ar592.
8. Robertson LP, Davis MJ. A longitudinal study of disease activity and functional status in a hospital cohort of patients with ankylosing spondylitis. *Rheumatology.* 2004;43(12):1565–1568. https://doi.org/10.1093/rheumatology/keh386.
9. Brophy S, Pavy S, Lewis P, et al. Inflammatory eye, skin, and bowel disease in spondyloarthritis: genetic, phenotypic, and environmental factors. *J Rheumatol.* 2001;28(12):2667–2673.
10. Gao X, Wendling D, Botteman MF, Carter JA, Rao S, Cifaldi M. Clinical and economic burden of extra-articular manifestations in ankylosing spondylitis patients treated with anti-tumor necrosis factor agents. *J Med Econ.* 2012;15(6):1054–1063. https://doi.org/10.3111/13696998.2012.692341.
11. Stolwijk C, Van Tubergen A, Castillo-Ortiz JD, Boonen A. Prevalence of extra-articular manifestations in patients with ankylosing spondylitis: a systematic review and meta-analysis. *Ann Rheum Dis.* 2015;74(1):65–73. https://doi.org/10.1136/annrheumdis-2013-203582.
12. Robinson PC, Claushuis TAM, Cortes A, et al. Genetic Dissection of acute anterior uveitis reveals similarities and differences in associations observed with ankylosing spondylitis. *Arthritis Rheumatol.* 2015;67(1):140–151. https://doi.org/10.1002/art.38873.
12a. Khan MA, Haroon M, Rosenbaum JT. Acute anterior uveitis and spondyloarthritis: more than meets the eye. *Curr Rheumatol Rep.* 2015;17(9):59. https://doi.org/10.1007/s11926-015-0536-x.
12b. Sharma SM, Jackson D. Uveitis and spondyloarthropathies. *Best Pract Res Clin Rheumatol.* 2017;31(6):846–862. https://doi.org/110.1016/j.berh.2018.08.002. Epub 2018 Oct 25.
13. van der Linden S. Valkenburg HA, Cats A. Evaluation of diagnostic criteria for ankylosing spondylitis. A proposal for modification of the New York criteria. *Arthritis Rheum.* 1984;27(4):361–368. https://doi.org/10.1002/art.v27.
14. de Winter JJ, van Mens LJ, van der Heijde D, Landewé R, Baeten DL. Prevalence of peripheral and extra-articular disease in ankylosing spondylitis versus non-radiographic axial spondyloarthritis: a meta-analysis. *Arthritis Res Ther.* 2016;18(1). https://doi.org/10.1186/s13075-016-1093-z.
15. Rudwaleit M, Haibel H, Baraliakos X, et al. The early disease stage in axial spondylarthritis: results from the German spondyloarthritis inception cohort. *Arthritis Rheum.* 2009;60(3):717–727. https://doi.org/10.1002/art.24483.
16. Varkas G, Cypers H, Vastesaeger N, et al. The association of extra-articular manifestations with disease duration in axial spa: results from the (Be-) giant cohort and the aspect study. *Ann Rheum Dis.* 2016;75(suppl 2). 87 LP-87 http://ard.bmj.com/content/75/Suppl_2/87.2.abstract.
17. Essers I, Ramiro S, Stolwijk C, et al. Characteristics associated with the presence and development of extra-articular manifestations in ankylosing spondylitis: 12-year results from OASIS. *Rheumatol (United Kingdom).* 2014;54(4):633–640. https://doi.org/10.1093/rheumatology/keu388.

18. Stolwijk C, Essers I, Van Tubergen A, et al. The epidemiology of extra-articular manifestations in ankylosing spondylitis: a population-based matched cohort study. *Ann Rheum Dis.* 2015;74(7):1373–1378. https://doi.org/10.1136/annrheumdis-2014-205253.

19. Gritz DC, Wong IG. Incidence and prevalence of uveitis in Northern California: the Northern California epidemiology of uveitis study. *Ophthalmology.* 2004;111(3):491–500. https://doi.org/10.1016/j.ophtha.2003.06.014.

20. Thorne JE, Suhler E, Skup M, et al. Prevalence of noninfectious uveitis in the United States: a claims-based analysis. *JAMA Ophthalmol.* 2016;134(11):1237–1245. https://doi.org/10.1001/jamaophthalmol.2016.3229.

21. Rosenbaum JT. Characterization of uveitis associated with spondyloarthritis. *J Rheumatol.* 1989;16(6):792–796.

22. Monnet D, Breban M, Hudry C, Dougados M, Brézin AP. Ophthalmic findings and frequency of extraocular manifestations in patients with HLA-B27 uveitis: a study of 175 cases. *Ophthalmology.* 2004;111(4):802–809. https://doi.org/10.1016/j.ophtha.2003.07.011.

23. Chung YM, Liao HT, Lin KC, et al. Prevalence of spondyloarthritis in 504 Chinese patients with HLA-B27-associated acute anterior uveitis. *Scand J Rheumatol.* 2009;38(2):84–90. https://doi.org/10.1080/03009740802385423.

24. Muñoz-Fernández S, De Miguel E, Cobo-Ibáñez T, et al. Enthesis inflammation in recurrent acute anterior uveitis without spondylarthritis. *Arthritis Rheum.* 2009;60(7):1985–1990. https://doi.org/10.1002/art.24636.

25. Juanola X, Loza Santamaría E, Cordero-Coma M. Description and prevalence of spondyloarthritis in patients with anterior uveitis: the SENTINEL interdisciplinary collaborative project. *Ophthalmology.* 2016;123(8):1632–1636. https://doi.org/10.1016/j.ophtha.2016.03.010.

26. Pato E, Banares A, Jover JA, et al. Undiagnosed spondyloarthropathy in patients presenting with anterior uveitis. *J Rheumatol.* 2000;27(9):2198–2202.

27. Fernández-Melón J, Muñoz-Fernández S, Hidalgo V, et al. Uveitis as the initial clinical manifestation in patients with spondyloarthropathies. *J Rheumatol.* 2004;31(3):524–527. https://doi.org/0315162X-31-753 [pii].

28. Haroon M, O'Rourke M, Ramasamy P, Murphy CC, FitzGerald O. A novel evidence-based detection of undiagnosed spondyloarthritis in patients presenting with acute anterior uveitis: the DUET (Dublin Uveitis Evaluation Tool). *Ann Rheum Dis.* 2015;74(11):1990–1995. https://doi.org/10.1136/annrheumdis-2014-205358.

29. Banares A, Hernandez-Garcia C, Fernandez-Gutierrez B, Jover JA. Eye involvement in the spondyloarthropathies. *Rheum Dis Clin N Am.* 1998;24(4):771–784. https://doi.org/10.1016/S0889-857X(05)70041-7.

30. Gran JT, Skomsvoll JF. The outcome of ankylosing spondylitis: a study of 100 patients. *Br J Rheumatol.* 1997;36(7):766–771. https://doi.org/10.1093/rheumatology/36.7.766.

31. Canoui-Poitrine F, Kemta Lekpa F, Farrenq V, et al. Prevalence and factors associated with uveitis in spondyloarthropathies patients in France: results from the EXTRA observational survey. *Arthritis Care Res.* 2012. https://doi.org/10.1002/acr.21616.

32. Sampaio-Barros PD, Conde RA, Bonfiglioli R, Bértolo MB, Samara AM. Characterization and outcome of uveitis in 350 patients with spondyloarthropathies. *Rheumatol Int.* 2006;26(12):1143–1146. https://doi.org/10.1007/s00296-006-0203-7.

33. Chen C-H, Lin K-C, Chen H-A, et al. Association of acute anterior uveitis with disease activity, functional ability and physical mobility in patients with ankylosing spondylitis: a cross-sectional study of Chinese patients in Taiwan. *Clin Rheumatol.* 2007;26(6):953–957. https://doi.org/10.1007/s10067-006-0403-2.

34. Collantes E, Zarco P, Muñoz E, et al. Disease pattern of spondyloarthropathies in Spain: description of the first national registry (REGISPONSER) - extended report. *Rheumatology.* 2007;46(8):1309–1315. https://doi.org/10.1093/rheumatology/kem084.

35. Gehlen M, Regis KC, Skare TL. Demographic, clinical, laboratory and treatment characteristics of spondyloarthritis patients with and without acute anterior uveitis. *Sao Paulo Med J.* 2012;130(3):141–144. http://ovidsp.ovid.com/ovidweb.cgi?T=JS&PAGE=reference&D=med7&NEWS=N&AN=22790545.

36. Rosenbaum JT, Smith JR. Anti-TNF therapy for eye involvement in spondyloarthropathy. *Clin Exp Rheumatol.* 2002;20(6 suppl 28).

37. Zeboulon N, Dougados M, Gossec L. Prevalence and characteristics of uveitis in the spondyloarthropathies: a systematic literature review. *Ann Rheum Dis.* 2008;67(7):955–959. https://doi.org/10.1136/ard.2007.075754.

38. Max R, Lorenz HM, Mackensen F. Ocular involvement in spondyloarthropathies: HLA B27 associated uveitis. *Zeitschrift fu¨r Rheumatol.* 2010;69(5):397–402. https://doi.org/10.1007/s00393-009-0576-6.

39. Rosenbaum JT. Uveitis in spondyloarthritis including psoriatic arthritis, ankylosing spondylitis, and inflammatory bowel disease. *Clin Rheumatol.* 2015;34(6):999–1002. https://doi.org/10.1007/s10067-015-2960-8.

40. Brewerton DA, Hart FD, Nicholls A, Caffrey M, James DCO, Sturrock RD. Ankylosing spondylitis and Hl-A 27. *Lancet.* 2018;301(7809):904–907. https://doi.org/10.1016/S0140-6736(73)91360-3.

41. Baggia S, Lyons JL, Angell E, et al. A novel model of bacterially-induced acute anterior uveitis in rats and the lack of effect from HLA-B27 expression. *J Investig Med.* 1997;45(5):295–301. http://www.ncbi.nlm.nih.gov/pubmed/9250003.

42. Maksymowych W, Russell A. Polymorphism in the LMP2 gene influences the relative risk for acute anterior uveitis in unselected patients with ankylosing spondylitis. *Clin Investig Med Méd Clin Exp.* 1995;18(1):42–46.

43. Ruutu M, Thomas G, Steck R, et al. β-Glucan triggers spondylarthritis and Crohn's disease-like ileitis in SKG mice. *Arthritis Rheum.* 2012;64(7):2211–2222. https://doi.org/10.1002/art.34423.

44. Kezic JM, Glant TT, Rosenbaum JT, Rosenzweig HL. Neutralization of IL-17 ameliorates uveitis but damages photoreceptors in a murine model of spondyloarthritis. *Arthritis Res Ther.* 2012;14(1). https://doi.org/10.1186/ar3697.

45. Kezic JM, Davey MP, Glant TT, Rosenbaum JT, Rosenzweig HL. Interferon-γ regulates discordant mechanisms of uveitis versus joint and axial disease in a murine model resembling spondylarthritis. *Arthritis Rheum.* 2012;64(3):762–771. https://doi.org/10.1002/art.33404.

46. Petty RE, Johnston W, McCormick AQ, Hunt DWC, Rootman J, Rollins DF. Uveitis and arthritis induced by adjuvant: clinical, immunologic and histologic characteristics. *J Rheumatol.* 1989;16(4):499–505.

47. Fiorelli VMB, Bhat P, Foster CS. Nonsteroidal anti-inflammatory therapy and recurrent acute anterior uveitis. *Ocul Immunol Inflamm.* 2010;18(2):116–120. https://doi.org/10.3109/09273941003587558.

48. Levinson RD, Rosenbaum JT. Nonsteroidal anti-inflammatory drugs for prophylaxis of acute anterior uveitis. *Ocul Immunol Inflamm.* 2010;18(2):69–71. https://doi.org/10.3109/09273941003768224.

48a. Kim MJ, Lee EE, Lee EY, et al. Preventive effect of tumor necrosis factor inhibitors versus nonsteroidal anti-inflammatory drugs on uveitis in patients with ankylosing spondylitis. *Clin Rheumatol.* 2018;37(10):2763–2770. https://doi.org/10.1007/s10067-018-4249-1. Epub 2018 Aug 4.

48b. Zu Hoerste MM, Walscheid K, Tappeiner C, et al. The effect of methotrexate and sulfasalazine on the course of HLA-B27-positive anterior uveitis: results from a retrospective cohort study. *Graefes Arch Clin Exp Ophthalmol.* 2018;256(10):1985–1992. https://doi.org/10.1007/s00417-018-4082-x. Epub 2018 Aug 1.

49. Colombel J-F, Schwartz DA, Sandborn WJ, et al. Adalimumab for the treatment of fistulas in patients with Crohn's disease. *Gut.* 2009;58(7):940–948. https://doi.org/10.1136/gut.2008.159251.

50. Benitez-Del-Castillo JM, Garcia-Sanchez J, Iradier T, Bañares A. Sulfasalazine in the prevention of anterior uveitis associated with ankylosing spondylitis. *Eye.* 2000;14(3a):340–343. https://doi.org/10.1038/eye.2000.84.

51. Clegg DO, Reda DJ, Abdellatif M. Comparison of sulfasalazine and placebo for the treatment of axial and peripheral articular manifestations of the seronegative spondylarthropathies: a Department of Veterans Affairs Cooperative Study. *Arthritis Rheum.* 1999;42(11):2325–2329. https://doi.org/10.1002/1529-0131(199911)42:11<2325::AID-ANR10>3.0.CO;2-C.

52. Braun J, Baraliakos X, Listing J, Sieper J. Decreased incidence of anterior uveitis in patients with ankylosing spondylitis treated with the anti-tumor necrosis factor agents infliximab and etanercept. *Arthritis Rheum.* 2005;52(8):2447–2451. https://doi.org/10.1002/art.21197.

53. Lie E, Lindström U, Zverkova-Sandström T, et al. Tumour necrosis factor inhibitor treatment and occurrence of anterior uveitis in ankylosing spondylitis: results from the Swedish biologics register. *Ann Rheum Dis.* 2017;76(9):1515–1521. https://doi.org/10.1136/annrheumdis-2016-210931.

54. Rudwaleit M, Rødevand E, Holck P, et al. Adalimumab effectively reduces the rate of anterior uveitis flares in patients with active ankylosing spondylitis: results of a prospective open-label study. *Ann Rheum Dis.* 2009;68(5):696–701. https://doi.org/10.1136/ard.2008.092585.

55. Rudwaleit M, Rosenbaum JT, Landewé R, et al. Observed incidence of uveitis following certolizumab pegol treatment in patients with axial spondyloarthritis. *Arthritis Care Res.* 2016;68(6):838–844. https://doi.org/10.1002/acr.22848.

56. Calvo-Río V, Blanco R, Santos-Gómez M, et al. Golimumab in refractory uveitis related to spondyloarthritis. Multicenter study of 15 patients. *Semin Arthritis Rheum.* 2016;46(1):95–101. https://doi.org/10.1016/j.semarthrit.2016.03.002.

57. Wendling D, Paccou J, Berthelot J-M, et al. New onset of uveitis during anti-tumor necrosis factor treatment for rheumatic diseases. *Semin Arthritis Rheum.* 2011;41(3):503–510. https://doi.org/10.1016/j.semarthrit.2011.05.005.

58. Sieper J, Koenig A, Baumgartner S, et al. Analysis of uveitis rates across all etanercept ankylosing spondylitis clinical trials. *Ann Rheum Dis.* 2010;69(1):226–229. https://doi.org/10.1136/ard.2008.103192.

58a. Taban M, Dupps WJ, Mandell B, Perez VL. Etanercept (enbrel)-associated inflammatory eye disease: case report and review of the literature. *Ocul Immunol Inflamm.* 2006;14(3):145–150.

58b. Kakkassery V, Mergler S, Pleyer U. Anti-TNF-alpha treatment: a possible promoter in endogenous uveitis? observational report on six patients: occurrence of uveitis following etanercept treatment. *Curr Eye Res.* 2010;35(8):751–756. https://doi.org/10.3109/02713683.2010.486520.

59. Lim LL, Fraunfelder FW, Rosenbaum JT. Do tumor necrosis factor inhibitors cause uveitis? A registry-based study. *Arthritis Rheum.* 2007;56(10):3248–3252. https://doi.org/10.1002/art.22918.

60. Dick AD, Tugal-Tutkun I, Foster S, et al. Secukinumab in the treatment of noninfectious uveitis: results of three randomized, controlled clinical trials. *Ophthalmology.* 2013;120(4):777–787. https://doi.org/10.1016/j.ophtha.2012.09.040.

61. Smolen JS, Schöls M, Braun J, et al. Treating axial spondyloarthritis and peripheral spondyloarthritis, especially psoriatic arthritis, to target: 2017 update of recommendations by an international task force. *Ann Rheum Dis.* 2018;77(1):3–17. https://doi.org/10.1136/annrheumdis-2017-211734.

62. De Vos M, Mielants H, Cuvelier C, Elewaut A, Veys E. Long-term evolution of gut inflammation in patients with spondyloarthropathy. *Gastroenterology*. 1996;110(6):1696–1703. https://doi.org/10.1053/gast.1996.v110.pm8964393.

63. Orchard TR, Wordsworth BP, Jewell DP. Peripheral arthropathies in inflammatory bowel disease: their articular distribution and natural history. *Gut*. 1998;42(3):387–391. https://doi.org/10.1136/gut.42.3.387.

64. Orchard TR. Management of arthritis in patients with inflammatory bowel disease. *Gastroenterol Hepatol*. 2012;8(5):327–329. http://www.ncbi.nlm.nih.gov/pubmed/22933865.

65. van der Horst-Bruinsma IE, Nurmohamed MT, Landewé RBM. Comorbidities in patients with spondyloarthritis. *Rheum Dis Clin N Am*. 2012;38(3):523–538. https://doi.org/10.1016/j.rdc.2012.08.010.

66. Dequeker J, Grillet B, De Clerck L, Rutgeerts P, Geboes K. Ileocolonoscopy and spondarthritis. *Rheumatology*. 1988;27(3):246–247. https://doi.org/10.1093/rheumatology/27.3.246.

67. Mielants H, Veys EM, Goemaere S, Goethals K, Cuvelier C, De Vos M. Gut inflammation in the spondyloarthropathies: clinical, radiologic, biologic and genetic features in relation to the type of histology. A prospective study. *J Rheumatol*. 1991;18(10):1542–1551. http://www.ncbi.nlm.nih.gov/pubmed/1765980.

68. Van Praet L, Van Den Bosch FE, Jacques P, et al. Microscopic gut inflammation in axial spondyloarthritis: a multiparametric predictive model. *Ann Rheum Dis*. 2013;72(3):414–417. https://doi.org/10.1136/annrheumdis-2012-202135.

69. Van Praet L, Jans L, Carron P, et al. Degree of bone marrow oedema in sacroiliac joints of patients with axial spondyloarthritis is linked to gut inflammation and male sex: results from the GIANT cohort. *Ann Rheum Dis*. 2014;73(6):1186–1189. https://doi.org/10.1136/annrheumdis-2013-203854.

70. de Vries M, van der Horst-Bruinsma I, van Hoogstraten I, et al. pANCA, ASCA, and OmpC antibodies in patients with ankylosing spondylitis without inflammatory bowel disease. *J Rheumatol*. 2010;37(11):2340–2344. https://doi.org/10.3899/jrheum.100269.

71. Cypers H, Varkas G, van Den Bosch F, et al. U. Microscopic bowel inflammation in spondyloarthritis as a baseline predictor of anti-tnf response. *Arthritis Rheumatol*. 2015;670:2453–2454.

72. Cypers H, Varkas G, Beeckman S, et al. Elevated calprotectin levels reveal bowel inflammation in spondyloarthritis. *Ann Rheum Dis*. 2016;75(7):1357–1362. https://doi.org/10.1136/annrheumdis-2015-208025.

73. Costello ME, Ciccia F, Willner D, et al. Brief Report: intestinal dysbiosis in ankylosing spondylitis. *Arthritis Rheumatol*. 2015;67(3):686–691. https://doi.org/10.1002/art.38967.

74. Nagalingam NA, Kao JY, Young VB. Microbial ecology of the murine gut associated with the development of dextran sodium sulfate-induced colitis. *Inflamm Bowel Dis*. 2011;17(4):917–926. https://doi.org/10.1002/ibd.21462.

75. Viladomiu M, Kivolowitz C, Abdulhamid A, et al. IgA-coated E. Coli enriched in Crohn's disease spondyloarthritis promote TH17-dependent inflammation. *Sci Transl Med*. 2017;9(376). https://doi.org/10.1126/scitranslmed.aaf9655.

76. Martínez-gonzález O, Cantero-hinojosa J, Paule-sastre P, Gómez-magán JC, Salvatierra-ríos D. Intestinal permeability in patients with ankylosing spondylitis and their healthy relatives. *Rheumatology*. 1994;33(7):644–647. https://doi.org/10.1093/rheumatology/33.7.644.

77. Olivieri I, Cantini F, Castiglione F, et al. Italian Expert Panel on the management of patients with coexisting spondyloarthritis and inflammatory bowel disease. *Autoimmun Rev*. 2014;13(8):822–830. https://doi.org/10.1016/j.autrev.2014.04.003.

78. Evans JMM, McMahon AD, Murray FE, McDevitt DG, MacDonald TM. Non-steroidal anti-inflammatory drugs are associated with emergency admission to hospital for colitis due to inflammatory bowel disease. *Gut*. 1997;40(5):619–622. https://doi.org/10.1136/gut.40.5.619.

79. Bonner GF, Walczak M, Kitchen L, Bayona M. Tolerance of nonsteroidal antiinflammatory drugs in patients with inflammatory bowel disease. *Am J Gastroenterol*. 2000;95(8):1946–1948. https://doi.org/10.1111/j.1572-0241.2000.02263.x.

80. Bonner GF, Fakhri A, Vennamaneni SR. A long-term cohort study of nonsteroidal anti-inflammatory drug use and disease activity in outpatients with inflammatory bowel disease. *Inflamm Bowel Dis*. 2004;10(6):751–757. http://www.ncbi.nlm.nih.gov/pubmed/15626893.

81. Van Assche G, Dignass A, Panes J, et al. The second European evidence-based Consensus on the diagnosis and management of Crohn's disease: definitions and diagnosis. *J Crohns Colitis*. 2010;4(1):7–27. https://doi.org/10.1016/j.crohns.2009.12.003.

82. Van Der Heijde D, Ramiro S, Landewé R, et al. 2016 update of the ASAS-EULAR management recommendations for axial spondyloarthritis. *Ann Rheum Dis*. 2017;76(6):978–991. https://doi.org/10.1136/annrheumdis-2016-210770.

83. Ward MM, Deodhar A, Akl EA, et al. American College of rheumatology/spondylitis association of America/spondyloarthritis research and treatment network 2015 recommendations for the treatment of ankylosing spondylitis and nonradiographic axial spondyloarthritis. *Arthritis Rheumatol*. 2016;68(2):282–298. https://doi.org/10.1002/art.39298.

84. De Cruz P, Kamm M, Hamilton AL, et al. P342 Adalimumab prevents post-operative Crohn's disease recurrence and is superior to thiopurines: early results from the prospective POCER study. *J Crohns Colitis*. 2012;6(suppl 1):S146. https://doi.org/10.1016/S1873-9946(12)60361-4.

85. Sands BE, Anderson FH, Bernstein CN, et al. Infliximab maintenance therapy for fistulizing crohn's disease. *N Engl J Med*. 2004;350(9):876–885. https://doi.org/10.1056/NEJMoa030815.

86. Present DH, Rutgeerts P, Targan S, et al. Infliximab for the treatment of fistulas in patients with Crohn's disease. *N Engl J Med*. 1999;340(18):1398–1405. https://doi.org/10.1056/NEJM199905063401804.

87. Sandborn WJ, Stenson WF, Brynskov J, et al. Safety of celecoxib in patients with ulcerative colitis in remission: a randomized, placebo-controlled, pilot study. *Clin Gastroenterol Hepatol*. 2006;4(2):203–211. https://doi.org/10.1016/j.cgh.2005.12.002.

88. Sutherland L, Macdonald JK. Oral 5-aminosalicylic acid for induction of remission in ulcerative colitis. *Cochrane Database Syst Rev*. 2006;(2):CD000543. https://doi.org/10.1002/14651858.CD000543.pub3.

89. Velayos FS, Loftus EV, Jess T, et al. Predictive and protective factors associated with colorectal cancer in ulcerative colitis: a case-control study. *Gastroenterology*. 2006;130(7):1941–1949. https://doi.org/10.1053/j.gastro.2006.03.028.

90. Braun J, Baraliakos X, Listing J, et al. Differences in the incidence of flares or new onset of inflammatory bowel diseases in patients with ankylosing spondylitis exposed to therapy with anti-tumor necrosis factor alpha agents. *Arthritis Rheum*. 2007;57(4):639–647. https://doi.org/10.1002/art.22669.

91. Van Der Heijde D, Kivitz A, Schiff MH, et al. Efficacy and safety of adalimumab in patients with ankylosing spondylitis: results of a multicenter, randomized, double-blind, placebo-controlled trial. *Arthritis Rheum*. 2006;54(7):2136–2146. https://doi.org/10.1002/art.21913.

92. Sandborn WJ, Hanauer SB, Katz S, et al. Etanercept for active Crohn's disease: a randomized, double-blind, placebo-controlled trial. *Gastroenterology*. 2001;121(5):1088–1094. https://doi.org/10.1053/gast.2001.28674.

93. Song IH, Appel H, Haibel H, et al. New onset of Crohn's disease during treatment of active ankylosing spondylitis with etanercept. *J Rheumatol*. 2008;35(3):532–536. https://doi.org/08/13/0122 [pii].

94. Deodhar AA, Schreiber S, Gandhi K, Fox T, Gaillez C, Karyekar C. No increased risk of inflammatory bowel disease among secukinumab-treated patients with moderate to severe psoriasis, psoriatic arthritis, or ankylosing spondylitis: data from 14 phase 2 and phase 3 clinical studies. In: *Arthritis & Rheumatology*. Vol. 68. Hoboken: Wiley 111 River St; 2016:07030–5774, NJ USA.

95. Sandborn WJ, Feagan BG, Rutgeerts P, et al. Vedolizumab as induction and maintenance therapy for crohn's disease. *N Engl J Med*. 2013;369(8):711–721. https://doi.org/10.1056/NEJMoa1215739.

96. Lin L, Liu X, Wang D, Zheng C. Efficacy and safety of antiintegrin antibody for inflammatory bowel disease: a systematic review and meta-analysis. *Medicine (Baltim)*. 2015;94(10):e556. https://doi.org/10.1097/MD.0000000000000556.

97. Rubin D, Feagan B, Dryden G, et al. P-105 the effect of vedolizumab on extraintestinal manifestations in patients with Crohn's disease in GEMINI 2. *Inflamm Bowel Dis*. 2016;22:S42–S43. https://doi.org/10.1097/01.MIB.0000480260.28955.65.

98. Bethge J, Meffert S, Ellrichmann M, Conrad C, Nikolaus S, Schreiber S. Combination therapy with vedolizumab and etanercept in a patient with pouchitis and spondylarthritis. *BMJ Open Gastroenterol*. 2017;4(1):e000127. https://doi.org/10.1136/bmjgast-2016-000127.

99. Varkas G, Thevissen K, De Brabanter G, et al. An induction or flare of arthritis and/or sacroiliitis by vedolizumab in inflammatory bowel disease: a case series. *Ann Rheum Dis*. 2017;76(5):878–881. https://doi.org/10.1136/annrheumdis-2016-210233.

100. Feagan BG, Greenberg GR, Wild G, et al. Treatment of ulcerative colitis with a humanized antibody to the alpha4beta7 integrin. *N Engl J Med*. 2005;352(24):2499–2507. https://doi.org/10.1056/NEJMoa042982.

101. Elewaut D, De Keyser F, Van Den Bosch F, et al. Enrichment of T cells carrying β7 integrins in inflamed synovial tissue from patients with early spondyloarthropathy, compared to rheumatoid arthritis. *J Rheumatol*. 1998;25(10):1932–1937.

102. Morales-Ducret J, Wayner E, Elices MJ, Alvaro-Gracia JM, Zvaifler NJ, Firestein GS. Alpha 4/beta 1 integrin (VLA-4) ligands in arthritis. Vascular cell adhesion molecule-1 expression in synovium and on fibroblast-like synoviocytes. *J Immunol*. 1992;149(4):1424–1431. http://www.ncbi.nlm.nih.gov/pubmed/1380043.

103. Poddubnyy D, Hermann KGA, Callhoff J, Listing J, Sieper J. Ustekinumab for the treatment of patients with active ankylosing spondylitis: results of a 28-week, prospective, open-label, proof-of-concept study (TOPAS). *Ann Rheum Dis*. 2014;73(5):817–823. https://doi.org/10.1136/annrheumdis-2013-204248.

104. Feagan BG, Sandborn WJ, Gasink C, et al. Ustekinumab as induction and maintenance therapy for crohn's disease. *N Engl J Med*. 2016;375(20):1946–1960. https://doi.org/10.1056/NEJMoa1602773.

105. Sandborn WJ, Ghosh S, Panes J, Vranic I, Wang W, Niezychowski W. A phase 2 study of Tofacitinib, an oral janus kinase inhibitor, inpatients with crohn's disease. *Clin Gastroenterol Hepatol*. 2014;12(9). https://doi.org/10.1016/j.cgh.2014.01.029.

106. Sandborn WJ, Ghosh S, Panes J, et al. Tofacitinib, an oral janus kinase inhibitor, in active ulcerative colitis. *N Engl J Med*. 2012;367(7):616–624. https://doi.org/10.1056/NEJMoa1112168.

107. Van Der Heijde D, Deodhar A, Wei JC, et al. Tofacitinib in patients with ankylosing spondylitis: a phase II, 16-week, randomised, placebo-controlled, dose-ranging study. *Ann Rheum Dis*. 2017;76(8):1340–1347. https://doi.org/10.1136/annrheumdis-2016-210322.

108. Korman AM, Hill D, Alikhan A, Feldman SR. Impact and management of depression in psoriasis patients. *Expert Opin Pharmacother*. 2016;17(2):147–152. https://doi.org/10.1517/14656566.2016.1128894.

109. Hrehorów E, Salomon J, Matusiak L, Reich A, Szepietowski JC. Patients with psoriasis feel stigmatized. *Acta Derm Venereol*. 2012;92(1):67–72. https://doi.org/10.2340/00015555-1193.

110. Rapp SR, Feldman SR, Exum ML, Fleischer AB, Reboussin DM. Psoriasis causes as much disability as other major medical diseases. *J Am Acad Dermatol*. 1999;41(3):401–407. https://doi.org/10.1016/S0190-9622(99)70112-X.

111. Gladman DD, Antoni C, Mease P, Clegg DO, Nash O. Psoriatic arthritis: epidemiology, clinical features, course, and outcome. *Ann Rheum Dis*. 2005Vol 64. https://doi.org/10.1136/ard.2004.032482.

112. Lavie F, Salliot C, Dernis E, et al. Prognosis and follow-up of psoriatic arthritis with peripheral joint involvement: development of recommendations for clinical practice based on published evidence and expert opinion. *Jt Bone Spine*. 2009;76(5):540–546. https://doi.org/10.1016/j.jbspin.2009.03.003.

113. Goupille P. Psoriatic arthritis. *Joint Bone Spine*. 2005;72:466–470. https://doi.org/10.1016/j.jbspin.2005.10.006.

114. Gupta AK, Ellis CN, Siegel MT, et al. Sulfasalazine improves psoriasis: a double-blind analysis. *Arch Dermatol*. 1990;126(4):487–493. https://doi.org/10.1001/archderm.1990.01670280071013.

115. Gossec L, Smolen JS, Gaujoux-Viala C, et al. European league against rheumatism recommendations for the management of psoriatic arthritis with pharmacological therapies. *Ann Rheum Dis*. 2012;71(1):4–12. https://doi.org/10.1136/annrheumdis-2011-200350.

116. Van Der Horst Bruinsma IE, Nurmohamed MT. Management and evaluation of extra-articular manifestations in spondyloarthritis. *Ther Adv Musculoskelet Dis*. 2012;4(6):413–422. https://doi.org/10.1177/1759720X12458372.

117. Papp KA, Langley RG, Sigurgeirsson B, et al. Efficacy and safety of secukinumab in the treatment of moderate-to-severe plaque psoriasis: a randomized, double-blind, placebo-controlled phase II dose-ranging study. *Br J Dermatol*. 2013;168(2):412–421. https://doi.org/10.1111/bjd.12110.

118. Schafer PH, Parton A, Gandhi AK, et al. Apremilast, a cAMP phosphodiesterase-4 inhibitor, demonstrates anti-inflammatory activity in vitro and in a model of psoriasis. *Br J Pharmacol*. 2010;159(4):842–855. https://doi.org/10.1111/j.1476-5381.2009.00559.x.

119. Gottlieb a B, Strober B, Krueger JG, et al. An open-label, single-arm pilot study in patients with severe plaque-type psoriasis treated with an oral anti-inflammatory agent, apremilast. *Curr Med Res Opin*. 2008;24(5):1529–1538. https://doi.org/10.1185/030079908X301866.

120. Papp K, Cather JC, Rosoph L, et al. Efficacy of apremilast in the treatment of moderate to severe psoriasis: a randomised controlled trial. *Lancet*. 2012;380(9843):738–746. https://doi.org/10.1016/S0140-6736(12)60642-4.

121. Papp KA, Kaufmann R, Thaçi D, Hu C, Sutherland D, Rohane P. Efficacy and safety of apremilast in subjects with moderate to severe plaque psoriasis: results from a phase II, multicenter, randomized, double-blind, placebo-controlled, parallel-group, dose-comparison study. *J Eur Acad Dermatol Venereol*. 2013;27(3). https://doi.org/10.1111/j.1468-3083.2012.04716.x.

122. Pathan E, Abraham S, Van Rossen E, et al. Efficacy and safety of apremilast, an oral phosphodiesterase 4 inhibitor, in ankylosing spondylitis. *Ann Rheum Dis*. 2013;72(9):1475–1480. https://doi.org/10.1136/annrheumdis-2012-201915.

123. Papp KA, Krueger JG, Feldman SR, et al. Tofacitinib, an oral Janus kinase inhibitor, for the treatment of chronic plaque psoriasis: long-term efficacy and safety results from 2 randomized phase-III studies and 1 open-label long-term extension study. *J Am Acad Dermatol*. 2016;74(5):841–850. https://doi.org/10.1016/j.jaad.2016.01.013.

124. Papp KA, Menter MA, Abe M, et al. Tofacitinib, an oral Janus kinase inhibitor, for the treatment of chronic plaque psoriasis: results from two randomized, placebo-controlled, phase III trials. *Br J Dermatol*. 2015;173(4):949–961. https://doi.org/10.1111/bjd.14018.

125. Bachelez H, Van De Kerkhof PCM, Strohal R, et al. Tofacitinib versus etanercept or placebo in moderate-to-severe chronic plaque psoriasis: a phase 3 randomised non-inferiority trial. *Lancet*. 2015;386(9993):552–561. https://doi.org/10.1016/S0140-6736(14)62113-9.

126. Papp KA, Menter A, Strober B, et al. Efficacy and safety of tofacitinib, an oral Janus kinase inhibitor, in the treatment of psoriasis: a Phase 2b randomized placebo-controlled dose-ranging study. *Br J Dermatol*. 2012;167(3):668–677. https://doi.org/10.1111/j.1365-2133.2012.11168.x.

127. Ports WC, Khan S, Lan S, et al. A randomized phase 2a efficacy and safety trial of the topical Janus kinase inhibitor tofacitinib in the treatment of chronic plaque psoriasis. *Br J Dermatol*. 2013;169(1):137–145. https://doi.org/10.1111/bjd.12266.

128. Levin AA, Gottlieb AB. Specific targeting of interleukin-23p19 as effective treatment for psoriasis. *J Am Acad Dermatol*. 2014;70(3):555–561. https://doi.org/10.1016/j.jaad.2013.10.043.

129. Papp KA, Langley RG, Lebwohl M, et al. Efficacy and safety of ustekinumab, a human interleukin-12/23 monoclonal antibody, in patients with psoriasis: 52-week results from a randomised, double-blind, placebo-controlled trial (PHOENIX 2). *Lancet*. 2008;371(9625):1675–1684. https://doi.org/10.1016/S0140-6736(08)60726-6.

130. Leonardi CL, Kimball AB, Papp KA, et al. Efficacy and safety of ustekinumab, a human interleukin-12/23 monoclonal antibody, in patients with psoriasis: 76-week results from a randomised, double-blind, placebo-controlled trial (PHOENIX 1). *Lancet*. 2008;371(9625):1665–1674. https://doi.org/10.1016/S0140-6736(08)60725-4.

131. Campa M, Mansouri B, Warren R, Menter A. A review of biologic therapies targeting IL-23 and IL-17 for use in moderate-to-severe plaque psoriasis. *Dermatol Ther*. 2016;6(1):1–12. https://doi.org/10.1007/s13555-015-0092-3.

132. Reich K, Armstrong AW, Foley P, et al. Efficacy and safety of guselkumab, an anti-interleukin-23 monoclonal antibody, compared with adalimumab for the treatment of patients with moderate to severe psoriasis with randomized withdrawal and retreatment: results from the phase III, double-blind, p. *J Am Acad Dermatol.* 2017;76(3):418–431. https://doi.org/10.1016/j.jaad.2016.11.042.

133. Blauvelt A, Papp KA, Griffiths CEM, et al. Efficacy and safety of guselkumab, an anti-interleukin-23 monoclonal antibody, compared with adalimumab for the continuous treatment of patients with moderate to severe psoriasis: results from the phase III, double-blinded, placebo- and active comparator–. *J Am Acad Dermatol.* 2017;76(3):405–417. https://doi.org/10.1016/j.jaad.2016.11.041.

134. Langley RG, Tsai TF, Flavin S, et al. Efficacy and safety of guselkumab in patients with psoriasis who have an inadequate response to ustekinumab: Results of the randomized, double-blind, phase III NAVIGATE trial. *Br J Dermatol.* 2018. Published January 2017 http://doi.wiley.com/10.1111/bjd.15750.

135. Deodhar AA, Gottlieb AB, Boehncke WH, et al. Efficacy and safety results of Guselkumab, an anti-IL23 monoclonal antibody, in patients with active psoriatic arthritis over 24 weeks: a phase 2a, randomized, double-blind, placebo-controlled study. *Arthritis Rheumatol.* 2016;68:4359–4361. https://doi.org/10.1002/art.39977.

136. Wendling D, Balblanc JC, Briançon D, et al. Onset or exacerbation of cutaneous psoriasis during TNFα antagonist therapy. *Jt Bone Spine.* 2008;75(3):315–318. https://doi.org/10.1016/j.jbspin.2007.06.011.

137. Ko JM, Gottlieb AB, Kerbleski JF. Induction and exacerbation of psoriasis with TNF-blockade therapy: a review and analysis of 127 cases. *J Dermatol Treat.* 2009;20(2):100–108. https://doi.org/10.1080/09546630802441234.

138. Wollina U, Hansel G, Koch A, Schönlebe J, Köstler E, Haroske G. Tumor necrosis factor-alpha inhibitor-induced psoriasis or psoriasiform exanthemata: first 120 cases from the literature including a series of six new patients. *Am J Clin Dermatol.* 2008;9(1):1–14. https://doi.org/911 [pii].

139. Collamer AN, Guerrero KT, Henning JS, Battafarano DF. Psoriatic skin lesions induced by tumor necrosis factor antagonist therapy: a literature review and potential mechanisms of action. *Arthritis Rheum.* 2008;59(7):996–1001. https://doi.org/10.1002/art.23835.

140. Moustou A-E, Matekovits A, Dessinioti C, Antoniou C, Sfikakis PP, Stratigos AJ. Cutaneous side effects of anti–tumor necrosis factor biologic therapy: a clinical review. *J Am Acad Dermatol.* 2009;61(3):486–504. https://doi.org/10.1016/j.jaad.2008.10.060.

141. de Gannes GC, Ghoreishi M, Pope J, et al. Psoriasis and pustular dermatitis triggered by TNF-α inhibitors in patients with rheumatologic conditions. *Arch Dermatol.* 2007;143(2):223–231. https://doi.org/10.1001/archderm.143.2.223.

142. Nestle FO, Conrad C, Tun-Kyi A, et al. Plasmacytoid predendritic cells initiate psoriasis through interferon-α production. *J Exp Med.* 2005;202(1):135–143. https://doi.org/10.1084/jem.20050500.

143. Nestle FO, Gilliet M. Defining upstream elements of psoriasis pathogenesis: an emerging role for interferon α. *J Investig Dermatol.* 2005;125(5). https://doi.org/10.1111/j.0022-202X.2005.23923.x.

144. Gilliet M, Conrad C, Geiges M, et al. Psoriasis triggered by toll-like receptor 7 agonist imiquimod in the presence of dermal plasmacytoid dendritic cell precursors. *Arch Dermatol.* 2004;140(12):1490–1495. https://doi.org/10.1001/archderm.140.12.1490.

145. Migliore A, Broccoli S, Bizzi E, Laganà B. Indirect comparison of the effects of anti-TNF biological agents in patients with Ankylosing Spondylitis by means of a Mixed Treatment Comparison performed on efficacy data from published randomised, controlled trials. *J Med Econ.* 2012;15(3):473–480. https://doi.org/10.3111/13696998.2012.660255.

146. McLeod C, Bagust A, Boland A, et al. Adalimumab, etanercept and infliximab for the treatment of ankylosing spondylitis: a systematic review and economic evaluation. *Health Technol Assess.* 2007;11(28):1–158.

147. Madá M, Barbosa MM, Almeida AM, et al. Treatment of ankylosing spondylitis with TNF blockers: a meta-analysis. *Rheumatol Int.* 2013;33(9):2199–2213. https://doi.org/10.1007/s00296-013-2772-6.

148. Ren L, Li J, Luo R, Tang R, Zhu S, Wan L. Efficacy of antitumor necrosis factor(α) agents on patients with ankylosing spondylitis. *Am J Med Sci.* 2013;346(6):455–461. https://doi.org/10.1097/MAJ.0b013e3182926a23.

149. Scallon B, Cai A, Solowski N, et al. Binding and functional comparisons of two types of tumor necrosis factor antagonists. *J Pharmacol Exp Ther.* 2002;301(2):418–426. https://doi.org/10.1124/jpet.301.2.418.

150. Arora T, Padaki R, Liu L, et al. Differences in binding and effector functions between classes of TNF antagonists. *Cytokine.* 2009;45(2):124–131. https://doi.org/10.1016/j.cyto.2008.11.008.

151. Ueda N, Tsukamoto H, Mitoma H, et al. The cytotoxic effects of certolizumab pegol and golimumab mediated by transmembrane tumor necrosis factorα. *Inflamm Bowel Dis.* 2013;19(6):1224–1231. https://doi.org/10.1097/MIB.0b013e318280b169.

152. Nesbitt A, Fossati G, Bergin M, et al. Mechanism of action of certolizumab pegol (CDP870): in vitro comparison with other anti-tumor necrosis factor α agents. *Inflamm Bowel Dis.* 2007;13(11):1323–1332. https://doi.org/10.1002/ibd.20225.

153. Mitoma H, Horiuchi T, Tsukamoto H, et al. Mechanisms for cytotoxic effects of anti-tumor necrosis factor agents on transmembrane tumor necrosis factor ??-expressing cells: comparison among infliximab, etanercept, and adalimumab. *Arthritis Rheum.* 2008;58(5):1248–1257. https://doi.org/10.1002/art.23447.

154. Kaymakcalan Z, Sakorafas P, Bose S, et al. Comparisons of affinities, avidities, and complement activation of adalimumab, infliximab, and etanercept in binding to soluble and membrane tumor necrosis factor. *Clin Immunol.* 2009;131(2):308–316. https://doi.org/10.1016/j.clim.2009.01.002.

155. Biancheri P, Brezski RJ, Di Sabatino A, et al. Proteolytic cleavage and loss of function of biologic agents that neutralize tumor necrosis factor in the mucosa of patients with inflammatory bowel disease. *Gastroenterology.* 2015;149(6):1564–1574.e3. https://doi.org/10.1053/j.gastro.2015.07.002.

156. Lymphotoxin RNH. TNF: how it all began-A tribute to the travelers. *Cytokine Growth Factor Rev.* 2014;25(2):83–89. https://doi.org/10.1016/j.cytogfr.2014.02.001.

157. Mitoma H, Horiuchi T, Tsukamoto H, Ueda N. Molecular mechanisms of action of anti-TNF-α agents – comparison among therapeutic TNF-α antagonists. *Cytokine.* 2018;101:56–63. https://doi.org/10.1016/j.cyto.2016.08.014.

158. Keck KM, Choi D, Savage LM, Rosenbaum JT. Insights into uveitis in association with spondyloarthritis from a large patient survey. *J Clin Rheumatol.* 2014;20(3):141–145. https://doi.org/10.1097/RHU.0000000000000087.

159. Deodhar A, Gensler LS, Sieper J, et al. Three Multicenter, Randomized, Double–Blind, Placebo–Controlled Studies Evaluating the Efficacy and Safety of Ustekinumab in Axial Spondyloarthritis. *Arthritis Rheumatol.* (2019). https://doi.org/10.1002/art.40728.

160. Mease P. Ustekinumab Fails to Show Efficacy in a Phase III Axial Spondyloarthritis Program: The Importance of Negative Results. *Arthritis Rheumatol.* 2019. https://doi.org/10.1002/art.40759.

161. Baeten D, Østergaard M, Wei JC, et al. Risankizumab, an IL-23 inhibitor, for ankylosing spondylitis: results of a randomised, double-blind, placebo-controlled, proof-of-concept, dose-finding phase 2 study Annals of the Rheumatic Diseases. 2018;77:1295–1302.

CHAPTER 12

Comorbidities*

MICHAEL M. WARD, MD, MPH

Although axial spondyloarthritis (axSpA) principally affects the musculoskeletal system, a number of other conditions can develop that are either directly or indirectly related to the inflammation or skeletal damage present in this disease. These comorbidities involve the cardiovascular, pulmonary, renal, reproductive, and nervous systems, as well as several noninflammatory musculoskeletal complications. This chapter focuses on comorbidities other than iritis, psoriasis, and inflammatory bowel diseases; these manifestations are addressed elsewhere. Comorbidities include conditions that are common but which have increased prevalence in patients with axSpA and conditions that are relatively uncommon and more specific to axSpA (Box 12.1).

Most of the literature on comorbidities in axSpA relates specifically to patients with ankylosing spondylitis (AS), and therefore, generalization to patients with axSpA other than AS should be done with caution. Additionally, these comorbidities rarely affect children with SpA, and therefore, this discussion applies only to adults. Conditions that have not been found to occur at higher frequencies in patients with AS, such as malignancies, are not specifically addressed. Lastly, adverse effects of medications are not included here.

CARDIOVASCULAR DISEASES

Aortitis and valvular heart disease. Aortitis involving the aortic root and leading to aortic insufficiency is among the most common serious comorbidities associated with AS. The aortitis is manifested by intimal proliferation and adventitial scarring, focused at the level of the valve.[1] Inflammation is localized primarily behind and above the sinuses of Valsalva and may extend to the interventricular septum, but only rarely extends distally to the ascending aorta.[1] Scarring typically develops in

the groove between the aortic valve and anterior mitral leaflet, forming a characteristic ridge or bump beneath the aortic valve seen on echocardiography, which can damage the anterior mitral leaflet.[2] Aortic valve leaflets are also thickened and shortened, which along with scarring at the base of the commissures leads to valvular incompetence. Commonly, the vaso vasora are affected by a chronic inflammatory infiltrate, with pathology similar to that of syphilitic aortitis.[1] Aneurysms due to aortitis in other parts of the ascending, descending, or abdominal aorta are rare.[3] The etiology of aortitis in AS is unknown. Although some studies had suggested an association with HLA-B27 independent of rheumatic disease, this association has not been confirmed.[4-6] Recent studies in animal models suggest that aortitis may be related to resident T cells that are responsive to interleukin-23, similar to T cells present in entheses.[7,8]

On echocardiography, up to 82% of unselected patients with AS have been found to have some structural abnormalities, although most of these are subclinical.[9-11] Aortic insufficiency has been reported in 0%–34% of patients, whereas mitral insufficiency has been reported in 5%–74%.[2,9-17] Valvular insufficiency on echocardiography is typically mild and may not become clinically manifest. The prevalence of clinically evident valvular heart disease in AS has been reported to range from 1% to 12%.[15,18,19] Valvular heart disease may rarely be the initial presentation of axial spondyloarthritis, but in most cases it develops after many years of AS.[6,13,19-21] No risk factors other than increasing age and duration of AS have been identified.

The course of valvular insufficiency in AS is typically slowly progressive. It may lead to congestive heart failure, stroke, or death if valve replacement or repair is delayed.[9] Rarely, fulminant aortic insufficiency may occur.[22] It is not clear if treatment with tumor necrosis factor-alpha inhibitor (TNFi) alters the frequency or severity of aortitis or valvular disease in AS, although aortitis has been reported to develop during treatment with etanercept.[23]

*This work was supported by the Intramural Research Program, National Institute of Arthritis and Musculoskeletal and Skin Diseases, National Institutes of Health.

Axial Spondyloarthritis. https://doi.org/10.1016/B978-0-323-56800-5.00012-6

BOX 12.1
Common and Uncommon Comorbidities Associated With Axial Spondyloarthritis.

	Common	Uncommon
Cardiovascular	Valvular heart disease	Aortitis
	Conduction abnormalities	Third-degree heart block
	Diastolic dysfunction	
	Atherosclerotic heart disease	
Pulmonary	Restrictive lung disease	Apical fibrobullous disease
	Sleep apnea	
Renal	Urolithiasis	Amyloidosis
		IgA nephropathy
Genitourinary	Prostatitis	
	Erectile dysfunction	
	Varicocele	
Musculoskeletal	Vertebral osteoporosis	
	Vertebral compression fractures	
Neurologic		Spinal cord injury
		Atlantoaxial subluxation
		Cauda equina syndrome
Others	Depression	
	Chronic widespread pain	

Conduction disturbances. Extension of inflammation and scarring from the aortic root to the interventricular septum can lead to atrioventricular conduction blocks, bundle branch blocks, and fascicular blocks.[5] Conduction disturbances may affect up to 35% of patients, depending on the types of conduction abnormalities considered.[17,19,21,24–27] Abnormalities may be intermittent. Third-degree heart block, the most serious conduction block, affects 0%–9% of patients.[19,21,25–27] Electrophysiologic studies localize the block to the suprahisian atrioventricular node in most patients.[28] Treatment with a permanent pacemaker is effective for patients with symptomatic bradycardia.

In surveys of men with permanent pacemakers but without known spondyloarthritis, the prevalence of AS was 3%–8%, much higher than expected in the general population.[29–31] These results support an association between symptomatic conduction disturbances and AS. However, evidence from well-controlled epidemiologic studies of the relative risk of conduction abnormalities in patients with AS is quite limited.[17,32]

Myocardial dysfunction. The most common abnormality of myocardial function in AS is diastolic dysfunction, most often due to decreased left ventricular relaxation.[33,34] In studies of patients with AS who did not have clinical or electrocardiographic evidence of heart disease or valvular disease, the prevalence of diastolic dysfunction ranged from 12% to 53%.[17,33–39] The number of patients included in these studies ranged from 21 to 100. In comparison with matched controls without AS, measures of left ventricular filling were generally only mildly decreased, indicating subtle abnormalities in diastolic function.[34–39] The cause of diastolic dysfunction in AS is unclear, but mild diffuse increases in myocardial connective tissue have been implicated.[35]

Echocardiographic studies have not found an increased risk of left ventricular systolic dysfunction in AS.[33,34,37,38] Early reports noted a high frequency of dilated cardiomyopathy in patients with AS, but this condition has not been a feature of recent cohorts.[40–42] Infiltrative cardiomyopathy due to secondary amyloidosis is extremely rare.[43]

Atherosclerotic cardiovascular disease. Risks of acute myocardial infarction and stroke are modestly higher among patients with AS than age- and sex-matched controls. A recent metaanalysis of longitudinal studies reported the odds of myocardial infarction to be 60% higher (odds ratio 1.60; 95% confidence interval 1.32, 1.93) in AS, and the odds of stroke to be 50% higher (odds ratio 1.50; 95% confidence interval 1.39, 1.62).[44] There was substantial heterogeneity in risks of myocardial infarction among studies. In two studies, relative risks were higher among women than men with AS.[45,46]

Population-based studies have also reported slightly increased risks of diagnoses of ischemic heart disease (relative prevalence 1.18 to 1.51) and cerebrovascular disease (relative prevalence 1.25) in patients with AS compared with controls, although a study from Sweden reported the risk of ischemic heart disease to be more than twice as high in persons with AS.[46–48] Cardiovascular disease is the main cause of death in AS, accounting for 40%–50% of deaths.[49,50] Risks of cardiovascular mortality are 40% higher among patients with AS than persons without AS.[50,51]

Subclinical atherosclerosis has also been reported to be more prevalent among patients with AS than controls in many, but not all, studies.[52-54] Increased carotid intima-media thickness has been a more common finding in AS than increases in carotid plaque. Subclinical atherosclerosis is less marked among patients with persistently low disease activity or on treatment with TNFi, suggesting an etiologic role for systemic inflammation.[54,55] A 6-month controlled trial of golimumab showed no effect on carotid intima-media thickness but was likely too short to observe any effects.[56]

Increased risks of atherosclerotic cardiovascular diseases in AS raise the question of whether traditional cardiovascular risk factors are more common among these patients.[57] Hypertension is the risk factor most consistently reported to be more common among patients with AS than controls.[48,57-61] This may be due to use of nonsteroidal antiinflammatory drugs (NSAIDs). Although most studies have not found diabetes mellitus to be more prevalent in AS, the risk of metabolic syndrome is twice as high in patients with AS than controls.[52,58,59,62] Whether rates of smoking are higher among patients with AS is not known, and the potential contribution of decreased physical activity to atherosclerotic disease in AS is unclear. Although hyperlipidemia is not more prevalent in AS, depressed levels of high-density lipoprotein, which correlated with increased disease activity, have been found.[52,59,63] Although systemic inflammation has been implicated in the increased risk of atherosclerotic disease in AS, the relative contributions of traditional risk factors and inflammation to this comorbidity remain unclear.

The effects of medications on the risk of atherosclerotic events in AS have not been widely studied. NSAIDs likely are associated with increased risk, based on data in patients with other conditions.[64] A population-based study of medical records from the United Kingdom reported a slightly increased risk of ischemic heart disease among patients with AS with any NSAID use (hazard ratio 1.36), with a much higher risk with use of cyclooxygenase-2 specific drugs (hazard ratio 3.0).[46] Associations between NSAID use and cardiac events were not reported. In contrast, a claims-based study reported that, among elderly patients with AS, use of traditional NSAIDs was protective of cardiovascular mortality, whereas use of cyclooxygenase-2 inhibitors was neutral.[51] A Swedish study of patients with spondyloarthritis reported no increased risk of either acute cardiac events or cerebrovascular events with use of etoricoxib or celecoxib

relative to traditional NSAIDs.[65] Whether use of TNFi alters the risk of cardiovascular events in axSpA has not been reported. Treatment with statins has been associated with a lower risk of mortality in AS, but it is not clear that this effect differs from that seen in the general population.[66]

PULMONARY DISEASES

Restrictive lung disease. The most common pulmonary manifestation of AS is restrictive lung disease, resulting from limitations in chest wall motion due to costovertebral fusion, costosternal fusion, and thoracic vertebral fusion.[67] Normal ventilation relies on anteroposterior expansion of the chest by respiratory and intercostal muscle contraction to move the ribs and sternum and by inferior diaphragmatic excursion. The former has a greater role when ventilatory demands are higher. With thoracic fusion in chronic AS, the loss of rib motion and deconditioning of respiratory muscles progressively result in reduced ability to increase the anteroposterior chest diameter and an increased reliance increasing reliance on diaphragmatic breathing.[68-70] Consequently, ventilation during times of higher demand tends to be affected first by restrictive lung disease in AS. If a patient does not regularly do physical activity, respiratory compromise may go unrecognized because diaphragmatic breathing may be sufficient to meet low demands. In addition to restriction due to thoracic fusion, acute symptoms affecting the anterior chest wall, costovertebral joints, or upper spine may cause splinting and temporary limitations in ventilation.

The classical defect in pulmonary function testing in AS is restrictive lung disease, with low forced vital capacity and normal or high total lung capacity or residual volume.[67] Diffusing capacity is normal in the absence of other lung pathologies. Estimates of the prevalence of restrictive lung disease in cross-sectional studies of unselected samples range from 15% to 57% (Table 12.1).[71-85] Because this prevalence will be influenced by the age composition and chronicity of each cohort, a more informative analysis would be the actuarial prevalence as a function on the duration of AS. However, it is clear that restrictive lung disease is common. The degree of restrictive defect on pulmonary function testing has also been consistently correlated with restriction of chest expansion and limitations in spinal motion.[80,82,86-88]

Restrictive lung defects are largely asymptomatic but can complicate other acute lung insults, such as infections, mechanical ventilation, or secondary lung

TABLE 12.1

Proportion of Patients With Ankylosing Spondylitis With Restrictive Defects on Pulmonary Function Testing

References	Number	Mean Age	PULMONARY FUNCTION TEST PATTERN (%)		
			Restrictive	Obstructive	Mixed
Casserly, 1997[71]	26	44.8	23.1	11.5	
Turetschek, 2000[72]	21	43.0	57.0	0	
Aggrawal, 2001[73]	17	28.2	35.3	0	
Kiris, 2003[74]	28	30.8	42.8	0	
Senocak, 2003[75]	20	40.0	30.0	10.0	
El-Maghraoui, 2004[76]	55	37.6	34.5	3.6	
Altin, 2005[77]	38	43.0	21.0	13.1	
Baser, 2006[78]	26	33.0	30.7	0	
Ayhan-Ardic, 2006[79]	20	47.4	20.0	5.0	
Dincer, 2007[80]	36	30.6	33.3	2.8	5.6
Sampaio-Barros, 2007[81]	46	40.1	52.0	0	13.0
Berdal, 2012[82]	147	48.5	18.4	10.2	
Özdemir, 2012[83]	20	37.1	15.0	5.0	
Brambila-Tapia, 2013[84]	61	39.0	57.4	0	
Yuksekkaya, 2014[85]	20	45.7	30.0	20.0	

diseases such as emphysema. For this reason, avoidance of smoking to reduce the likelihood of obstructive lung disease is critical in patients with AS.

The degree to which restrictive lung disease may contribute to exercise limitations in patients with AS is unresolved.[80,82,87–90] Although some studies suggest that peripheral muscle deconditioning is the primary factor contributing to exercise limitations in AS, other studies implicate impaired respiratory muscle function, which is a consequence of chest wall limitations.[68,91,92] Respiratory muscle exercises, particularly focused on increasing maximal inspiratory pressure, can increase aerobic capacity and forced vital capacity.[93,94] Treatment with TNFi has also been associated with short-term (12-week) improvements in lung function in one clinical trial in patients with AS.[95] These results indicate that part of the restrictive lung disease is related to acute inflammation, improvement of which can lead to better chest wall mechanics in the short term. Whether these effects are sustained over the long term is unknown.

Parenchymal lung diseases. Very few patients have clinically evident pulmonary disease associated with AS. Historically, the most specific pulmonary manifestation of AS has been apical fibrobullous disease, which in the 1970s was reported to affect 1.2% of patients.[96] In this condition, apical infiltrates and nodules slowly progress to fibrosis and cavity formation, most often bilaterally, mimicking the apical disease associated with tuberculosis. The etiology of this condition is unknown. Apical fibrobullous disease first develops after many years of AS and is largely asymptomatic, although cough, dyspnea, and spontaneous pneumothorax may occur.[97,98] Fungal or mycobacterial superinfection of the cavities can result in worsening symptoms, including hemoptysis. Clinical focus on apical fibrobullous disease has waned in recent years, which may suggest a decrease in prevalence. However, a survey from Taiwan in the 1990s to mid-2000s reported a prevalence of apical fibrobullous disease of 1%.[99]

A wide variety of other parenchymal diseases have been described in AS, including interstitial lung disease, fibrosing alveolitis, bronchiolitis obliterans, bronchiectasis, and centrilobular emphysema, often in case reports or uncontrolled case series.[71,72,74–81,83,85] Whether these conditions cooccur with AS more often than expected by chance is not clear. Lung abnormalities on high-resolution computed tomography scans have been reported in 40%–95% of patients.[71,72,74–81,83,85]

The most common abnormalities are nonspecific interstitial changes, interlobular septal thickening, linear septal thickening, nodules, bronchial wall thickening, and emphysema. In one small controlled series, the prevalence of interstitial lung disease was 20% among patients with AS and 5% among controls.[79] Although the frequency of imaging abnormalities was higher among those with more longstanding AS, abnormalities were also detected in the first 5–10 years of AS.[74,76,78,83] Longitudinal follow-up studies of these imaging abnormalities have not been reported, so their potential clinical consequences are unclear.

Obstructive sleep apnea. In two small series, obstructive sleep apnea was found in 2 of 17 (11.7%) subjects and 7 of 31 (22.6%) subjects with AS, which is more than three times the expected frequency in the population.[100,101] Age was the main risk factor in one study, while the other noted that both affected subjects were obese and middle-aged. Alterations in neck anatomy due to cervical spine disease or bulbar compromise have been speculated to be potential causes.[100,102] However, a third study did not find sleep-disordered breathing to be more frequent in patients with AS, and more studies are needed to establish this link.[103] Sleep apnea may be only one of many sleep problems that contribute to fatigue in AS.[104]

RENAL DISEASES

Secondary amyloidosis. Serum amyloid A, an acute phase reactant, can cause organ dysfunction when chronically elevated levels are deposited extracellularly in tissues.[105] The most common sites of deposition are the kidney, liver, and spleen.[105] Rarely, malabsorption due to gastrointestinal involvement, adrenal insufficiency, peripheral neuropathy, and cardiomyopathy may also occur. In the kidney, amyloid fibril deposition is most prominent in the glomeruli, resulting in the loss of permselectivity and consequent proteinuria. Renal amyloidosis can be asymptomatic and only detected by finding proteinuria on laboratory testing, although nephrotic syndrome is not uncommon. Kidney biopsy that demonstrates amyloid deposition on Congo red staining is required for a definite diagnosis. Severe amyloid deposition can sufficiently compromise kidney function to cause end-stage renal disease.

Most evidence for the presence of secondary amyloidosis in AS comes from case reports and small case series.[106,107] In recent larger cohort studies, the prevalence of clinically evident renal amyloidosis in patients with AS has been reported to be 1.1% among 730 patients in Turkey, 0.14% of 681 patients in South

Korea, and 0.1% of 8616 patients in an administrative medical claims study from Canada.[108–110] The frequency of subclinical amyloidosis is likely somewhat higher, as up to 7% of asymptomatic patients have been found with amyloid deposits on subcutaneous fat pad biopsies.[111,112] Renal amyloidosis is more prevalent among those with longer durations of AS, older age, higher measures of systemic inflammation, and perhaps in those with peripheral arthritis.[108,110] Treatment with TNFi has resulted in improvement in proteinuria and renal function.[109,113]

The frequency with which renal amyloidosis results in end-stage renal disease in patients with AS is unclear, but anecdotally is uncommon.[114] Renal transplantation is an effective treatment, but amyloidosis may recur in the transplanted kidney. Examination of temporal trends suggests that the impact of secondary amyloidosis on outcomes in AS has decreased over time, reflecting improved control of inflammation. Secondary amyloidosis was the cause of death in 70% of patients followed in the 1960s but in only 2% followed in the 1980s.[49,115] It is not clear if the frequency of renal amyloidosis in AS has decreased in recent years with the advent of more effective therapies, but this would be expected.

IgA nephropathy. IgA nephropathy is a chronic glomerulopathy caused by the deposition of IgA-containing immune complexes in the glomerular mesangium.[116] The immune complexes preferentially involve serum IgA1 that has been poorly O-galactosylated, which may be pathogenetically important. Immune complex deposition results in mesangial cell proliferation, release of proinflammatory and profibrotic mediators, complement activation, podocyte injury, and eventually tubulointerstitial injury.[116] Its clinical presentation is typically with nephritic- or nephrotic-range proteinuria, microscopic hematuria, and hypertension. Although often slowly progressive, the 10-year risk of end-stage renal disease may exceed 15%.[117]

IgA nephropathy has been implicated as being associated with AS based on numerous case reports of the coexistence of these two uncommon diseases.[118] In case series, the proportion of patients with AS who had IgA nephropathy ranged from 0% to 3.1%.[109,119–123] However, no epidemiologic studies have been done to establish whether IgA nephropathy occurs more frequently in patients with AS than without AS. Nonetheless, suspicion of an association is supported by similar cooccurrences of IgA nephropathy and inflammatory bowel diseases, which share certain genetic markers and elevated serum IgA levels in patients with AS.[124,125]

Urolithiasis. Patients with AS are at increased risk for urolithiasis. In a large population-based study of administrative data from Sweden, risk of urolithiasis was 2.1 times higher among patients with AS than controls.[126] 4% of AS patients and 1.8% of controls had urolithiasis before, or during, observation. Those at greatest risk were men and those with concomitant inflammatory bowel disease, prior stone disease, or TNFi users (considered as a marker of severe AS). A similar study from Taiwan reported a much weaker association between urolithiasis and AS, with an adjusted hazard ratio of 1.19 (95% confidence interval 1.01, 1.40).[127] Reasons for this difference are not clear.

The association between urolithiasis and AS has also been examined in smaller clinical studies, which have generally found a twofold higher risk of urolithiasis among patients with AS than controls, whether the diagnosis of kidney stones was based on clinical history or ultrasound testing.[128-131] Absolute frequencies of urolithiasis in patients with AS varied widely, in part because of geographic variation in rates of urolithiasis, but were greater than 10% in many series. The increased risk in AS is thought to be due to alterations in calcium homeostasis, and possibly subclinical ileal disease, analogous to the mechanisms that lead to urolithiasis in patients with inflammatory bowel diseases.[132] These hypotheses presume that most stones in AS are calcium oxalate stones, but the frequency of stones by chemical composition has not been reported. Because urolithiasis is associated with osteopenia, osteoporotic fractures, and poor bone remodeling, patients with urolithiasis should be considered for bone mineral density testing.[133] In one small study, there was no association between urolithiasis and spinal fusion.[134] Treatment is not different from that of patients without AS. However, patients with AS more often need urologic intervention.[135]

GENITOURINARY CONDITIONS AND PREGNANCY

Male genitourinary conditions. Past literature on associations between urogenital inflammation and infection and AS is confounded by lack of a clear distinction between reactive arthritis and AS. However, recent studies suggest a possible association with AS. A nationwide survey in Iceland found that 27% of men with AS reported having a history of prostatitis.[136] Prostatitis and urethritis, often associated with Chlamydia infections, were each found in 13% of patients with AS in a clinical study from Germany.[137] Varicoceles are also more common among men with AS, possibly induced because of frequent Valsalva maneuvers during episode of low back pain.[138-140]

Sexual dysfunction. Men with AS generally report more problems with erectile function, orgasmic function, sexual drive, intercourse satisfaction, and overall satisfaction than men without AS on validated questionnaires such as the International Index of Erectile Function.[141,142] Estimates of the prevalence of erectile dysfunction range from 4.7% to 35%.[143-146] Sexual dysfunction is directly correlated with the severity of inflammatory symptoms and depression.[144-147] Although data are limited, women with AS generally report no greater problems with sexual functioning than women without AS, except possibly for less sexual desire and arousal.[142,148,149] Because most studies are from referral centers, these findings may reflect only more severely affected patients. In a recent survey of 379 patients with axial SpA, 82% reported little or no effect of their health condition on sexual activity.[150]

Pregnancy. AS does not affect fertility. Inflammatory symptoms do not clearly improve during pregnancy, as is common in women with rheumatoid arthritis, and mechanical back pain often worsens late in pregnancy.[151-153] Worsening of low back pain postpartum is common in relation to bending over and lifting the infant. Risks of obstetrical complications are not different in women with AS and women without AS, although delivery by Caesarean section is more often used in women with AS.[154,155] Women with AS may be at higher risk for preterm delivery.[155]

OSTEOPOROSIS AND FRACTURES

Osteoporosis. Vertebral osteoporosis has long been recognized as a common feature affecting the ankylosed spine. Osteoporosis in this setting has been traditionally attributed to both immobility and mechanical off-loading of vertebral trabecular bone by perivertebral ossification and bridging syndesmophytes.[156] Importantly, low vertebral bone density has also been repeatedly found in patients with early AS and who are physically active and without syndesmophytes.[157-193] In studies of lumbar spine bone mineral density (BMD), a median of 31% of patients had osteopenia and 16.1% had osteoporosis (Table 12.2). Similarly, in studies that reported BMD at the femoral neck, a median of 38.1% of patients had osteopenia and 10.9% had osteoporosis at this site.

The presence of low vertebral BMD early in AS has implicated inflammation as a mediator of this process. In many cross-sectional studies, acute phase reactants

TABLE 12.2

Bone Mineral Density and Osteoporosis in Patients With Ankylosing Spondylitis. Sex-Stratified Results are Provided When Available. Proportions With Osteopenia or Osteoporosis are Based on T Scores of Bone Mineral Density

References	Number/ Sex	Mean Age	Mean Duration	LUMBAR SPINE BMD or Z score[a]	Osteo-penia (%)	Osteopo-rosis (%)	FEMORAL NECK BMD or Z score[a]	Osteop-enia (%)	Osteop-orosis (%)
Will[156b]	25/M	33	11.5	0.82 vs. 0.91			0.83 vs. 0.92		
Devogelaer[157b]	60/M	39	15.0	−0.73					
Bronson[158]	19/M	50.5	25.2	0.68 vs. 0.86			0.73 vs. 0.82	57.9	10.5
Donnelly[159]	62/M	43.5	16.3	−0.58			−0.94		
	25/F	44.8	16.6	+0.78			−0.43		
Mullaji[160]	16/M	36.6	8.7	0.89 vs. 0.98			0.76 vs. 0.87		
	6/F	36.7	6.8	0.90 vs. 1.09			0.76 vs. 0.87		
Lee[161]	14/M	43.9	9.8	−0.63			−0.96		
Meirelles[162]	30	37.0	17.0	0.97 vs. 1.08	23	27	0.80 vs. 0.91	31	45
El Maghraoui[163]	80	36.7	8.7		31	18.7		41.2	13.7
Juanola[164]	18/F	36.7	15.1	−0.19			−0.03		
Toussirot[165]	71	39.1	10.6	1.08 vs. 1.18	32.4	14.1	0.97 vs. 1.04	22.5	4.2
Dos Santos[166]	39/M	37.6	8.4	1.08 vs. 1.23					
Speden[167]	66/F	43.4	21.5		18	8		52	6
Franck[168]	190/M	50.4	–	1.05 vs. 1.03			0.57 vs. 0.63		
	74/F	48.0	–	1.01 vs. 1.04			0.61 vs. 0.69		
Lange[169]	49	38.7	13.9		18.3	6.1			
Karberg[170]	103	40.0	9.3		31	14		52	24
Aydin[171]	58/M	38.2	9.3					43.1	15.5
Baek[172]	76/M	28.1	9.4		42.1	7.9		14.5	1.3
Kim[173]	60	32.1	5.5		37	19		41	33
Jun[174]	68/M	30.7	7.1	0.94 vs. 1.01			0.78 vs. 0.87		
Borman[175]	32/M	39.1	14.8		34.3	34.3			
Sarikaya[176]	26	44.3	–				0.75 vs. 0.85	76.9	

Continued

TABLE 12.2
Bone Mineral Density and Osteoporosis in Patients With Ankylosing Spondylitis. Sex-Stratified Results are Provided When Available. Proportions With Osteopenia or Osteoporosis are Based on T Scores of Bone Mineral Density—cont'd

References	Number/ Sex	Mean Age	Mean Duration	LUMBAR SPINE BMD or Z score[a]	Osteo-penia (%)	Osteoporosis (%)	FEMORAL NECK BMD or Z score[a]	Osteopenia (%)	Osteoporosis (%)
Ghozlani[177]	80	38.9	10.8	−1.2					
Başkan[178]	100	39.9	10.5	0.73 vs. 0.84		32	0.81 vs. 0.89		
Kaya[179]	55	35.8	11.0		32.7	23.6		43.6	10.9
Arends[180]	128	41.0	14		32.0	7.0		32.8	1.5
Van der Wei-jden[181]	130	38.0	0.7		30.8	7.7		28.5	2.3
Muntean[182]	44/M	41	13.3		22.7	25.0		38.1	21.4
Vasdev[183]	80/M	32.9	8.1			28.8			11.5
Grazio[184]	80	52.3	21.8		20.0	25.0		47.5	22.5
Korczowska[185]	43/M	–	–					51.1	4.6
Klingberg[186]	117/M	–	–		6.8	6.0		21.3	5.1
	87/F	–	–		17.2	16.1		27.6	4.6
Taylan[187]	55	36	10	0.9 vs. 1.0			0.8 vs. 0.9		
Ulu[188]	59	34.3	4.5			32.2		45.7	
Wang[189]	504	29.1	7.7			3.2			9.2
Nazir[190]	25	25.0	5.1		32	36		36	20
Magrey[191]	101	45.6	–		41.9	4.3		26.8	9.6
Gamez-Nava[192]	50/M	45	–	1.18 vs. 1.17			0.97 vs. 1.09		
	28/F	48	–	1.13 vs. 1.10			0.95 vs. 1.02		

[a]Bone mineral density (BMD) values are expressed as AS versus controls in g/cm^2.
[b]By dual photon absorptiometry. All other studies used dual-energy X-ray absorptiometry.

were among the most important correlates of low vertebral bone density.[163,166,168,173,174,176,177,180,181,184,186,191] In prospective studies, bone loss over 2–5 years was greater in patients with more persistent systemic inflammation, as reflected by high erythrocyte sedimentation rates or C-reactive protein levels.[189,193,194] Additionally, the presence of bone marrow edema on magnetic resonance imaging of the spine or sacroiliac joints has been associated with low vertebral BMD, further supporting a role for inflammation.[195,196] These associations are consistent with the known actions of interleukin-1,

interleukin-6, TNF-alpha, and interleukin-17 in promoting osteoclastogenesis and bone resorption and inhibiting osteoblasts.[197] Low body mass index and hip arthritis may also be risk factors for low vertebral BMD.[159,177,181,186,188]

Syndesmophytes, disc calcification, and facet joint fusion can result in falsely high BMD readings on conventional dual-energy X-ray absorptiometry studies of the lumbar spine done in the anteroposterior projection.[157,158,161,169,186] Although valid readings may be obtained in patients without perivertebral ossification on plain radiographs, when these changes are present, either a lateral projection of the lumbar spine should be used or assessment of BMD should be based on measures at the hip. Alternatively, quantitative computed tomography can be used to measure volumetric BMD of vertebral trabecular bone.

Measures to prevent and treat low BMD should include repletion of vitamin D stores, adequate dietary calcium intake, and weight-bearing exercise. Few data are available on the effectiveness of bisphosphonates in the treatment of low BMD in patients with AS, and generalization from the literature on the treatment of postmenopausal osteoporosis is needed.[198-200] There is no consensus on indications for treatment, although experts recommend bisphosphonates in the setting of severe osteoporosis or fractures.[201-204] TNFi may also increase BMD in AS. In a metaanalysis largely of observational studies, lumbar BMD increased 5% over 1 year and total hip BMD increased 1.8%.[205] Patients treated with TNFi had a gain in lumbar BMD over 1 year of 2.8% relative to untreated patients. The durability of these increases is uncertain.

Vertebral compression fractures. Two types of vertebral fractures can occur: compression fractures and traumatic fractures. Traumatic fractures are discussed below in the section on neurologic comorbidities, given their associated risk of spinal cord injury.

Vertebral compression fractures may cause focal back pain, which typically abates over time. Vertebral fracture should therefore be considered when evaluating patients with AS who present with new back symptoms. However, up to three-fourths of vertebral compression fractures may be asymptomatic and detected only as reductions in the height of the vertebral body on imaging.[206,207] Compression fractures may exacerbate hyperkyphosis in AS and are associated with increased functional limitations.[206,208] Although any vertebral level may be involved, compression fractures most commonly affect the midthoracic vertebrae (Fig. 12.1).[159,177,207-211] Multiple vertebrae may be affected. Vertebral deformities can be difficult to detect on lateral thoracic radiographs, and newer screening methods such as morphometric X-ray absorptiometry may be useful.

Estimates of the prevalence of vertebral compression fractures in AS vary based on whether clinically evident or morphometric fractures are assessed, the number of vertebrae examined, and the composition of the AS cohort. In clinical cohorts, the proportion of patients with at least one vertebral fracture ranged from 10% to 41%.[159,174,177,188,207,209-213] Vertebral fractures were more common in older patients and those with

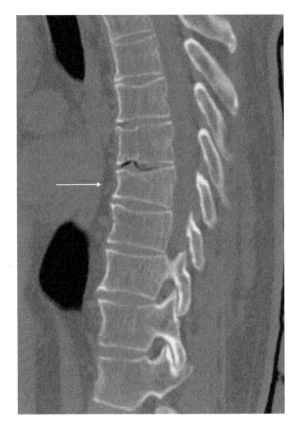

FIG. 12.1 Thoracic spine computed tomography scan of a 60-year-old man with ankylosing spondylitis showing a compression fracture of T8.

longer durations of AS, low body mass index or weight, more extensive spinal fusion, and in some studies, low hip BMD.[174,177,188,207,209,211,212]

In epidemiologic studies, patients with AS had higher risks of clinically recognized vertebral fractures than controls without AS. In a cohort study from Spain, the risk was twice as high among patients with AS.[214] In case-control studies from Denmark and the United Kingdom, odds ratios of the association between AS and clinical vertebral fractures were 5.42 and 3.26, respectively.[215,216] A US study reported the risk of radiologically identified vertebral fractures to be 7.6 times higher in patients with AS compared with those without AS.[217]

Appendicular fractures. The risk of hip, forearm, or other nonvertebral fractures is not increased in patients with AS.[214-217] This contrast with the increased risk of vertebral fractures provides additional circumstantial support for the hypothesis that local inflammation contributes to vertebral osteoporosis.

NEUROLOGIC DISORDERS

Spinal cord injury. The combination of multilevel vertebral fusion and osteoporosis makes the spine of these patients particularly vulnerable to fracture, even with low-energy trauma such as ground-level falls. Fractures can occur through the vertebral bodies or calcified disc spaces. When posterior elements are fused, fractures may also occur through the pedicles and posterior arch, occasionally at levels adjacent to the vertebral body fracture, leading to disruption of the spinal column.[218] Because fractures also tend to transect fused perivertebral ligaments, the adjacent vertebral segments become unstable, and this, with dislocation, can compress the spinal cord.

The subaxial cervical and cervicothoracic regions are the most common locations for traumatic spine fractures in AS, with C5–C7 levels most frequently involved.[219] Multilevel fractures can occur. Hyperextension injuries are responsible for three-fourths of traumatic vertebral fractures in AS.[220] Pain that is present at rest and worsened with movement is common. Delay in diagnosis occurs in 15%–40% of patients, due to a low index of suspicion given the often minor trauma, confounding by preexisting back symptoms, and imaging difficulty.[219] Plain radiographs often fail to demonstrate fractures, particularly in the crowded posterior elements and in the presence of osteopenia, because the cervicothoracic junction is obscured by shoulders and clavicles. An increase in spine angulation may provide a clue to the presence of a fracture. Computed tomography and magnetic resonance imaging are often needed to evaluate fully for the presence of vertebral fractures.[218,219,221]

Neurologic deficits have been reported in 16%–91% of patients with traumatic spine fractures, whereas paraplegia may occur in 10%–20%.[219,220] Movement of the patient with a new spine fracture must be done with extreme care to avoid worsening injury to the spinal cord. The cornerstone of treatment is immobilization of the spine. Nonoperative immobilization with braces or halos is typically reserved for patients with nondisplaced fractures and those with severe comorbidities.[219,220] Surgical immobilization, most often with posterior instrumentation, is indicated for patients with neurologic deficits, unstable fractures, or epidural hematomas.[219] In the first three postoperative months, 27% of surgically treated patients had neurologic improvement, whereas 59% were stable and 13% deteriorated.[220] Later improvement was less common.

Mortality in the first year after traumatic spine fracture ranges from 6% to 32%.[219,220] Patients at highest risk for mortality are those with spinal cord injury, particularly in the cervical spine. Lumbar fractures are rarely associated with mortality. Common complications are pneumonia, respiratory insufficiency, thromboembolic disease, and wound infections.[220]

Spinal pseudarthrosis may develop as a consequence of fracture through both a calcified disc and fused posterior elements.[222,223] Nonunion is thought to occur because movement persists at this level but not at adjacent fused vertebral levels. Radiographically similar lesions may develop as a result of inflammation in the disc space (i.e., Andersson lesions) with either fractured posterior elements or open facet joints, both of which promote more movement at the affected disc level. On radiographs, vertebral endplates are typically blurred and irregular, suggesting osteolysis, with sclerosis extending into the adjacent vertebral bodies. Focal pain that is relieved by lying supine is typical. Myelopathy may result from spinal cord compression at the unstable segment. Treatment is with immobilization or surgical fusion.[222,223]

Atlantoaxial subluxation. Atlantoaxial subluxation has long been recognized as a potential complication of AS, despite the fact that cervical fusion, including atlantodental fusion, can also occur. In case series, 13%–21% of patients with AS were found to have atlantoaxial subluxation, primarily with anterior subluxation.[224-227] As is the case in rheumatoid arthritis, atlantoaxial subluxation in AS is due to odontoid pannus formation and subsequent ligamentous instability.[228,229] Although atlantoaxial subluxation can develop early in AS, it more commonly occurs in patients with advanced AS and in association with ossification of the posterior longitudinal ligament.[224] Other risk factors include peripheral arthritis and elevated C-reactive protein levels.[224,227]

Most patients with atlantoaxial subluxation are asymptomatic but can present with severe neck pain, spasm, and occipital headache. A high index of suspicion aids to prompt diagnosis in patients who may also have inflammatory neck pain due to AS. Myelopathy has been reported in only 2% of cases, likely because prophylactic surgery is done in cases with progressive subluxation.[224,227,230]

Cauda equina syndrome. Cauda equina syndrome is a rare complication of AS characterized by slowly progressive bilateral lower extremity and perineal sensory loss and sphincter dysfunction.[231] It typically occurs in patients with longstanding AS. Some patients present with neuropathic pain, but others may be unaware of the presence or extent of sensory loss. Sensory loss ascends the legs and can progress to involve the buttocks, genital, and perianal regions, giving "saddle anesthesia." In some patients, lower extremity weakness develops subsequent to the sensory loss. Bladder involvement usually manifests as urinary retention with overflow incontinence, whereas bowel dysfunction may manifest as either retention or incontinence. Erectile dysfunction is common. Characteristic lesions on lumbosacral magnetic resonance imaging include widening of the dural sac, dural diverticulae that erode the vertebral laminae and pedicles, or less commonly, the posterior border of the vertebral body, and adhesions involving the lumbosacral nerve roots.[232]

The etiology of cauda equina syndrome in AS is unknown. Proposed causes include chronic inflammation resulting in arachnoiditis, vasculitis of the vaso vasora of the nerve roots, and elevated intrathecal pressure.[232] There is no consensus on the most appropriate treatment.[233] Antiinflammatory treatment may help with pain control but not neurologic dysfunction. Improvement with infliximab treatment has been reported in one case.[234] Lumboperitoneal shunts and laminectomy to relieve intrathecal pressure have been used, with unclear benefit.[233] If cauda equina syndrome begins as an inflammatory process that progresses to a mechanical complication, the most appropriate treatment may depend on whether the patient is seen early or later in the course.

OTHER CONDITIONS

Depression. As is the case for many chronic conditions, patients with AS are at increased risk for depression. In clinical cohorts, 12%–59% of patients reported high levels of depressive symptoms on self-report questionnaires (median 30%).[235–240] In three large population-based studies, the likelihood of a clinical diagnosis of depression was modestly higher among patients with AS than controls, with risks of 1.34, 1.63, and 1.72.[241–243] Women with AS and those with lower levels of formal education are more likely to have depression than men and those who are more well educated.[235,238,240,241] Pain, functional limitations, fatigue, sleep disturbances, and concerns with body image and work ability contribute to the potential for depressive symptoms.[236–238,240,244,245] Improvement in physical symptoms following treatment with TNFi has been associated with improvements in depression, supporting a link between physical and mental health.[246] However, depression may not solely be reactive, and dedicated antidepressive treatment may be warranted.

Chronic widespread pain. Chronic widespread pain, or fibromyalgia, may be present in 4%–18% of men and up to 50% of women with AS or axSpA.[247–255] The presence of chronic widespread pain is associated with worse symptoms, functioning, and quality of life.[247–250,253–255] In some patients, it can be difficult to differentiate inflammatory from noninflammatory symptoms, and diffuse enthesial tenderness may be confused with tender points.[256] Commonly, acute phase reactants are normal despite active AS and are not helpful in this setting unless elevated. Fatigue and sleep disturbance occur in both conditions. Therefore, there is the potential for misdiagnosis of axSpA in patients with chronic widespread pain, particularly when imaging abnormalities are not present, and particularly in women. Self-report measures, such as the Bath AS Disease Activity Index and Bath AS Functional Index, are not disease-specific and are often increased in patients with chronic widespread pain.[257,258] Chronic widespread pain can confound the assessment of disease activity in AS and can decrease the responses of patients with AS to treatment with TNFi.[259] Specific treatment of chronic widespread pain is indicated if found to be present.

REFERENCES

1. Bulkley BH, Roberts WC. Ankylosing spondylitis and aortic regurgitation. *Circulation.* 1973;48:1014–1027.
2. Tucker CR, Fowles RE, Calin A, Popp RL. Aortitis in ankylosing spondylitis: early detection of aortic root abnormalities with two dimensional echocardiography. *Am J Cardiol.* 1982;49:680–686.
3. Grewal GS, Leipsic J, Klinkhoff AV. Abdominal aortitis in HLA-B27+ spondyloarthritis: case report with 5-year follow-up and literature review. *Semin Arthritis Rheum.* 2014;44:305–308.
4. Bergfeldt L, Insulander P, Lindblom D, Möller E, Edhag O. HLA-B27: an important genetic risk factor for lone aortic regurgitation and severe conduction system abnormalities. *Am J Med.* 1988;85:12–18.
5. Bergfeldt L. HLA-B27-associated cardiac disease. *Ann Intern Med.* 1997;127:621–629.
6. Qaiyumi S, Hassan ZU, Toone E. Seronegative spondyloarthropathies in lone aortic insufficiency. *Arch Intern Med.* 1985;145:822–824.
7. Sherlock JP, Joyce-Shaikh B, Turner SP, et al. IL-23 induces spondyloarthropathy by acting on ROR-γt+ CD3+CD4-CD8- entheseal resident T cells. *Nat Med.* 2012;18:1069–1076.
8. Reinhardt A, Yevsa T, Worbs T, et al. Interleukin-23-dependent γ/δ t cells produce interleukin-17 and accumulate in the enthesis, aortic valve, and ciliary body in mice. *Arthritis Rheumatol.* 2016;68:2476–2486.
9. Roldan CA, Chavez J, Wiest PW, Qualls CR, Crawford MH. Aortic root disease and valve disease associated with ankylosing spondylitis. *J Am Coll Cardiol.* 1998;32:1397–1404.

10. Park SH, Sohn IS, Joe BH, et al. Early cardiac valvular changes in ankylosing spondylitis: a transesophageal echocardiography study. *J Cardiovasc Ultrasound*. 2012;20:30–36.

11. Klingberg E, Sveälv BG, Täng MS, Bech-Hanssen O, Forsblad-d'Elia H, Bergfeldt L. Aortic regurgitation is common in ankylosing spondylitis: time for routine echocardiography evaluation? *Am J Med*. 2015;128:1244–1250.

12. Thomas D, Hill W, Geddes R, et al. Early detection of aortic dilatation in ankylosing spondylitis using echocardiography. *Aust N Z J Med*. 1982;12:10–13.

13. O'Neill TW, King G, Graham IM, Molony J, Bresnihan B. Echocardiographic abnormalities in ankylosing spondylitis. *Ann Rheum Dis*. 1992;51:652–654.

14. Arnason JA, Patel AK, Rahko PS, Sundstrom WR. Transthoracic and transesophageal echocardiographic evaluation of the aortic root and subvalvular structures in ankylosing spondylitis. *J Rheumatol*. 1996;23:120–123.

15. Gran JT, Skomsvoll JF. The outcome of ankylosing spondylitis: a study of 100 patients. *Rheumatology*. 1997;36:766–771.

16. Alves MG, Espirito-Santo J, Queiroz MV, Madeira H, Macieira-Coelho E. Cardiac alterations in ankylosing spondylitis. *Angiology*. 1988;39:567–571.

17. Brunner F, Kunz A, Weber U, Kissling R. Ankylosing spondylitis and heart abnormalities: do cardiac conduction disorders, valve regurgitation and diastolic dysfunction occur more often in male patients with diagnosed ankylosing spondylitis for over 15 years than in the normal population? *Clin Rheumatol*. 2006;25:24–29.

18. Graham DC, Smythe HA. The carditis and aortitis of ankylosing spondylitis. *Bull Rheum Dis*. 1958;9: 171–174.

19. Kinsella TD, Johnson LG, Sutherland RI. Cardiovascular manifestations of ankylosing spondylitis. *CMAJ*. 1974;111:1309–1311.

20. Eversmeyer WH, Rosenstock D, Biundo JJ. Aortic insufficiency with mild ankylosing spondylitis in black men. *JAMA*. 1978;240:2652–2653.

21. Sukenik S, Pras A, Buskila D, Katz A, Snir Y, Horowitz J. Cardiovascular manifestations of ankylosing spondylitis. *Clin Rheumatol*. 1987;6:588–592.

22. Demoulin JC, Lespagnard J, Bertholet M, Soumagne D. Acute fulminant aortic regurgitation in ankylosing spondylitis. *Am Heart J*. 1983;105:859–861.

23. Verhoeven F, Bossert M, Lohse-Walliser A, Balblanc JC. Aortitis during etanercept therapy for ankylosing spondylitis: finding the culprit. *Joint Bone Spine*. 2012;79:524–526.

24. Thomsen NH, Hørslev-Petersen K, Beyer JM. Ambulatory 24-hour continuous electrocardiographic monitoring in 54 patients with ankylosing spondylitis. *Eur Heart J*. 1986;7:240–246.

25. Forsblad-d'Elia H, Wallberg H, Klingberg E, et al. Cardiac conduction system abnormalities in ankylosing spondylitis: a cross-sectional study. *BMC Musculoskeletal Dis*. 2013;14:237.

26. Dik VK, Peters MJ, Dijkmans PA, et al. The relationship between disease-related characteristics and conduction disturbances in ankylosing spondylitis. *Scand J Rheumatol*. 2010;39:38–41.

27. Bergfeldt L, Edhag O, Vallin H. Cardiac conduction disturbances, an underestimated manifestation in ankylosing spondylitis. *J Intern Med*. 1982;212:217–224.

28. Bergfeldt L, Vallin H, Edhag O. Complete heart block in HLA B27 associated disease. Electrophysiological and clinical characteristics. *Br Heart J*. 1984;51:184–188.

29. Bergfeldt L, Edhag O, Vedin L, Vallin H. Ankylosing spondylitis: an important cause of severe disturbances of the cardiac conduction system: prevalence among 223 pacemaker-treated men. *Am J Med*. 1982;73:187–191.

30. Bergfeldt L. HLA B27-associated rheumatic diseases with severe cardiac bradyarrhythmias: clinical features and prevalence in 223 men with permanent pacemakers. *Am J Med*. 1983;75:210–215.

31. Peeters AJ, Ten Wolde S, Sedney MI, de Vries RR, Dijkmans BA. Heart conduction disturbance: an HLA-B27 associated disease. *Ann Rheum Dis*. 1991;50:348–350.

32. Møller P. Atrioventricular conduction time in ankylosing spondylitis. *J Intern Med*. 1985;217:85–88.

33. Crowley JJ, Donnelly SM, Tobin M, et al. Doppler echocardiographic evidence of left ventricular diastolic dysfunction in ankylosing spondylitis. *Am J Cardiol*. 1993;71:1337–1340.

34. Gould BA, Turner J, Keeling DH, Hickling P, Marshall AJ. Myocardial dysfunction in ankylosing spondylitis. *Ann Rheum Dis*. 1992;51:227–232.

35. Brewerton D, Goddard D, Moore R, et al. The myocardium in ankylosing spondylitis: a clinical, echocardiographic, and histopathological study. *Lancet*. 1987;329:995–998.

36. Caliskan M, Erdogan D, Gullu H, et al. Impaired coronary microvascular and left ventricular diastolic functions in patients with ankylosing spondylitis. *Atherosclerosis*. 2008;196:306–312.

37. Yildirir A, Aksoyek S, Calguneri M, Oto A, Kes S. Echocardiographic evidence of cardiac involvement in ankylosing spondylitis. *Clin Rheumatol*. 2002;21:129–134.

38. Sun JP, Khan MA, Farhat AZ, Bahler RC. Alterations in cardiac diastolic function in patients with ankylosing spondylitis. *Int J Cardiol*. 1992;37:65–72.

39. Okan T, Sari I, Akar S, et al. Ventricular diastolic function of ankylosing spondylitis patients by using conventional pulsed wave Doppler, myocardial performance index and tissue Doppler imaging. *Echocardiography*. 2008;25:47–56.

40. Takkunen J, Vuopala U, Isomäki H. Cardiomyopathy in ankylosing spondylitis. I. Medical history and results of clinical examination in a series of 55 patients. *Ann Clin Res*. 1970;2:106–112.

41. Ribeiro P, Morley KD, Shapiro LM, Garnett RA, Hughes GR, Goodwin JF. Left ventricular function in patients with ankylosing spondylitis and Reiter's disease. *Eur Heart J*. 1984;5:419–422.

42. Nagyhegyi G, Nadas I, Banyai F, et al. Cardiac and cardiopulmonary disorders in patients with ankylosing spondylitis and rheumatoid arthritis. *Clin Exp Rheumatol.* 1988;6:17–26.

43. Fujito T, Inoue T, Hoshi K, et al. Systemic amyloidosis following ankylosing spondylitis associated with congestive heart failure. *Jpn Heart J.* 1995;36:681–688.

44. Mathieu S, Pereira B, Soubrier M. Cardiovascular events in ankylosing spondylitis: an updated meta-analysis. *Semin Arthritis Rheum.* 2015;44:551–555.

45. Peters MJ, Visman I, Nielen MM, et al. Ankylosing spondylitis: a risk factor for myocardial infarction? *Ann Rheum Dis.* 2010;69:579–581.

46. Essers I, Stolwijk C, Boonen A, et al. Ankylosing spondylitis and risk of ischaemic heart disease: a population-based cohort study. *Ann Rheum Dis.* 2016;75: 203–209.

47. Szabo SM, Levy AR, Rao SR, et al. Increased risk of cardiovascular and cerebrovascular diseases in individuals with ankylosing spondylitis: a population-based study. *Arthritis Rheumatol.* 2011;63:3294–3304.

48. Bremander A, Petersson IF, Bergman S, Englund M. Population-based estimates of common comorbidities and cardiovascular disease in ankylosing spondylitis. *Arthritis Care Res.* 2011;63:550–556.

49. Bakland G, Gran JT, Nossent JC. Increased mortality in ankylosing spondylitis is related to disease activity. *Ann Rheum Dis.* 2011;70:1921–1925.

50. Prati C, Claudepierre P, Pham T, Wendling D. Mortality in spondylarthritis. *Joint Bone Spine.* 2011;78: 466–470.

51. Haroon NN, Paterson JM, Li P, Inman RD, Haroon N. Patients with ankylosing spondylitis have increased cardiovascular and cerebrovascular mortality: a population-based study. *Ann Intern Med.* 2015;163:409–416.

52. Mathieu S, Gossec L, Dougados M, Soubrier M. Cardiovascular profile in ankylosing spondylitis: a systematic review and meta-analysis. *Arthritis Care Res.* 2011;63:557–563.

53. Gonzalez-Juanatey C, Vazquez-Rodriguez TR, Miranda-Filloy JA, et al. The high prevalence of subclinical atherosclerosis in patients with ankylosing spondylitis without clinically evident cardiovascular disease. *Medicine.* 2009;88:358–365.

54. Arida A, Protogerou AD, Konstantonis G, et al. Subclinical atherosclerosis is not accelerated in patients with ankylosing spondylitis with low disease activity: new data and metaanalysis of published studies. *J Rheumatol.* 2015;42:2098–2105.

55. van Sijl AM, van Eijk IC, Peters MJ, et al. Tumour necrosis factor blocking agents and progression of subclinical atherosclerosis in patients with ankylosing spondylitis. *Ann Rheum Dis.* 2015;74:119–123.

56. Tam LS, Shang Q, Kun EW, et al. The effects of golimumab on subclinical atherosclerosis and arterial stiffness in ankylosing spondylitis—a randomized, placebo-controlled pilot trial. *Rheumatology.* 2014;53:1065–1074.

57. Peters MJ, van der Horst-Bruinsma IE, Dijkmans BA, Nurmohamed MT. Cardiovascular risk profile of patients with spondylarthropathies, particularly ankylosing spondylitis and psoriatic arthritis. *Semin Arthritis Rheum.* 2004;34:585–592.

58. Han C, Robinson Jr DW, Hackett MV, Paramore LC, Fraeman KH, Bala MV. Cardiovascular disease and risk factors in patients with rheumatoid arthritis, psoriatic arthritis, and ankylosing spondylitis. *J Rheumatol.* 2006;33:2167–2172.

59. Papadakis JA, Sidiropoulos PI, Karvounaris SA, et al. High prevalence of metabolic syndrome and cardiovascular risk factors in men with ankylosing spondylitis on anti-TNFalpha treatment: correlation with disease activity. *Clin Exp Rheumatol.* 2009;27:292–298.

60. Kang JH, Chen YH, Lin HC. Comorbidity profiles among patients with ankylosing spondylitis: a nationwide population-based study. *Ann Rheum Dis.* 2010;69:1166–1168.

61. Ahmed N, Prior JA, Chen Y, Hayward R, Mallen CD, Hider SL. Prevalence of cardiovascular-related comorbidity in ankylosing spondylitis, psoriatic arthritis and psoriasis in primary care: a matched retrospective cohort study. *Clin Rheumatol.* 2016;35: 3069–3073.

62. Mok CC, Ko GT, Ho LY, Yu KL, Chan PT, To CH. Prevalence of atherosclerotic risk factors and the metabolic syndrome in patients with chronic inflammatory arthritis. *Arthritis Care Res.* 2011;63:195–202.

63. Van Halm VP, Van Denderen JC, Peters MJ, et al. Increased disease activity is associated with a deteriorated lipid profile in patients with ankylosing spondylitis. *Ann Rheum Dis.* 2006;65:1473–1477.

64. Bally M, Dendukuri N, Rich B, et al. Risk of acute myocardial infarction with NSAIDs in real world use: Bayesian meta-analysis of individual patient data. *BMJ.* 2017;357:j1909.

65. Kristensen LE, Jakobsen AK, Askling J, Nielsson FX, Jacobsson LT. Safety of etoricoxib, celecoxib and non-selective NSAIDs in ankylosing spondylitis and other spondyloarthritis patients: a Swedish national population based cohort study. *Arthritis Care Res.* 2015;67: 1137–1149.

66. Oza A, Lu N, Schoenfeld SR, et al. Survival benefit of statin use in ankylosing spondylitis: a general population-based cohort study. *Ann Rheum Dis.* 2017;76:1737–1742.

67. Donath J, Miller A. Restrictive chest wall disorders. *Semin Respir Crit Care Med.* 2009;30:275–292.

68. Vanderschueren D, Decramer M, Van den Daele P, Dequeker J. Pulmonary function and maximal transrespiratory pressures in ankylosing spondylitis. *Ann Rheum Dis.* 1989;48:632–635.

69. Sahin G, Calikoğlu M, Ozge C, et al. Respiratory muscle strength but not BASFI score relates to diminished chest expansion in ankylosing spondylitis. *Clin Rheumatol.* 2004;23:199–202.

70. Ragnarsdottir M, Geirsson AJ, Gudbjornsson B. Rib cage motion in ankylosing spondylitis patients: a pilot study. *Spine J.* 2008;8:505–509.

71. Casserly IP, Fenlon HM, Breatnach E, Sant SM. Lung findings on high-resolution computed tomography in idiopathic ankylosing spondylitis-correlation with clinical findings, pulmonary function testing and plain radiography. *Br J Rheumatol.* 1997;36:677–682.

72. Turetschek K, Ebner W, Fleischmann D, et al. Early pulmonary involvement in ankylosing spondylitis: assessment with thin-section CT. *Clin Radiol.* 2000;55:632–636.

73. Aggarwal AN, Gupta D, Wanchu A, Jindal SK. Use of static lung mechanics to identify early pulmonary involvement in patients with ankylosing spondylitis. *J Postgrad Med.* 2001;47:89–94.

74. Kiris A, Ozgocmen S, Kocakoc E, Ardicoglu O, Ogur E. Lung findings on high resolution CT in early ankylosing spondylitis. *Eur J Radiol.* 2003;47:71–76.

75. Şenocak Ö, Manisalı M, Özaksoy D, Sevinç C, Akalın E. Lung parenchyma changes in ankylosing spondylitis: demonstration with high resolution CT and correlation with disease duration. *Eur J Radiol.* 2003;45:117–122.

76. El-Maghraoui A, Chaouir S, Abid A, et al. Lung findings on thoracic high-resolution computed tomography in patients with ankylosing spondylitis. Correlations with disease duration, clinical findings and pulmonary function testing. *Clin Rheumatol.* 2004;23:123–128.

77. Altin R, Ozdolap S, Savranlar A, et al. Comparison of early and late pleuropulmonary findings of ankylosing spondylitis by high-resolution computed tomography and effects on patients' daily life. *Clin Rheumatol.* 2005;24:22–28.

78. Baser S, Cubukcu S, Ozkurt S, Sabir N, Akdag B, Diri E. Pulmonary involvement starts in early stage ankylosing spondylitis. *Scand J Rheumatol.* 2006;35:325–327.

79. Ayhan-Ardic FF, Oken O, Yorgancioglu ZR, Ustun N, Gokharman FD. Pulmonary involvement in lifelong non-smoking patients with rheumatoid arthritis and ankylosing spondylitis without respiratory symptoms. *Clin Rheumatol.* 2006;25:213–218.

80. Dincer U, Cakar E, Kiralp MZ, Bozkanat E, Kilac H, Dursun H. The pulmonary involvement in rheumatic diseases: pulmonary effects of ankylosing spondylitis and its impact on functionality and quality of life. *Tohoku J Exp Med.* 2007;212:423–430.

81. Sampaio-Barros PD, Cerqueira EM, Rezende SM, et al. Pulmonary involvement in ankylosing spondylitis. *Clin Rheumatol.* 2007;26:225–230.

82. Berdal G, Halvorsen S, van der Heijde D, Mowe M, Dagfinrud H. Restrictive pulmonary function is more prevalent in patients with ankylosing spondylitis than in matched population controls and is associated with impaired spinal mobility: a comparative study. *Arthritis Res Ther.* 2012;14:R19. https://doi.org/10.1186/ar3699.

83. Ozdemir O, Gülsün Akpınar M, Inanıcı F, Hasçelik HZ. Pulmonary abnormalities on high-resolution computed tomography in ankylosing spondylitis: relationship to disease duration and pulmonary function testing. *Rheumatol Int.* 2012;32:2031–2036.

84. Brambila-Tapia AJ, Rocha-Muñoz AD, Gonzalez-Lopez L, et al. Pulmonary function in ankylosing spondylitis: association with clinical variables. *Rheumatol Int.* 2013;33:2351–2358.

85. Yuksekkaya R, Almus F, Celıkyay F, et al. Pulmonary involvement in ankylosing spondylitis assessed by multidetector computed tomography. *Pol J Radiol.* 2014;79:156–163.

86. Feltelius N, Hedenstrom H, Hillerdal G, Hallgren R. Pulmonary involvement in ankylosing spondylitis. *Ann Rheum Dis.* 1986;45:736–740.

87. Fisher LR, Cawley MI, Holgate ST. Relation between chest expansion, pulmonary function, and exercise tolerance in patients with ankylosing spondylitis. *Ann Rheum Dis.* 1990;49:921–925.

88. Sahin G, Guler H, Calikoglu M, Sezgin M. A comparison of respiratory muscle strength, pulmonary function tests and endurance in patients with early and late stage ankylosing spondylitis. *Z Rheumatol.* 2006;65:535–538.

89. Hsieh L-F, Wei JC, Lee H-Y, Chuang C, Jiang J, Chang K-C. Aerobic capacity and its correlates in patients with ankylosing spondylitis. *Int J Rheum Dis.* 2016;19:490–499.

90. Özdemýr O, Inanici F, Hasçelik Z. Reduced vital capacity leads to exercise intolerance in patients with ankylosing spondylitis. *Eur J Phys Rehabil Med.* 2011;47:391–397.

91. Carter R, Riantawan P, Banham SW, Sturrock RD. An investigation of factors limiting aerobic capacity in patients with ankylosing spondylitis. *Respir Med.* 1999;93:700–708.

92. van der Esch M, van't Hul AJ, Heijmans M, Dekker J. Respiratory muscle performance as a possible determinant of exercise capacity in patients with ankylosing spondylitis. *Aust J Physiother.* 2004;50:41–45.

93. Drăgoi RG, Amaricai E, Drăgoi M, Popoviciu H, Avram C. Inspiratory muscle training improves aerobic capacity and pulmonary function in patients with ankylosing spondylitis: a randomized controlled study. *Clin Rehabil.* 2016;30:340–346.

94. So MW, Heo HM, San Koo B, Kim YG, Lee CK, Yoo B. Efficacy of incentive spirometer exercise on pulmonary functions of patients with ankylosing spondylitis stabilized by tumor necrosis factor inhibitor therapy. *J Rheumatol.* 2012;39:1854–1858.

95. Dougados M, Braun J, Szanto S, et al. Efficacy of etanercept on rheumatic signs and pulmonary function tests in advanced ankylosing spondylitis: results of a randomised double-blind placebo-controlled study (SPINE). *Ann Rheum Dis.* 2011;70:799–804.

96. Rosenow E, Strimlan CV, Muhm JR, Ferguson RH. Pleuropulmonary manifestations of ankylosing spondylitis. *Mayo Clin Proc.* 1977;52:641–649.

97. Boushea DK, Sundstrom WR. The pleuropulmonary manifestations of ankylosing spondylitis. *Semin Arthritis Rheum*. 1989;18:277–281.

98. Lee CC, Lee SH, Chang IJ, et al. Spontaneous pneumothorax associated with ankylosing spondylitis. *Rheumatology*. 2005;44:1538–1541.

99. Ho HH, Lin MC, Yu KH, Wang CM, Wu YJ, Chen JY. Pulmonary tuberculosis and disease-related pulmonary apical fibrosis in ankylosing spondylitis. *J Rheumatol*. 2009;36:355–360.

100. Erb N, Karokis D, Delamere JP, Cushley MJ, Kitas GD. Obstructive sleep apnoea as a cause of fatigue in ankylosing spondylitis. *Ann Rheum Dis*. 2003;62:183–184.

101. Solak Ö, Fidan F, Dündar Ü, et al. The prevalence of obstructive sleep apnoea syndrome in ankylosing spondylitis patients. *Rheumatology*. 2009;48:433–435.

102. Yamamoto J, Okamoto Y, Shibuya E, Nishimura M, Kawakami Y. Obstructive sleep apnea syndrome induced by ossification of the anterior longitudinal ligament with ankylosing spondylitis. *Nihon Kokyuki Gakkai Zasshi*. 2000;38:413–416.

103. Abdulaziez O, Asaad T. Sleep problems in ankylosing spondylitis: polysomnographic pattern and disease related variables. *Egypt Rheumatol*. 2012;34:59–65.

104. Leverment S, Clarke E, Wadeley A, Sengupta R. Prevalence and factors associated with disturbed sleep in patients with ankylosing spondylitis and non-radiographic axial spondyloarthritis: a systematic review. *Rheumatology Int*. 2017;37:257–271.

105. Lachmann HJ, Goodman HJB, Gilbertson JA, et al. Natural history and outcome in systemic AA amyloidosis. *N Engl J Med*. 2007;356:2361–2371.

106. Strobel ES, Fritschka E. Renal diseases in ankylosing spondylitis: review of the literature illustrated by case reports. *Clin Rheumatol*. 1998;17:524–530.

107. Kovacsovics-Bankowski M, Zufferey P, So AK, Gerster JC. Secondary amyloidosis: a severe complication of ankylosing spondylitis. Two case-reports. *Joint Bone Spine*. 2000;67:129–133.

108. Dönmez S, Pamuk ÖN, Pamuk GE, Aydoğdu E, Inman R. Secondary amyloidosis in ankylosing spondylitis. *Rheumatol Int*. 2013;33:1725–1729.

109. Lee SH, Lee EJ, Chung SW, et al. Renal involvement in ankylosing spondylitis: prevalence, pathology, response to TNF-a blocker. *Rheumatol Int*. 2013;33:1689–1692.

110. Levy AR, Szabo SM, Rao SR, Cifaldi M, Maksymowych WP. Estimating the occurrence of renal complications among persons with ankylosing spondylitis. *Arthritis Care Res*. 2014;66:440–445.

111. Singh G, Kumari N, Aggarwal A, Krishnani N, Misra R. Prevalence of subclinical amyloidosis in ankylosing spondylitis. *J Rheumatol*. 2007;34:371–373.

112. Gratacos J, Orellana C, Sanmarti R, et al. Secondary amyloidosis in ankylosing spondylitis. A systematic survey of 137 patients using abdominal fat aspiration. *J Rheumatol*. 1997;24:912–915.

113. Pamuk ÖN, Kalyoncu U, Aksu K, et al. A multicenter report of biologic agents for the treatment of secondary amyloidosis in Turkish rheumatoid arthritis and ankylosing spondylitis patients. *Rheumatol Int*. 2016;36:945–953.

114. Immonen K, Finne P, Grönhagen-Riska C, et al. A marked decline in the incidence of renal replacement therapy for amyloidosis associated with inflammatory rheumatic diseases - data from nationwide registries in Finland. *Amyloid*. 2011;18:25–28.

115. Lehtinen K. Mortality and causes of death in 398 patients admitted to hospital with ankylosing spondylitis. *Ann Rheum Dis*. 1993;52:174–176.

116. Yeo SC, Cheung CK, Barratt J. New insights into the pathogenesis of IgA nephropathy. *Pediatr Nephrol*. 2017. https://doi.org/10.1007/s00467-017-3699-z.

117. D'Amico G. Natural history of idiopathic IgA nephropathy and factors predictive of disease outcome. *Semin Nephrol*. 2004;24:179–196.

118. Lai KN, Li PK, Hawkins B, Lai FM. IgA nephropathy associated with ankylosing spondylitis: occurrence in women as well as men. *Ann Rheum Dis*. 1989;48:435–437.

119. van de Laar MAFJ, Bernelot Moens HJ, van der Korst JK. Absence of an association between ankylosing spondylitis and IgA nephropathy. *Ann Rheum Dis*. 1989;48:262–263.

120. Jones DW, Mansell MA, Samuell CT, Isenberg DA. Renal abnormalities in ankylosing spondylitis. *Br J Rheumatol*. 1987;26:341–345.

121. Swaak AJ, Frankfort I, Menon RS, Pekelharing JM, Planten O. Absence of IgA nephropathy in patients with ankylosing spondylitis. *Rheumatol Int*. 1986;6:145–149.

122. Wall BA, Agudelo CA, Pisko EJ. Increased incidence of recurrent hematuria in ankylosing spondylitis: a possible association with IgA nephropathy. *Rheumatol Int*. 1984;4:27–29.

123. Ben TC, Ajlani H, Ben MF, Ben AT, Ben MH, Khedher A. Renal involvement in ankylosing spondylitis: concerning 210 cases. *Rev Med Interne*. 2005;26:966–969.

124. Kiryluk K, Li Y, Scolari F, et al. Discovery of new risk loci for IgA nephropathy implicates genes involved in immunity against intestinal pathogens. *Nat Genet*. 2014;46:1187–1196.

125. Montenegro V, Monteiro RC. Elevation of serum IgA in spondyloarthropathies and IgA nephropathy and its pathogenic role. *Curr Opin Rheumatol*. 1999;11:265–272.

126. Jakobsen AK, Jacobsson LT, Patschan O, Askling J, Kristensen LE. Is nephrolithiasis an unrecognized extra-articular manifestation in ankylosing spondylitis? A prospective population-based Swedish national cohort study with matched general population comparator subjects. *PLoS One*. 2014;9(11):e113602. https://doi.org/10.1371/journal.pone.0113602.eCollection 2014.

127. Shih MT, Tang SH, Cha TL, Wu ST, Chiang JH, Chen WC. The risk of nephrolithiasis among patients with ankylosing spondylitis: a population-based cohort study. *Arch Rheumatol*. 2016;31:346–352.

128. Korkmaz C, Ozcan A, Akçar N. Increased frequency of ultrasonographic findings suggestive of renal stones in patients with ankylosing spondylitis. *Clin Exp Rheumatol.* 2005;23:389–392.

129. Fallahi S, Jamshidi AR, Gharibdoost F, et al. Urolithiasis in ankylosing spondylitis: correlation with Bath ankylosing spondylitis disease activity index (BASDAI), Bath ankylosing spondylitis functional index (BASFI) and Bath ankylosing spondylitis metrology index (BASMI). *Caspian J Intern Med.* 2012;3:508–513.

130. Resorlu M, Gokmen F, Resorlu H, et al. Prospective evaluation of the renal morphology and vascular resistance in patients with ankylosing spondylitis. *Med Ultrason.* 2015;17:180–184.

131. Canales BK, Leonard SM, Singh JA, et al. Spondyloarthropathy: an independent risk factor for kidney stones. *J Endourol.* 2006;20:542–546.

132. Gönüllü E, Bilge NŞ.Y., Cansu DU, et al. Risk factors for urolithiasis in patients with ankylosing spondylitis: a prospective case-control study. *Urolithiasis.* 2017;45:353–357.

133. Incel NA, Gökoğlu F, Nacir B, Incel N. Bone and stone in ankylosing spondylitis: osteoporosis and urolithiasis. *Clin Rheumatol.* 2006;25:667–670.

134. Lui NL, Carty A, Haroon N, Shen H, Cook RJ, Inman RD. Clinical correlates of urolithiasis in ankylosing spondylitis. *J Rheumatol.* 2011;38:1953–1956.

135. Jakobsen AK, Jacobsson LT, Patschan O, Hopfgarten T, Askling J, Kristensen LE. Surgical interventions for nephrolithiasis in ankylosing spondylitis and the general population. *Scand J Urol.* 2015;49:486–491.

136. Geirsson AJ, Eyjolfsdottir H, Bjornsdottir G, Kristjansson K, Gudbjornsson B. Prevalence and clinical characteristics of ankylosing spondylitis in Iceland - a nationwide study. *Clin Exp Rheumatol.* 2010;28:333–340.

137. Lange U, Berliner M, Weidner W, Schiefer HG, Schmidt KL, Federlin K. Ankylosing spondylitis and urogenital infection: diagnosis of urologic infection and correlation with rheumatologic findings. *Z Rheumatol.* 1996;55:249–255.

138. Ozgocmen S, Kocakoc E, Kiris A, Ardicoglu A, Ardicoglu O. Incidence of varicoceles in patients with ankylosing spondylitis evaluated by physical examination and color duplex sonography. *Urology.* 2002;59:919–922.

139. Hamidi C, Batmaz I, Gümüş H, et al. The association between varicocele and ankylosing spondylitis via color duplex sonography. *Mod Rheumatol.* 2014;24:162–165.

140. Chiu H-Y, Wang I-T, Huang W-F, Tsia Y-W, Tsai T-F. Risk of varicocele in patients with rheumatoid arthritis, ankylosing spondylitis, and psoriatic disease: a population-based case-control study. *Scand J Rheumatol.* 2017;46:411–413.

141. Fan D, Liu L, Ding N, et al. Male sexual dysfunction and ankylosing spondylitis: a systematic review and metaanalysis. *J Rheumatol.* 2015;42:252–257.

142. Liu YF, Dong H, Chen Z, Wang YU, Tu SH. Impact of ankylosing spondylitis on sexual function: a systematic review and meta-analysis. *Exp Ther Med.* 2015;9:1501–1507.

143. Gordon D, Beastall GH, Thomson JA, Sturrock RD. Androgenic status and sexual function in males with rheumatoid arthritis and ankylosing spondylitis. *QJM.* 1986;60:671–679.

144. Pirildar T, Müezzinoğlu T, Pirildar Ş.. Sexual function in ankylosing spondylitis: a study of 65 men. *J Urol.* 2004;171:1598–1600.

145. Bal S, Bal K, Turan Y, et al. Sexual functions in ankylosing spondylitis. *Rheumatol Int.* 2011;31:889–894.

146. Özkorumak E, Karkucak M, Civil F, Tiryaki A, Özden G. Sexual function in male patients with ankylosing spondylitis. *Int J Impot Res.* 2011;23:262–267.

147. Cakar E, Dincer U, Kiralp MZ, et al. Sexual problems in male ankylosing spondylitis patients: relationship with functionality, disease activity, quality of life, and emotional status. *Clin Rheumatol.* 2007;26:1607–1613.

148. Demir SE, Rezvani A, Ok S. Assessment of sexual functions in female patients with ankylosing spondylitis compared with healthy controls. *Rheumatol Int.* 2013;33:57–63.

149. Sariyildiz MA, Batmaz I, Inanir A, et al. The impact of ankylosing spondylitis on female sexual functions. *Int J Impot Res.* 2013;25:104–108.

150. Berg KH, Rohde G, Prøven A, et al. Exploring the relationship between demographic and disease-related variables and perceived effect of health status on sexual activity in patients with axial spondyloarthritis: associations found only with non-disease variables. *Scand J Rheumatol.* 2017;46:461–467.

151. Østensen M, Fuhrer L, Mathieu R, Seitz M, Villiger PM. A prospective study of pregnant patients with rheumatoid arthritis and ankylosing spondylitis using validated clinical instruments. *Ann Rheum Dis.* 2004;63:1212–1217.

152. Lui NL, Haroon N, Carty A, et al. Effect of pregnancy on ankylosing spondylitis: a case-control study. *J Rheumatol.* 2011;38:2442–2444.

153. Ostensen M, Ostensen H. Ankylosing spondylitis--the female aspect. *J Rheumatol.* 1998;25:120–124.

154. Giovannopoulou E, Gkasdaris G, Kapetanakis S, Kontomanolis E. Ankylosing spondylitis and pregnancy: a literature review. *Curr Rheumatol Rev.* 2017;13:162–169.

155. Jakobsson GL, Stephansson O, Askling J, Jacobsson LT. Pregnancy outcomes in patients with ankylosing spondylitis: a nationwide register study. *Ann Rheum Dis.* 2016;75:1838–1842.

156. Will R, Bhalla A, Palmer R, Ring F, Calin A. Osteoporosis in early ankylosing spondylitis: a primary pathological event? *Lancet.* 1989;334:1483–1485.

157. Devogelaer JP, Maldague B, Malghem J, Deuxchaisnes D, Nagant C. Appendicular and vertebral bone mass in ankylosing spondylitis. A comparison of plain radiographs with single-and dual-photon absorptiometry and with quantitative computed tomography. *Arthritis Rheumatol.* 1992;35:1062–1067.

158. Bronson WD, Walker SE, Hillman LS, Keisler D, Hoyt T, Allen SH. Bone mineral density and biochemical markers of bone metabolism in ankylosing spondylitis. *J Rheumatol.* 1998;25:929–935.

159. Donnelly S, Doyle DV, Denton A, Rolfe I, McCloskey EV, Spector TD. Bone mineral density and vertebral compression fracture rates in ankylosing spondylitis. *Ann Rheum Dis.* 1994;53:117–121.

160. Mullaji AB, Upadhyay SS, Ho EK. Bone mineral density in ankylosing spondylitis. DEXA comparison of control subjects with mild and advanced cases. *Bone Joint Lett J.* 1994;76:660–665.

161. Lee YL, Schlotzhauer T, Ott SM, et al. Skeletal status of men with early and late ankylosing spondylitis. *Am J Med.* 1997;103:233–241.

162. Meirelles ES, Borelli A, Camargo OP. Influence of disease activity and chronicity on ankylosing spondylitis bone mass loss. *Clin Rheumatol.* 1999;18:364–368.

163. El Maghraoui A, Borderie D, Cherruau B, Edouard R, Dougados M, Roux C. Osteoporosis, body composition, and bone turnover in ankylosing spondylitis. *J Rheumatol.* 1999;26:2205–2209.

164. Juanola XA, Mateo LO, Nolla JM, Roig-Vilaseca DA, Campoy ES, Roig-Escofet DA. Bone mineral density in women with ankylosing spondylitis. *J Rheumatol.* 2000;27:1028–1031.

165. Toussirot E, Michel F, Wendling D. Bone density, ultrasound measurements and body composition in early ankylosing spondylitis. *Rheumatology.* 2001;40: 882–888.

166. Dos Santos FP, Constantin AR, Laroche MI, et al. Whole body and regional bone mineral density in ankylosing spondylitis. *J Rheumatol.* 2001;28:547–549.

167. Speden DJ, Calin AI, Ring FJ, Bhalla AK. Bone mineral density, calcaneal ultrasound, and bone turnover markers in women with ankylosing spondylitis. *J Rheumatol.* 2002;29:516–521.

168. Franck H, Meurer T, Hofbauer LC. Evaluation of bone mineral density, hormones, biochemical markers of bone metabolism, and osteoprotegerin serum levels in patients with ankylosing spondylitis. *J Rheumatol.* 2004;31:2236–2241.

169. Lange U, Kluge A, Strunk J, Teichmann J, Bachmann G. Ankylosing spondylitis and bone mineral density—what is the ideal tool for measurement? *Rheumatol Int.* 2005;26:115–120.

170. Karberg K, Zochling J, Sieper J, Felsenberg D, Braun J. Bone loss is detected more frequently in patients with ankylosing spondylitis with syndesmophytes. *J Rheumatol.* 2005;32:1290–1298.

171. Aydin T, Karacan İ., Demir SE, Sahin Z. Bone loss in males with ankylosing spondylitis: its relation to sex hormone levels. *Clin Endocrinol.* 2005;63:467–469.

172. Baek HJ, Kang SW, Lee YJ, et al. Osteopenia in men with mild and severe ankylosing spondylitis. *Rheumatol Int.* 2005;26:30–34.

173. Kim HR, Kim HY, Lee SH. Elevated serum levels of soluble receptor activator of nuclear factors-κB ligand (sRANKL) and reduced bone mineral density in patients with ankylosing spondylitis (AS). *Rheumatology.* 2006;45:1197–1200.

174. Jun JB, Joo KB, Her MY, et al. Femoral bone mineral density is associated with vertebral fractures in patients with ankylosing spondylitis: a cross-sectional study. *J Rheumatol.* 2006;33:1637–1641.

175. Borman P, Bodur H, Bingöl N, Bingöl S, Bostan EE. Bone mineral density and bone turnover markers in a group of male ankylosing spondylitis patients: relationship to disease activity. *J Clin Rheumatol.* 2001;7:315–321.

176. Sarikaya S, Basaran A, Tekin Y, Ozdolap S, Ortancil O. Is osteoporosis generalized or localized to central skeleton in ankylosing spondylitis? *J Clin Rheumatol.* 2007;13:20–24.

177. Ghozlani I, Ghazi M, Nouijai A, et al. Prevalence and risk factors of osteoporosis and vertebral fractures in patients with ankylosing spondylitis. *Bone.* 2009;44:772–776.

178. Başkan BM, Doğan YP, Sivas F, Bodur H, Özoran K. The relation between osteoporosis and vitamin D levels and disease activity in ankylosing spondylitis. *Rheumatol Int.* 2010;30:375–381.

179. Kaya A, Ozgocmen S, Kamanli A, Ardicoglu O. Bone loss in ankylosing spondylitis: does syndesmophyte formation have an influence on bone density changes? *Med Princ Pract.* 2009;18:470–476.

180. Arends S, Spoorenberg A, Bruyn GA, et al. The relation between bone mineral density, bone turnover markers, and vitamin D status in ankylosing spondylitis patients with active disease: a cross-sectional analysis. *Osteoporos Int.* 2011;22:1431–1439.

181. Van der Weijden MA, Van Denderen JC, Lems WF, Heymans MW, Dijkmans BA, van der Horst-Bruinsma IE. Low bone mineral density is related to male gender and decreased functional capacity in early spondylarthropathies. *Clin Rheumatol.* 2011;30:497–503.

182. Muntean L, Rojas-Vargas M, Font P, et al. Relative value of the lumbar spine and hip bone mineral density and bone turnover markers in men with ankylosing spondylitis. *Clin Rheumatol.* 2011;30:691–695.

183. Vasdev V, Bhakuni D, Garg MK, Narayanan K, Jain R, Chadha D. Bone mineral density in young males with ankylosing spondylitis. *Int J Rheum Dis.* 2011;14:68–73.

184. Grazio S, Kusić Z, Cvijetić S, et al. Relationship of bone mineral density with disease activity and functional ability in patients with ankylosing spondylitis: a cross-sectional study. *Rheumatol Int.* 2012;32:2801–2808.

185. Korczowska I, Przepiera-Bedzak H, Brzosko M, Lacki JK, Trefler J, Hrycaj P. Bone tissue metabolism in men with ankylosing spondylitis. *Adv Med Sci.* 2011;56:264–269.

186. Klingberg E, Lorentzon M, Mellström D, et al. Osteoporosis in ankylosing spondylitis-prevalence, risk factors and methods of assessment. *Arthritis Res Ther.* 2012;14:R108.

187. Taylan A, Sari I, Akinci B, et al. Biomarkers and cytokines of bone turnover: extensive evaluation in a cohort of patients with ankylosing spondylitis. *BMC Musculoskel Dis.* 2012;1:191.

188. Ulu MA, Batmaz İ., Dilek B, Çevik R. Prevalence of osteoporosis and vertebral fractures and related factors in patients with ankylosing spondylitis. *Chin Med J (Engl).* 2014;127:2740–2747.

189. Wang DM, Zeng QY, Chen SB, Gong Y, Hou ZD, Xiao ZY. Prevalence and risk factors of osteoporosis in patients with ankylosing spondylitis: a 5-year follow-up study of 504 cases. *Clin Exp Rheumatol.* 2015;33:465–470.

190. Nazir L, Rehman S, Riaz A, Saeed M, Perveen T. Frequency of low bone mineral density in spondyloarthropathy presenting at a tertiary care hospital. *J Pak Med Assoc.* 2015;65:973–977.

191. Magrey MN, Lewis S, Khan MA. Utility of DXA scanning and risk factors for osteoporosis in ankylosing spondylitis—a prospective study. *Semin Arthritis Rheum.* 2016;46:88–94.

192. Gamez-Nava JI, de la Cerda-Trujillo LF, Vazquez-Villegas ML, et al. Association between bone turnover markers, clinical variables, spinal syndesmophytes and bone mineral density in Mexican patients with ankylosing spondylitis. *Scand J Rheumatol.* 2016;45:480–490.

193. Maillefert JF, Aho LS, El Maghraoui A, Dougados M, Roux C. Changes in bone density in patients with ankylosing spondylitis: a two-year follow-up study. *Osteoporos Int.* 2001;12:605–609.

194. Gratacos J, Collado A, Pons F, et al. Significant loss of bone mass in patients with early, active ankylosing spondylitis: a followup study. *Arthritis Rheum.* 1999;42:2319–2324.

195. Briot K, Durnez A, Paternotte S, Miceli-Richard C, Dougados M, Roux C. Bone oedema on MRI is highly associated with low bone mineral density in patients with early inflammatory back pain: results from the DESIR cohort. *Ann Rheum Dis.* 2013;72:1914–1919.

196. Wang D, Hou Z, Gong Y, Chen S, Lin L, Xiao Z. Bone edema on magnetic resonance imaging is highly associated with low bone mineral density in patients with ankylosing spondylitis. *PLoS One.* 2017;12:e0189569.

197. Briot K, Geusens P, Bultink IE, Lems WF, Roux C. Inflammatory diseases and bone fragility. *Osteoporos Int.* 2017;28:3301–3314.

198. Viapiana O, Gatti D, Idolazzi L, et al. Bisphosphonates vs infliximab in ankylosing spondylitis treatment. *Rheumatology.* 2014;53:90–94.

199. Khabbazi A, Noshad H, Gafarzadeh S, Hajialiloo M, Kolahi S. Alendronate effect on the prevention of bone loss in early stages of ankylosing spondylitis: a randomized, double-blind, placebo-controlled pilot study. *Iran Red Crescent Med J.* 2014;16:e18022.

200. Kang KY, Ju JH, Park S-H, Kim H-Y. The paradoxical effects of TNF inhibitors on bone mineral density and radiographic progression in patients with ankylosing spondylitis. *Rheumatology.* 2013;52:718–726.

201. Bessant R, Keat A. How should clinicians manage osteoporosis in ankylosing spondylitis? *J Rheumatol.* 2002;29:1511–1519.

202. Sidiropoulos PI, Hatemi G, Song IH, et al. Evidence-based recommendations for the management of ankylosing spondylitis: systematic literature search of the 3E Initiative in Rheumatology involving a broad panel of experts and practising rheumatologists. *Rheumatology.* 2008;47:355–361.

203. Briot K, Roux C. Inflammation, bone loss and fracture risk in spondyloarthritis. *RMD Open.* 2015;1(1): e000052.

204. Hinze AM, Louie GH. Osteoporosis management in ankylosing spondylitis. *Curr Treatm Opt Rheumatol.* 2016;2:271–282.

205. Haroon NN, Sriganthan J, Al Ghanim N, Inman RD, Cheung AM. Effect of TNF-alpha inhibitor treatment on bone mineral density in patients with ankylosing spondylitis: a systematic review and meta-analysis. *Semin Arthritis Rheum.* 2014;44:155–161.

206. Nevitt MC, Ettinger B, Black DM, et al. The association of radiographically detected vertebral fractures with back pain and function: a prospective study. *Ann Intern Med.* 1998;128:793–800.

207. Klingberg E, Geijer M, Göthlin J, et al. Vertebral fractures in ankylosing spondylitis are associated with lower bone mineral density in both central and peripheral skeleton. *J Rheumatol.* 2012;39:1987–1995.

208. Vosse D, van der Heijde DM, Landewé R, et al. Determinants of hyperkyphosis in patients with ankylosing spondylitis. *Ann Rheumatic Dis.* 2006;65: 770–774.

209. Montala N, Juanola X, Collantes E, et al. Prevalence of vertebral fractures by semiautomated morphometry in patients with ankylosing spondylitis. *J Rheumatol.* 2011;38:893–897.

210. Van der Weijden MA, Van der Horst-Bruinsma IE, van Denderen JC, Dijkmans BA, Heymans MW, Lems WF. High frequency of vertebral fractures in early spondylarthropathies. *Osteoporos Int.* 2012;23:1683–1690.

211. Geusens P, De Winter L, Quaden D, et al. The prevalence of vertebral fractures in spondyloarthritis: relation to disease characteristics, bone mineral density, syndesmophytes and history of back pain and trauma. *Arthritis Res Ther.* 2015;17:294.

212. Mitra D, Elvins DM, Speden DJ, Collins AJ. The prevalence of vertebral fractures in mild ankylosing spondylitis and their relationship to bone mineral density. *Rheumatology.* 2000;39:85–89.

213. Sivri A, Kilinç Ş, Gökçe-Kustal Y, Ariyürek M. Bone mineral density in ankylosing spondylitis. *Clin Rheumatol.* 1996;15:51–54.

214. Muñoz–Ortego J, Vestergaard P, Rubio JB, et al. Ankylosing spondylitis is associated with an increased risk of vertebral and nonvertebral clinical fractures: a population-based cohort study. *J Bone Miner Res.* 2014;29:1770–1776.

215. Prieto-Alhambra D, Muñoz-Ortego J, De Vries F, et al. Ankylosing spondylitis confers substantially increased risk of clinical spine fractures: a nationwide case-control study. *Osteoporos Int.* 2015;26:85–91.

216. Vosse D, Landewé R, van der Heijde D, van der Linden S, van Staal TP, Geusens P. Ankylosing spondylitis and the risk of fracture: results from a large primary care-based nested case-control study. *Ann Rheum Dis.* 2009;68:1839–1842.

217. Cooper C, Carbone L, Michet CJ, Atkinson EJ, O'Fallon WM, Melton 3rd LJ. Fracture risk in patients with ankylosing spondylitis: a population based study. *J Rheumatol.* 1994;21:1877–1882.

218. Wang YF, Teng MM, Chang CY, Wu HT, Wang ST. Imaging manifestations of spinal fractures in ankylosing spondylitis. *AJNR Am J Neuroradiol.* 2005;26:2067–2076.

219. Rustagi T, Drazin D, Oner C, et al. Fractures in spinal ankylosing disorders: a narrative review of disease and injury types, treatment techniques, and outcomes. *J Orthop Trauma.* 2017;31:S57–S74.

220. Westerveld L, Verlaan JJ, Oner FC. Spinal fractures in patients with ankylosing spinal disorders: a systematic review of the literature on treatment, neurological status and complications. *Eur Spine J.* 2009;18:145–156.

221. Hitchon PW, From AM, Brenton MD, Glaser JA, Torner JC. Fractures of the thoracolumbar spine complicating ankylosing spondylitis. *J Neurosurg.* 2002;97:218–222.

222. Bron JL, de Vries MK, Snieders MN, van der Horst-Bruinsma IE, Van Royen BJ. Discovertebral (Andersson) lesions of the spine in ankylosing spondylitis revisited. *Clin Rheumatol.* 2009;28:883–892.

223. Fang DA, Leong JC, Ho EK, Chan FL, Chow SP. Spinal pseudarthrosis in ankylosing spondylitis. Clinicopathological correlation and the results of anterior spinal fusion. *J Bone Joint Surg Br.* 1988;70:443–447.

224. Ramos-Remus C, Gomez-Vargas A, Guzman-Guzman JL, et al. Frequency of atlantoaxial subluxation and neurologic involvement in patients with ankylosing spondylitis. *J Rheumatol.* 1995;22:2120–2125.

225. Lee HS, Kim TH, Yun HR, et al. Radiologic changes of cervical spine in ankylosing spondylitis. *Clin Rheumatol.* 2001;20:262–266.

226. Lee JY, Kim JI, Park JY, et al. Cervical spine involvement in longstanding ankylosing spondylitis. *Clin Exp Rheumatol.* 2005;23:331–338.

227. Lee JS, Lee S, Bang SY, et al. Prevalence and risk factors of anterior atlantoaxial subluxation in ankylosing spondylitis. *J Rheumatol.* 2012;39:2321–2326.

228. Rajak R, Wardle P, Rhys-Dillon C, Martin JC. Odontoid pannus formation in a patient with ankylosing spondylitis causing atlanto-axial instability. *BMJ Case Rep.* 2012;2012. bcr1120115178.

229. Singh S, Balakrishnan C, Maheshwari S. Pannus and enthesitis in the atlanto-axial region in ankylosing spondylitis. *Int J Rheum Dis.* 2005;8:138–140.

230. Ramos-Remus C, Gomez-Vargas A, Hernandez-Chavez A, Gamez-Nava JI, Gonzalez-Lopez L, Russell AS. Two year followup of anterior and vertical atlantoaxial subluxation in ankylosing spondylitis. *J Rheumatol.* 1997;24:507–510.

231. Russell ML, Gordon DA, Ogryzlo MA, McPhedran RS. The cauda equina syndrome of ankylosing spondylitis. *Ann Intern Med.* 1973;78:551–554.

232. Liu C-C, Lin Y-C, Lo C-P, Chang T-P. Cauda equina syndrome and dural ectasia: rare manifestations in chronic ankylosing spondylitis. *Br J Radiol.* 2011;84:e123–e125.

233. Ahn NU, Ahn UM, Nallamshetty L, et al. Cauda equina syndrome in ankylosing spondylitis (the CES-AS syndrome): meta-analysis of outcomes after medical and surgical treatments. *J Spinal Disord.* 2001;14:427–433.

234. Cornec D, Pensec VD, Joulin SJ, Saraux A. Dramatic efficacy of infliximab in cauda equina syndrome complicating ankylosing spondylitis. *Arthritis Rheumatol.* 2009;60:1657–1660.

235. Barlow JH, Macey SJ, Struthers GR. Gender, depression, and ankylosing spondylitis. *Arthritis Rheumatol.* 1993;6:45–51.

236. Martindale J, Smith J, Sutton CJ, Grennan D, Goodacre L, Goodacre JA. Disease and psychological status in ankylosing spondylitis. *Rheumatology.* 2006;45:1288–1293.

237. Baysal Ö, Durmuş B, Ersoy Y, et al. Relationship between psychological status and disease activity and quality of life in ankylosing spondylitis. *Rheumatol Int.* 2011;31:795–800.

238. Ward MM. Health-related quality of life in ankylosing spondylitis: a survey of 175 patients. *Arthritis Care Res.* 1999;12:247–255.

239. Hyphantis T, Kotsis K, Tsifetaki N, et al. The relationship between depressive symptoms, illness perceptions and quality of life in ankylosing spondylitis in comparison to rheumatoid arthritis. *Clin Rheumatol.* 2013;32:635–644.

240. Jiang Y, Yang M, Lv Q, et al. Prevalence of psychological disorders, sleep disturbance and stressful life events and their relationships with disease parameters in Chinese patients with ankylosing spondylitis. *Clin Rheumatol.* 2018;37:407–414.

241. Meesters JJ, Bremander A, Bergman S, Petersson IF, Turkiewicz A, Englund M. The risk for depression in patients with ankylosing spondylitis: a population-based cohort study. *Arthritis Res Ther.* 2014;16:418.

242. Wu JJ, Penfold RB, Primatesta P, et al. The risk of depression, suicidal ideation, and suicide attempt in patients with psoriasis, psoriatic arthritis or ankylosing spondylitis. *J Eur Acad Dermatol Venereol.* 2017;31:1168–1175.

243. Shen CC, Hu LY, Yang AC, Kuo BI, Chiang YY, Tsai SJ. Risk of psychiatric disorders following ankylosing spondylitis: a nationwide population-based retrospective cohort study. *J Rheumatol.* 2016;43:625–631.

244. Dumus D, Sarisoy G, Alayli G, et al. Psychiatric symptoms in ankylosing spondylitis: their relationship with disease activity, functional capacity, pain and fatigue. *Compr Psychiatry.* 2015;62:170–177.

245. Batmaz I, Sarıyıldız MA, Dilek B, Bez Y, Karakoç M, Cevik R. Sleep quality and associated factors in ankylosing spondylitis: relationship with disease parameters, psychological status and quality of life. *Rheumatol Int.* 2013;33:1039–1045.

246. Ertenli I, Ozer S, Kiraz S, et al. Infliximab, a TNF-alpha antagonist treatment in patients with ankylosing spondylitis: the impact on depression, anxiety and quality of life level. *Rheumatol Int.* 2012;32:323–330.

247. Aloush V, Ablin JN, Reitblat T, Caspi D, Elkayam O. Fibromyalgia in women with ankylosing spondylitis. *Rheumatol Int.* 2007;27:865–868.

248. Azevedo VF, Paiva ED, Felippe LR, Moreira RA. Occurrence of fibromyalgia in patients with ankylosing spondylitis. *Rev Bras Reumatol.* 2010;50:646–650.

249. Almodóvar R, Carmona L, Zarco P, et al. Fibromyalgia in patients with ankylosing spondylitis: prevalence and utility of the measures of activity, function and radiological damage. *Clin Exp Rheumatol.* 2010;28:S33–S39.

250. Salaffi F, De Angelis R, Carotti M, Gutierrez M, Sarzi-Puttini P, Atzeni F. Fibromyalgia in patients with axial spondyloarthritis: epidemiological profile and effect on measures of disease activity. *Rheumatol Int.* 2014;34:1103–1110.

251. Slobodin G, Reyhan I, Avshovich N, et al. Recently diagnosed axial spondyloarthritis: gender differences and factors related to delay in diagnosis. *Clin Rheumatol.* 2011;30:1075–1080.

252. Haliloglu S, Carlioglu A, Akdeniz D, Karaaslan Y, Kosar A. Fibromyalgia in patients with other rheumatic diseases: prevalence and relationships with disease activity. *Rheumatol Int.* 2014;34:1275–1280.

253. Dean LE, Macfarlane GJ, Jones GT. Five potentially modifiable factors predict poor quality of life in ankylosing spondylitis: results from the Scotland Registry for Ankylosing Spondylitis. *J Rheumatol.* 2018;45:62–69.

254. Macfarlane GJ, Barnish MS, Pathan E, et al. The co-occurrence and characteristics of patients with axial spondyloarthritis who meet criteria for fibromyalgia: results from a UK national register (BSRBR-AS). *Arthritis Rheumatol.* 2017;69:2144–2150.

255. Mease P. Fibromyalgia, a missed comorbidity in spondyloarthritis: prevalence and impact on assessment and treatment. *Curr Opin Rheumatol.* 2017;29:304–310.

256. Roussou E, Ciurtin C. Clinical overlap between fibromyalgia tender points and enthesitis sites in patients with spondyloarthritis who present with inflammatory back pain. *Clin Exp Rheumatol.* 2012;30(Suppl. 74):24–30.

257. Heikkilä S, Ronni S, Kautiainen HJ, Kauppi MJ. Functional impairment in spondyloarthropathy and fibromyalgia. *J Rheumatol.* 2002;29:1415–1419.

258. Altan L, Sivrioğlu Y, Ercan I. Can bath ankylosing spondylitis disease activity index be affected by accompanying fibromyalgia or depression? *Arch Rheumatol.* 2015;30:34–39.

259. Kristensen LE, Karlsson JA, Englund M, Petersson IF, Saxne T, Geborek P. Presence of peripheral arthritis and male sex predicting continuation of anti-tumor necrosis factor therapy in ankylosing spondylitis: an observational prospective cohort study from the south Swedish arthritis treatment group register. *Arthritis Care Res.* 2010;62:1362–1369.

CHAPTER 13

Nonpharmacologic Management of Axial Spondyloarthritis

SALIH ÖZGÖÇMEN, MD

Axial spondyloarthritis (ax-SpA) defines a chronic progressive inflammatory disease with predominant involvement in the axial skeleton. The new classification criteria developed by Assessment in Spondyloarthritis International Society (ASAS) include two major advances: first, SpA was classified based on predominant symptoms (axial or peripheral); second, magnetic resonance imaging (MRI) was introduced allowing detection of sacroiliitis at the early stages of the disease.[1] Therefore, this term comprises the spectrum of axSpA including classical AS on one end and nonradiographic axial spondyloarthritis (nr-axSpA) on the other end.[2,3] Ankylosing spondylitis is the prototype of axSpA, and most of the patients may eventually develop structural damage in the axial skeleton. Formation of syndesmophytes leading to ankylosis of the spine is characteristic for AS and associated with decreased physical functions, disability, and lower quality of life. Functional limitations and the burden of disease are quite similar between patients with radiographic and those with nonradiographic axial SpA.[4,5] Individuals with axial SpA effect at early adulthood and patients live with the disease relatively longer than some other inflammatory joint diseases during their entire life. Therefore the impact of the disease on different aspects of life like functioning and health can be substantial.[6,7]

The ASAS published recommendations for the management of AS in 2006 and updated in 2010 and 2016.[8–10] In the last updated version of the recommendations, there are two novelties: first, the recommendations focused on the whole spectrum of axSpA rather than patients with radiographic axSpA (AS), and second, the term bDMARDs was used covering IL-17 pathway inhibiting therapy, which has become available for the treatment of patients with radiographic axSpA.[9] The panel recommends a multidisciplinary and patient-centered approach, which combines pharmacologic and nonpharmacologic modalities in the management of patients with axSpA. Education of patients about axSpA, exercising on a regular basis, encouraging patients to stop smoking, and physical therapy are considered as the key nonpharmacologic modalities in the management. The primary goal of treating a patient with axSpA is to maximize health-related quality of life, which could be achieved by controlling disease activity, preventing structural damage, and improving/maintaining physical functions and social participations.[9] Similarly, physical therapy is strongly recommended in adult patients with active or stable AS, by the expert panel of American College of Rheumatology/Spondylitis Association of America/Spondyloarthritis Research and Treatment Network. In addition, participation in formal group or individual self-management education is conditionally recommended in adult patients with AS by the same panel.[11]

Physiotherapy (also referred to as physical therapy) is one of the leading components of nonpharmacologic management in axSpA. The primary aim of physiotherapy is to help patients to maintain, recover, or improve their physical abilities. Exercise is the leading modality used in physiotherapy interventions, but there are other physical modalities such as heat, cold, electrotherapy, or manual techniques. Physiotherapy is usually conducted by a physiotherapist, a specially trained practitioner who often works as a part of multidisciplinary team in the rehabilitation process of patients with axSpA. Educating about axSpA and encouraging patients for maintaining proper posture, physical activity, exercising on a regular basis and smoking cessation are important. Appropriate assessment of anthropometric measurements and outcome variables and monitoring disease-related outcome data is recommended to document efficacy of physiotherapy interventions.[12] The ASAS group recommended a core set of domains for the assessment and monitoring of physiotherapy interventions[13] (Table 13.1). In addition to these core domains, patients can be individually assessed by other measures, such as monitoring range of motion

TABLE 13.1

Core Set of Domains for the Assessment of Physical Therapy Interventions Proposed by Assessment of SpondyloArthritis International Society (ASAS)

Domain	Instrument
Physical function	Bath Ankylosing Spondylitis Functional Index (BASFI)
Pain	NRS/VAS (spinal pain/at night due to AS/last week)
Spinal mobility	Chest expansion Modified Schober Occiput to wall Cervical rotation Lateral spinal flexion or Bath Ankylosing Spondylitis Metrology Index (BASMI)
Spinal stiffness	NRS/VAS (duration of morning stiffness/spine/last week)
Patient global	NRS/VAS (global disease activity/ last week)
Fatigue	Fatigue question Bath Ankylosing Spondylitis Disease Activity Index (BASDAI)

NRS, numeric rating scale.

in the effected joint or documenting health-related quality of life data by means of validated and widely used outcome measures. Ankylosing spondylitis quality-of-life questionnaire (ASQoL) may be used to assess QoL. In addition, newly validated ASAS Health Index (ASAS HI) measures functioning and health in patients with spondyloarthritis (SpA) across 17 aspects of health and 9 environmental factors (EFs).[6]

While prescribing exercise or at startup of physiotherapy programs, patients should be entirely evaluated for musculoskeletal findings to apply most suitable interventions and prevent undesired effect of any intervention.[14] Patients should be evaluated for painful enthesitis, inflammation of the tendons, ligaments, and periarticular structures, or limited motions of the spine and peripheral joints. Stretching and endurance exercise or other hands-on techniques may aggravate pain at enthesis or cause entrapments, rupture of ligaments or tendons, or even fractures particularly in the ankylosed and osteoporotic bone structures. Previous surgeries such as corrective osteotomy, joint prosthesis, or presence of metallic implants, pacemakers as well as cardiopulmonary

status of the patients should be carefully evaluated before physiotherapy. Some of the electrophysical agents (i.e., shortwave diathermy) are contraindicated in patients with metallic implants or those with pacemakers.

Not all patients with axSpA have restricted mobility; those who are in the early stage or do not have structural damage may eventually have normal range of motion and have no physical or social restriction in their daily lives particularly in pain-free periods. However, patients with active inflammation on sacroiliac MRI, smoking, or elevated CRP are more prone to develop structural damage and evolving radiographic axSpA.[15]

EXERCISE

In the past two decades, tremendous progress has been made in the treatment of axSpA. TNFα-blocking agents have been shown effective in the treatment of axSpA in all stages of the disease (in early or nonradiographic cases and in totally ankylosed advanced cases). Recently, secukinumab, the monoclonal antibody that neutralizes IL-17A, has been approved for the treatment of AS, and this provides an opportunity for the treatment of patients who have failed TNFα-inhibiting therapies or have contraindications for TNF blockers. However, robust data are still lacking, demonstrating that these biologics prevent the development of syndesmophytes. A combination of biologic therapy and exercise has synergistic effects and benefits documented regarding pain, physical functions, respiratory capacity, cardiovascular risk, and health-related quality of life.[16] Therefore, exercise and physical therapy is still considered as an important integral part of management in patients with axSpA. Patients should be encouraged to perform lifelong exercise on a regular basis, and physical therapy interventions can be considered according to the patients' clinical status, needs, and expectations.

Despite the fact that exercise is one of the mostly studied nonpharmacologic management modalities in patients with AS, there are some difficulties to obtain robust conclusions from these studies. Heterogeneity of exercise protocols (i.e., type of exercises, duration, frequency, and concomitant medical treatments differing across studies) is a major problem. In addition, small sample size, variation in the study populations regarding demographic or clinical characteristics, high rates of withdrawal, short follow-up periods, underreported adherence rates, and difficulties in blinding are other problems in exercise trials.

BOX 13.1
Quantity and Intensity of the Exercises

Exercise Type	Frequency (Days/Week)	Intensity	Duration
Cardiorespiratory (aerobic)	3–5	Moderate to vigorous (for most adults) Light to moderate (in deconditioned persons)	20–60 min (150 min/week)
Muscle strength (resistance)	2–3	Resistance equivalent to 60%–80% of an individual's one repetition maximal effort 8–12 repetitions (for most adults) 15–20 repetitions (to improve muscle endurance)	2–4 sets (for most adults)
Flexibility (stretching)	2–3	Stretch to point of slight discomfort	10–30 s × 4 repetitions (for most adults)

Despite some efforts, there is still no consensus on evidence-based recommendations for exercise prescription in AS yet; therefore, these guidelines published by the American College of Sports Medicine can be referred to and adapted as indicated when prescribing exercise for patients with axSpA.

Adapted from Garber CE, Blissmer B, Deschenes MR, Franklin BA, Lamonte MJ, Lee IM, Nieman DC, Swain DP. American College of Sports Medicine: Exercise Recommendations. American College of Sports Medicine position stand. Quantity and quality of exercise for developing and maintaining cardiorespiratory, musculoskeletal, and neuromotor fitness in apparently healthy adults: guidance for prescribing exercise. *Med Sci Sports Exerc* 2011;43(7):1334–1359.

In the literature, several exercise programs have been described for AS. Individualized home exercise programs are one of the assessed programs and allow patients to do exercises in their homes. Home exercises has advantages such as being performed independently and in the home and thus is, cost-effective, and able to be done in their spare time. These exercises are prescribed according to predefined protocols of instructions or patients' special needs and are performed unsupervised and deprived of social integration and motivation. Supervised individual exercises can be performed at home or at a physiotherapy facility under supervision of a qualified instructor who is usually a physiotherapist. Supervised programs allow patient education, increase motivation and adherence, and improve self-efficacy. In addition, the instructor can observe the patients and ensure that exercise techniques are performed correctly. Supervised group-based exercises are suitable for patients who have difficulty adhering to regular exercises and need motivation. Group-based programs allow a social environment for the patients and can also be commenced as an inpatient program. In-patient programs usually consist of 2–4 weeks of intensive exercise including posture, flexibility, and strengthening. Special programs such as aerobic or pulmonary exercises or other physiotherapy modalities such as electrotherapy and hydrotherapy can be included. Some countries have balneotherapy or spa therapy facilities, which can be commenced. In addition to thermal baths, mineral waters, and pool exercises, some other techniques such as mud packs or massage therapies can be used.

In the literature, there is no consensus for the quantity and intensity of exercise in axSpA; however, American College of Sports Medicine guidelines can be referred to and adapted as indicated to prescribe exercise in axSpA (Box 13.1).

Home-Based Exercises

Home-based exercise is one of the important exercise programs used for the management of AS. Most of the earlier studies assessed supervised exercises and largely focused on improvements on the spinal range of motions. However, a number of studies assessing effect of supervised or unsupervised exercise programs on symptoms and measures of health status increased in consistence with the new advances in disease assessment and monitoring tools. In a prospective longitudinal study consisting of 220 patients with AS effect of unsupervised recreational exercise in addition to the specific back exercises on pain, stiffness and functional disability was assessed. Beneficial effects were documented only in patients who performed exercises more than 200 min per week or back exercises at least 5 days per week. In subgroup patients who had AS for 15 years or less, more frequent exercise was associated with reduced severity of pain and stiffness but no change in functional disability. In addition, the frequency of back exercises was not associated with any of the study measures in this subgroup. In contrast, more frequent back exercises were associated with improvements in both pain and functional disability in patients with AS more than 15 years. The important result arising from this study is that long-term and consistent back exercises (at least 30 min per day and 5 days per week) may help stabilize or decrease rate of progression in functional disability in AS.[17] Likewise, another study underscores the importance of consistency, showing that patients with AS who perform moderate, consistent exercise can have long-term beneficial effects on functional capacity and disease activity.[18] Home-based exercises had superiority to standard care or no intervention regarding physical functions, quality-of-life measures, and disease activity in patients with AS.[19–21] Furthermore, improvement in respiratory muscle strength and pulmonary functions after 12 weeks of home exercise program has been documented.[21]

Recently the feasibility of structured education and home exercise program was compared in a nationwide study conducted in Spain.[22] A large number of patients with AS were included in the study; one group underwent an educational session followed by a physiotherapist-guided structured practice session for exercises and physical activity program, which was invited to be implemented at home. The nonintervention group followed the pharmacologic and nonpharmacologic managements recommended by rheumatologist in charge. Although the differences between primary and secondary outcome measures were small, the educational group showed better improvements in disease activity, physical function, and quality-of-life measures in comparison with control group after 6 months. In addition, patients in the educational group significantly increased their knowledge about the disease and its treatments and practiced more regular exercise than controls.[22] Despite positive perceptions, low compliance with the exercise programs or adherence to exercises, which is one of the greatest challenges in AS management, is frequently underscored in studies.[22,23]

Patients with AS have been compared with population controls in regard to parameters of physical fitness and demonstrated that patients had significantly decreased flexibility and cardiorespiratory fitness.[24] Ancillary results from the same study showed promising effects on emotional distress, fatigue, and ability to do a full day's activities in patients with axSpA.[25] A pilot study showed that high-intensity endurance and strength exercise improved disease activity (ASDAS, BASDAI) and reduced CV risk factors (VO_2 peak, resting HR, total body fat, abdominal fat, and waist circumference) in axSpA patients with active disease.[26] In another study, cardiovascular training on cardiovascular fitness and perceived disease activity has been investigated in patients with AS.[27] The intervention group received a 12-week supervised Nordic waking training for 30 min twice a week using individually monitored, moderate-intensity heart rate levels. The control group received an attention control intervention consisting of monthly 2.5-hour discussion groups on coping strategies and techniques of mindfulness-based stress reduction led by a psychologist. All of the participants also attended a weekly 1-hour exercise group (focused on spinal flexibility) supervised by a physiotherapist. Cardiovascular fitness levels in the training group were significantly higher than the control patients after 3 months. As a secondary outcome, peripheral joint pain scores were lower in the training group than the control group. Cardiovascular fitness exercises along with spinal flexibility exercises increase physical fitness and reduce peripheral pain in patients with AS.[27]

Supervised Group Exercises

Supervised group physiotherapy is one of the most studied exercise modalities in patients with AS and has been suggested to be better than home exercises in the most recent Cochrane analysis.[28] In supervised programs, patients can receive support from therapists or other participants and may be a booster for the motivation to exercise. Global posture reeducation (GPR) program is a physical therapy method focusing on postural symmetry, stretching or strengthening of muscles to maintain proper posture. Although the level of evidence is moderate to low, beneficial effects of GPR method in spinal mobility, physical functions, disease activity, and pulmonary functions have been shown in patients with AS.[21,29–32]

Supervised group exercises may consist of special exercise methods such as Pilates, which is an effective therapeutic method for patients with musculoskeletal disorders of the spine. Patients with AS who underwent Pilates (1-hour, three times per week, for 12 weeks) showed better improvement in physical functions compared with patients who received standard care.[33] Multimodal exercise programs, a combination of Pilates, McKenzie, and Heckscher methods versus step-aerobic and pulmonary exercises, were compared in patients with AS. Patients who received complex training combining Pilates, McKenzie, and Heckscher methods showed significant improvements in pain, lumbar spinal mobility, BASFI, BASDAI, and BASMI scores.[34] Tai chi is a combination of physical exercise and relaxation techniques originating in ancient China and helps to enhance mental and physical health. Some beneficial effects of Tai chi on disease activity and flexibility have been reported in a study with a small number of patients with AS.[35]

Water-Based or Aquatic Therapies

Aquatic therapy refer to treatments and exercises performed in water for physical rehabilitation, relaxation, fitness, and other therapeutic gains. Aquatic physical therapy is a widely used therapeutic modality in all age groups with various disabilities or disorders and had some advantages. Aquatic therapies or water-based therapies increase muscle relaxation and peripheral circulation through the use of warm water. Muscle strengthening may be better achieved with the resistance of water, and reduction of gravitational forces and painful joints can easily perform range of motion or stretching exercises through pain-reducing effect of warm water. In addition, swimming on a regular basis may help to improve respiratory functions and thoracic mobility. Swimming improves pulmonary functions and aerobic capacity as well as quality-of-life parameters in patients with AS, however, do not have superiority to land exercises.[36]

Balneotherapy or spa therapy have a long traditional background in some countries. Balneotherapy is defined as the use of baths containing thermal mineral waters from natural springs at a temperature of at least 20°C and with a mineral content of at least 1 g/L.[37] Balneotherapy in patients with AS has been assessed in several studies showing improvement in most of the outcome measures compared with conventional exercises and standard care groups.[38-42]

In-Patient Programs

The effect of in-patient programs has been assessed in several studies. In-patient programs have some advantages: that is, able to give more than one session of program per day and intensive programs with multiple modalities, including comprehensive education. There is evidence that young patients and patients in the early stages of the disease benefitted more from in-patient rehabilitation programs.[43-45] For a continuous efficacy of in-patient programs, it is strictly advised that patients should continue their independent home exercise programs.[46,47] A 3-week intensive in-patient rehabilitation program (consisting of individualized combination of exercises in the gym, in a hot water pool, and outdoor physical activities) had sustained improvement over a 1-year period in terms of significant reductions in disease activity and pain and improved function and

well-being.[48] On the other hand, another study showed declining efficacy over time in a similar in-patient rehabilitation program, which assessed responses by ASAS response criteria.[44] A 4-week comprehensive team rehabilitation in a warm climate resulted in improved physical functions, general health, and pain which was maintained for up to 1 year in most of the patients with various rheumatic disorders including AS.[49] The role of climate in the treatment efficacy has been assessed by comparing 4-week in-patient rehabilitation program given in Mediterranean and Norwegian settings. Response to rehabilitation program was similar in both settings; however, improvements in health status and spinal mobility measures were higher and sustained longer when the rehabilitation was performed in a Mediterranean country rather than in Norway.[50]

Concurrent Treatments With Tumor Necrosis Factor Alpha Inhibitors and Exercise

In the past 15 years, TNFα-blocking therapies dramatically improved disease course and also promoted new advancements in early diagnosis, assessment, and monitoring in patients with axSpA. Despite recent pharmacologic developments, exercise and physiotherapy did not lose significance; moreover, it enhanced its existence in the management of patients with axSpA. Recent reports underscored the synergistic effect of concurrent use of exercise or rehabilitation techniques with TNFα-blocking therapies.[16,51] The effect of combination therapy with rehabilitation and anti-TNF agent (etanercept) has been evaluated in a pilot study.[52] The results revealed that a combination of intensive rehabilitation and anti-TNF treatment improved physical function, disability, and quality of life in patients with active AS. Another controlled study assessed the efficacy of a 2-week course of combined treatment with rehabilitation plus spa versus no intervention in AS. Patients were under treatment with TNF inhibitors (etanercept or infliximab) for at least 3 months and continued during the study and throughout the follow-up period. The combined treatment group had long-term clinical improvements; however, there is no change in outcome measures in the control group.[39] A recent study compared rehabilitation program (rehabilitation group), educational-behavioral program (educational group), and no intervention in patients with AS who were stable under treatment with TNF inhibitors. The exercise group demonstrated better improvement in BASDAI and some anthropometric measurements compared with educational program and no intervention groups.[53] A recent metaanalysis reviewed five studies with a total of 221 participants and concluded that concurrent intervention with exercise and TNF inhibitor therapy significantly improves disease activity, physical functions, and anthropometric measures.[16] This conclusion is also in accordance with the evidence suggesting synergistic effect of combining rehabilitation with TNF inhibitor treatments in patients with AS.[51] As a result of comprehensive review of interventional studies, the most effective rehabilitation appears to be supervised or in-patient programs with an educational component.[51]

Some Practical Points on Exercise in axSpA

Considering the potentially debilitating nature of axSpA, exercise and physiotherapy should start as soon as the disease is diagnosed. Individualized exercise programs are better if accompanied with an educational program. Supervised exercises along with an educational program are one of the better ways to motivate and encourage the patient for physical activity and lifelong exercising on a regular basis. The assessment and monitoring of the patients with appropriate measures is necessary to tailor the most suitable exercises and also to be aware for the changing needs and safety concerns for exercise prescription. Severity of musculoskeletal involvement, mobility and balance, cardiopulmonary status, and established osteoporosis are important aspects for safety concerns. There is evidence for the synergistic effect and additional benefits of exercises in patients who are under successful treatment with TNF-blocking agents. Individualized exercise prescription targeting primarily the spinal mobility and maintaining appropriate posture and mobility of peripheral joints is essential (Box 13.2). An exercise program can include stretching, strengthening, cardiopulmonary, and physical fitness components. Patients can be encouraged for recreational and safe sports activities. Quantity and intensity of exercises should be tailored according to the patient's individual needs, findings on assessment, and lifestyle; however, consistency is also an important factor.

Electrotherapeutic Modalities and Thermotherapy Physical Agents

Electrotherapy or thermotherapy physical agents are used as part of a rehabilitation program that mainly helps to reduce pain and muscle spasms. These agents are noninvasive interventions and relatively safe (a very few adverse effects and contraindications), easily and rapidly administered modalities (portable, i.e., transcutaneous electrical nerve stimulation [TENS] or can be found at home, i.e., ice packs). Studies on the effectiveness of electrotherapy and thermotherapy in

the management of SpA are scanty. However, the use of these electrophysical agents and thermotherapies in the management of SpA is largely promoted by the experience gained from their use in other rheumatic disorders.

The efficacy of TENS in patients with AS was assessed in a sham-controlled double-blind trial with a small number of patients, and improvement in pain and stiffness was noted in favor of TENS group.[54]

The efficacy of whole-body hyperthermia using a new modality called infrared sauna has been assessed in patients with AS and RA. Improvement in pain, stiffness, and fatigue achieved, however, did not reach statistically significant levels.[55] Another small study demonstrated prolonged decrease in proinflammatory cytokine levels (TNFα, IL1β, and IL6) in patients with AS who underwent whole-body hyperthermy.[56] Recently, efficacy of therapeutic ultrasound (US) in the management of patients with AS was assessed in a sham-controlled randomized double-blind study. In the intervention and sham groups, therapeutic US/sham US was applied on both sides of spinal paravertebral muscles at cervical, thoracic, and lumbar levels. All of the patients received 2 weeks of supervised exercises (consisting of postural exercises, strengthening and stretching exercises of back and pelvic muscles, and breathing exercises) followed by 4 weeks of individual home exercises with a similar protocol. Therapeutic US group had superiority over sham group in physical functions, patient and physician's global assessment at week 2, and disease activity and quality of life at week 6.[57]

PATIENT EDUCATION

Patient education is an important integral part of the management in patients with axSpA.[9] Patient education can be explained as an interactive process between patient and the healthcare provider. The education program comprises all educational activities provided for the patient, enhancing patients' understanding of the disease, coping strategies, and supporting adherence to both pharmacologic and nonpharmacologic managements.[58] Patient education interventions have been well assessed in patients with RA, and it is documented that patient education achieved short-term improvements in knowledge, pain, coping behavior, disability, and depression.[59–62] Patient education can be given as a group intervention or individually. In this communication era, various methods of patient education became available through online communication services, web-based platforms, and smartphone applications.

BOX 13.2
Samples of Specific Exercises for Patients With axSpA. Patients are Advised to Do the Individually
Prescribed Exercises by Their Healthcare Provider on a Regular Basis

Stretch out

Cat-back and sway back

Knee to chest

Bridging

Pelvic rotation

Abdominal strengthening

Brid-dog

Extension in lying

Continued

Neck flexion, extension, and rotation

Thoracic lateral flexion and rotation

Hamstring and quadriceps stretching

Anterior chest wall stretching

Deep breathing

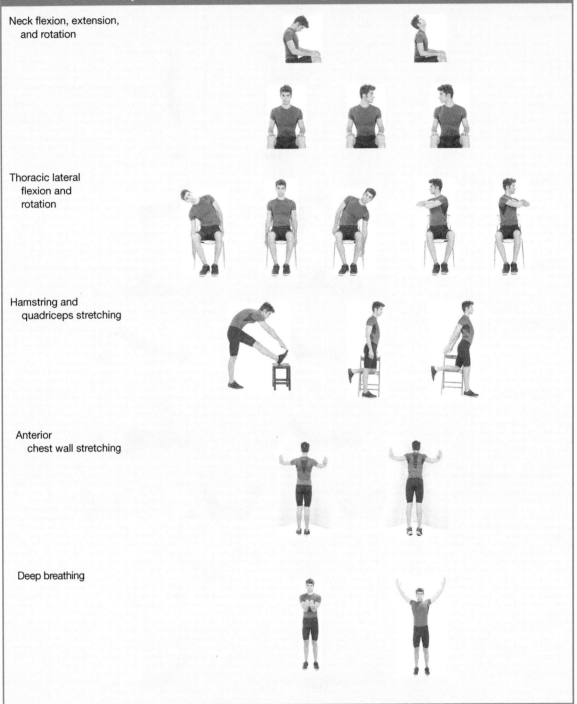

In a randomized nationwide study, patients who had a structured education program before unsupervised home exercise program had slightly better outcome measures including BASDAI, BASFI, patient global, and ASQoL.[22] Supervised exercises and in-patient programs with an educational component have been suggested as an effective approach in the rehabilitation of patients with AS.[51,63] Studies showed that patients with AS want to know more about the exercise, fatigue, pain, joint dysfunction, and the ways to improve activities of daily living.[64,65] A latest research showed that almost half of the patients with SpA considered that they need education concerning self-help, feelings, and disease process. This study also revealed that educational needs were reported more by women and patients with active disease.[66] Internet and new communication ways are considered as possible resources by the patients, however, mentioned as less reliable resources.[66] In recent years, ASAS/EULAR AS treatment recommendations have been translated into a language that can be easily understood by patients.[67] This was an international collaborative study consisting of patients and rheumatologists; the patient-friendly version has been translated into different languages, which serve to further disseminate the recommendations.[68,69]

Ankylosing spondylitis patient organizations are currently present in more than 25 countries. These organizations and self-help groups contribute to increased awareness about the disease promote shared experiences, enhance participation, and improve coping with the disease. A German study showed that patients who are members of a patient society had more information about the disease, better functional levels, and fewer missed days at work than nonmembers.[70]

COMPLEMENTARY AND ALTERNATIVE MEDICINE OR INTEGRATIVE HEALTH

CAM is considered as a group of diverse medical and healthcare systems, practices, and products that are not generally considered part of conventional medicine.[71] The *"complementary"* and *"alternative"* terms have different connotations. If a nonmainstream practice is used *together with* conventional medicine, it is considered *"complementary."* If a nonmainstream practice is used *in place of* conventional medicine, it is considered *"alternative."* People usually use CAM to improve their health and well-being or to relieve symptoms related to their chronic illnesses or to minimize side effects of any conventional treatments used for their diseases. Commonly used CAM therapies included nonvitamin, nonmineral, natural products; chiropractic

care; meditation; deep breathing exercises; yoga; massage; and diet-based therapies.[71] CAM is most often used to treat back pain or back problems, head or chest colds, neck pain or neck problems, joint pain or stiffness, and anxiety or depression. Nearly, 80% of patients with RA have used a form of CAM during the course of their disease,[72] and 94.7% of patients with AS reported previous or current use of CAM.[73] Women with AS were more likely to use dietary CAM, and patients with university education and higher disease activity were more likely to be attending a CAM practitioner. Nearly 83% of patients with AS were currently using CAM and almost 50% used four or more forms of CAM.[73]

ACUPUNCTURE

Acupuncture is one of the oldest forms of therapy, has its roots in ancient China, and is developed along with other ancient Chinese medicine. After its use in the western world, styles and forms of acupuncture are developed. It is still unclear what is the underlying mechanism in the action of acupuncture; however, gate control theory of pain has been suggested as an explanation in the effect of acupuncture in pain relief. There is also evidence for different mechanisms in the analgesic effect or neuroendocrine regulation such as stimulation of endorphins and serotonin or acetylcholine release in the central nervous system.[74] Although efficacy of acupuncture has been assessed in some of the musculoskeletal disorders, robust evidence for its use in axSpA is lacking. Recent Cochrane review for use of acupuncture in nonspecific low-back pain suggested that there is evidence of pain relief, and functional improvement compared with no treatment or sham therapy is, however, observed only immediately after the intervention or at the short-term follow-up. The use of acupuncture in low-back pain is featured as an addition to conventional treatments to better enhance pain relief and functional improvement.[75]

MASSAGE THERAPY

Massage therapy is one of the oldest healthcare practices. It is defined as the manipulation of the soft tissues of the body using a group of manual techniques to help mental relaxation, decrease muscle tension, and reduce pain or to reinforce blood or lymphatic circulation. The most recent Cochrane review on massage therapy for nonspecific low-back pain suggests modest benefits regarding pain relief and return to normal physical functions when combined with exercise and education.[76] According to this Cochrane analysis, massage therapy improved pain but not function when compared with inactive controls in the short-term follow-up in acute low-back pain. In subacute and chronic LBP, massage therapy improved pain and functional outcomes in the short-term but not in the long-term follow-up compared with inactive controls. Moreover, massage therapy improved pain in short- and long-term follow-ups but did not improve function at any follow-up when compared with active controls. The evidence level was very low in this review related to a small number of patients in studies or methodological flaws.[76] Data on the efficacy of massage in the management of AS are scanty, mostly case presentations discussed massage therapy in AS. A recent study compared deep tissue and traditional massage in a small group of patients with AS.[77] Patients were randomized into two groups and received a 30-min session of deep tissue massage or therapeutic massage daily for 2 weeks practiced by two licensed therapists. Similar improvements were noted in outcome measures except for BAS-DAI and pain, which improved in favor of deep tissue massage. The results were encouraging despite small amount of improvement in most of the outcome measures in this pilot study.[77]

CHIROPRACTIC TREATMENTS

The World Federation of Chiropractic defined chiropractic as a health profession interested in the diagnosis, treatment, and prevention of mechanical disorders of the musculoskeletal system and the effects of these disorders on the function of the nervous system and general health. Nearly, 40%–60% of patients attending to chiropractors present with low-back pain.[78] In a recent Cochrane review combined chiropractic, interventions for low-back pain were analyzed. Combined chiropractic interventions (rather than spinal manipulation therapy alone) provide short- and medium-term relief for pain and disability for individuals with acute and subacute low-back pain when compared with other treatments. However, it is difficult to reach robust conclusions since the evidence base shows small and clinically not relevant effect sizes and high risk of bias in the analyzed studies.[78] Spinal manipulations should be avoided in patients with AS or axSpA, particularly those with osteoporosis, established syndesmophytes, or atlantoaxial instability because of the high risk of potential harm. Seronegative spondyloarthropathies, ankylosing spondylitis characterized by episodes of acute inflammation, demineralization, and ligamentous

laxity with anatomic subluxation or dislocation presented as *absolute contraindications* for high-velocity trust procedures according to the clinical guidelines for spinal manipulation in neuropathic practice by College of Neuropathic Physicians of British Columbia and clinical guidelines for chiropractic in Canada.[79]

Natural Health Products and Nutritional Supplements

Nonvitamin, nonmineral natural products are the most commonly used CAM therapy among adults in the United States according to the results of 2007 National Health Interview Survey (NHIS), conducted by the Centers for Disease Control and Prevention's (CDC) National Center for Health Statistics (NCHS).[71] In patients with AS, most commonly used form of CAM was dietary forms (72.1%) and fish oil (26.7%) was the most commonly reported dietary form despite lack of a robust evidence for its efficacy.[73] Green tea (25.3%), vitamin supplements (24.0%), and glucosamine (21.3%) were other forms preferred by the patients. More than half of the patients (56.4%) reported slight or no benefit of dietary CAM and only 11.2% were initiated by a CAM practitioner.[73]

A natural health product and traditional Chinese medicine *Tripterygium wilfordii* (also known as thunder god vine) has been suggested to be effective in a case study consisting of 12 patients with AS.[80] This product has been assessed in the treatment of autoimmune and inflammatory diseases; however, it has a very low therapeutic index. A recent study assessed the efficacy of *Kunxian* capsules in patients with AS in a double-blind, placebo-controlled study.[81] The main component in this medicine was *triprolide*, which is extracted from the genus *Tripterygium* plant *Tripterygium hypoglaucum*. Patients received *Kunxian* capsules or placebo for 12 weeks. The primary endpoint (ASAS 20 response) was significantly higher in the *Kunxian* group (37.1%), compared with placebo (12.1%) as well as ASAS 40 responses, which were also higher than placebo group (22.9% vs. 11.0%, respectively) at week 12. Some side effects such as mild to moderate liver toxicity, decreased WBC or platelets, and gastrointestinal discomfort were reported in this study.[81]

A recent Cochrane review analyzing herbal medicines in patients with RA, underscored possible side effects associated with *Tripterygium* plant extracts may include painful periods in women, decreased fertility in men, insufficient urine excretion, and increased rate of infections.[82]

Another Cochrane review analyzed 14 studies examining six herbal medications to treat nonspecific low-back pain.[83] The results indicate that Devil's claw (*Harpagophytum procumbens*), white willow bark (*Salix alba*), cayenne (*Capsicum frutescens*) topical plaster, comfrey (*Symphytum officinale* L.), Brazilian arnica (*Solidago chilensis*) ointments, and lavender essential oil applied by acupressure were shown to reduce pain more than placebo, although the quality of evidence was considered to be low to moderate.[83] The reported adverse effects were mild consisting of transient GI complaints, which were described for oral intake of Devil's claw and white willow bark.

Regarding various forms of natural health product remedies, a number of issues should be considered. First, pooling of data from these studies is very difficult related to factors such as variations in treatment protocols, various ways of administration, or forms (whole, powder, extract, standardized mixture) of drugs. Secondly, the quality and preparation of such products is not necessarily under strict control of a regulatory body; therefore, bioavailability and pharmacodynamics of these products are vague. Lastly, there is a risk of potential interaction between conventional treatments and natural health products, particularly if used without proper guidance from a trained healthcare provider.

In conclusion, successful management of AS requires a comprehensive approach that includes a variety of nonpharmacological strategies comprising physiotherapy and exercise, as well as self-management and patient education. There is little data regarding the use of nonpharmacological treatments in patients with axSpA which includes nr-axSpA; however, the results in AS could be extrapolated for patients with axSpA. Benefits of conventional exercise protocols (flexibility, stretching, postural exercises, and cardiovascular exercises) have been well documented. A standardized form of rehabilitation is not yet clear; however, there is evidence in favor of patient-centered rehabilitation strategies which include supervised exercises supported with an educational component. Combination of TNFα; blockers with a rehabilitation and/ or spa program may have synergistic effects and provide enhanced efficacy. Self-management and patient education strategies are also an important component of nonpharmacological management.

REFERENCES

1. Rudwaleit M, van der Heijde D, Landewe R, et al. The development of Assessment of SpondyloArthritis international Society classification criteria for axial spondyloarthritis (part II): validation and final selection. *Ann Rheum Dis.* 2009;68(6):777–783.

2. Ozgocmen S, Khan MA. Current concept of spondyloarthritis: special emphasis on early referral and diagnosis. *Curr Rheumatol Rep.* 2012;14(5):409–414.

3. Sieper J, Poddubnyy D. Axial spondyloarthritis. *Lancet.* 2017;390(10089):73–84.

4. Boonen A, Sieper J, van der Heijde D, et al. The burden of non-radiographic axial spondyloarthritis. *Semin Arthritis Rheum.* 2015;44(5):556–562.

5. de Winter JJ, van Mens LJ, van der Heijde D, Landewe R, Baeten DL. Prevalence of peripheral and extra-articular disease in ankylosing spondylitis versus non-radiographic axial spondyloarthritis: a meta-analysis. *Arthritis Res Ther.* 2016;18:196.

6. Kiltz U, van der Heijde D, Boonen A, et al. Measuring impairments of functioning and health in patients with axial spondyloarthritis by using the ASAS Health Index and the Environmental Item Set: translation and cross-cultural adaptation into 15 languages. *RMD Open.* 2016;2(2):e000311.

7. van Echteld I, Cieza A, Boonen A, et al. Identification of the most common problems by patients with ankylosing spondylitis using the international classification of functioning, disability and health. *J Rheumatol.* 2006;33(12):2475–2483.

8. Braun J, van den Berg R, Baraliakos X, et al. 2010 update of the ASAS/EULAR recommendations for the management of ankylosing spondylitis. *Ann Rheum Dis.* 2011;70(6):896–904.

9. van der Heijde D, Ramiro S, Landewe R, et al. 2016 update of the ASAS-EULAR management recommendations for axial spondyloarthritis. *Ann Rheum Dis.* 2017;76(6):978–991.

10. Zochling J, van der Heijde D, Burgos-Vargas R, et al. ASAS/EULAR recommendations for the management of ankylosing spondylitis. *Ann Rheum Dis.* 2006;65(4):442–452.

11. Ward MM, Deodhar A, Akl EA, et al. American College of Rheumatology/spondylitis association of America/spondyloarthritis research and treatment network 2015 recommendations for the treatment of ankylosing spondylitis and nonradiographic axial spondyloarthritis. *Arthritis Rheumatol.* 2016;68(2):282–298.

12. Passalent LA, Ozgocmen S. Non-pharmacological management in axial spondyloarthritis. In: Robert I, Joachim S, eds. *Oxford Textbook of Axial Spondyloarthritis.* Oxford: Oxford University Press; 2016:175–187.

13. van der Heijde D, van der Linden S, Bellamy N, Calin A, Dougados M, Khan MA. Which domains should be included in a core set for endpoints in ankylosing spondylitis? Introduction to the ankylosing spondylitis module of OMERACT IV. *J Rheumatol.* 1999;26(4):945–947.

14. Ozgocmen S, Akgul O, Altay Z, et al. Expert opinion and key recommendations for the physical therapy and rehabilitation of patients with ankylosing spondylitis. *Int J Rheum Dis.* 2012;15(3):229–238.

15. Poddubnyy D, Haibel H, Listing J, et al. Baseline radiographic damage, elevated acute-phase reactant levels, and cigarette smoking status predict spinal radiographic progression in early axial spondylarthritis. *Arthritis Rheum.* 2012;64(5):1388–1398.

16. Liang H, Li WR, Zhang H, Tian X, Wei W, Wang CM. Concurrent intervention with exercises and stabilized tumor necrosis factor inhibitor therapy reduced the disease activity in patients with ankylosing spondylitis: a meta-analysis. *Medicine (Baltim)*. 2015;94(50):e2254.

17. Uhrin Z, Kuzis S, Ward MM. Exercise and changes in health status in patients with ankylosing spondylitis. *Arch Intern Med*. 2000;160(19):2969–2975.

18. Santos H, Brophy S, Calin A. Exercise in ankylosing spondylitis: how much is optimum? *J Rheumatol*. 1998;25(11):2156–2160.

19. Aytekin E, Caglar NS, Ozgonenel L, Tutun S, Demiryontar DY, Demir SE. Home-based exercise therapy in patients with ankylosing spondylitis: effects on pain, mobility, disease activity, quality of life, and respiratory functions. *Clin Rheumatol*. 2012;31(1):91–97.

20. Durmus D, Alayli G, Cil E, Canturk F. Effects of a home-based exercise program on quality of life, fatigue, and depression in patients with ankylosing spondylitis. *Rheumatol Int*. 2009;29(6):673–677.

21. Durmus D, Alayli G, Uzun O, et al. Effects of two exercise interventions on pulmonary functions in the patients with ankylosing spondylitis. *Joint Bone Spine*. 2009;76(2):150–155.

22. Rodriguez-Lozano C, Juanola X, Cruz-Martinez J, et al. Outcome of an education and home-based exercise programme for patients with ankylosing spondylitis: a nationwide randomized study. *Clin Exp Rheumatol*. 2013;31(5):739–748.

23. Passalent LA. Physiotherapy for ankylosing spondylitis: evidence and application. *Curr Opin Rheumatol*. 2011;23(2):142–147.

24. Halvorsen S, Vollestad NK, Fongen C, et al. Physical fitness in patients with ankylosing spondylitis: comparison with population controls. *Phys Ther*. 2012;92(2):298–309.

25. Sveaas SH, Berg IJ, Fongen C, Provan SA, Dagfinrud H. High-intensity cardiorespiratory and strength exercises reduced emotional distress and fatigue in patients with axial spondyloarthritis: a randomized controlled pilot study. *Scand J Rheumatol*. 2017:1–5.

26. Ortancil O, Sarikaya S, Sapmaz P, Basaran A, Ozdolap S. The effect(s) of a six-week home-based exercise program on the respiratory muscle and functional status in ankylosing spondylitis. *J Clin Rheumatol*. 2009;15(2):68–70.

27. Niedermann K, Sidelnikov E, Muggli C, et al. Effect of cardiovascular training on fitness and perceived disease activity in people with ankylosing spondylitis. *Arthritis Care Res*. 2013;65(11):1844–1852.

28. Dagfinrud H, Kvien TK, Hagen KB. Physiotherapy interventions for ankylosing spondylitis. *Cochrane Database Syst Rev*. 2008;(1):CD002822.

29. Fernandez-de-Las-Penas C, Alonso-Blanco C, Alguacil-Diego IM, Miangolarra-Page JC. One-year follow-up of two exercise interventions for the management of patients with ankylosing spondylitis: a randomized controlled trial. *Am J Phys Med Rehabil*. 2006;85(7):559–567.

30. Fernandez-de-Las-Penas C, Alonso-Blanco C, Morales-Cabezas M, Miangolarra-Page JC. Two exercise interventions for the management of patients with ankylosing spondylitis: a randomized controlled trial. *Am J Phys Med Rehabil*. 2005;84(6):407–419.

31. Silva EM, Andrade SC, Vilar MJ. Evaluation of the effects of Global Postural Reeducation in patients with ankylosing spondylitis. *Rheumatol Int*. 2012;32(7):2155–2163.

32. Teodori RM, Negri JR, Cruz MC, Marques AP. Global Postural Re-education: a literature review. *Rev Bras Fisioter*. 2011;15(3):185–189.

33. Altan L, Korkmaz N, Dizdar M, Yurtkuran M. Effect of Pilates training on people with ankylosing spondylitis. *Rheumatol Int*. 2012;32(7):2093–2099.

34. Rosu MO, Topa I, Chirieac R, Ancuta C. Effects of Pilates, McKenzie and Heckscher training on disease activity, spinal motility and pulmonary function in patients with ankylosing spondylitis: a randomized controlled trial. *Rheumatol Int*. 2014;34(3):367–372.

35. Lee EN, Kim YH, Chung WT, Lee MS. Tai chi for disease activity and flexibility in patients with ankylosing spondylitis–a controlled clinical trial. *Evid Based Complement Altern Med*. 2008;5(4):457–462.

36. Karapolat H, Eyigor S, Zoghi M, Akkoc Y, Kirazli Y, Keser G. Are swimming or aerobic exercise better than conventional exercise in ankylosing spondylitis patients? A randomized controlled study. *Eur J Phys Rehabil Med*. 2009;45(4):449–457.

37. Pittler MH, Karagulle MZ, Karagulle M, Ernst E. Spa therapy and balneotherapy for treating low back pain: meta-analysis of randomized trials. *Rheumatology*. 2006;45(7):880–884.

38. Altan L, Bingol U, Aslan M, Yurtkuran M. The effect of balneotherapy on patients with ankylosing spondylitis. *Scand J Rheumatol*. 2006;35(4):283–289.

39. Ciprian L, Lo Nigro A, Rizzo M, et al. The effects of combined spa therapy and rehabilitation on patients with ankylosing spondylitis being treated with TNF inhibitors. *Rheumatol Int*. 2013;33(1):241–245.

40. Codish S, Dobrovinsky S, Abu Shakra M, Flusser D, Sukenik S. Spa therapy for ankylosing spondylltis at the Dead Sea. *Isr Med Assoc J*. 2005;7(7):443–446.

41. Colina M, Ciancio G, Garavini R, Conti M, Trotta F, Govoni M. Combination treatment with etanercept and an intensive spa rehabilitation program in active ankylosing spondylitis. *Int J Immunopathol Pharmacol*. 2009;22(4):1125–1129.

42. Van Tubergen A, Boonen A, Landewe R, et al. Cost effectiveness of combined spa-exercise therapy in ankylosing spondylitis: a randomized controlled trial. *Arthritis Rheumatol*. 2002;47(5):459–467.

43. Band DA, Jones SD, Kennedy LG, et al. Which patients with ankylosing spondylitis derive most benefit from an inpatient management program? *J Rheumatol*. 1997;24(12):2381–2384.

44. Lubrano E, D'Angelo S, Parsons WJ, et al. Effectiveness of rehabilitation in active ankylosing spondylitis assessed by the ASAS response criteria. *Rheumatology*. 2007;46(11):1672–1675.

45. Viitanen JV, Suni J, Kautiainen H, Liimatainen M, Takala H. Effect of physiotherapy on spinal mobility in ankylosing spondylitis. *Scand J Rheumatol.* 1992;21(1):38–41.

46. Bulstrode SJ, Barefoot J, Harrison RA, Clarke AK. The role of passive stretching in the treatment of ankylosing spondylitis. *Br J Rheumatol.* 1987;26(1):40–42.

47. Helliwell PS, Abbott CA, Chamberlain MA. A randomised trial of three different physiotherapy regimes in ankylosing spondylitis. *Physiotherapy.* 1996;82:85–90.

48. Kjeken I, Bo I, Ronningen A, et al. A three-week multidisciplinary in-patient rehabilitation programme had positive long-term effects in patients with ankylosing spondylitis: randomized controlled trial. *J Rehabil Med.* 2013;45(3):260–267.

49. Ajeganova S, Wornert M, Hafstrom I. A four-week team-rehabilitation programme in a warm climate decreases disability and improves health and body function for up to one year: a prospective study in Swedish patients with inflammatory joint diseases. *J Rehabil Med.* 2016;48(8):711–718.

50. Staalesen Strumse YA, Nordvag BY, Stanghelle JK, et al. Efficacy of rehabilitation for patients with ankylosing spondylitis: comparison of a four-week rehabilitation programme in a Mediterranean and a Norwegian setting. *J Rehabil Med.* 2011;43(6):534–542.

51. Lubrano E, Spadaro A, Amato G, et al. Tumour necrosis factor alpha inhibitor therapy and rehabilitation for the treatment of ankylosing spondylitis: a systematic review. *Semin Arthritis Rheum.* 2015;44(5):542–550.

52. Lubrano E, D'Angelo S, Parsons WJ, et al. Effects of a combination treatment of an intensive rehabilitation program and etanercept in patients with ankylosing spondylitis: a pilot study. *J Rheumatol.* 2006;33(10):2029–2034.

53. Masiero S, Poli P, Bonaldo L, et al. Supervised training and home-based rehabilitation in patients with stabilized ankylosing spondylitis on TNF inhibitor treatment: a controlled clinical trial with a 12-month follow-up. *Clin Rehabil.* 2013;28(6):562–572.

54. Gemignani G, Olivieri I, Ruju G, Pasero G. Transcutaneous electrical nerve stimulation in ankylosing spondylitis: a double-blind study. *Arthritis Rheumatol.* 1991;34(6):788–789.

55. Oosterveld FG, Rasker JJ, Floors M, et al. Infrared sauna in patients with rheumatoid arthritis and ankylosing spondylitis. A pilot study showing good tolerance, short-term improvement of pain and stiffness, and a trend towards long-term beneficial effects. *Clin Rheumatol.* 2009;28(1):29–34.

56. Tarner IH, Muller-Ladner U, Uhlemann C, Lange U. The effect of mild whole-body hyperthermia on systemic levels of TNF-alpha, IL-1beta, and IL-6 in patients with ankylosing spondylitis. *Clin Rheumatol.* 2009;28(4):397–402.

57. Silte Karamanlioglu D, Aktas I, Ozkan FU, Kaysin M, Girgin N. Effectiveness of ultrasound treatment applied with exercise therapy on patients with ankylosing spondylitis: a double-blind, randomized, placebo-controlled trial. *Rheumatol Int.* 2016;36(5):653–661.

58. Zangi HA, Ndosi M, Adams J, et al. EULAR recommendations for patient education for people with inflammatory arthritis. *Ann Rheum Dis.* 2015;74(6):954–962.

59. Astin JA, Beckner W, Soeken K, Hochberg MC, Berman B. Psychological interventions for rheumatoid arthritis: a meta-analysis of randomized controlled trials. *Arthritis Rheum.* 2002;47(3):291–302.

60. Christie A, Jamtvedt G, Dahm KT, Moe RH, Haavardsholm EA, Hagen KB. Effectiveness of nonpharmacological and nonsurgical interventions for patients with rheumatoid arthritis: an overview of systematic reviews. *Phys Ther.* 2007;87(12):1697–1715.

61. Niedermann K, Fransen J, Knols R, Uebelhart D. Gap between short- and long-term effects of patient education in rheumatoid arthritis patients: a systematic review. *Arthritis Rheum.* 2004;51(3):388–398.

62. Riemsma RP, Taal E, Kirwan JR, Rasker JJ. Systematic review of rheumatoid arthritis patient education. *Arthritis Rheum.* 2004;51(6):1045–1059.

63. Kasapoglu Aksoy M, Birtane M, Tastekin N, Ekuklu G. The effectiveness of structured group education on ankylosing spondylitis patients. *J Clin Rheumatol.* 2017;23(3):138–143.

64. Cooksey R, Brophy S, Husain MJ, Irvine E, Davies H, Siebert S. The information needs of people living with ankylosing spondylitis: a questionnaire survey. *BMC Musculoskelet Disord.* 2012;13:243.

65. Kang R, Passalent L, Morton R, et al. Utilization of an informational needs assessment to develop an education program for patients with ankylosing spondylitis and related axial spondyloarthritis. *Ann Rheum Dis.* 2013;72:1037–1038.

66. Haglund E, Bremander A, Bergman S, Larsson I. Educational needs in patients with spondyloarthritis in Sweden - a mixed-methods study. *BMC Musculoskelet Disord.* 2017;18(1):335.

67. Kiltz U, van der Heijde D, Mielants H, Feldtkeller E, Braun J, group PEpi. ASAS/EULAR recommendations for the management of ankylosing spondylitis: the patient version. *Ann Rheum Dis.* 2009;68(9):1381–1386.

68. Kiltz U, Feldtkeller E, Braun J. [German patient version of the ASAS/EULAR recommendations for the management of ankylosing spondylitis]. *Z Rheumatol.* 2010;69(2):171–174, 176-179.

69. Ozgocmen S, Duruoz MT. Turkish translation and patient evaluation of the ASAS/EULAR recommendations-patient version for the management of ankylosing spondylitis. *Turk J Rheumatol Turk Romatoloji Dergisi.* 2009;24(4):190–195.

70. Song IH, Brenneis C, Hammel L, et al. Ankylosing spondylitis self-help organisations - do members differ from non-members? *Joint Bone Spine.* 2016;83(3):295–300.

71. Barnes PM, Bloom B, Nahin RL. Complementary and alternative medicine use among adults and children: United States, 2007. *Natl Health Stat Rep.* 2008;(12):1–23.

72. Rose G. Why do patients with rheumatoid arthritis use complementary therapies? *Muscoskel Care.* 2006;4(2):101–115.

73. Chatfield SM, Dharmage SC, Boers A, et al. Complementary and alternative medicines in ankylosing spondylitis: a cross-sectional study. *Clin Rheumatol.* 2009;28(2):213–217.

74. Yu JS, Zeng BY, Hsieh CL. Acupuncture stimulation and neuroendocrine regulation. *Int Rev Neurobiol.* 2013;111:125–140.

75. Furlan AD, van Tulder MW, Cherkin DC, et al. Acupuncture and dry-needling for low back pain. *Cochrane Database Syst Rev.* 2005;(1):CD001351.

76. Furlan AD, Brosseau L, Imamura M, Irvin E. Massage for low back pain. *Cochrane Database Syst Rev.* 2002;(2):CD001929.

77. Romanowski MW, Spiritovic M, Rutkowski R, Dudek A, Samborski W, Straburzynska-Lupa A. Comparison of deep tissue massage and therapeutic massage for lower back pain, disease activity, and functional capacity of ankylosing spondylitis patients: a randomized clinical pilot study. *Evid Based Complement Altern Med.* 2017;2017:9894128.

78. Walker BF, French SD, Grant W, Green S. Combined chiropractic interventions for low-back pain. *Cochrane Database Syst Rev.* 2010;(4):C1D005427.

79. Clinical guidelines for spinal manipulation in neuropathic practice by College of Neuropathic Physicians of British Colombia. www.cnpbc.bc.ca/wp-content/uploads/QAC-Manipulation.pdf.

80. Ji W, Li J, Lin Y, et al. Report of 12 cases of ankylosing spondylitis patients treated with Tripterygium wilfordii. *Clin Rheumatol.* 2010;29(9):1067–1072.

81. Li Q, Li L, Bi L, et al. Kunxian capsules in the treatment of patients with ankylosing spondylitis: a randomized placebo-controlled clinical trial. *Trials.* 2016;17(1):337.

82. Cameron M, Gagnier JJ, Chrubasik S. Herbal therapy for treating rheumatoid arthritis. *Cochrane Database Syst Rev.* 2011;(2):CD002948.

83. Oltean H, Robbins C, van Tulder MW, Berman BM, Bombardier C, Gagnier JJ. Herbal medicine for low-back pain. *Cochrane Database Syst Rev.* 2014;12:CD004504.

CHAPTER 14

Pharmacologic Nonbiologic Treatment of Axial Spondyloarthritis

FABIAN PROFT, MD • DENIS PODDUBNYY, MD, MSC (EPI)

INTRODUCTION

Under the umbrella term spondyloarthritis (SpA), a group of chronic inflammatory autoimmune diseases are encompassed. They share frequent clinical, pathophysiologic, and genetic features,[1,2] as involvement of the axial skeleton (sacroiliac joints and spine), characteristic peripheral manifestations (dactylitis, enthesitis, and asymmetric mono- or oligoarthritis predominantly affecting the lower extremities), and specific extraarticular manifestations, such as psoriasis, acute anterior uveitis, and inflammatory bowel disease (IBD),[2,3] as well as association with the MHC class I human leukocyte antigen-B27 (HLA-B27).[3–5] Considering the leading manifestation, two major SpA subgroups can be defined: axial SpA with predominant involvement of the sacroiliac joints and/or spine and peripheral SpA with predominant peripheral manifestations—arthritis, enthesitis, and dactylitis. In the past two decades, the concept of axial SpA as one disease with two subsets (with radiographic changes in the sacroiliac joints [=ankylosing spondylitis/AS or radiographic axial spondyloarthritis] and without [=nonradiographic axial spondyloarthritis/nr-axSpA]) has arisen.[6–9] Nonradiographic and radiographic axial SpA share common epidemiologic, clinical, and genetic characteristics,[4,10–15] which supports the concept of axial SpA as one disease with two stages.[3,10]

In this chapter, we will focus on the pharmacologic but nonbiologic treatment options for axial SpA.

TREATMENT OF AXIAL SPA

In the past years, the major treatment objective in spondyloarthritis has been defined as clinical remission/inactive disease of musculoskeletal (arthritis, dactylitis, enthesitis, and axial disease) and extraarticular manifestations.[16] Moreover, stopping—or at least slowing—the radiographic progression of the spine, and also in the sacroiliac joints, is a desirable long-term treatment outcome and remains a high ranked topic on the "research agenda." Axial SpA is presently an important focus of rheumatology research, and promising preliminary results suggest that other therapeutic compounds will be available in the near future,[17] but their place in the treatment algorithm still has to be defined.

The current versions of the leading international and evidence-based management recommendations for axial spondyloarthritis (Assessment of Spondylo-Arthritis International Society [ASAS] and European League Against Rheumatism [EULAR] recommendations from 2017[18] and treatment recommendations from the American College of Rheumatology [ACR]/Spondylitis Association of America [SAA]/SPARTAN from 2016[19]) are mainly analogic and differ only in few points related to the interpretation of the existing literature. Therefore, we present in this chapter the international treatment recommendations for pharmacologic but nonbiologic therapies of axial SpA and highlight the similarities and differences in these transatlantic approaches and the evidence for accomplishing the abovementioned treatment goals (Fig. 14.1).

Nonsteroidal Antiinflammatory Drugs

Despite the tremendous advancement in understanding the underlying pathogenesis and treatment with the introduction of tumor necrosis factor inhibitors (TNFi),[15,20–26] interleukin-17 inhibitor(s) (IL-17i),[27] and other new treatment options on the horizon,[17] nonsteroidal antiinflammatory drugs (NSAIDs) remain the cornerstone of pharmacologic treatment in axial SpA. According to either of the abovementioned recommendations, first-line therapies for patients with axial SpA are nonsteroidal antiinflammatory drugs (NSAIDs), including selective cyclooxygenase-2 (COX-2) antagonists up to the maximal (tolerated) dosage, along with continuous exercise/physiotherapy and education of the patients.[18,19]

Axial Spondyloarthritis. https://doi.org/10.1016/B978-0-323-56800-5.00014-X

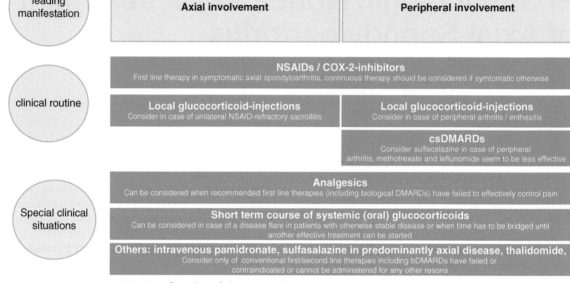

FIG. 14.1 Overview of pharmacologic, nonbiologic treatment of axial SpA.

ASAS/EULAR

Patients suffering from pain and stiffness should use an NSAID as first-line drug treatment up to the maximum dose, taking risks and benefits into account. For patients who respond well to NSAIDs continuous use is preferred if symptomatic otherwise.[18]

ACR/SAA/SPARTAN

In adults with active AS, we strongly recommend treatment with NSAIDs over no treatment with NSAIDs.[19]

We conditionally recommend continuous treatment with NSAIDs over on-demand treatment with NSAIDs.[19]

We do not recommend any particular NSAID as the preferred choice.[19]

Because nonradiographic axial SpA has only recently been defined, the literature on treatment of this condition is limited. Therefore, the panel relied on the AS literature as the basis for most recommendations, ... These recommendations were the same as for AS.[19]

These recommendations are based on the evidence that NSAIDs are effective in reducing pain and stiffness in patients with radiographic axial SpA (AS).[28–37] There are no robust data from placebo-controlled randomized clinical trials (RCTs) for their use in the nonradiographic form of axial SpA, but observational studies[38–40] and clinical experience clearly support their efficacy in the entire group of patients with axial SpA. Thus it is assumed that NSAIDs are similarly effective in patients with the nonradiographic form of axial SpA.[18,19] With regard to clinical efficacy, there seems to be no class difference between the nonselective COX antagonists and the selective COX-2 inhibitors,[29–32,37] even though a recent metaanalysis of NSAID treatment in 3410 AS patients suggested a possible advantage of etoricoxib over some other NSAIDs in reducing pain.[41] With regard to an interindividual variation in treatment response to NSAIDs, it is advisable to administer at least one other NSAID after failure of the first NSAID to achieve the predefined treatment target.[18] Short symptom duration at the time point of treatment initiation seems to predict a better response to NSAIDs: the ASAS partial remission rate after 6 months of naproxen treatment was achieved in 35% of the axial SpA patients with early disease (symptom duration <3 years), who were either NSAID-naive or had not been treated with more than two-thirds of the maximum recommended dose of an NSAID 2 weeks before initial screening, but it was only 12% in another trial of patients with long-standing AS.[30] In addition to the effect of NSAIDs on pain and stiffness, an effect on reduction of objective signs of inflammation could be demonstrated for C-reactive protein (CRP)[30] as well as for bone marrow edema on magnetic resonance imaging (MRI) in axial SpA.[30,42,43] This leads to the conclusion that the clinical symptomatic benefit of NSAIDs may be not only due to an analgesic effect but also determined by an antiinflammatory capacity of these drugs.

Besides control of symptoms related to active inflammation, preventing structural damage in the spine (reduction of radiographic spinal progression) is a highly desirable long-term treatment outcome in axial SpA.[16] Whether NSAIDs have the ability to decrease the radiographic progression in the spine over time still remains a matter of debate.[44-47] The existing data are discrepant and this question has to be further evaluated.[18] An earlier study suggested that NSAIDs, specifically celecoxib, might possess not only a symptomatic efficacy but also disease-modifying properties in AS, slowing progression of structural damage in the spine if taken continuously.[48] This effect seemed to be stronger in patients with elevated CRP-levels,[49] which was supported by data from an observation cohort study.[38] However, for the nonselective COX inhibitor diclofenac, such effect could not be shown in a more recently conducted trial.[50] Whether continuous therapy with a selective COX-2 inhibitor (celecoxib) added to a TNFi-therapy is beneficial in AS patients with risk factors for syndesmophyte progression (elevated CRP or existing syndesmophytes at baseline) is currently under investigation in a prospective randomized controlled trial (RCT).[51]

Safety aspects should always be taken into account when starting NSAIDs, especially when long-term treatment is anticipated.[18] To date, there are no prospective RCTs investigating the long-term efficacy and safety of NSAIDs in AS patients (except two trials with focus on radiographic spinal progression mentioned above, although none were placebo or non-NSAID controlled). It has been shown that AS is associated with an increased mortality,[52-54] particularly associated with higher disease activity.[55] Data from observational studies have suggested a protective effect of NSAID intake in AS patients in terms of overall mortality and cardiovascular risk.[52,55] This might be explained by the reduction of the underlying systemic inflammation through NSAID usage. It should be taken into account, however, that large studies performed in patients with other forms of arthritis showed an increased cardiovascular risk associated with NSAID treatment.[56,57] Although a recent study suggested no differences between celecoxib, ibuprofen, and naproxen concerning cardiovascular events,[58] a large metaanalysis of NSAID treatment showed no significant differences between selective COX-2 inhibitors and traditional NSAIDs but suggested that naproxen can be associated with lower cardiovascular risk.[56] Selective COX-2 inhibitors on the other hand have a better gastrointestinal safety profile when compared with traditional NSAIDs,[58] especially in high-risk patients.[59]

Analgesics
ASAS/EULAR

Analgesics, such as paracetamol- (like) drugs, might be considered for residual pain after previously recommended treatments have failed, are contraindicated and/or poorly tolerated.[18]

Formal evidence that nonnarcotic analgesics are effective in reducing pain in axial SpA is missing. However, based on expert opinions, extrapolations from other diseases causing painful conditions, and data from one small RCT, which tested the add-on effect of tramadol to an NSAID (acetaminophen) in AS patients and showed a significantly higher ASAS20 response rate in the treatment group,[60] the use of nonnarcotic analgesics is recommended in situations, where preferred therapies (including biologic DMARDs) have failed to effectively control the pain or cannot be used because of contraindications/intolerability.[18]

Considering concerns about narcotic addiction in society, development of analgesics, which work via nonnarcotic mechanisms, will be increasingly important; several of such therapies are in development and should be tested in axial SpA.

Glucocorticoids
ASAS/EULAR

Glucocorticoid injections directed to the local site of musculoskeletal inflammation may be considered. Patients with axial disease should not receive long-term treatment with systemic glucocorticoids.[18]

ACR/SAA/SPARTAN

In adults with active AS, we strongly recommend against treatment with systemic glucocorticoids.[19]

In adults with AS and isolated active sacroiliitis despite treatment with NSAIDs, we conditionally recommend treatment with locally administered parenteral glucocorticoids over no treatment with local glucocorticoids.[19]

In adults with AS with stable axial disease and active enthesitis despite treatment with NSAIDs, we conditionally recommend using treatment with locally administered parenteral glucocorticoids over no treatment with local glucocorticoids. Peri-tendon injections of Achilles, patellar, and quadriceps tendons should be avoided.[19]

In adults with AS with stable axial disease and active peripheral arthritis despite treatment with NSAIDs, we conditionally recommend using treatment with locally administered parenteral glucocorticoids over no treatment with local glucocorticoids.[19]

Concerning glucocorticoid use, a differentiation needs to be made between topical use of glucocorticoid for treatment of acute anterior uveitis, local injections for treating arthritis/enthesitis, and systemic treatments (including differentiation between short- and long-term uses).

Only one RCT has investigated the effect of systemic prednisolone in AS patients. The 50% improvement of BASDAI (=Bath Ankylosing Spondylitis Disease Activity Index after 2 weeks) has been observed in 33% of patients treated with oral prednisolone 50 mg/d for 2 weeks as compared with only 8% response rate in placebo-treated patients, although this difference was statistically nonsignificant ($P = .16$). Furthermore, a significant improvement in the ASDAS (=Ankylosing Spondylitis Disease Activity Score) was observed.[61] This may justify a short-term course of oral glucocorticoids as a possible treatment option in special clinical situations,[18] such as treatment of an acute disease flare in patients with otherwise stable disease or when time has to be bridged until another effective treatment can be started.

Considering side effects of a long-term glucocorticoid treatment and lack of any data showing a benefit of such treatment in axial SpA, a long-term glucocorticoid therapy is not recommended.[18,19]

The effect of intravenous glucocorticoids in AS has not been investigated in prospective RCTs until now, but an open-label trial[62] and observational data reported[63-65] some clinical improvement. In consideration of the availability of other efficacious treatment modalities and the lack of controlled trials, intravenous high-dose glucocorticoids cannot be recommended for a wide routine use.

The use of local corticosteroid injections in case of predominant peripheral manifestations (arthritis/enthesitis)[18,19] of SpA or isolated unilateral sacroiliitis[19] is recommended as a therapeutic option by both international guidelines, even though controlled trials are also missing for peripheral injections in this indication. Thus, this recommendation is mainly based on clinical experience, expert opinion, and extrapolated results from other rheumatic diseases such as rheumatoid arthritis,[66-68] whereas the effect of sacroiliac glucocorticoid injections has a good level of evidence (1b), with one placebo-controlled trial showing significant superiority of glucocorticoid injections, lasting for up

to 6 months.[69] These results are supported by open-label data.[70]

Conventional Synthetic Disease-Modifying Antirheumatic Drugs
ASAS/EULAR

Patients with purely axial disease should normally not be treated with csDMARDs; sulfasalazine may be considered in patients with peripheral arthritis.[18]

ACR/SAA/SPARTAN

In adults with active AS despite treatment with NSAIDs, we conditionally recommend against treatment with SAARDs[19] (=slow-acting antirheumatic drugs=csDMARDs).

In adults with active AS despite treatment with NSAIDs and who have contraindications to TNFi, we conditionally recommend treatment with a SAARD over treatment with a non-TNFi biologic agent.[19]

According to either of the abovementioned recommendations, csDMARDs do not play a major role in the treatment algorithm of axial SpA and are reserved mostly as an option for patients with peripheral arthritis.[18,19] These guidelines are based on the evidence that csDMARDs, in general, are not efficacious in the treatment of axial involvement of AS patients but might have some beneficial effect in patients with peripheral joint involvement (arthritis).[71-79] A Cochrane review revealed no meaningful effect of sulfasalazine (SSZ) in reducing pain, disease activity, radiographic progression, or improving physical function/spinal mobility in AS patients.[76,80] In axial SpA patients with concomitant peripheral arthritis, SSZ treatment showed moderate efficacy,[81,82] while no effect on peripheral enthesitis as a manifestation of axial SpA could be demonstrated.[83]

In line with an open-label trial in active AS patients that showed no benefit of MTX therapy (20 mg MTX per week for 12 weeks) for axial manifestations,[74] a Cochrane systematic review found no benefit of MTX in the treatment of AS.[75] There is also no evidence in support of use of MTX for the treatment of peripheral manifestations of axial SpA,[75] as only one trial in AS addressing the effect of MTX on these manifestations showed a nonsignificant trend toward improvement of peripheral arthritis,[74] whereas this could not be confirmed by other trials.[84,85] Concerning the effect of MTX on peripheral enthesitis in axial SpA, the literature is scarce,[75,86] but the existing data do not support administration of MTX in these patients.[74] Nevertheless, MTX is sometimes used in clinical practice for the treatment of peripheral arthritis/enthesitis in axial SpA, which is driven by the derived results from other indications as rheumatoid arthritis (RA)[87–90] and to a lesser degree psoriatic arthritis (PsA).[91–93]

Leflunomide (LFL) is not recommended for treatment of axial manifestations of axial SpA,[77,78] although there might be some beneficial effects on peripheral arthritis in patients with axial SpA. One open-label study, which assessed the effect on peripheral arthritis in AS patients, showed a significant improvement in a small subgroup (n = 10) with peripheral arthritis.[77] A further validation of these preliminary findings has not been pursued. The effect of LFL on peripheral enthesitis in axial SpA has not been systematically investigated.

Data concerning the use of azathioprine (AZA) in axial SpA are limited. Although one case report describes good clinical response in a refractory AS patient of intravenous loading with AZA followed by oral AZA therapy,[94] results from the only available RCT showed low response rates and a significant withdrawal rate because of side effects.[95]

Results from the only controlled trial of treatment with systemic gold in AS do not support the administration of this historical drug in axial SpA, as no effect on axial manifestations was observed under treatment with auranofin.[96] The sample size was too small to assess an effect on peripheral manifestations.

The use of cyclosporine for peripheral arthritis associated with ankylosing spondylitis is advocated only by one anecdotal case report;[97] data from RCTs are lacking and therefore cannot be recommended.

Targeted Synthetic Disease-Modifying Antirheumatic Drugs

As no tsDMARD has the formal approval in the indication axial SpA or AS, neither of the international treatment recommendations directly address their application in these patients. Nevertheless, the nomenclature "targeted synthetic disease-modifying antirheumatic drugs (tsDMARD)" has been established, especially in relation to RA and PsA.[18] This group includes small molecules such as JAK inhibitors and the phosphodiesterase (PDE)-4-inhibitor apremilast. Two JAK inhibitors (tofacitinib and baricitinib) have been approved for RA. Recently, tofacitinib also obtained FDA approval for PsA. A phase-II placebo-controlled dose-ranging RCT of tofacitinib in AS demonstrated a statistically higher than placebo ASAS20 response rate for the dosage of 5 mg twice daily (80.8% vs. 41.2%; $P < .001$), whereas the differences from placebo did not reach statistical significance for 2 and 10 mg twice a day.[98] Therefore, further studies are needed to confirm the efficacy of tofacitinib in axial SpA.

In the near future, phase II/III data on selective JAK-1 inhibitors (upadacitinib and filgotinib) in AS will be available, as these trials are currently ongoing.

Apremilast, an oral PDE-4-inhibitor, has approval for the treatment of psoriasis vulgaris (Pso) and PsA and was also tested in AS. In a proof of concept study (n = 38), apremilast 30 mg twice a day showed a numerical (although statistically not significant) reduction for BASDAI, BASFI (Bath Ankylosing Spondylitis Functional Index), and BASMI (=Bath Ankylosing Spondylitis Metrology Index).[99] However, the preliminary results of the phase III double-blind placebo-controlled trial (ClinicalTrials.gov Identifier: NCT01583374) showed no benefit over placebo with regard to the primary endpoint (ASAS20 response rate at week 16: 32.5% for apremilast, 36.6% for placebo), and therefore the future of this mode of action in axial SpA is uncertain.

Other Nonbiologic Treatment Options

Besides the abovementioned treatment options, a broad range of other pharmacologic treatment modalities have been investigated in axial SpA with conflicting results. The data on intravenous (iv) bisphosphonate pamidronate in AS patients is inconsistent,[100–104] resulting in a lack of a clear recommendation for its use in axial SpA.[18,19] Pamidronate showed a dose-dependent effect in AS in a double-blind RCT; patients who received 60 mg of pamidronate iv monthly for 6 months had significantly better clinical outcomes (BASDAI, BASFI, BASMI) than those who received pamidronate 10 mg monthly, whereas no statistical significant differences were seen in acute phase reactants (CRP/erythrocyte sedimentation rate [ESR]) between the two groups.[102] In an open-label trial with a rather small sample size (n = 30), high-dose pamidronate demonstrated similar clinical response rates as the TNFi golimumab, although golimumab was more effective in reduction of objective signs of inflammation (inflammation on MRI, CRP, ASDAS-CRP).[105] Hence, in particular situations, for example, when biologic DMARDs (bDMARDs, i.e., TNFi and IL-17i in axial SpA) are contraindicated or cannot be used in axial SpA patients not responding to conventional therapies, pamidronate might be a therapeutic option.[19] Nonetheless, oral bisphosphonates appear to be ineffective in AS.

One uncontrolled study evaluated the effect of radium chloride in AS patients and showed moderate to good results in reducing pain, disease activity, and improving function with a reasonable safety profile.[106] These findings have not been confirmed so far in prospective RCTs.

The data concerning the application of thalidomide in refractory AS patients seem promising,[107-110] but toxicity is substantial and teratogenic effects and potential side effects (e.g., peripheral neuropathy),[111] which lead to high rates of treatment withdrawal to be taken into account. Therefore, thalidomide might be used in the same situation as pamidronate: contraindications to or unavailability of bDMARDs in axial SpA patients not responding to conventional therapies.

Despite some anecdotal case reports claiming good response to antimalarial medications in AS,[112] no good evidence for the application of antimalarial drugs in AS exists.[113]

Intravenous cyclophosphamide might be efficacious in very active AS patients with predominant peripheral arthritis,[114,115] but as data from RCTs are missing and the potential side effects have to be taken into account, this treatment modality has only a subordinated place in the treatment algorithm of axial SpA.

The intake of probiotics was not superior to placebo in an RCT of (axial and peripheral) spondyloarthritis[116] and therefore cannot be recommended.

SUMMARY

- Despite the recent advances in the treatment of axial SpA with the introduction of biologic DMARDs and other new treatment options on the horizon, nonsteroidal antiinflammatory drugs (NSAIDs) remain the first option of pharmacologic treatment in axial SpA.
- Different NSAIDs (including selective COX-2 inhibitors) seem to be similarly effective in axial SpA and the treatment decision has to be made on an individual basis, taking potential benefits and risks into account.
- Whether NSAIDs have the ability to decrease radiographic progression in the spine in axial SpA still remains a matter of debate.
- Patients with axial disease should not receive long-term treatment with systemic glucocorticoids; short-term courses of high-dose oral glucocorticoids might be an option in particular clinical situations.
- Local steroid injections should be considered in case of predominant peripheral manifestations (arthritis/enthesitis) or isolated unilateral sacroiliitis.
- csDMARDs are usually not effective in reduction of axial symptoms but can be considered in case of peripheral arthritis as a manifestation of axial SpA; sulfasalazine is the preferred csDMARD.
- tsDMARDs are not formally approved for the indication axial SpA thus far; a JAK inhibitor tofacitinib showed promising results in a phase II study; phase III studies with several JAK inhibitors are underway now.

REFERENCES

1. Raychaudhuri SP, Deodhar A. The classification and diagnostic criteria of ankylosing spondylitis. *J Autoimmun.* 2014;48-49:128-133.
2. Rudwaleit M, van der Heijde D, Landewe R, et al. The Assessment of SpondyloArthritis International Society classification criteria for peripheral spondyloarthritis and for spondyloarthritis in general. *Ann Rheum Dis.* 2011;70:25-31.
3. Sieper J, Poddubnyy D. Axial spondyloarthritis. *Lancet.* 2017;390(10089):73-84.
4. Reveille JD, Weisman MH. The epidemiology of back pain, axial spondyloarthritis and HLA-B27 in the United States. *Am J Med Sci.* 2013;345:431-436.
5. Reveille JD, Ball EJ, Khan MA. HLA-B27 and genetic predisposing factors in spondyloarthropathies. *Curr Opin Rheumatol.* 2001;13:265-272.
6. Rudwaleit M, Khan MA, Sieper J. The challenge of diagnosis and classification in early ankylosing spondylitis: do we need new criteria? *Arthritis Rheum.* 2005; 52:1000-1008.
7. Rudwaleit M, Haibel H, Baraliakos X, et al. The early disease stage in axial spondylarthritis: results from the German spondyloarthritis inception cohort. *Arthritis Rheum.* 2009;60:717-727.
8. Rudwaleit M, Sieper J. [Early diagnosis of spondyloarthritis with special attention to the axial forms]. *Z Rheumatol.* 2005;64:524-530.
9. Rudwaleit M, van der Heijde D, Khan MA, Braun J, Sieper J. How to diagnose axial spondyloarthritis early. *Ann Rheum Dis.* 2004;63:535-543.
10. Poddubnyy D, Sieper J. Similarities and differences between nonradiographic and radiographic axial spondyloarthritis: a clinical, epidemiological and therapeutic assessment. *Curr Opin Rheumatol.* 2014;26:377-383.
11. Strand V, Rao SA, Shillington AC, Cifaldi MA, McGuire M, Ruderman EM. Prevalence of axial spondyloarthritis in United States rheumatology practices: assessment of SpondyloArthritis International Society criteria versus rheumatology expert clinical diagnosis. *Arthritis Care Res.* 2013;65:1299-1306.
12. Song IH, Weiss A, Hermann KG, et al. Similar response rates in patients with ankylosing spondylitis and nonradiographic axial spondyloarthritis after 1 year of treatment with etanercept: results from the ESTHER trial. *Ann Rheum Dis.* 2013;72:823-825.
13. Kiltz U, Baraliakos X, Karakostas P, et al. Do patients with non-radiographic axial spondylarthritis differ from patients with ankylosing spondylitis? *Arthritis Care Res.* 2012;64:1415-1422.
14. Ciurea A, Scherer A, Exer P, et al. Tumor necrosis factor alpha inhibition in radiographic and nonradiographic axial spondyloarthritis: results from a large observational cohort. *Arthritis Rheum.* 2013;65:3096-3106.
15. Landewe R, Braun J, Deodhar A, et al. Efficacy of certolizumab pegol on signs and symptoms of axial spondyloarthritis including ankylosing spondylitis: 24-week results

of a double-blind randomised placebo-controlled Phase 3 study. *Ann Rheum Dis.* 2014;73:39–47.

16. Smolen JS, Schols M, Braun J, et al. Treating axial spondyloarthritis and peripheral spondyloarthritis, especially psoriatic arthritis, to target: 2017 update of recommendations by an international task force. *Ann Rheum Dis.* 2018;77(1):3–17.

17. Rademacher J, Poddubnyy D. Emerging drugs for the treatment of axial spondyloarthritis. *Expert Opin Emerg Drugs.* 2018;23(1):83–96.

18. van der Heijde D, Ramiro S, Landewe R, et al. 2016 update of the ASAS-EULAR management recommendations for axial spondyloarthritis. *Ann Rheum Dis.* 2017;76:978–991.

19. Ward MM, Deodhar A, Akl EA, et al. American College of rheumatology/spondylitis association of America/ spondyloarthritis research and treatment network 2015 recommendations for the treatment of ankylosing spondylitis and nonradiographic axial spondyloarthritis. *Arthritis Rheumatol.* 2016;68:282–298.

20. Braun J, Brandt J, Listing J, et al. Treatment of active ankylosing spondylitis with infliximab: a randomised controlled multicentre trial. *Lancet.* 2002;359:1187–1193.

21. van der Heijde D, Kivitz A, Schiff MH, et al. Efficacy and safety of adalimumab in patients with ankylosing spondylitis: results of a multicenter, randomized, double-blind, placebo-controlled trial. *Arthritis Rheum.* 2006;54:2136–2146.

22. Davis Jr JC, Van Der Heijde D, Braun J, et al. Recombinant human tumor necrosis factor receptor (etanercept) for treating ankylosing spondylitis: a randomized, controlled trial. *Arthritis Rheum.* 2003;48:3230–3236.

23. Inman RD, Davis Jr JC, Heijde D, et al. Efficacy and safety of golimumab in patients with ankylosing spondylitis: results of a randomized, double-blind, placebo-controlled, phase III trial. *Arthritis Rheum.* 2008;58:3402–3412.

24. Maksymowych WP, Dougados M, van der Heijde D, et al. Clinical and MRI responses to etanercept in early nonradiographic axial spondyloarthritis: 48-week results from the EMBARK study. *Ann Rheum Dis.* 2016;75:1328–1335.

25. Sieper J, van der Heijde D, Dougados M, et al. Efficacy and safety of adalimumab in patients with non-radiographic axial spondyloarthritis: results of a randomised placebo-controlled trial (ABILITY-1). *Ann Rheum Dis.* 2013; 72:815–822.

26. Sieper J, van der Heijde D, Dougados M, et al. A randomized, double-blind, placebo-controlled, sixteen-week study of subcutaneous golimumab in patients with active nonradiographic axial spondyloarthritis. *Arthritis Rheumatol.* 2015;67:2702–2712.

27. Baeten D, Sieper J, Braun J, et al. Secukinumab, an Interleukin-17A inhibitor, in ankylosing spondylitis. *N Engl J Med.* 2015;373:2534–2548.

28. Dougados M, Gueguen A, Nakache JP, et al. Ankylosing spondylitis: what is the optimum duration of a clinical study? A one year versus a 6 weeks non-steroidal anti-inflammatory drug trial. *Rheumatology.* 1999;38:235–244.

29. van der Heijde D, Baraf HS, Ramos-Remus C, et al. Evaluation of the efficacy of etoricoxib in ankylosing spondylitis: results of a fifty-two-week, randomized, controlled study. *Arthritis Rheum.* 2005;52:1205–1215.

30. Sieper J, Klopsch T, Richter M, et al. Comparison of two different dosages of celecoxib with diclofenac for the treatment of active ankylosing spondylitis: results of a 12-week randomised, double-blind, controlled study. *Ann Rheum Dis.* 2008;67:323–329.

31. Barkhuizen A, Steinfeld S, Robbins J, West C, Coombs J, Zwillich S. Celecoxib is efficacious and well tolerated in treating signs and symptoms of ankylosing spondylitis. *J Rheumatol.* 2006;33:1805–1812.

32. Kroon FP, van der Burg LR, Ramiro S, et al. Nonsteroidal antiinflammatory drugs for axial spondyloarthritis: a Cochrane review. *J Rheumatol.* 2016;43:607–617.

33. Balazcs E, Sieper J, Bickham K, et al. A randomized, clinical trial to assess the relative efficacy and tolerability of two doses of etoricoxib versus naproxen in patients with ankylosing spondylitis. *BMC Musculoskelet Disord.* 2016;17:426.

34. Sieper J, Rudwaleit M, Lenaerts J, et al. Partial remission in ankylosing spondylitis and non-radiographic axial spondyloarthritis in treatment with infliximab plus naproxen or naproxen alone: associations between partial remission and baseline disease characteristics. *Rheumatology.* 2016;55:1946–1953.

35. Peloso PM, Gammaitoni A, Smugar SS, Wang H, Moore AR. Longitudinal numbers-needed-to-treat (NNT) for achieving various levels of analgesic response and improvement with etoricoxib, naproxen, and placebo in ankylosing spondylitis. *BMC Musculoskelet Disord.* 2011;12:165.

36. Sturrock RD, Hart FD. Double-blind cross-over comparison of indomethacin, flurbiprofen, and placebo in ankylosing spondylitis. *Ann Rheum Dis.* 1974;33:129–131.

37. Dougados M, Behier JM, Jolchine I, et al. Efficacy of celecoxib, a cyclooxygenase 2-specific inhibitor, in the treatment of ankylosing spondylitis: a six-week controlled study with comparison against placebo and against a conventional nonsteroidal antiinflammatory drug. *Arthritis Rheum.* 2001;44:180–185.

38. Poddubnyy D, Rudwaleit M, Haibel H, et al. Effect of non-steroidal anti-inflammatory drugs on radiographic spinal progression in patients with axial spondyloarthritis: results from the German Spondyloarthritis Inception Cohort. *Ann Rheum Dis.* 2012;71:1616–1622.

39. Baraliakos X, Kiltz U, Peters S, et al. Efficiency of treatment with non-steroidal anti-inflammatory drugs according to current recommendations in patients with radiographic and non-radiographic axial spondyloarthritis. *Rheumatology.* 2017;56:95–102.

40. Sieper J, Lenaerts J, Wollenhaupt J, et al. Efficacy and safety of infliximab plus naproxen versus naproxen alone in patients with early, active axial spondyloarthritis: results from the double-blind, placebo-controlled INFAST study, Part 1. *Ann Rheum Dis.* 2014;73:101–107.

41. Wang R, Dasgupta A, Ward MM. Comparative efficacy of non-steroidal anti-inflammatory drugs in ankylosing spondylitis: a Bayesian network meta-analysis of clinical trials. *Ann Rheum Dis.* 2016;75:1152–1160.

42. Poddubnyy D, Listing J, Sieper J. Brief report: course of active inflammatory and fatty lesions in patients with early axial spondyloarthritis treated with infliximab plus naproxen as compared to naproxen alone: results from the infliximab as first line therapy in patients with early active axial spondyloarthritis trial. *Arthritis Rheumatol.* 2016;68:1899–1903.

43. Gaidukova IE, Rebrov AP, Nam IF, Kirsanova NV. Etoricoxib in the treatment of active sacroiliitis in patients with axial spondyloarthritis, including ankylosing spondylitis. *Ter Arkh.* 2014;86:42–47.

44. Dubash S, McGonagle D, Marzo-Ortega H. New advances in the understanding and treatment of axial spondyloarthritis: from chance to choice. *Ther Adv Chronic Dis.* 2018;9:77–87.

45. Poddubnyy D, Sieper J. Mechanism of new bone formation in axial spondyloarthritis. *Curr Rheumatol Rep.* 2017;19:55.

46. Neerinckx B, Lories RJ. Structural disease progression in axial spondyloarthritis: still a cause for concern? *Curr Rheumatol Rep.* 2017;19:14.

47. Magrey MN, Khan MA. The paradox of bone formation and bone loss in ankylosing spondylitis: evolving new concepts of bone formation and future trends in management. *Curr Rheumatol Rep.* 2017;19:17.

48. Wanders A, Heijde D, Landewe R, et al. Nonsteroidal antiinflammatory drugs reduce radiographic progression in patients with ankylosing spondylitis: a randomized clinical trial. *Arthritis Rheum.* 2005;52:1756–1765.

49. Kroon F, Landewe R, Dougados M, van der Heijde D. Continuous NSAID use reverts the effects of inflammation on radiographic progression in patients with ankylosing spondylitis. *Ann Rheum Dis.* 2012;71:1623–1629.

50. Sieper J, Listing J, Poddubnyy D, et al. Effect of continuous versus on-demand treatment of ankylosing spondylitis with diclofenac over 2 years on radiographic progression of the spine: results from a randomised multicentre trial (ENRADAS). *Ann Rheum Dis.* 2016;75:1438–1443.

51. Proft F, Muche B, Listing J, Rios-Rodriguez V, Sieper J, Poddubnyy D. Study protocol: COmparison of the effect of treatment with Nonsteroidal anti-inflammatory drugs added to anti-tumour necrosis factor a therapy versus anti-tumour necrosis factor a therapy alone on progression of StrUctural damage in the spine over two years in patients with ankyLosing spondylitis (CONSUL) - an open-label randomized controlled multicenter trial. *BMJ Open.* 2017;7:e014591.

52. Haroon NN, Paterson JM, Li P, Inman RD, Haroon N. Patients with ankylosing spondylitis have increased cardiovascular and cerebrovascular mortality: a population-based study. *Ann Intern Med.* 2015;163:409–416.

53. Zochling J, Braun J. Mortality in ankylosing spondylitis. *Clin Exp Rheumatol.* 2008;26:S80–S84.

54. Exarchou S, Lie E, Lindstrom U, et al. Mortality in ankylosing spondylitis: results from a nationwide population-based study. *Ann Rheum Dis.* 2016;75:1466–1472.

55. Bakland G, Gran JT, Nossent JC. Increased mortality in ankylosing spondylitis is related to disease activity. *Ann Rheum Dis.* 2011;70:1921–1925.

56. Coxib, traditional NTC, Bhala N, et al. Vascular and upper gastrointestinal effects of non-steroidal anti-inflammatory drugs: meta-analyses of individual participant data from randomised trials. *Lancet.* 2013;382:769–779.

57. Schjerning Olsen AM, Fosbol EL, Gislason GH. The impact of NSAID treatment on cardiovascular risk - insight from Danish observational data. *Basic Clin Pharmacol Toxicol.* 2014;115:179–184.

58. Nissen SE, Yeomans ND, Solomon DH, et al. Cardiovascular safety of celecoxib, naproxen, or ibuprofen for arthritis. *N Engl J Med.* 2016;375:2519–2529.

59. Chan FKL, Ching JYL, Tse YK, et al. Gastrointestinal safety of celecoxib versus naproxen in patients with cardiothrombotic diseases and arthritis after upper gastrointestinal bleeding (CONCERN): an industry-independent, double-blind, double-dummy, randomised trial. *Lancet.* 2017;389:2375–2382.

60. Chang JK, Yu CT, Lee MY, et al. Tramadol/acetaminophen combination as add-on therapy in the treatment of patients with ankylosing spondylitis. *Clin Rheumatol.* 2013;32:341–347.

61. Haibel H, Fendler C, Listing J, Callhoff J, Braun J, Sieper J. Efficacy of oral prednisolone in active ankylosing spondylitis: results of a double-blind, randomised, placebo-controlled short-term trial. *Ann Rheum Dis.* 2014;73:243–246.

62. Gaydukova IZ, Rebrov AP, Poddubnyi DA. Efficacy and safety of intravenous methylprednisolone in the treatment of patients with active ankylosing spondylitis: results of a 12-week, prospective, open-label, pilot (METALL) study. *Ter Arkh.* 2015;87:47–52.

63. Mintz G, Enriquez RD, Mercado U, Robles EJ, Jimenez FJ, Gutierrez G. Intravenous methylprednisolone pulse therapy in severe ankylosing spondylitis. *Arthritis Rheum.* 1981;24:734–736.

64. Peters ND, Ejstrup L. Intravenous methylprednisolone pulse therapy in ankylosing spondylitis. *Scand J Rheumatol.* 1992;21:134–138.

65. Yoshida S, Motai Y, Hattori H, Yoshida H, Torikai K. A case of HLA-B27 negative ankylosing spondylitis treated with methylprednisolone pulse therapy. *J Rheumatol.* 1993;20:1805–1806.

66. Axelsen MB, Eshed I, Horslev-Petersen K, et al. A treat-to-target strategy with methotrexate and intra-articular triamcinolone with or without adalimumab effectively reduces MRI synovitis, osteitis and tenosynovitis and halts structural damage progression in early rheumatoid arthritis: results from the OPERA randomised controlled trial. *Ann Rheum Dis.* 2015;74:867–875.

67. Hetland ML, Stengaard-Pedersen K, Junker P, et al. Aggressive combination therapy with intra-articular

glucocorticoid injections and conventional disease-modifying anti-rheumatic drugs in early rheumatoid arthritis: second-year clinical and radiographic results from the CIMESTRA study. *Ann Rheum Dis.* 2008;67:815–822.

68. Ammitzboll-Danielsen M, Ostergaard M, Fana V, et al. Intramuscular versus ultrasound-guided intratenosynovial glucocorticoid injection for tenosynovitis in patients with rheumatoid arthritis: a randomised, double-blind, controlled study. *Ann Rheum Dis.* 2017;76:666–672.

69. Maugars Y, Mathis C, Berthelot JM, Charlier C, Prost A. Assessment of the efficacy of sacroiliac corticosteroid injections in spondylarthropathies: a double-blind study. *Br J Rheumatol.* 1996;35:767–770.

70. Althoff CE, Bollow M, Feist E, et al. CT-guided corticosteroid injection of the sacroiliac joints: quality assurance and standardized prospective evaluation of long-term effectiveness over six months. *Clin Rheumatol.* 2015;34:1079–1084.

71. Zochling J, van der Heijde D, Dougados M, Braun J. Current evidence for the management of ankylosing spondylitis: a systematic literature review for the ASAS/EULAR management recommendations in ankylosing spondylitis. *Ann Rheum Dis.* 2006;65:423–432.

72. van den Berg R, Baraliakos X, Braun J, van der Heijde D. First update of the current evidence for the management of ankylosing spondylitis with non-pharmacological treatment and non-biologic drugs: a systematic literature review for the ASAS/EULAR management recommendations in ankylosing spondylitis. *Rheumatology.* 2012;51:1388–1396.

73. Chen J, Liu C. Is sulfasalazine effective in ankylosing spondylitis? A systematic review of randomized controlled trials. *J Rheumatol.* 2006;33:722–731.

74. Haibel H, Brandt HC, Song IH, et al. No efficacy of subcutaneous methotrexate in active ankylosing spondylitis: a 16-week open-label trial. *Ann Rheum Dis.* 2007;66:419–421.

75. Chen J, Veras MM, Liu C, Lin J. Methotrexate for ankylosing spondylitis. *Cochrane Database Syst Rev.* 2013:CD004524.

76. Chen J, Lin S, Liu C. Sulfasalazine for ankylosing spondylitis. *Cochrane Database Syst Rev.* 2014:CD004800.

77. Haibel H, Rudwaleit M, Braun J, Sieper J. Six months open label trial of leflunomide in active ankylosing spondylitis. *Ann Rheum Dis.* 2005;64:124–126.

78. van Denderen JC, van der Paardt M, Nurmohamed MT, de Ryck YM, Dijkmans BA, van der Horst-Bruinsma IE. Double blind, randomised, placebo controlled study of leflunomide in the treatment of active ankylosing spondylitis. *Ann Rheum Dis.* 2005;64:1761–1764.

79. Braun J, Zochling J, Baraliakos X, et al. Efficacy of sulfasalazine in patients with inflammatory back pain due to undifferentiated spondyloarthritis and early ankylosing spondylitis: a multicentre randomised controlled trial. *Ann Rheum Dis.* 2006;65:1147–1153.

80. Chen J, Liu C. Sulfasalazine for ankylosing spondylitis. *Cochrane Database Syst Rev.* 2005:CD004800.

81. Braun J, Pavelka K, Ramos-Remus C, et al. Clinical efficacy of etanercept versus sulfasalazine in ankylosing spondylitis subjects with peripheral joint involvement. *J Rheumatol.* 2012;39:836–840.

82. Clegg DO, Reda DJ, Abdellatif M. Comparison of sulfasalazine and placebo for the treatment of axial and peripheral articular manifestations of the seronegative spondylarthropathies: a Department of Veterans Affairs cooperative study. *Arthritis Rheum.* 1999;42:2325–2329.

83. Song IH, Hermann K, Haibel H, et al. Effects of etanercept versus sulfasalazine in early axial spondyloarthritis on active inflammatory lesions as detected by whole-body MRI (ESTHER): a 48-week randomised controlled trial. *Ann Rheum Dis.* 2011;70:590–596.

84. Gonzalez-Lopez L, Garcia-Gonzalez A, Vazquez-Del-Mercado M, Munoz-Valle JF, Gamez-Nava JI. Efficacy of methotrexate in ankylosing spondylitis: a randomized, double blind, placebo controlled trial. *J Rheumatol.* 2004;31:1568–1574.

85. Altan L, Bingol U, Karakoc Y, Aydiner S, Yurtkuran M, Yurtkuran M. Clinical investigation of methotrexate in the treatment of ankylosing spondylitis. *Scand J Rheumatol.* 2001;30:255–259.

86. Kehl AS, Corr M, Weisman MH. Review: enthesitis: new insights into pathogenesis, diagnostic modalities, and treatment. *Arthritis Rheumatol.* 2016;68:312–322.

87. Smolen JS, Landewe R, Bijlsma J, et al. EULAR recommendations for the management of rheumatoid arthritis with synthetic and biological disease-modifying antirheumatic drugs: 2016 update. *Ann Rheum Dis.* 2017;76:960–977.

88. Weinblatt ME. Efficacy of methotrexate in rheumatoid arthritis. *Br J Rheumatol.* 1995;34(suppl 2):43–48.

89. van Dongen H, van Aken J, Lard LR, et al. Efficacy of methotrexate treatment in patients with probable rheumatoid arthritis: a double-blind, randomized, placebo-controlled trial. *Arthritis Rheum.* 2007;56:1424–1432.

90. Visser K, van der Heijde D. Optimal dosage and route of administration of methotrexate in rheumatoid arthritis: a systematic review of the literature. *Ann Rheum Dis.* 2009;68:1094–1099.

91. Coates LC, Kavanaugh A, Ritchlin CT, Committee GTG. Systematic review of treatments for psoriatic arthritis: 2014 update for the GRAPPA. *J Rheumatol.* 2014;41:2273–2276.

92. Coates LC, Kavanaugh A, Mease PJ, et al. Group for research and assessment of psoriasis and psoriatic arthritis 2015 treatment recommendations for psoriatic arthritis. *Arthritis Rheumatol.* 2016;68:1060–1071.

93. Gossec L, Smolen JS, Ramiro S, et al. European League against Rheumatism (EULAR) recommendations for the management of psoriatic arthritis with pharmacological therapies: 2015 update. *Ann Rheum Dis.* 2016;75:499–510.

94. Durez P, Horsmans Y. Dramatic response after an intravenous loading dose of azathioprine in one case of severe and refractory ankylosing spondylitis. *Rheumatology.* 2000;39:182–184.

95. Dougados M, Dijkmans B, Khan M, Maksymowych W, van der Linden S, Brandt J. Conventional treatments for ankylosing spondylitis. *Ann Rheum Dis.* 2002;61(suppl 3). iii40–50.

96. Grasedyck K, Schattenkirchner M, Bandilla K. The treatment of ankylosing spondylitis with auranofin (Ridaura). *Z Rheumatol.* 1990;49:98–99.

97. Geher P, Gomor B. Repeated cyclosporine therapy of peripheral arthritis associated with ankylosing spondylitis. *Med Sci Monit.* 2001;7:105–107.

98. van der Heijde D, Deodhar A, Wei JC, et al. Tofacitinib in patients with ankylosing spondylitis: a phase II, 16-week, randomised, placebo-controlled, dose-ranging study. *Ann Rheum Dis.* 2017;76:1340–1347.

99. Pathan E, Abraham S, Van Rossen E, et al. Efficacy and safety of apremilast, an oral phosphodiesterase 4 inhibitor, in ankylosing spondylitis. *Ann Rheum Dis.* 2013;72:1475–1480.

100. Haibel H, Brandt J, Rudwaleit M, Soerensen H, Sieper J, Braun J. Treatment of active ankylosing spondylitis with pamidronate. *Rheumatology.* 2003;42:1018–1020.

101. Grover R, Shankar S, Aneja R, Marwaha V, Gupta R, Kumar A. Treatment of ankylosing spondylitis with pamidronate: an open label study. *Ann Rheum Dis.* 2006; 65:688–689.

102. Maksymowych WP, Jhangri GS, Fitzgerald AA, et al. A six-month randomized, controlled, double-blind, dose-response comparison of intravenous pamidronate (60 mg versus 10 mg) in the treatment of nonsteroidal antiinflammatory drug-refractory ankylosing spondylitis. *Arthritis Rheum.* 2002;46:766–773.

103. Cairns AP, Wright SA, Taggart AJ, Coward SM, Wright GD. An open study of pulse pamidronate treatment in severe ankylosing spondylitis, and its effect on biochemical markers of bone turnover. *Ann Rheum Dis.* 2005;64: 338–339.

104. Viapiana O, Gatti D, Idolazzi L, et al. Bisphosphonates vs infliximab in ankylosing spondylitis treatment. *Rheumatology.* 2014;53:90–94.

105. Mok CC, Li OC, Chan KL, Ho LY, Hui PK. Effect of golimumab and pamidronate on clinical efficacy and MRI inflammation in axial spondyloarthritis: a 48-week open randomized trial. *Scand J Rheumatol.* 2015;44:480–486.

106. Alberding A, Stierle H, Brandt J, Braun J. Effectiveness and safety of radium chloride in the treatment of ankylosing spondylitis. Results of an observational study. *Z Rheumatol.* 2006;65:245–251.

107. Choudhury MR, Hassan MM, Kabir ME, Rabbani MG, Haq SA, Rahman MK. An open label clinical trial of thalidomide in NSAIDs refractory ankylosing spondylitis. *Mod Rheumatol.* 2018:1–3.

108. Wei JC, Chan TW, Lin HS, Huang F, Chou CT. Thalidomide for severe refractory ankylosing spondylitis: a 6-month open-label trial. *J Rheumatol.* 2003;30:2627–2631.

109. Huang F, Gu J, Zhao W, Zhu J, Zhang J, Yu DT. One-year open-label trial of thalidomide in ankylosing spondylitis. *Arthritis Rheum.* 2002;47:249–254.

110. Breban M, Gombert B, Amor B, Dougados M. Efficacy of thalidomide in the treatment of refractory ankylosing spondylitis. *Arthritis Rheum.* 1999;42:580–581.

111. Xue HX, Fu WY, Cui HD, Yang LL, Zhang N, Zhao LJ. High-dose thalidomide increases the risk of peripheral neuropathy in the treatment of ankylosing spondylitis. *Neural Regen Res.* 2015;10:814–818.

112. Granier S, Waxman J. A case of ankylosing spondylitis treated with hydroxychloroquine. *J Clin Rheumatol.* 1995; 1:136.

113. Williamson L, Illingworth H, Smith D, Mowat A. Oral quinine in ankylosing spondylitis: a randomized placebo controlled double blind crossover trial. *J Rheumatol.* 2000;27:2054–2055.

114. Sadowska-Wroblewska M, Garwolinska H, Maczynska-Rusiniak B. A trial of cyclophosphamide in ankylosing spondylitis with involvement of peripheral joints and high disease activity. *Scand J Rheumatol.* 1986;15:259–264.

115. Fricke R, Petersen D. Treatment of ankylosing spondylitis with cyclophosphamide and azathioprine. *Verh Dtsch Ges Rheumatol.* 1969;1:189–195.

116. Jenks K, Stebbings S, Burton J, Schultz M, Herbison P, Highton J. Probiotic therapy for the treatment of spondyloarthritis: a randomized controlled trial. *J Rheumatol.* 2010;37:2118–2125.

CHAPTER 15

Biologic Treatment of Axial Spondyloarthritis

FILIP VAN DEN BOSCH, MD, PHD • PHILIPPE CARRON, MD, PHD • PHILIP MEASE, MD, MACR

DISCLOSURES

Filip Van den Bosch has received speaker and/or consultancy fees from AbbVie, Bristol-Myers Squibb, Celgene, Eli Lilly, Galapagos, Janssen, Merck, Novartis, Pfizer, and UCB.

Philippe Carron has received speaker and/or consultancy fees from AbbVie, Bristol-Myers Squibb, Celgene, Janssen, Merck, Novartis, Pfizer, and UCB.

Philip Mease has received research grants, consultation fees, and/or speaker honoraria: Abbvie, Amgen, Boehringer Ingelheim, Bristol Myers, Celgene, Galapagos, Genentech, Gilead, Janssen, Lilly, Novartis, Pfizer, SUN Pharma, UCB.

INTRODUCTION AND BACKGROUND

Until about two decades ago, the management of AS was rather limited: patients were educated about the chronic nature of the inflammation in the spine and were advised to perform exercises in combination with (supervised) physical therapy. The only available pharmacologic treatments were nonsteroidal antiinflammatory drugs (NSAIDs), which provided fast symptomatic relief, however, with a fast relapse of symptoms after discontinuation. In contrast to rheumatoid arthritis (RA), conventional synthetic (cs) disease-modifying antirheumatic drugs (DMARDs) have no proven long-term benefit in AS and "clinical remission" was utopic in those days. The treatment paradigm of AS changed dramatically because of the advent of biologic DMARDs (bDMARDs) at the end of the previous millennium, with the first agents (infliximab, etanercept) targeting the proinflammatory cytokine tumor necrosis factor-alpha (TNFα). The first clinical trials in the 1990s focused on patients with active RA and demonstrated a rapid improvement in signs and symptoms,[1] consequent amelioration of physical function and quality of life, and finally also retardation of structural damage (erosions, joint space narrowing) as a consequence of inhibition of chronic uncontrolled inflammation.

Around the same time, promising efficacy was also demonstrated with the anti-TNFα monoclonal antibody infliximab in patients with active Crohn disease.[2] The link between (subclinical) inflammatory bowel disease and multiple diseases of the SpA concept on one hand (reviewed in Van Praet et al.[3]), and the demonstration of TNFα in sacroiliac joint biopsy specimens on the other hand,[4] sparked the interest to investigate TNF blockade in (axial) SpA. German investigators[5,6] performed the first investigator-initiated trials in the specific SpA subgroup of AS patients, demonstrating a fast symptomatic improvement after infliximab administration. At the same time, a Belgian research group provided preliminary evidence that infliximab was also efficacious in the broader SpA concept.[7,8] In the following years, the experience with etanercept[9] and infliximab was further expanded with large phase 3 trial programs in AS (as well as PsA[10]), and evidence for the efficacy of other members of the TNF inhibitor class (adalimumab, golimumab) gradually accumulated.

Although the major improvements observed in AS patients were of course a blessing for patients with longstanding disease and already apparent structural damage, it also uncovered an increasing unmet need: given the well-recognized long delay in AS patients between symptom onset and diagnosis, a growing group of patients with early axial inflammatory disease was denied effective treatment, simply because an arbitrary cutoff for radiographic sacroiliitis (at least bilateral grade 2 or at least unilateral grade 3) could not (yet) be demonstrated on conventional X-rays. This prompted the Assessment in SpondyloArthritis International Society (ASAS) to start the development of new classification criteria for the broader concept of axSpA, including early forms without definitive structural damage. These early disease stages are now commonly referred to as "nonradiographic axial SpA" (nr-axSpA). The availability of magnetic resonance imaging (MRI), which can detect active inflammation of the sacroiliac joints before structural lesions are seen

Axial Spondyloarthritis. https://doi.org/10.1016/B978-0-323-56800-5.00015-1

on plain radiographs, has further strengthened this clinical concept of early disease. In summary, while before the publication of the ASAS axSpA classification criteria in 2009, the focus was primarily on trials in patients fulfilling mNY criteria for AS, there was an increased recognition of the importance of the nr-axSpA population after publication of the criteria and a need to demonstrate efficacy of biologics in this population as well as in AS. Post 2009, both separate and combined trials of biologics in nr-axSpA and AS (e.g., certolizumab) were conducted. Evolving treatment recommendations (discussed in Chapter 16) also gradually reflected this broader patient population. At the same time, the therapeutic armamentarium also progressively broadened with—besides TNFi—also newer agents targeting other inflammatory cytokines, such as the ones involved in the Th17 axis. In this chapter, we will discuss the different biologic treatments available to patients with axSpA, as well as treatment strategies to optimally utilize these agents.

BIOLOGIC DMARD TREATMENT OPTIONS IN AXIAL SPONDYLOARTHRITIS

Over the past 20 years, basic researchers in the field of SpA have identified a significant number of potential culprit immune cells and cytokines. Although some of these showed interesting data in animal data or in vitro experiments, in reality, the most convincing test whether a particular proinflammatory mediator plays a role in axSpA is to determine whether targeted therapies against the putative mediator are effective in controlling the disease. Three mediators have been demonstrated to play a role in AS based on that criterion.[11] The first

group of medications shown to control disease activity in some patients with AS was NSAIDs, suggesting that cyclooxygenase-2-dependent inflammation was important in maintaining disease activity.[12] Subsequently, therapeutic trials have focused on those patients whose disease activity is resistant to NSAIDs. A key insight in the pathogenesis was the discovery of the important role played by proinflammatory cytokines such as tumor necrosis factor (TNF).[4,13] bDMARDs are proteins developed by biotechnological techniques, which can block inflammatory cytokines via different mechanisms (Fig. 15.1): most frequently, this is achieved by designing monoclonal antibodies against the cytokine or its receptors (generic drug name ending in "-mab"); an alternative way is the construction of a molecule consisting of a soluble cytokine receptor coupled to the constant fragment (Fc) of an immunoglobulin (generic drug name ending in "-cept"); finally, there is also the possibility to design receptor antagonists.

However, despite the impressive efficacy of TNF-blocking agents in clinical trials and real-world evidence, some patients do not or only partially respond to TNF antagonism. This might be attributable to lower levels of TNF expression, the involvement of other proinflammatory cytokines, and/or the development of neutralizing antibodies against the TNF-blocking agent during treatment. It is clear that despite the likely importance of TNF, many of the cellular and molecular mechanisms in AS remain unknown,[11] with multiple reports supporting the view that the T-helper (Th)-17 axis plays an important role.[14–16]

If one wants to study the efficacy of a new drug, it is of course important to define relevant outcomes, to evaluate

Selective Cytokine Blockade

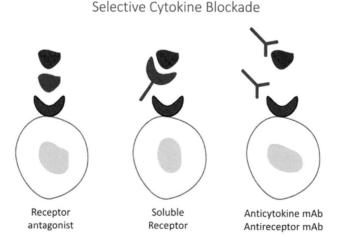

FIG. 15.1 Several types of mechanisms to block inflammatory cytokines.

patients in a standardized way, and to capture all aspects of the disease. In a disease such as axSpA, outcomes may vary substantially because of the heterogenic presentation. In 1999, the Assessment of Spondyloarthritis International Society (ASAS)—under Outcome Measures in Rheumatoid Arthritis Clinical Trials (OMERACT) auspices—defined a core set of variables to be measured in patients with AS, by applying the OMERACT filter for use in clinical trials and daily practice[17,18]: for the specific setting of "disease-controlling antirheumatic treatment," which would include the broad group of bDMARDs, important domains were identified and specific instruments to be used in clinical trials were selected: these are reviewed in Chapter 9. In the next paragraphs, we will discuss biologic agents that target TNF, IL17, and IL12/23, as well as some preliminary data regarding drugs with other mode of action. Effect on signs and symptoms (assessed by BASDAI, ASAS 20/40 responses, and more recently ASDAS) and potential retardation of structural damage (evaluated by the mSASSS score of conventional X-rays of cervical and lumbar spine) will be systematically described.

TNF Inhibitors

In most countries worldwide, there are currently five approved original TNF inhibitors (TNFi) for the treatment of patients with active AS. Of these, four are monoclonal antibodies directed against TNFα (infliximab, adalimumab, golimumab, and certolizumab), with the fifth (etanercept) being a soluble receptor composed of the TNF p75 receptor fused to human IgG1. In Europe and a number of other countries worldwide (but as yet not in the United States), adalimumab, certolizumab, etanercept, and golimumab have also been approved for patients with nr-axSpA. In phase 3 studies, clinically important responses (ASAS 40% response rate) have been demonstrated in 39% up to 48% of patients with AS, with comparable responses (35%–60%) in nr-axSpA (Fig. 15.2).[19-23] The improvement in signs and symptoms of axial inflammation has been consistently associated with significant decreases in objective measures of inflammation, such as C-reactive protein or inflammatory lesions on MRI of the sacroiliac joints and/or spine. Despite the fact that there are no formal clinical trials on peripheral arthritis in axSpA patients, there is little doubt that TNFi also have efficacy on these manifestations with peripheral joint involvement, which is corroborated by the convincing efficacy of these drugs in peripheral psoriatic arthritis.[10] Finally, agents targeting TNF are also efficacious for the treatment of extraarticular manifestations, with relatively comparable efficacy of all agents on psoriatic skin disease, but a differential effect on gut and eye disease, where etanercept is not (gut) or less effective (eye) than TNF-blocking monoclonal antibodies[24,25] Based on these data, TNFi are indicated in axSpA patients with persistently active spinal disease (defined as BASDAI ≥4 or ASDAS ≥2.1), which have failed adequate NSAID therapy (for at least 4 weeks); for the indication of nr-axSpA, the additional presence of objective measures of inflammation (either elevated CRP or inflammation on MRI of the sacroiliac joints) is mandatory for the European approval.

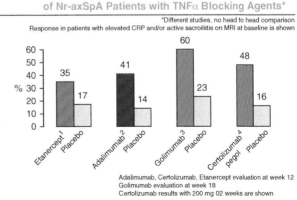

ASAS 40 Response after 24 Weeks of Treatment of AS Patients with TNFα Blocking Agents*

*Different studies, no head to head comparison

ASAS 40 Response after 12 (16) Weeks of Treatment of Nr-axSpA Patients with TNFα Blocking Agents*

*Different studies, no head to head comparison
Response in patients with elevated CRP and/or active sacroiliitis on MRI at baseline is shown

Adalimumab, Certolizumab, Etanercept evaluation at week 12
Golimumab evaluation at week 18
Certolizumab results with 200 mg 02 weeks are shown

1. van der Heijde D et al Arthritis Rheum 2005;52:582-91
2. Davis JC et al Ann Rheum Dis 2005;64:1557-62
3. van der Heijde D et al. Arthritis Rheum 2006;54:2136-45
4. Inman RD et al Arthritis Rheum 2008;58:3402 12
5. Landewé et al Ann Rheum Dis 2014;73:39-47

1. Dougados M et al Arthritis Rheumatol 2014;66:2091-102:Pfizer date on file
2. Sieper J et al Ann Rheum Dis 2013;72:815-22
3. Sieper J et al Arthritis Rheumatol 2015
4. Landewé et al Ann Rheum Dis 2014;73:39-47

FIG. 15.2 ASAS 40% responses with TNFi in patients with AS and nr-axSpA.

Recently, biosimilars have also entered the field of rheumatology. A "biosimilar" is defined by the World Health Organization (WHO) as a "biotherapeutic product" which is similar in terms of quality, safety and efficacy to an already licensed reference biotherapeutic product (REF: World Health Organization. Expert Committee on Biological Standardization. Guidelines on evaluation of similar biotherapeutic products. Geneva, 2009. http://www.who.int/biologicals/areas/biological); "similarity" is defined as the "absence of a relevant difference in the parameter of interest." CT-P13 has an identical amino acid sequence to infliximab and is produced in the same type of cell line; it exhibits highly similar in vitro and in vivo pharmacodynamics, binding specificities and affinities, and other biologic characteristics.[26,27] CT-P13 has shown equivalent clinical efficacy to the innovator infliximab in a small number of clinical trials, including the PLANETAS (program evaluating the autoimmune disease investigational drug CT-P13 in AS patients) trial, a randomized phase 1 trial in 250 patients with active AS.[27] In this trial, treatment with CT-P13 demonstrated equivalent efficacy to infliximab up to week 30 (ASAS 40% response rate of 52% and 47%, OR 1.19, 95% CI 0.70–2.00). Multiple other response measures were also comparable, and there were no differences detected in immunogenicity or safety. Follow-up of the PLANETAS trial provided evidence for sustained efficacy of the biosimilar up to 54 weeks, as well as preliminary data on switching between the biooriginator and the biosimilar.[28,29] The initial trials of CT-P13 were the first clinical trials comparing a biosimilar with an innovator biologic agent for a rheumatic disease.[30] Comparable results regarding equivalent efficacy up to 52 weeks and switching are now also available for SB4 and reference product etanercept in RA.[31,32] The worldwide availability of these agents will depend on regulatory requirements in different regions and local patent laws and patent expiration dates.[30]

Given the link between control of inflammation and inhibition of structural damage (erosions, joint space narrowing) that has been observed with all TNFi in RA and PsA, the initial results regarding retardation of structural damage in AS were rather disappointing. Because of the slow rate of radiographic progression as measured by the mSASSS score, randomized, placebo-controlled trials are not considered ethical in axSpA. Initial comparison of the radiographic progression after 2 years of TFNi therapy (infliximab, etanercept, and adalimumab) to a historical cohort not exposed to bDMARDs could not demonstrate a significant difference (Fig. 15.3).

However, based on the association between disease activity (ASDAS) and subsequent structural damage in AS patients,[33] there is now accumulating circumstantial evidence that TNFi may inhibit syndesmophyte formation after a longer period of time (≥4 years) via the inhibition of inflammatory activity.[34–36]

Regarding safety, the major advantage of the TNFi class is the fact that these agents have been commercially available for almost 20 years with a vast amount of real-world registry data; this is probably the major driver for the statement on the choice of the first bDMARD in the ASAS/EULAR treatment recommendations for axSpA that "current practice is to start with TNFi therapy." Infection remains the most common adverse effect, with data suggesting a somewhat higher risk in the first 6–12 months of treatment; for general infections, no relevant differences are observed between agents. In daily practice, it is important to take other risk factors for infection into account (age, presence of comorbidities, concomitant medication, etc.). A well-known risk is the reactivation of latent tuberculosis, which seems to be higher in patients using monoclonal antibodies, compared with etanercept. However, the recommendation of appropriate TB prevention procedures has largely overcome this problem. Finally, regarding malignancies, the current evidence seems to suggest that there is no significant increase in the risk of solid cancers in patients using TNFi compared with bDMARD-naïve patients. Data on lymphoma also seem to be reassuring, especially because SpA—in contrast to RA—does not seem to be associated with an inherent higher a priori risk.

Predictors of Response to TNFi Treatment in axSpA

It is relevant to identify predictors before start of treatment, which are able to identify patients that will have a beneficial response to biologic therapy in axSpA patients, especially considering the economic burden and potential side effects of these agents. Although the majority of AS patients respond very well to TNF-blocking therapy, a significant proportion of patients have to withdraw from treatment because of inefficacy or adverse events. In clinical practice, the reported 1-year and 2-year treatment survival rates are 70%–85% and 60%–75%, respectively.[72–75]

The presence of inflammation at baseline was found to be an important independent predictor of achieving response to TNF-blocking therapy in almost all studies in AS patients. Increased levels of CRP or ESR were predictive for BASDAI50, ASAS20, ASAS40, ASAS partial remission, and AS Disease Activity Score (ASDAS)

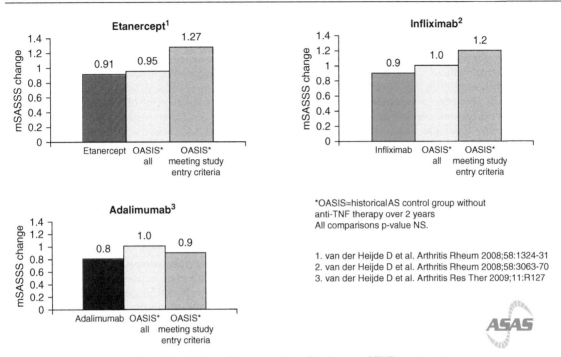

FIG. 15.3 Radiographic progression after 2 years of TNFi treatment.

major improvement,[72,73,76–83] as well as for continuation of TNFα-blocking therapy.[72–74,84] The presence of peripheral arthritis was also identified as a predictor of both response (BASDAI50 and ASAS20) and treatment continuation.[72,75] Higher Berlin MRI spine score (reflecting the extent of bone marrow edema) was shown to be predictive for BASDAI50 response.[85] In patients with nr-axSpA, a baseline SPARCC MRI score ≥2 for either the SI joint or the spine was associated with better response after 12 weeks of adalimumab.[20] These results clearly indicate that axSpA patients with active inflammatory disease are more likely to benefit from TNFi therapy than patients with chronic, less inflammatory disease. The ASDAS, a composite score of patient-reported measures and acute phase reactants, was found to be an independent predictor of ASAS20 and ASAS40 response.[72] Furthermore, clinical responders had significantly higher ASDAS scores at baseline than nonresponders.[86] Multiple studies have identified a better functional status as an independent baseline predictor of clinical response to TNFi treatment. Lower Bath AS Functional Index (BASFI) score (indicating better physical function) was found to be related to

BASDAI50, ASAS20, ASAS40, and ASAS partial remission.[73,76,78–81] In addition, lower Bath AS Metrology Index (BASMI)[81] and lower modified Schober test (reflecting less severe restriction of spinal mobility) were predictive for ASAS partial remission and BASDAI50 response, respectively.[72] Younger age was identified as a predictor of BASDAI50, ASAS20, ASAS40, and ASAS partial remission,[72,73,80,81] and shorter disease duration was related to BASDAI50 and ASAS40 response.[76] The fact that younger AS patients with shorter disease duration and better functional status respond better to TNFi may indicate that less structural damage has occurred and more acute inflammation is present in these patients.[76] Male sex was found to be predictive for both response (BASDAI50, ASAS20, and ASAS40)[72] and treatment continuation.[72–75] Two studies[80,81] that included a very large number of patients in their analyses identified HLA-B27 positivity as a predictor of BASDAI50, ASAS40, and ASAS partial remission. It is unclear whether this predictive value can be explained by the fact that HLA-B27 positivity results in earlier diagnosis or that the disease biology differs between HLA-B27-positive and HLA-B27-negative patients.[80]

Until now, no biomarker or a set of biomarkers have been found to predict clearly the response to TNFi. For evaluating TNFi, not only the response regarding disease activity but also the effect on disease-related quality of life and radiographic outcome is important. A first step has been taken to create a prediction model that provides a potential basis for patient selection for TNFα-blocking therapy. Age, BASFI, enthesitis, CRP, and HLA-B27 were associated with outcomes in AS. Their combined use enables adequate prediction of outcome resulting from anti-TNF and conventional therapy in various AS sub-populations.[80] The development of such a prediction model may lead to a more robust instrument to support physicians to make evidence-based decisions to start anti-TNFα treatment in daily clinical practice.

IL17 Inhibitors

Serum concentrations of IL-23 and IL-17 have been found to be high in patients with AS.[37] Macrophages from patients with AS in response to lipopolysaccharide produce high levels of IL-23.[38] IL-17-positive cells in AS facet joints also have been demonstrated.[39] In addition to AS and PsA, high levels of IL-17 in the synovial fluid of patients with reactive arthritis and undifferentiated SpA have been reported.[40]

Currently, several agents blocking IL-17 are available (secukinumab) or still under investigation (ixekizumab, brodalumab, and bimekizumab). Given the importance of the IL-17/IL-23 axis in SpA, this pathway became an obvious novel therapeutic target. Secukinumab and ixekizumab target IL-17A, bimekizumab targets IL-17A and IL-17F, whilst brodalumab targets the IL-17 receptor, thus inhibiting all forms of IL-17. Secukinumab and ixekizumab are approved for the treatment of psoriasis and psoriatic arthritis and brodalumab is approved for the treatment of psoriasis.

Two placebo controlled phase III trials in AS (MEASURE 1 and 2) were recently reported, showing positive responses, regardless of prior anti-TNFα exposure.[16,41,42] In the MEASURE 2 trial, 43.2% of subjects treated with secukinumab 150mg monthly achieved ASAS40 responses in the TNFi naive group and 25% in the TNFi experienced group at week 16 and was sustained over time.[43] These studies also demonstrated significant improvement in other key domains of AS including physical function and quality of life. Prevention of structural damage is a long-term treatment goal in AS. The mean change in mSASSS through 2 years of secukinumab therapy was 0.30 (SD 2.53) overall and 0.38 -0.52 among patients with known predictors of radiographic progression at baseline, such as syndesmophytes or elevated CRP.[43] The 4-year follow up data has just been published

and it shows sustained efficacy of secukinumab, and 79% of patients showed no radiographic progression (mSASSS change from baseline <2).[43a] The low overall rate of progression seen with secukinumab is very encouraging but requires further exploration in long-term controlled studies before definite conclusions can be reached on whether anti-IL-17A therapy is effective in inhibiting mSASSS progression in patients with AS.

Secukinumab showed an acceptable safety profile over 622.5 patient-years of exposure, with no new safety signals or unexpected safety findings compared with the first 52 weeks 16 or with the safety profile reported in PsA and psoriasis.[44,45] The incidence of AEs was higher with 150mg than with 75mg, driven primarily by nonserious infections. The most common AEs with secukinumab were nasopharyngitis, diarrhea, headache, upper respiratory tract infections, and pharyngitis. Serious infections were infrequent in both secukinumab groups. Candida infections, a known risk with IL-17 inhibitors given the role of IL-17 in mucosal defense,[46] were infrequent (0.7 cases per 100 patient-years of secukinumab exposure), mild, and clinically manageable with antifungals. No dose dependence was observed for other safety risks. Crohn disease was reported as a nonserious AE in four patients in the 75mg group (of whom two had a history of Crohn disease and one had a history of a polyp and colon adenoma) and one patient in the 150mg group, equivalent to 0.8 cases per 100 patient-years of secukinumab exposure.[43]

Ixekizumab has also demonstrated significant improvement in AS (also known as radiographic AxSpA in these studies).[46a,46b] In the COAST-V trial, in patients naive to biologic agents, ASAS 40 responses were demonstrated in 52%, 48%, and 18% in subjects treated with 80 mg ixekizumab every 2 week, 4 weeks and placebo at 16 weeks.[46a] In the COAST-W study of patients previously treated with 1 or 2 anti-TNF agents, the same dose regimen also showed significant ASAS 40 improvements.[46b] Similar to secukinumab, other key domains such as function and quality of life also improved in both studies.

Bimekizumab, targeting both IL-17A and IL-17F, is currently under study.

IL23 Inhibitors

Knowledge of the involvement of the IL-23/Th17 pathway in SpA comes from limited clinical investigations. It has been reported that polymorphisms in the receptor for IL-23 are associated with AS, and thus, IL-23 and its receptor system are likely to play a critical role in the disease susceptibility and the pathogenic of AS.[47]

Ustekinumab is a humanized monoclonal antibody directed against the shared p40 subunit of IL

23 and IL12. In a phase III placebo-controlled RCT in PsA (PSUMMIT2), ustekinumab led to significant and sustained clinical improvement in both skin and joint symptoms (including TNFi-experienced patients).[48] The efficacy and safety of ustekinumab was also evaluated in a prospective, open-label, proof-of-concept study in AS patients, showing high ASAS40 response (in 65%) at week 24.[14] A phase III, multicenter, randomized, double-blind, placebo-controlled study evaluating the efficacy and safety of ustekinumab in the treatment of subjects with active axSpA was stopped because neither dose of ustekinumab achieved the study's primary or major secondary endpoints.[49] Furthermore, treatment with risankizumab, a monoclonal antibody that selectively inhibits IL-23 by specifically targeting the p19 subunit, did not meet the study primary endpoint and showed no evidence of clinically meaningful improvements compared with placebo in patients with active AS, suggesting that IL-23 may not be a relevant driver of disease pathogenesis and symptoms in AS.[50] Tildrakizumab, another selective interleukin IL-23 p19 inhibitor, is currently being studied, and no efficacy data are available.

Other Agents

Biologic drugs targeting other cytokines or cytokine receptors such as IL-1 and IL-6, or controlling B and T lymphocytes, have been tested in small uncontrolled or controlled trials in SpA. Trials on anakinra,[51,52] abatacept,[53] rituximab,[54,55] tocilizumab,[56] and sarilumab[57] have shown no consistent efficacy. Small immunomodulating molecules, such as JAK inhibitors (e.g., tofacitinib, baricitinib, upadacitinib, and filgotinib)—interfering with intracellular proinflammatory pathways—may be promising new treatment options, and tofacitinib has yielded initial positive results in phase II trials with AS patients.[58]

AREAS OF SPECIAL INTEREST

Treatment Paradigms

The concept of treat to target

The 2017 updated EULAR recommendations for axSpA and PsA focus on a treat-to-target strategy.[59] They indicate that treat-to-target should be the standard and general approach to care of SpA. The targets to be achieved within 3–6 months of starting therapy are defined as "remission" or, alternatively, "low or minimal disease activity." Patients should be assessed regularly and, if the target is not attained, treatment should be escalated to the next phase of the algorithm. The ASDAS for axial SpA is recommended. Shared decision-making between the clinician and the patient is seen as pivotal to the

process. The task force defined the treatment target for SpA as remission or low disease activity and developed a large research agenda to further advance the field.

Although no treat-to-target study has yet been performed in axial SpA, it is deemed that such an approach could also improve outcomes in axial SpA, given the correlation of damage progression with disease activity.[33,60] Currently, a trial on treatment to target in axSpA is being performed (TICOSPA, NCT03043846).

The Concept of Treat to Remission and Withdrawal of Treatment Tapering and TNF blockade discontinuation strategies in axial SpA

Published data indicate that a tapering strategy for anti-TNF therapy is successful in maintaining remission or low disease activity (LDA) in most patients with axial spondyloarthritis (Table 15.1).[61–68] In addition, trials were set up to evaluate the efficacy of an anti-TNF discontinuation strategy for maintaining low disease activity or remission in patients with axSpA (mainly AS) after achieving this state with a standard dose of anti-TNF therapy. In most cases, discontinuation of anti-TNF therapy led to the appearance of flare within a few months in most cases (Table 15.2).[69–74] In rheumatoid arthritis, there is accumulating evidence for a so-called "window of opportunity," referring to the existence of a transient time frame in which the disease is more susceptible to treatment.[75] It was shown that response to treatment was markedly higher in early forms of axial disease with high rates of clinical remission.[76] However, given the observation of a higher chance of obtaining remission or low disease activity with biologic treatment in an early stage of the disease,[76] one could speculate that there is at least also a possibility of a "window of opportunity" for drug-free remission in axial SpA. Moreover, in ongoing trials in axial Spa, there is a marked interest in the exploration of a therapy withdrawal strategy upon induction of clinical remission by a TNF-blocking agent in more early stages of the disease to achieve biologic-free remission or even the ultimate goal of therapy, drug-free remission, resembling recovery (ClinicalTrials.gov: NCT01808118 [adalimumab]; NCT02509026 [etanercept]; NCT02505542 [certolizumab pegol]; NCT02407223 [ustekinumab]).

Immunogenicity—How Much of a Problem Is This in axSpA and Should It Be Addressed?

Because biologic agents are proteins, there is the potential that the human immune system could perceive them as foreign proteins and generate antidrug antibodies (ADAbs) directed against them, leading to

TABLE 15.1
Tapering Strategies in axSpA Patients

	Lee et al.[61]	Navarro-Compán et al.[62]	Paccou et al.[63]	Cantini et al.[64]	Morck et al.[65]	Borras-Blasco et al.[66]	De Stefano et al.[67]	Zavada et al.[68]
Patients with tapering	109	16	49	22	19	8	21	53
Age, years	35	43	45	37	40	–	44	41
Male (%)	90	87	79	79	74	–	76	75
Disease duration, years	9	8	14	13	8	–	3	9
Synthetic DMARDs (%)	94	31	10	–	100	–	–	11
Anti-TNF	ETA	ETA	ADA (5), ETA (17), INF(25)	ETA	INF	ETA	ETA	ADA ETA or INF
Remission maintenance (%)	–	–	ml2: 80% ADA, 53% ETA, 81% INF	86	–	100	67	75
Most frequent regimen	25 mg/12 d	25 mg/w	40 mg/3 w	50 mg/2 w	3 mg/kg/8 w	25 mg/w	25 mg/2 w	Increasing interval

d, days; *w*, weeks.

formation of immune complexes of the therapeutic protein and ADAbs.[77] These complexes may result in increased clearance and reduced serum levels of the biologic agent and/or may have a neutralizing effect on target binding, resulting in reduced or loss of effect or rarely, adverse effects such as infusion reactions. Fortunately, development of ADAbs is not common and only rarely neutralizing. Some drugs may be more immunogenic than others, e.g., infliximab because of the mouse component of its molecular construct. The phenomenon is rather well-described rheumatoid arthritis (RA), where it has been shown that concomitant use of methotrexate (MTX), even in small doses such as 10 mg/week, may abrogate the formation of ADAbs. Thus, it is generally recommended that MTX be used in conjunction with infliximab, for example, to prevent immunogenicity. Often, this strategy is used with adalimumab as well. This practice is more controversial in axSpA, because there is not an intrinsic reason to use MTX, as it does not seem to be helpful for disease treatment, unlike its potential utility in RA, and thus would not be routinely used as a background medication. In patients with AS, ADAbs have been described with infliximab[78] and adalimumab.[79]

Is it important to consider immunogenicity in axSpA and might there be a role for use of MTX to abrogate ADAbs in this disease? So far, there are no direct data to support the concept that addition of csDMARDs, such as MTX, could decrease the titer of ADAbs in patients with axSpA, and the scarce evidence comes from registry data on drug survival of TNFi. Data from the Swedish national biologics registry ARTIS on 1365 AS patients initiating a TNFi between 2003 and 2010 suggested a better 5-year retention rate to the first TNFi in patients on csDMARD comedication at baseline.[80] In an accompanying editorial, a number of issues that make interpretation of this type of data difficult were pointed out[81]: confounding by indication; no direct measurement of efficacy or safety, but instead a "proxy" of this combination, being TNFi retention; and the use of several types of csDMARDs and TNFi, which in turn might have been dependent on several factors, such as start date of the treatment and perceived beliefs about the relative potency of some TNFi. In contrast, a prospective cohort study from the Rheumatic Diseases Portuguese Register on 954 SpA patients starting treatment with a first TNFi between 2001 and 2014 demonstrated a high rate of long-term

TABLE 15.2
Discontinuation Strategies in axSpA

	Brandt et al.[70]	Baraliakos et al.[71]	Song et al.[72]	Deng et al.[73]	Haibel et al.[74]
Number of patients, AS/nr-axSpA	26/0	42/0	6vsll	111/0	0/24
Patients who discontinued	26	42	17	111 (thalidomide vs. SSZ or NSAID)	24
Control group	No	No	No	No	No
Follow-up, weeks	36	52	52	52	52
Age, years	37	40	34	18–57	38
Male	77	65	71	–	45
Disease duration, years	Mean (s.d.) 14(9)	Mean (s.d.) 15(9)	All patients <5 symptom duration	Mean 9	Adalimumab, mean 7; placebo mean 8
HLA-B27+	89	–	94	100	67
Peripheral arthritis	–	–	–	–	30
Anti-TNF	ETA	INF	ETA	ETA	ADA
Time on anti-TNF, months	3	36	11	2.5	12
Definition to discontinue anti-TNF	>20% improvement in BASDAI	All patients	ASASpr and remission on MRI	ASAS20 response	ASAS40 response
Flare definition	BASDAI ≥4 and PhyGV≥4	BASDAI ≥4 and PhyGV ≥4	Increment in BASDAI of 2 units versus baseline	Increment in BASDAI of 2 units or 80% of BASDAI before treatment	Loss of ASAS40 versus baseline
Number patients with flare	75% at 12 weeks, 100% at 36 weeks	24% at wl2, 98% at w48	76% at w52	79% at w52	79% at w52
Time to flare, weeks	Mean (s.d.) 6.2 (3.0)	Mean (s.d.) 17(8)	Mean 24	Mean (s.d.) 14(9)	Mean (s.d.) 15(5.5)

TNFi retention (63% of patients after 5 years), with no measurable effect of comedication with csDMARDs,[82] neither in the prediction analysis (with baseline and time-varying covariates) nor in the dedicated propensity-adjusted analysis with a focus on confounding by indication. A recent publication focused on the prevalence of ADAbs in patients with inflammatory arthritis (among them 294 with SpA) that experienced secondary failure to TNFi[83]: 20% of the study population tested positive for ADAbs, which was associated in 81% of patients with undetectable serum drug levels (the lack of a control group [patients with persistent good response were excluded]), and the fact that immunogenicity could not explain all cases of treatment failure calls for caution in the interpretation of these data. In the absence of a well-designed and appropriately powered RCT that would randomize patients to either monotherapy with a bDMARD or combination therapy of a biologic plus a csDMARD, the current management recommendations should be followed ("patients with purely axial disease should normally not be treated with csDMARDs").[84]

Are There Any Differences in Consideration of Treatment of AS Versus nr-axSpA?

Ankylosing Spondylitis Versus Nonradiographic Axial Spondyloarthritis

In axial SpA, anti-TNF agents are also effective in the early stages not fulfilling the modified New York criteria for AS now commonly called nr-axSpA.[19–23] One of these trials included patients both with AS and with nr-axSpA and reported similar clinical response rates in each subgroup.[20] However, it should be emphasized that all patients in this trial had to have elevated CRP levels and/or sacroiliitis on MRI for inclusion into the study. Based on the positive results of these studies, three TNF inhibitors have been approved for the treatment of nr-axSpA by the European Medicines Agency (EMA), but not by the Food and Drug Administration (FDA). Notably, their approval in Europe for the indication of nr-axSpA is restricted to patients with evidence of sacroiliitis on MRI and/or elevated CRP.[85]

Although studies of TNF inhibitors conducted among AS patients reported a better clinical response in patients with shorter disease,[86] it is of note that the difference between the treatment and placebo groups for ASAS20, ASAS40, and ASAS PR (partial remission) responses obtained in the nr-axSpA trials was not greater than that in AS trials and was even somewhat lower (Table 15.3). The mean disease durations in two of these nr-axSpA trials were ≤2.5 years.[21,22] Also remarkable is that in the Swiss registry, the ASAS40 response rate to anti-TNF agents at 1 year was significantly better in patients with AS than in those with nr-axSpA (48.1% vs. 29.6%; $P = .02$), despite a mean disease duration of 12.2 years for patients with AS versus 6.1 years for those with nr-axSpA.[87] Thus, it seems like there are differences between patients with AS and those with nr-ax SpA in their clinical response to TNF blockers, particularly in the absence of objective signs of inflammation.[88] The probability of achieving a BASDAI50 response in classical AS patients with normal CRP and short disease duration (≤5 years) was estimated to be as high as 65%, based on a combined analysis of the data from two early RCTs on infliximab and etanercept.[86] In contrast, in the nr-axSpA trials with adalimumab and etanercept, ASAS40 response rates at week 12 obtained in patients with normal CRP levels at baseline were only minimally greater in the active treatment arms as compared with the placebo arms (27% vs. 18% and 20.7% vs. 12.5%, respectively).[19,22] Of note, the mean disease duration in the adalimumab trial was 10.1 years versus only 2.5 years in the etanercept trial (Table 15.3).

Subgroup interaction analyses in the adalimumab trial in nr-axSpA (ABILITY 1 trial) showed significant treatment interactions with ASAS40 response as an outcome for symptom duration (<5 years), age (<40 years), and elevated baseline CRP status. In addition, a significant interaction with treatment was observed between the continuous SPARCC sacroiliac (SI) joint scores at baseline and ASAS40 response at week 12. Finally, patients with either a positive MRI or an elevated CRP at baseline demonstrated a greater response to adalimumab compared with placebo in contrast to patients who had negative MRI of the SI joints and spine and a normal CRP at baseline, although the interaction was not statistically significant.[19]

Nonradiographic Axial Spondyloarthritis With Short Symptom Duration

Some trials of early axSpA included patients both with AS and with nr-axSpA, provided that they fulfilled the inclusion criterion for disease duration. The first RCT showing that TNF inhibitors are effective for reducing clinical and imaging evidence of disease activity in patients with MRI-determined early axSpA was conducted with infliximab.[76] The study included 40 patients with recent onset inflammatory back pain (≤3 years duration; mean 15.3 months), who were positive for HLA-B27 and had MRI evidence of sacroiliitis. Four study patients met the mNY criteria for AS. At week 16, an impressively high ASAS partial remission response of 55.6% was obtained in the infliximab group, whereas the corresponding figure in the placebo group was only 12.5%. In another trial on early axSpA (INFAST), efficacy of the combination infliximab and naproxen was compared with naproxen monotherapy.[23] Patients with a symptom duration ≤3 years and who were not refractory to NSAID treatment were included. All patients were required to fulfill the imaging arm of the ASAS criteria for inclusion, with active inflammation of the SI joints. As expected, a higher proportion of patients in the infliximab plus naproxen group achieved ASAS partial remission (61.9%; 65/105) at week 28 than in the group with naproxen monotherapy (35.3%; 18/51). Of the 156 patients in the INFAST study, 94 (60.2%) had AS (with radiographic sacroiliitis) according to the mNY criteria. A very recent posthoc analysis of this study has demonstrated larger treatment effects of infliximab plus naproxen in AS patients as compared with those observed in nr-axSpA patients.[89] After 28 weeks of treatment with infliximab plus naproxen versus naproxen monotherapy in the AS group, the ASAS20, ASAS40, and ASAS partial remission response rates were 86.9% versus 72.7%, 86.9%

TABLE 15.3

Patient Baseline Characteristics and ASAS Response Rates in Randomized Placebo-Controlled Trials With TNF Inhibitors Conducted in AS and nr-axSpA

	AS TRIALS								
	BASELINE CHARACTERISTICS						**RESPONSE RATES (%) IN PLACEBO/ACTIVE TREATMENT GROUPS**		
	Male, %	**Age, Years**	**Disease Duration, Years**	**BASDAI**	**BASFI**	**CRP (mg/dL)**	**Time Points**	**ASAS 20**	**ASAS 40**	**ASAS PR**
ETN[91]	76	42	10.1	5.8	5.2	1.9	12 weeks	59/28	45/13[a]	21/8
							24 weeks	57/22	42/10[a]	17/4
INF[92]	78[b]	40[b]	7.7[b]	6.6[b]	5.7[b]	1.5[b]	12 weeks	NA[c]	NA[c]	NA
							24 weeks	61/19	47/12	22/1
ADA[93]	76	42	11.3	6.3	5.2	1.8	12 weeks	58/21	40/13	21/4
							24 weeks	51/18[d]	39/13	22/6
GLM[e], Ref. 94	72	38[b]	11[b]	6.8[b]	5.2[b]	1.0[b]	14 weeks	59/22	45/15[f]	23/5
							24 weeks	56/23[f]	44/15[f]	NA/NA
CZP[g], Ref. 20	73	42	9.1[b]	6.4	5.7	1.4[b]	12 weeks	64/37	50/19	20/2[h]
							24 weeks	70/33	59/16	25/7[h]

NONRADIOGRAPHIC AXIAL SpA TRIALS

ETN[22]	57	32	2.5	6.0	3.9	0.6	12 weeks	52/36	33/15	NA/NA
							24 weeks	NA/NA	NA/NA	NA/NA
ADA[19]	48	38	10.1	6.4	4.5	0.7	12 weeks	52/31	36/15	16/5
							24 weeks	NA/NA	NA/NA	NA/NA
GLM[21]	62	31	<1	6.6	5.3	1.5	16 weeks	71/40	57/23	33/18
							24 weeks	NA/NA	NA/NA	NA/NA
CZP[20]	48	37	5.5[2]	6.5	4.9	1.2[b]	12 weeks	63/40	47/16	29/6[h]
							24 weeks	71/24	45/14	35/10[h]

Unless stated otherwise, values represent the mean. *ADA*, adalimumab; *ASAS 20, ASAS 40, ASAS PR*, Assessment of SpondyloArthritis International Society criteria for 20% improvement, 40% improvement, and partial remission; *BASDAI*, Bath Ankylosing Spondylitis Disease Activity Index; *BASFI*, Bath Ankylosing Spondylitis Functional Index; *CRP*, C-reactive protein; *CZP*, certolizumab pegol; *ETN*, etanercept; *GLM*, golimumab; *INF*, infliximab; *TNF*, tumor necrosis factor; *NA*, not available.

[a]Numbers represent ASAS 50 response rates.

[b]Median value.

[c]Response rates for infliximab and placebo at week 12 are almost identical to those achieved at week 24 as shown in Fig. 15.2 of the cited publication.

[d]Numbers are retrieved from the abstract presented at the ACR (*Arthritis Rheum*. 2006;54(Suppl. 9):792).

[e]Response rates in the golimumab 50 mg arm.

[f]Numbers are retrieved from the abstract presented at the ACR (*Arthritis Rheum*. 2007;56(Suppl. 12):4236).

[g]Response rates in the CZP 400 mg every 4 weeks arm.

[h]Numbers are retrieved from the abstract presented at the ACR (*Arthritis Rheum*. 2012;64(Suppl. 10):777).

versus 54.5%, and 70.5% versus 33.3%, respectively, whereas the corresponding response rates in the nr-axSpA group were 72.5 versus 68.8%, 60.0% versus 50.3%, and 50.0% versus 37.3%, respectively.[89] Efficacy of etanercept on clinical and imaging evidence of disease activity relative to sulfasalazine was studied in the ESTHER trial, which also included a mixed population of axSpA patients.[90] ASAS partial remission was achieved by 50% of the patients in the etanercept group and by 19% in the sulfasalazine group. The inclusion criteria used in these studies of early axSpA, such as brief symptom duration and presence of inflammatory lesions on MRI, may account for the very good clinical response rates obtained with etanercept, which were higher not only than those observed in AS trials[20,91–94] but also than those observed in the nr-axSpA trials.[19–22]

Recently, two RCTs with TNFi were performed in peripheral SpA.[95,96] The ABILITY 2 trial focused on already established disease, whereas the CRESPA study dealt with very early disease to explore the window of opportunity and to evaluate drug-free clinical remission after an induction therapy with golimumab. In the ABILITY 2 study, the efficacy and safety of adalimumab was evaluated in 165 patients with active nonpsoriatic pSpA fulfilling the peripheral ASAS classification criteria with a mean symptom duration around 7 years. In this trial, efficacy was evaluated with newly designed peripheral SpA Remission Criteria (pSpARC), with as a primary endpoint a 40% improvement. At week 12, a greater proportion of patients receiving adalimumab achieved this pSpARC40 response compared with patients receiving placebo (39% vs. 20%). In the CRESPA study that included patients with a mean symptom duration of only 5 weeks, the pSpARC40 response was achieved in 57.5% of patients treated with golimumab versus 20% in the placebo group. In this early cohort, it was also observed that all other efficacy outcomes were better in patients with short symptom duration, compared with more longstanding disease. This concept was already established in axSpA, but these data are the first to also demonstrate this in peripheral SpA. Earlier work in peripheral SpA has demonstrated that most patients with more long-standing forms of the disease quickly relapse after withdrawal of TNFi therapy.[97] In contrast, a withdrawal strategy in the CRESPA study in patients achieving clinical remission with a first-line TNFi indicated that drug-free remission is an achievable target in early SpA in at least 50% of patients.[98]

CONCLUSION

The treatment of axSpA has undergone a complete revolution over the past two decades, mainly as a consequence of the introduction of biologic therapies targeting individual proinflammatory cytokines. Their success has set a new treatment standard, with an acceptable and manageable safety profile. Although the story is quite straightforward regarding efficacy on clinical signs and symptoms, there is still considerable debate as to the efficacy on retardation of structural damage, which is currently not taken into account as treatment recommendations suggest initiation of

bDMARD in axSpA patients with consistently elevated inflammatory disease activity.

Because we now have an increasing "toolbox" to treat axial disease, such as TNFi and IL17i, it becomes increasingly important to define and investigate treatment strategies that may inform us on the best way to use these new, very effective bDMARDs: these include treat-to-target strategies, as well as the more recent concept of treating to induce remission, followed by withdrawal of the biologic agent. Finally, there is an increasing need for validated prediction algorithms, which can inform the clinician about the best therapeutic choices in daily practice. It is clear that more work lies ahead of us, but the future is still looking bright.

REFERENCES

1. Elliott MJ, Maini RN, Feldmann M, et al. Randomised double-blind comparison of chimeric monoclonal antibody to tumour necrosis factor alpha (cA2) versus placebo in rheumatoid arthritis. *Lancet (London, England)*. 1994;344(8930):1105–1110.
2. van Dullemen HM, van Deventer SJ, Hommes DW, et al. Treatment of Crohn's disease with anti-tumor necrosis factor chimeric monoclonal antibody (cA2). *Gastroenterology*. 1995;109(1):129–135.
3. Van Praet L, Jacques P, Van den Bosch F, Elewaut D. The transition of acute to chronic bowel inflammation in spondyloarthritis. *Nat Rev Rheumatol*. 2012;8(5):288–295.
4. Braun J, Bollow M, Neure L, et al. Use of immunohistologic and in situ hybridization techniques in the examination of sacroiliac joint biopsy specimens from patients with ankylosing spondylitis. *Arthritis Rheum US*. 1995;38(4):499–505.
5. Braun J, Brandt J, Listing J, et al. Treatment of active ankylosing spondylitis with infliximab: a randomised controlled multicentre trial. *Lancet (London, England)*. 2002;359(9313):1187–1193.
6. Brandt J, Haibel H, Cornely D, et al. Successful treatment of active ankylosing spondylitis with the anti-tumor necrosis factor alpha monoclonal antibody infliximab. *Arthritis Rheum US*. 2000;43(6):1346–1352.
7. Van den Bosch F, Kruithof E, De Vos M, De Keyser F, Mielants H. Crohn's disease associated with spondyloarthropathy: effect of TNF-alpha blockade with infliximab on articular symptoms. *Lancet (London, England)*. 2000;356(9244):1821–1822.
8. Van Den Bosch F, Kruithof E, Baeten D, et al. Randomized double-blind comparison of chimeric monoclonal antibody to tumor necrosis factor alpha (infliximab) versus placebo in active spondylarthropathy. *Arthritis Rheum US*. 2002;46(3):755–765.
9. Gorman JD, Sack KE, Davis Jr JC. Treatment of ankylosing spondylitis by inhibition of tumor necrosis factor alpha. *N Engl J Med*. 2002;346(18):1349–1356.

10. Mease PJ. Biologic therapy for psoriatic arthritis. *Rheum Dis Clin N Am*. 2015;41(4):723–738.

11. Hreggvidsdottir HS, Noordenbos T, Baeten DL. Inflammatory pathways in spondyloarthritis. *Mol Immunol*. 2014;57(1):28–37.

12. Poddubnyy D, van der Heijde D. Therapeutic controversies in spondyloarthritis: nonsteroidal anti-inflammatory drugs. *Rheum Dis Clin N Am*. 2012;38(3):601–611.

13. Cope AP, Aderka D, Doherty M, et al. Increased levels of soluble tumor necrosis factor receptors in the sera and synovial fluid of patients with rheumatic diseases. *Arthritis Rheum*. 1992;35(10):1160–1169.

14. Poddubnyy D, Hermann KG, Callhoff J, Listing J, Sieper J. Ustekinumab for the treatment of patients with active ankylosing spondylitis: results of a 28-week, prospective, open-label, proof-of-concept study (TOPAS). *Ann Rheum Dis*. 2014;73(5):817–823.

15. Smith JA, Colbert RA. Review: the interleukin-23/interleukin-17 axis in spondyloarthritis pathogenesis: Th17 and beyond. *Arthritis Rheumatol*. 2014;66(2):231–241.

16. Baeten D, Sieper J, Braun J, et al. Secukinumab, an Interleukin-17A inhibitor, in ankylosing spondylitis. *N Engl J Med*. 2015;373(26):2534–2548.

17. van der Heijde D, Calin A, Dougados M, Khan MA, van der Linden S, Bellamy N. Selection of instruments in the core set for DC-ART, SMARD, physical therapy, and clinical record keeping in ankylosing spondylitis. Progress report of the ASAS Working Group. Assessments in Ankylosing Spondylitis. *J Rheumatol*. 1999;26(4): 951–954.

18. van der Heijde D, van der Linden S, Dougados M, Bellamy N, Russell AS, Edmonds J. Ankylosing spondylitis: plenary discussion and results of voting on selection of domains and some specific instruments. *J Rheumatol*. 1999;26(4):1003–1005.

19. Sieper J, van der Heijde D, Dougados M, et al. Efficacy and safety of adalimumab in patients with non-radiographic axial spondyloarthritis: results of a randomised placebo-controlled trial (ABILITY-1). *Ann Rheum Dis*. 2013;72(6): 815–822.

20. Landewe R, Braun J, Deodhar A, et al. Efficacy of certolizumab pegol on signs and symptoms of axial spondyloarthritis including ankylosing spondylitis: 24-week results of a double-blind randomised placebo-controlled Phase 3 study. *Ann Rheum Dis*. 2014;73(1):39–47.

21. Sieper J, van der Heijde D, Dougados M, et al. A randomized, double-blind, placebo-controlled, sixteen-week study of subcutaneous golimumab in patients with active nonradiographic axial spondyloarthritis. *Arthritis Rheumatol*. 2015;67(10):2702–2712.

22. Dougados M, van der Heijde D, Sieper J, et al. Symptomatic efficacy of etanercept and its effects on objective signs of inflammation in early nonradiographic axial spondyloarthritis: a multicenter, randomized, double-blind, placebo-controlled trial. *Arthritis Rheumatol*. 2014;66(8):2091–2102.

23. Sieper J, Lenaerts J, Wollenhaupt J, et al. Efficacy and safety of infliximab plus naproxen versus naproxen alone in patients with early, active axial spondyloarthritis: results from the double-blind, placebo-controlled INFAST study, Part 1. *Ann Rheum Dis*. 2014;73(1):101–107.

24. Jacques P, Van Praet L, Carron P, Van den Bosch F, Elewaut D. Pathophysiology and role of the gastrointestinal system in spondyloarthritides. *Rheum Dis Clin N Am*. 2012;38(3):569–582.

25. Carron P, Van Praet L, Jacques P, Elewaut D, Van den Bosch F. Therapy for spondyloarthritis: the role of extra-articular manifestations (eye, skin). *Rheum Dis Clin N Am*. 2012;38(3):583–600.

26. Yoo DH, Hrycaj P, Miranda P, et al. A randomised, double-blind, parallel-group study to demonstrate equivalence in efficacy and safety of CT-P13 compared with innovator infliximab when coadministered with methotrexate in patients with active rheumatoid arthritis: the PLANETRA study. *Ann Rheum Dis*. 2013;72(10):1613–1620.

27. Park W, Hrycaj P, Jeka S, et al. A randomised, double-blind, multicentre, parallel-group, prospective study comparing the pharmacokinetics, safety, and efficacy of CT-P13 and innovator infliximab in patients with ankylosing spondylitis: the PLANETAS study. *Ann Rheum Dis*. 2013;72(10):1605–1612.

28. Park W, Yoo DH, Jaworski J, et al. Comparable long-term efficacy, as assessed by patient-reported outcomes, safety and pharmacokinetics, of CT-P13 and reference infliximab in patients with ankylosing spondylitis: 54-week results from the randomized, parallel-group PLANETAS study. *Arthritis Res Ther*. January 20, 2016;18:25.

29. Park W, Yoo DH, Miranda P, et al. Efficacy and safety of switching from reference infliximab to CT-P13 compared with maintenance of CT-P13 in ankylosing spondylitis: 102-week data from the PLANETAS extension study. *Ann Rheum Dis*. 2017;76(2):346–354.

30. Kay J, Smolen JS. Biosimilars to treat inflammatory arthritis: the challenge of proving identity. *Ann Rheum Dis*. 2013;72(10):1589–1593.

31. Emery P, Vencovsky J, Sylwestrzak A, et al. A phase III randomised, double-blind, parallel-group study comparing SB4 with etanercept reference product in patients with active rheumatoid arthritis despite methotrexate therapy. *Ann Rheum Dis*. 2017;76(1):51–57.

32. Emery P, Vencovsky J, Sylwestrzak A, et al. 52-week results of the phase 3 randomized study comparing SB4 with reference etanercept in patients with active rheumatoid arthritis. *Rheumatology*. 2017;56(12):2093–2101.

33. Ramiro S, van der Heijde D, van Tubergen A, et al. Higher disease activity leads to more structural damage in the spine in ankylosing spondylitis: 12-year longitudinal data from the OASIS cohort. *Ann Rheum Dis*. 2014;73(8):1455–1461.

34. Baraliakos X, Haibel H, Listing J, Sieper J, Braun J. Continuous long-term anti-TNF therapy does not lead to an increase in the rate of new bone formation over 8 years

in patients with ankylosing spondylitis. *Ann Rheum Dis.* 2014;73(4):710–715.

35. Haroon N, Inman RD, Learch TJ, et al. The impact of tumor necrosis factor alpha inhibitors on radiographic progression in ankylosing spondylitis. *Arthritis Rheum US.* 2013;65(10):2645–2654.

36. Molnar C, Scherer A, Baraliakos X, et al. TNF blockers inhibit spinal radiographic progression in ankylosing spondylitis by reducing disease activity: results from the Swiss Clinical Quality Management cohort. *Ann Rheum Dis.* 2018;77(1):63–69.

37. Mei Y, Pan F, Gao J, et al. Increased serum IL-17 and IL-23 in the patient with ankylosing spondylitis. *Clin Rheumatol.* 2011;30(2):269–273.

38. Zeng L, Lindstrom MJ, Smith JA. Ankylosing spondylitis macrophage production of higher levels of interleukin-23 in response to lipopolysaccharide without induction of a significant unfolded protein response. *Arthritis Rheum US.* 2011;63(12):3807–3817.

39. Appel H, Maier R, Wu P, et al. Analysis of IL-17(+) cells in facet joints of patients with spondyloarthritis suggests that the innate immune pathway might be of greater relevance than the Th17-mediated adaptive immune response. *Arthritis Res Ther.* 2011;13(3):R95.

40. Singh AK, Misra R, Aggarwal A. Th-17 associated cytokines in patients with reactive arthritis/undifferentiated spondyloarthropathy. *Clin Rheumatol.* 2011;30(6):771–776.

41. Baeten D, Baraliakos X, Braun J, et al. Anti-interleukin-17A monoclonal antibody secukinumab in treatment of ankylosing spondylitis: a randomised, double-blind, placebo-controlled trial. *Lancet.* 2013;382(9906):1705–1713.

42. Sieper J, Deodhar A, Marzo-Ortega H, et al. Secukinumab efficacy in anti-TNF-naive and anti-TNF-experienced subjects with active ankylosing spondylitis: results from the MEASURE 2 Study. *Ann Rheum Dis.* 2017;76(3):571–592.

43. Braun J, Baraliakos X, Deodhar A, et al. Effect of secukinumab on clinical and radiographic outcomes in ankylosing spondylitis: 2-year results from the randomised phase III MEASURE 1 study. *Ann Rheum Dis.* 2017;76(6):1070–1077.

43a. Braun J, Baraliakos X, Deodhar A, et al. Secukinumab shows sustained efficacy and low structural progression in ankylosing spondylitis: 4-year results from the MEASURE 1 study. *Rheumatology (Oxford).* 2018 Dec 19. https://doi.org/10.1093/rheumatology/key375. [Epub ahead of print].

44. Langley RG, Elewski BE, Lebwohl M, et al. Secukinumab in plaque psoriasis–results of two phase 3 trials. *N Engl J Med.* 2014;371(4):326–338.

45. Mease PJ, McInnes IB, Kirkham B, et al. Secukinumab inhibition of Interleukin-17A in patients with psoriatic arthritis. *N Engl J Med.* 2015;373(14):1329–1339.

46. Puel A, Cypowyj S, Bustamante J, et al. Chronic mucocutaneous candidiasis in humans with inborn errors of interleukin-17 immunity. *Science (New York, NY).* 2011;332(6025):65–68.

46a. van der Heijde D, Cheng-Chung Wei J, Dougados M, et al. COAST-V study group. Ixekizumab, an interleu- kin-17A antagonist in the treatment of ankylosing spondylitis or radiographic axial spondyloarthritisin patients previously

untreated with biological dis- ease-modifying anti-rheumatic drugs (COAST-V): 16 week results of a phase 3 randomised, double-blind, active-controlled and placebo-controlled trial. *Lancet.* 2018;392(10163):2441–2451.

46b. Deodhar A, Poddubnyy D, Pacheco-Tena C, et al. Efficacy and safety of ixekizumab in the treatment of radiographic axial spondyloarthritis: 16 week results of a phase 3 randomized, double-blind, placebo controlled trial in patients with prior inadequate response or intolerance to tumor necrosis factor inhibitors. *Arthritis Rheumatol.* 20 October 2018. https://doi.org/10.1002/art.40753.

47. Australo-Anglo-American Spondyloarthritis C, Reveille JD, Sims AM, et al. Genome-wide association study of ankylosing spondylitis identifies non-MHC susceptibility loci. *Nat Genet.* 2010;42(2):123–127.

47a. van der Heijde D, Cheng-Chung Wei J, Dougados M, et al. COAST-V study group. Ixekizumab, an interleukin-17A antagonist in the treatment of ankylosing spondylitis or radiographic axial spondyloarthritis in patients previously untreated with biological disease-modifying anti-rheumatic drugs (COAST-V): 16 week results of a phase 3 randomised, double-blind, active-controlled and placebo-controlled trial. *Lancet.* 2018;392(10163):2441–2451.

47b. Deodhar A, Poddubnyy D, Pacheco-Tena C, et al. Efficacy and safety of ixekizumab in the treatment of radiographic axial spondyloarthritis: 16 week results of a phase 3 randomized, double-blind, placebo controlled trial in patients with prior inadequate response or intolerance to tumor necrosis factor inhibitors. *Arthritis Rheumatol.* 20 October 2018. https://doi.org/10.1002/art.40753.

48. Ritchlin C, Rahman P, Kavanaugh A, et al. Efficacy and safety of the anti-IL-12/23 p40 monoclonal antibody, ustekinumab, in patients with active psoriatic arthritis despite conventional non-biological and biological anti-tumour necrosis factor therapy: 6-month and 1-year results of the phase 3, multicentre, double-blind, placebo-controlled, randomised PSUMMIT 2 trial. *Ann Rheum Dis.* 2014;73(6):990–999.

49. *A Study to Evaluate the Efficacy and Safety of Ustekinumab in the Treatment of Anti-TNF(Alpha) Refractory Participants with Active Radiographic Axial Spondyloarthritis* (NCT02438787). Available from: ClinicalTrials.gov.

50. Baeten D, Ostergaard M, Wei JC, et al. Risankizumab, an IL-23 inhibitor, for ankylosing spondylitis: results of a randomised, double-blind, placebo-controlled, proof-of-concept, dose-finding phase 2 study. *Ann Rheum Dis.* 2018;77(9):1295–1302.

51. Tan AL, Marzo-Ortega H, O'Connor P, Fraser A, Emery P, McGonagle D. Efficacy of anakinra in active ankylosing spondylitis: a clinical and magnetic resonance imaging study. *Ann Rheum Dis.* 2004;63(9):1041–1045.

52. Haibel H, Rudwaleit M, Listing J, Sieper J. Open label trial of anakinra in active ankylosing spondylitis over 24 weeks. *Ann Rheum Dis.* 2005;64(2):296–298.

53. Song IH, Heldmann F, Rudwaleit M, et al. Treatment of active ankylosing spondylitis with abatacept: an open-label, 24-week pilot study. *Ann Rheum Dis.* 2011;70(6):1108–1110.

54. Song IH, Heldmann F, Rudwaleit M, et al. Different response to rituximab in tumor necrosis factor blocker-naive patients with active ankylosing spondylitis and in patients in whom tumor necrosis factor blockers have failed: a twenty-four-week clinical trial. *Arthritis Rheum.* 2010;62(5):1290–1297.

55. Song IH, Heldmann F, Rudwaleit M, et al. One-year follow-up of ankylosing spondylitis patients responding to rituximab treatment and re-treated in case of a flare. *Ann Rheum Dis.* 2013;72(2):305–306.

56. Sieper J, Porter-Brown B, Thompson L, Harari O, Dougados M. Assessment of short-term symptomatic efficacy of tocilizumab in ankylosing spondylitis: results of randomised, placebo-controlled trials. *Ann Rheum Dis.* 2014;73(1):95–100.

57. Sieper J, Braun J, Kay J, et al. Sarilumab for the treatment of ankylosing spondylitis: results of a Phase II, randomised, double-blind, placebo-controlled study (ALIGN). *Ann Rheum Dis.* 2015;74(6):1051–1057.

58. van der Heijde D, Deodhar A, Wei JC, et al. Tofacitinib in patients with ankylosing spondylitis: a phase II, 16-week, randomised, placebo-controlled, dose-ranging study. *Ann Rheum Dis.* 2017;76(8):1340–1347.

59. Smolen JS, Schols M, Braun J, et al. Treating axial spondyloarthritis and peripheral spondyloarthritis, especially psoriatic arthritis, to target: 2017 update of recommendations by an international task force. *Ann Rheum Dis.* July 06, 2017.

60. Poddubnyy D, Protopopov M, Haibel H, Braun J, Rudwaleit M, Sieper J. High disease activity according to the Ankylosing Spondylitis Disease Activity Score is associated with accelerated radiographic spinal progression in patients with early axial spondyloarthritis: results from the German SPondyloarthritis Inception Cohort. *Ann Rheum Dis.* 2016;75(12):2114–2118.

61. Lee J, Noh JW, Hwang JW, et al. Extended dosing of etanercept 25 mg can be effective in patients with ankylosing spondylitis: a retrospective analysis. *Clin Rheumatol.* 2010;29(10):1149–1154.

62. Navarro-Compan V, Moreira V, Ariza-Ariza R, Hernandez-Cruz B, Vargas-Lebron C, Navarro-Sarabia F. Low doses of etanercept can be effective in ankylosing spondylitis patients who achieve remission of the disease. *Clin Rheumatol.* 2011;30(7):993–996.

63. Paccou J, Bacle-Boutry MA, Solau-Gervais E, Bele-Philippe P, Flipo RM. Dosage adjustment of anti-tumor necrosis factor-alpha inhibitor in ankylosing spondylitis is effective in maintaining remission in clinical practice. *J Rheumatol.* 2012;39(7):1418–1423.

64. Cantini F, Niccoli L, Cassara E, Kaloudi O, Nannini C. Duration of remission after halving of the etanercept dose in patients with ankylosing spondylitis: a randomized, prospective, long-term, follow-up study. *Biologics.* 2013;7:1–6.

65. Morck B, Pullerits R, Geijer M, Bremell T, Forsblad-d'Elia H. Infliximab dose reduction sustains the clinical treatment effect in active HLAB27 positive ankylosing spondylitis: a two-year pilot study. *Mediat Inflamm.* 2013;2013:289845.

66. Borras-Blasco J, Gracia-Perez A, Rosique-Robles JD, Castera ME, Abad FJ. Clinical and economic impact of the use of etanercept 25 mg once weekly in rheumatoid arthritis, psoriatic arthropathy and ankylosing spondylitis patients. *Expert Opin Biol Ther.* 2014;14(2):145–150.

67. De Stefano R, Frati E, De Quattro D, Menza L, Manganelli S. Low doses of etanercept can be effective to maintain remission in ankylosing spondylitis patients. *Clin Rheumatol.* 2014;33(5):707–711.

68. Zavada J, Uher M, Sisol K, et al. A tailored approach to reduce dose of anti-TNF drugs may be equally effective, but substantially less costly than standard dosing in patients with ankylosing spondylitis over 1 year: a propensity score-matched cohort study. *Ann Rheum Dis.* 2016;75(1):96–102.

69. Navarro-Compan V, Plasencia-Rodriguez C, de Miguel E, et al. Anti-TNF discontinuation and tapering strategies in patients with axial spondyloarthritis: a systematic literature review. *Rheumatology.* 2016;55(7):1188–1194.

70. Brandt J, Khariouzov A, Listing J, et al. Six-month results of a double-blind, placebo-controlled trial of etanercept treatment in patients with active ankylosing spondylitis. *Arthritis Rheum.* 2003;48(6):1667–1675.

71. Baraliakos X, Listing J, Brandt J, et al. Clinical response to discontinuation of anti-TNF therapy in patients with ankylosing spondylitis after 3 years of continuous treatment with infliximab. *Arthritis Res Ther.* 2005;7(3):R439–R444.

72. Song IH, Althoff CE, Haibel H, et al. Frequency and duration of drug-free remission after 1 year of treatment with etanercept versus sulfasalazine in early axial spondyloarthritis: 2 year data of the ESTHER trial. *Ann Rheum Dis.* 2012;71(7):1212–1215.

73. Deng X, Zhang J, Zhang J, Huang F. Thalidomide reduces recurrence of ankylosing spondylitis in patients following discontinuation of etanercept. *Rheumatol Int.* 2013;33(6):1409–1413.

74. Haibel H, Heldmann F, Braun J, Listing J, Kupper H, Sieper J. Long-term efficacy of adalimumab after drug withdrawal and retreatment in patients with active non-radiographically evident axial spondyloarthritis who experience a flare. *Arthritis Rheum.* 2013;65(8):2211–2213.

75. van Nies JA, Tsonaka R, Gaujoux-Viala C, Fautrel B, van der Helm-van Mil AH. Evaluating relationships between symptom duration and persistence of rheumatoid arthritis: does a window of opportunity exist? Results on the Leiden early arthritis clinic and ESPOIR cohorts. *Ann Rheum Dis.* 2015;74(5):806–812.

76. Barkham N, Keen HI, Coates LC, et al. Clinical and imaging efficacy of infliximab in HLA-B27-Positive patients with magnetic resonance imaging-determined early sacroiliitis. *Arthritis Rheum.* 2009;60(4):946–954.

77. Strand V, Balsa A, Al-Saleh J, et al. Immunogenicity of biologics in chronic inflammatory diseases: a systematic review. *BioDrugs Clin Immunother Biopharm Gene Ther.* 2017;31(4):299–316.

78. de Vries MK, Wolbink GJ, Stapel SO, et al. Decreased clinical response to infliximab in ankylosing spondylitis is correlated with anti-infliximab formation. *Ann Rheum Dis.* 2007;66(9):1252–1254.

79. de Vries MK, Brouwer E, van der Horst-Bruinsma IE, et al. Decreased clinical response to adalimumab in ankylosing spondylitis is associated with antibody formation. *Ann Rheum Dis.* 2009;68(11):1787–1788.

80. Lie E, Kristensen LE, Forsblad-d'Elia H, et al. The effect of comedication with conventional synthetic disease modifying antirheumatic drugs on TNF inhibitor drug survival in patients with ankylosing spondylitis and undifferentiated spondyloarthritis: results from a nationwide prospective study. *Ann Rheum Dis.* 2015;74(6):970–978.

81. Landewe RB. Conventional DMARDs in axial spondyloarthritis: wishful–rather than rational–thinking!. *Ann Rheum Dis.* 2015;74(6):951–953.

82. Sepriano A, Ramiro S, van der Heijde D, et al. Effect of comedication with conventional synthetic disease-modifying antirheumatic drugs on retention of tumor necrosis factor inhibitors in patients with spondyloarthritis: a prospective cohort study. *Arthritis Rheumatol (Hoboken, NJ).* 2016;68(11):2671–2679.

83. Balsa A, Sanmarti R, Rosas J, et al. Drug immunogenicity in patients with inflammatory arthritis and secondary failure to tumour necrosis factor inhibitor therapies: the REASON study. *Rheumatology.* 2018;57(4):688–693.

84. van der Heijde D, Ramiro S, Landewe R, et al. 2016 update of the ASAS-EULAR management recommendations for axial spondyloarthritis. *Ann Rheum Dis.* 2017;76(6): 978–991.

85. Deodhar A, Reveille JD, van den Bosch F, et al. The concept of axial spondyloarthritis: joint statement of the spondyloarthritis research and treatment network and the Assessment of SpondyloArthritis international Society in response to the US Food and Drug Administration's comments and concerns. *Arthritis Rheumatol.* 2014;66(10):2649–2656.

86. Rudwaleit M, Listing J, Brandt J, Braun J, Sieper J. Prediction of a major clinical response (BASDAI 50) to tumour necrosis factor alpha blockers in ankylosing spondylitis. *Ann Rheum Dis.* 2004;63(6):665–670.

87. Ciurea A, Scherer A, Exer P, et al. Tumor necrosis factor alpha inhibition in radiographic and nonradiographic axial spondyloarthritis: results from a large observational cohort. *Arthritis Rheum.* 2013;65(12):3096–3106.

88. Akkoc N, Khan MA. Looking into the new ASAS classification criteria for axial spondyloarthritis through the other side of the glass. *Curr Rheumatol Rep.* 2015;17(6):515.

89. Sieper J, Rudwaleit M, Lenaerts J, et al. Partial remission in ankylosing spondylitis and non-radiographic axial spondyloarthritis in treatment with infliximab plus naproxen or naproxen alone: associations between partial remission and baseline disease characteristics. *Rheumatology.* 2016;55(11):1946–1953.

90. Song IH, Hermann K, Haibel H, et al. Effects of etanercept versus sulfasalazine in early axial spondyloarthritis on active inflammatory lesions as detected by whole-body MRI (ESTHER): a 48-week randomised controlled trial. *Ann Rheum Dis.* 2011;70(4):590–596.

91. Davis Jr JC, Van Der Heijde D, Braun J, et al. Recombinant human tumor necrosis factor receptor (etanercept) for treating ankylosing spondylitis: a randomized, controlled trial. *Arthritis Rheum.* 2003;48(11):3230–3236.

92. van der Heijde D, Dijkmans B, Geusens P, et al. Efficacy and safety of infliximab in patients with ankylosing spondylitis: results of a randomized, placebo-controlled trial (ASSERT). *Arthritis Rheum.* 2005;52(2):582–591.

93. van der Heijde D, Kivitz A, Schiff MH, et al. Efficacy and safety of adalimumab in patients with ankylosing spondylitis: results of a multicenter, randomized, double-blind, placebo-controlled trial. *Arthritis Rheum.* 2006;54(7): 2136–2146.

94. Inman RD, Davis Jr JC, Heijde D, et al. Efficacy and safety of golimumab in patients with ankylosing spondylitis: results of a randomized, double-blind, placebo-controlled, phase III trial. *Arthritis Rheum.* 2008;58(11): 3402–3412.

95. Mease P, Sieper J, Van den Bosch F, Rahman P, Karunaratne PM, Pangan AL. Randomized controlled trial of adalimumab in patients with nonpsoriatic peripheral spondyloarthritis. *Arthritis Rheumatol (Hoboken, NJ).* 2015;67(4):914–923.

96. Carron P, Varkas G, Cypers H, Van Praet L, Elewaut D, Van den Bosch F. Anti-TNF-induced remission in very early peripheral spondyloarthritis: the CRESPA study. *Ann Rheum Dis.* February 17, 2017.

97. Paramarta JE, Heijda TF, Baeten DL. Fast relapse upon discontinuation of tumour necrosis factor blocking therapy in patients with peripheral spondyloarthritis. *Ann Rheum Dis.* 2013;72(9):1581–1582.

98. Carron P, Varkas G, Renson T, Colman R, Elewaut D, Van den Bosch F. High rate of drug-free remission after induction therapy with golimumab in early peripheral spondyloarthritis. *Arthritis Rheumatol (Hoboken, NJ).* May 27, 2018.

CHAPTER 16

Treatment Guidelines for Axial Spondyloarthritis

SONAM KIWALKAR, MBBS • ATUL DEODHAR, MD, MRCP • JOACHIM SIEPER, MD, PHD

INTRODUCTION

The Institute of Medicine (IOM) in 2011 defined clinical practice guidelines as "Statements that include recommendations, intended to optimize patient care, that are informed by a systemic review of evidence and an assessment of the benefits and harms of alternative care options."

The process of development of treatment recommendations needs to be rigorous and evidence-based. Ideal recommendations would reduce inappropriate care, enable effective use of healthcare resources, prevent waste, and minimize geographical variations in clinical practices. The purpose of creating guidelines is to give patients the best possible treatment and improve outcomes, as well as to educate clinicians. Having said that, the approval and availability of pharmacologic agents, costs of healthcare, payers, and regulatory authorities differ from region to region. For guidelines to be successfully embraced by all stakeholders, they need to be region-specific. This would ensure that the guidelines share similar preferences and attitudes as the healthcare professionals invested in taking care of patients residing in their regions.

The main societies that have developed recommendations for axSpA include Assessment of SpondyloArthritis International Society/European League against Rheumatism (ASAS-EULAR), American College of Rheumatology/Spondylitis Association of America/Spondyloarthritis Research and Treatment Network (ACR/SAA/SPARTAN), Canadian Rheumatology Association and the Spondyloarthritis Research Consortium of Canada (CRA/SPARCC), British Society for Rheumatology/British Health Professionals in Rheumatology (BSR/BHPR), and other national societies. This chapter will focus on the two most widely publicized treatment recommendations for axSpA—those by ASAS-EULAR and by ACR/SAA/SPARTAN.

THE SCIENCE OF DEVELOPMENT OF GUIDELINES

Guidelines should inform clinicians about the quality of the underlying evidence and the strength of the recommendations. The following are some of the methods involved in the development of guidelines:

1. GRADE (Grading of Recommendations Assessment, Development and Evaluation)[3]:

    GRADE was developed by a widely representative group of international guideline developers. Their widespread adoption reflects its success as a rigorous, transparent, and user-friendly grading system. There are nine basic steps in development of guidelines by the GRADE methodology:

    a. Form a guideline panel

    b. Define the scope of the project (e.g., whether to include pediatric population, management of extraarticular manifestation, etc.)

    c. Ask precise clinical questions ("PICO"—population, intervention, comparison, and outcome—questions)

    d. Determine the critical outcomes of interest

    e. Summarize the evidence

    f. Determine the confidence in the effect estimates—quality of the evidence of each outcome

    g. Determine the quality of the body of evidence

    h. Make recommendations and determine the associated strength of each recommendation

The treatment recommendations developed by GRADE system are transparent, as every recommendation can be traced backward to reveal all these nine steps. The GRADE system classifies the quality of evidence in one of four levels—high, moderate, low, and very low (see Table 16.1).

Typically, a randomized controlled trial begins as a high-quality evidence, and a case control study begins as a low-quality evidence. The level of evidence can be downgraded depending on study limitations,

Axial Spondyloarthritis. https://doi.org/10.1016/B978-0-323-56800-5.00016-3

inconsistencies of results, and bias, whereas it can be upgraded if the treatment effect is large. The next step is to determine factors that define a strength of recommendation (see Table 16.2).

The voting group—ideally consisting of different members than those forming the literature review group—weighs the overall balance of desirable and undesirable consequences of intervention and variability of patient values and preferences. The strengths of this system are a clear distinction between determination of quality of evidence, rating of strength of recommendation, and a transparent process of moving from evidence to recommendation.

The guidelines development process by the American College of Rheumatology mandates

that the entire group of experts involved, as well as its subcomponents—the literature review panel, the voting panel, and the core group—all needs to have >51% "unconflicted" members, and the others need to disclose their conflicts.

2. The European League Against Rheumatism (EULAR) standardized Operating Procedures (SOP):
The goal of EULAR SOP is to describe the elements required for a project to develop recommendations. The following is a summary of the step-by-step approach:

   a. Define the stake holders that would be interested in the recommendations (e.g., rheumatologists, general practitioners, health professionals, policy makers, insurance companies, etc.).
   b. Establish a task force consisting of a convener, rheumatologist, fellows, clinical experts, health professionals, and patients. Each member of the task force must disclose potential conflicts of interest.
   c. Define research questions and specific clinical outcomes.
   d. Conduct a systemic literature review and analyze data.
   e. Assign a level of evidence using the GRADE or Oxford Center for Evidence-Based Medicine (OCEBM)[4] (see Table 16.3).
   f. Every recommendation is given a "grade." It can be seen in Table 16.4 that the level of evidence is clearly reflected through the grade of recommendation. This is one of the strengths of OCEBM.
   g. Prepare a manuscript.
   h. Dissemination of recommendations by an abstract or manuscript.

TABLE 16.1
Quality of Evidence and Definitions in GRADE Methodology

High quality	Further research is very unlikely to change our confidence in the estimate of effect
Moderate quality	Further research is likely to have an important impact on our confidence in the estimate of effect and may change the estimate
Low quality	Further research is likely to have an important impact on our confidence in the estimate of effect and is likely to change the estimate
Very low quality	Any estimate of effect is very uncertain

TABLE 16.2
Strength of Recommendations in GRADE

Strength	Interpretation	Implication for Clinicians	Implications for Policymakers
Strongly in favor	Almost all informed patients would choose to receive the intervention.	Should be accepted by most patients to whom it is offered.	Should be adopted as policy.
Conditionally in favor	Most informed patients would choose the intervention, but a sizable minority would not.	Large role for education and shared decision-making.	Requires stakeholder engagement and discussion.
Conditionally against	Most informed patients would not choose the intervention, but a small minority would.	Large role for education and shared decision-making.	Requires stakeholder engagement and discussion.
Strongly against	Most patients should not receive the intervention	Should not be offered to patients.	Should be adopted as policy

THE 2015 ACR/SAA/SPARTAN GUIDELINES

The ACR/SAA/SPARTAN developed recommendations primarily for US-based clinicians, and thus there is a majority of North American representation in the core committee, as well as in the literature review and the voting panel.[2] As per the Institute of Medicine (IOM), high-quality guidelines need to have multidisciplinary contributions and have a transparent development process. The ACR/SAA/SPARTAN used the GRADE methodology to formulate guidelines. Fig. 16.1 gives an overview of the layout of the methodology used.

Before publication, and following the final review of the draft, the recommendations were reviewed and ratified by the ACR Committee of Quality of Care, as well as the Board of Directors of the ACR, SAA, and SPARTAN organizations.[2]

TABLE 16.3
Oxford Center for Evidence-Based Medicine— Definition for the Levels of Evidence

Level	Trials for Therapy/Prevention/Harm
1a	Systematic reviews of randomized controlled trials
1b	Individual randomized controlled trials
2a	Systematic reviews of cohort studies
2b	Individual cohort studies
3a	Systematic reviews of case-control studies
3b	Individual case-control studies
4	Case series
5	Expert opinion without explicit critical appraisal, or based on physiology, bench research or "first principles"

TABLE 16.4
Oxford Center for Evidence-Based Medicine— Grades of Recommendation

Grade of Recommendation	Summarized Form
A	Consistent level 1 studies
B	Consistent level 2 or 3 studies, extrapolations from level 1 studies
C	Consistent level 4 studies, extrapolations from level 2 or 3 studies
D	Consistent level 5 studies

The ACR/SAA/SPARTAN recommendations are grouped for various stages and presentation of the disease. They developed different sets of questions for AS, nr-axSpA, and extraarticular manifestations (see Fig. 16.2). They differentiated recommendations for patients with stable disease and active disease. If symptoms were at an unacceptably bothersome level as reported by the patient, and judged by the examining clinician to be due to axSpA, the disease was qualified as an active disease. On the other hand, a stable disease was that which was symptomatic or causing symptoms that were bothersome, but an acceptable level as reported by the patient. Status of stable-disease required a minimum of 6 months of stability.

The committee chose to illustrate their treatment recommendations using flowcharts to suggest how various treatments (pharmacologic and nonpharmacologic) might be used in patients with active and stable axSpA. The flowchart is shown in Fig. 16.3.

Exercise formed the first step of treatment of both active and stable axSpA. Given the evidence of benefits of physical therapy, and the very low likelihood of harm, the panel judged this was a strong recommendation.[5,6] Unsupervised or home exercises are efficacious and are therefore recommended.[7–9] However, overall active physical therapy is proven to be more efficacious than unsupervised or home exercises.[9] Although aquatic therapy can be used by those with access to a swimming pool or hydrotherapy tub, land-based therapy was conditionally preferred because access to land-based therapy is often greater.[10–14]

The next step of management of axSpA is use of **non-steroidal antiinflammatory drugs (NSAIDs)**. This was a strong recommendation based on several placebo-controlled trials.[15–19] Although there was a serious risk of bias and imprecision in the trials, it was argued that the desirable consequences outweigh the undesirable effects for a large majority of the patients. It was conditionally recommended to base the decision of continuous versus need-based therapy on the severity (active or stable disease), intermittency of symptoms, comorbidities, and patient preferences. However, risk of depression and hypertension was greater in the continuous use group in one study.

Based on lack of head-to-head controlled trials, the panel recommended against designating any particular NSAID as the preferred treatment option. The choice of NSAID was to be based on consideration of the patient's history of NSAID use, risk factors, and comorbidities. If two NSAIDs are not effective in controlling pain and stiffness over a period of 1 month, or there is an incomplete response to at least two different NSAIDs over 2 months, escalation of therapy is warranted.

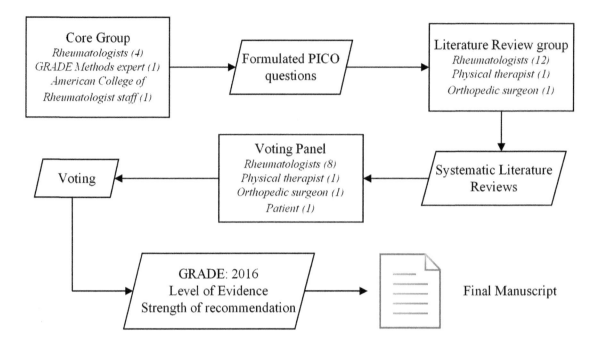

FIG. 16.1 2015: ACR/SAA/SPARTAN—overview of methodology.

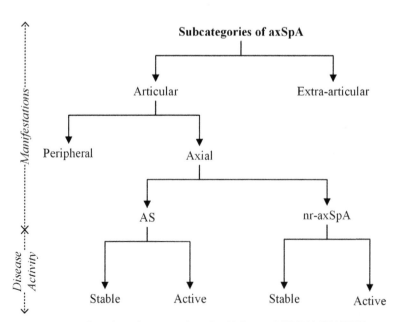

FIG. 16.2 Overview of presentation of guidelines—ACR/SAA/SPARTAN.

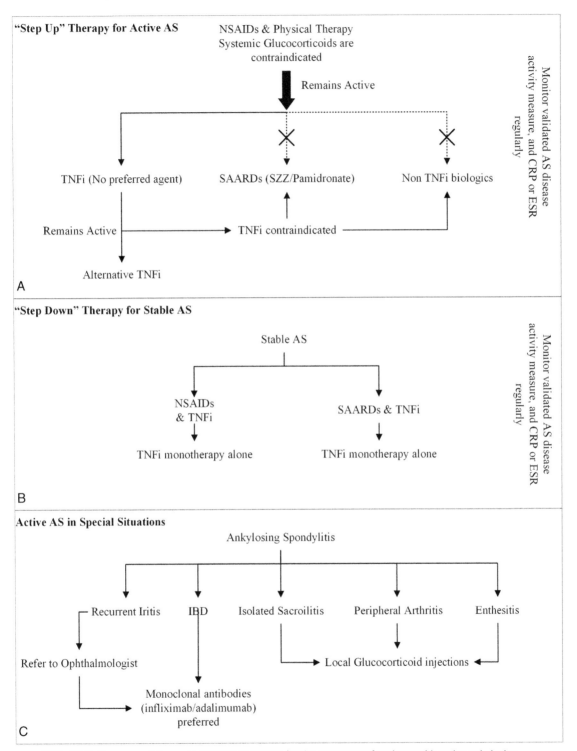

FIG. 16.3 Summary of the main recommendations for the treatment of patients with active ankylosing spondylitis (AS) (A) or stable AS (B). *CRP*, C-reactive protein; *ESR*, erythrocyte sedimentation rate; *GC*, glucocorticoid; *IBD*, inflammatory bowel disease; *NSAIDs*, nonsteroidal antiinflammatory drugs; *SSZ*, sulfasalazine; *TNFi*, tumor necrosis factor inhibitors; SAARDs, Slow acting anti-rheumatic drugs.

Escalation of therapy implies usage of **tumor necrosis factor inhibitors (TNFi)**. This was a strong recommendation based on 13 randomized control trials in AS patients.[20-32] Although data are sparse in other aspects of management of nr-axSpA, five randomized control trials were considered, which favor TNFi over placebo in such patients.[33-37] No TNFi agent is preferred over the other. Evidence stems from an indirect comparison showing similar ASAS 20 response criteria across all TNFi.[38-41] However, when considering treatment of extraarticular manifestations such as iritis or inflammatory bowel disease, the guidelines recommend use of monoclonal antibodies (such as infliximab and adalimumab) over soluble receptor TNFi.

The use of an alternative TNFi agent was recommended when the initial TNFi fails due to ineffectiveness.[42] The data suggested that a second TNFi can still be effective—although the level of efficacy may be lower than the first TNFi. IL-17 inhibitors such as secukinumab were not yet approved for the indication AS at the time of development and publication of these recommendations and are therefore not included.

Slow-acting antirheumatic drugs (SAARDs), such as sulfasalazine, methotrexate, pamidronate, were not recommended as a treatment for axSpA. If there are contraindications to TNFi, treatment with an SAARD was preferred over a non-TNF biologic. No studies have directly compared treatment responses between SAARD and non-TNF biologic agents. Thus, data to support this recommendation stem from indirect evidence. Data from small single arm trials comparing axSpA patients (only AS patients were investigated in these trials) before and after treatment with abatacept, rituximab, tocilizumab, and ustekinumab failed to demonstrate significant benefits.[43-48] High dose of pamidronate showed an improvement in BASDAI (Bath Ankylosing Spondylitis Disease Activity Index) scores. Sulfasalazine had a weak beneficial effect on spinal pain but not on other critical outcomes.[49-51] Given these indirect comparisons, the ACR/SAA/SPARTAN conditionally recommend SAARDs such as pamidronate and sulfasalazine over non-TNF biologics in a clinical scenario where there is a contraindication or toxicity to TNFi.

The panel strongly advocated against the use of **long-term systemic glucocorticoids** in patients with axSpA. This was based on data from three small case series, and a 2-week randomized control trial, which showed only modest improvements with glucocorticoids.[52-55]

It was agreed that there are no studies of **local glucocorticoid injections** for enthesitis or intraarticular injections for active peripheral arthritis in axSpA. The positive recommendation for this treatment was based on expert opinion and extrapolation from experiences from other rheumatologic conditions.[56,57] Given the risk of rupture, ACR/SAA/SPARTAN further specifically recommended against local injections in Achilles, patellar, and quadriceps tendons.[58] **Sulfasalazine** was an acceptable drug predominantly for **peripheral disease.** This was based on trials before 1996, in which the effect on concomitant peripheral arthritis favored sulfasalazine compared with placebo in ankylosing spondylitis patients.[50,51]

If a patient has **stable axSpA** and was on biologics along with an SAARD or NSAID, they advocated to stop the SAARD or NSAID (Fig. 16.3: panel B). They suggested to individualize this decision based on patient comorbidities and consider long-term gastrointestinal, renal, cardiac, and hematologic toxicities.[59]

The ACR/SAA/SPARTAN panel consisted of an ophthalmologist, and they had a few recommendations on comanaging patients with iritis and axSpA. Given the expertise of an ophthalmologist in managing **uveitis**, the panel agreed that the treatment by an ophthalmologist would decrease the severity, duration, and complications of iritis. Prompt treatment with topical glucocorticoids decreases the severity of episodes and decreases the likelihood of ocular complications.[60] Hence, the committee proposed at-home prescriptions to be made available for patients with recurrent iritis flares.

The guidelines panel agreed that **total hip arthroplasty** should be considered in patients with refractory pain or disability and radiographic evidence of structural damage. No high-quality data exist for elective **spinal corrective osteotomy.**[61] Consequently, ACR/SAA/SPARTAN conditionally recommend against elective spinal osteotomy except in rare circumstances and in specialized centers.

ACR/SAA/SPARTAN made several suggestions on screening individuals with axSpA for other comorbidities. Although they acknowledged that the quality of evidence supporting these recommendations was poor, they proposed the following:

1. Fall evaluation and counseling at clinic visits.
2. Screening for osteopenia and osteoporosis with a dual-energy X-ray absorptiometry (DEXA). They propose to consider patient demographics while making the decision of when to start screening and to determine the interval of screening.
3. Against screening for cardiac conduction defects with an electrocardiogram in asymptomatic individuals.
4. Against screening for valvular heart defects with echocardiogram in asymptomatic individuals.[62]

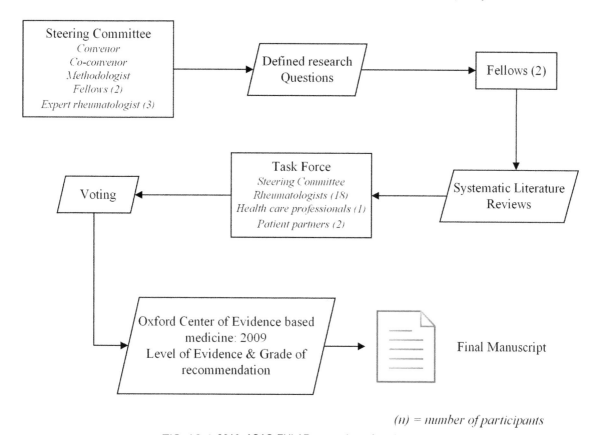

FIG. 16.4 2016: ASAS-EULAR—overview of methodology.

The following tools were recommended for monitoring disease activity:

1. Clinical composite scores such as BASDAI or ASDAS (Ankylosing Spondylitis Disease Activity Score)
2. Laboratory tests such as C-reactive protein (CRP) or erythrocyte sedimentation rate (ESR)

They also suggested that it would be more beneficial to monitor patients with active symptoms as a guide to managing their disease. Because it is difficult to set a "target" for a multifaceted disease such as axSpA, which has articular and extraarticular involvement, the committee recommended to strive toward a goal of stable disease where the patient reports symptoms to be at an acceptable level, which was not further defined.

2016 ASAS-EULAR RECOMMENDATIONS

In 2016, the ASAS group updated the 2010 ASAS-EULAR recommendations for the management of axSpA and the ASAS recommendation for use of TNF agents for axSpA into a single set.[63,64] The primary objective of the ASAS treatment guidelines was to develop an intervention-based guidance on the sequence of nonpharmacologic and pharmacologic management of patients with axSpA. The target population covered the whole group of axial SpA, including AS as well as nr-axSpA patients, according to the ASAS classification criteria for axSpA.[65]

The ASAS-EULAR guidelines were drafted according to EULAR Standardized Operating Procedures (SOP). The panel had rheumatologists, other healthcare professionals involved in the treatment of axSpA (e.g., physical therapists), and patient research partners, who contributed to the development of the recommendations. Potential conflicts of interest were stated for all panel members. Fig. 16.4 gives an overview of the layout of the methodology:

They used the Oxford Center for Evidence-Based Medicine (OCEBM) to allot a level of evidence and to assign a "grade" to the recommendations. Following the final review of the draft, the ASAS-EULAR recommendations were sanctioned by the EULAR Executive Committee and the ASAS Executive Committee.

The recommendations start with **overarching principles**, which are considered generic, implicit in nature, and serve as a basis for the state-of-the-art management of patients with axSpA. They included the following overarching principles:

1. Multidisciplinary approach—given the diversity of articular and extraarticular symptoms seen in axSpA.
2. Best possible care to maximize long-term health-related quality of life and prevention of progressive structural damage due to axSpA.
3. Optimal management with nonpharmacologic and pharmacologic treatment modalities.
4. Shared decision-making and patient education.
5. Cost consideration when one chooses between treatment modalities of similar efficacy and side effect profiles but with varying costs.

The panelists chose to illustrate their treatment recommendations using a flowchart. They suggest how various treatments (nonpharmacologic and pharmacologic) might be used in patients with axSpA. An overview of this intervention-based approach is shown in Fig. 16.5.

Exercise, patient education, and smoking cessation formed the initial treatment of axSpA. Similar to the ACR-SAA-SPARTAN recommendation, the panel judged this to be a strong recommendation. Active physical therapy was recommended over unsupervised or home exercises.[9]

An important first step before starting treatment of axSpA is to make sure that the clinical diagnosis of axSpA is correct. As shown in Fig. 16.5, the algorithm is divided into three phases. The phase I of pharmaceutical treatment is as follows: treatment of pain and stiffness of axSpA starts by using **nonsteroidal antiinflammatory drugs (NSAIDs)**. This is a strong recommendation based on several placebo-controlled trials. Pervious trial and observational evidence had suggested that the continuous use of NSAIDs reduced the progression of structural damage in the spine in comparison with on-demand use of NSAIDs. However, a recently published randomized control trial casts doubt on the potential structural benefits of NSAIDs on the spine.[66] Consequently, ASAS/EULAR agreed to base the intensity (doses, continuous vs. on demand) of therapy on the severity of symptoms only. **Disease activity** is assessed by using established disease activity scores: the BASDAI, which is a composite score based on five patients' reported outcome parameters alone, or the ASDAS, which contains four patients' reported outcome parameters plus an acute-phase reactant, preferably CRP, and which gives different weight to the different parameters.[65,67] If two NSAIDs are not effective

in controlling pain and stiffness over a period of at least 1 month, and the axial disease still remains active (ASDAS >2.1 or BASDAI >4), this step was to be followed by escalation of therapy to the next phase (phase II)—biologic agents.

According to the ASAS-EULAR recommendations, a **biologic agent** should only be considered as a next step if there is a radiographic sacroiliitis (according to the definition of AS) or MRI inflammation (subchondral bone marrow edema) in the SI joints or spine or if patients are CRP-elevated. It has been shown that patients with nr-axSpA (without radiographic sacroiliitis) show only a good response to TNF-blocker therapy if they are also MRI- or CRP-positive. A similar wording is also used for the label of TNF inhibitors for the indication of axSpA in the EU. The ASAS-EULAR recommendations state that, according to current practice, treatment with a biologic should start with **a TNF inhibitor** because much more experience is available with TNF inhibitors compared with the other biologic, **the IL-17 inhibitor secukinumab**, which has been found to show similar efficacy in the treatment of patients with AS. No study data are yet available for the treatment of nr-axSpA with secukinumab; clinical trials are ongoing. **Continuation of biologic therapy** was recommended if there was an improvement of ASDAS >1.1 or BASDAI >2 after 12 weeks.

The ASAS/EULAR recommendations do not recommend any specific TNFi agent over the other. They have additional comments when axSpA was associated with extraarticular manifestations. Monoclonal TNFi such as infliximab and adalimumab were preferred over etanercept when comanaging axSpA patients with uveitis or inflammatory bowel disease.

If the disease is found to be active after a trial of NSAIDs for 4 weeks and the symptoms are predominantly peripheral, local glucocorticoid intraarticular injections or sulfasalazine is recommended before considering a treatment with a biologic.

Phase III was to explore options when TNFi fail due to ineffectiveness (failure of improvement of ASDAS >1.1 or BASDAI >2 after 12 weeks) or are contraindicated due to toxicity.

In this case, the ASAS-EULAR recommended switching to another TNFi or IL-17i in the scenario that the initial TNFi fails. As shown in a trial published in 2016, IL-17i has proven efficacy in patients who have failed a TNFi.[68]

ASAS-EULAR also recommended starting directly with IL-17i when there is a contraindication or toxicity to TNFi.[68,69] In exceptional situations, where IL-17i cannot be used, the use of sulfasalazine or methotrexate

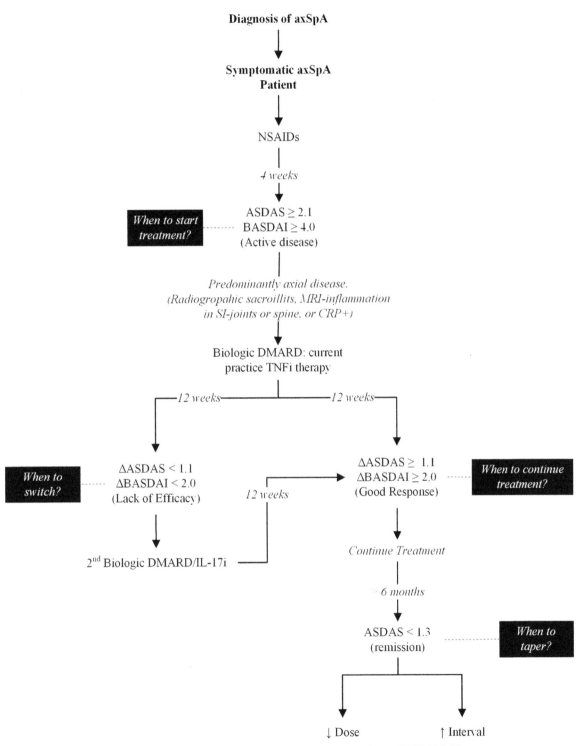

FIG. 16.5 Overview of presentation of recommendations—ASAS-EULAR.

might be considered, although such an approach would currently not be supported by data.[70-72]

If axSpA patients continue to be in remission (preferentially defined by an ASDAS <1.3 for at least 6 months), the next step was to **consider tapering of biologic agents**. There were two studies showing possibility of maintaining remission in patients with stable axSpA either with reducing the dose or with spacing out the interval of dose.[67,75] One of the newly added overarching principles of ASAS-EULAR in 2016 was "cost-effectiveness." They recognized the individual and societal costs of continuing biologics in stable axSpA patients and thus recommended to consider tapering biologics. They propose to use a shared decision-making approach when faced with this situation.

Additional topics of the ASAS-EULAR treatment recommendations were as follows:

1. Strongly advocating against the use of **long-term systemic glucocorticoids** in patients with axSpA. This was based on data from three small case series, and a 2-week randomized control trial, which showed only (modest) improvements with high-dosed glucocorticoids.
2. It was suggested that **total hip arthroplasty** should be considered in patients with refractory pain or disability and radiographic evidence of structural damage.
3. There are not much high-quality data that exist for elective **spinal corrective osteotomy**. Given some degree of restoration of range of motion achieved by patients with axSpA and kyphosis, the ASAS-EULAR conditionally recommended the surgery for improvement of quality of life; however, operations should only be conducted in experienced centers.
4. If a significant change in the course of the disease occurs, causes other than inflammation, such as a **spinal fracture**, should be considered before medical treatment is changed.

In a nutshell, the approach proposed by ASAS/EULAR fulfills one of the main goals of treatments recommendations, which is providing guidance for rheumatologist who are unsure to use biologic agents in a particular sequence.

COMPARISON OF THE ACR-SAA-SPARTAN AND THE ASAS-EULAR TREATMENT GUIDELINES FOR AXSPA

The Similarities

Both sets of recommendations, ACR/SAA/SPARTAN and ASAS-EULAR, strived to produce high-quality recommendations as per IOM, developed research

questions, followed by an in-depth systematic literature review, with a predefined voting and consensus process to finally develop a draft of their respective recommendations. Among others, ASAS-EULAR included the following three overarching principles: (1) multidisciplinary approach, (2) striving for best possible care, and (3) patient education. Both groups chose to illustrate their treatment recommendations using flowcharts. They suggest how various treatments (pharmacologic and nonpharmacologic) might be used in patients with axSpA. These flowcharts have been shown in Figs. 16.3 and 16.5. With the lack of head-to-head clinical trials comparing different treatment options and the optimal sequence of different therapies, about 80% of the guidelines by both groups were conditional recommendations.

Exercise was the first step of both the guidelines. NSAID treatment was the second step; if not efficacious after a month of trial, this was followed by TNFi to treat predominantly axial disease. On the other hand, if the disease is more peripheral, local corticosteroid injections and sulfasalazine were recommended as an alternative to TNFi. Neither ASAS-EULAR nor ACR/SAA/SPARTAN favored to incorporate methotrexate for peripheral arthritis.

Both panels strongly advocated against the use of long-term systemic glucocorticoids in patients with axSpA. Both panels agreed that total hip arthroplasty should be considered in patients with refractory pain or disability and radiographic evidence of structural damage.[73-75]

Both sets of recommendations included disease monitoring of axSpA patients with the following:

1. Clinical outcomes, e.g., composite indices for disease activity such as ASDAS or BASDAI
2. Laboratory tests such as CRP or ESR

ASDAS combines patient-reported outcomes and CRP into one index.[67] It has been shown that structural damage (syndesmophyte formation) goes hand-in-hand with disease activity as measured by ASDAS. Such a relationship between BASDAI and syndesmophyte formation has not been shown.[67] Thus, ASAS/EULAR prefers ASDAS to monitor disease activity. There are no studies to address the benefits of routine monitoring, which show improved patient outcomes, so neither body of recommendation commented on the frequency of monitoring. ASAS/EULAR recommendations further clarified the use of imaging for disease activity monitoring. MRI continues to be expensive, and there is currently no established benefit of treating residual inflammation on MRI in an asymptomatic individual. Regarding X-rays, it has not been shown yet clearly and without doubt that the therapeutic reduction of disease activity has an influence on structural damage of the SI joints and the spine (visible on X-rays). Therefore, neither MRI nor X-ray was preferred modality to monitor disease activity.

The Differences

The ACR/SAA/SPARTAN used the GRADE methodology, whereas the ASAS-EULAR used OCEBM to develop guidelines.

ACR/SAA/SPARTAN recommendations were grouped for various stages and presentation of the disease. They developed different sets of questions for AS, nr-axSpA, and extraarticular manifestations (see Figs. 16.2 and 16.3). The ASAS-EULAR committee developed a condensed flowchart to summarize the management of axSpA—both AS and nr-axSpA together (Fig. 16.5).

ACR/SAA/SPARTAN relies on patient symptoms and physician opinion, without trying to measure this by scores, to describe the disease as stable or active. Active disease was defined as symptoms at an unacceptably bothersome level as reported by the patient, and judged by the examining clinician to be due to axSpA. Stable disease is that which causes symptoms that are bothersome but at an acceptable level as reported by the patient. The decision of escalation of therapy was based on these clinical parameters. On the other hand, the ASAS-EULAR committee developed a step-up approach, where they mentioned the explicit conditions in which biologic agents should be started, continued, switched, and tapered. These conditions were defined by disease activity, measured by ASDAS or BASDAI.

ACR/SAA/SPARTAN do not mention use of IL-17i because the literature review in 2015 preceded the approval of IL-17i (secukinumab) in February 2016, while the 2016 ASAS-EULAR included IL-17i in the step-up approach to be used as an alternative to switching to another TNFi, when the initial TNFi fails.

ASAS-EULAR emphasized an important concept, which was newly added in the 2016 recommendations—treat to target. This implies that a treatment algorithm including escalation steps is guided by measuring disease activity with the aim to reach clinical remission or, if not possible, a status of low disease activity. This was based on the rationale that high disease activity leads to new syndesmophyte formation in patients with axSpA,[76] thus underscoring the importance to achieve remission or low disease activity. Furthermore, it was postulated that

attainment of a symptom-free state, which is always an important therapeutic aim, can better be reached if treating physicians are guided by measuring disease activity (target). Currently, remission has been defined best by reaching an ASDAS <1.3, according to an international task force on targeted therapies in spondyloarthritis.[77] In addition, because of lack of reliable data, ACR/SAA/SPARTAN did currently not comment on a treat-to-target strategy.

Other concepts that were introduced in the 2016 ASAS-EULAR updated guidelines were tapering of biologics and cost-effectiveness. The ACR/SAA/SPARTAN did not endorse tapering or stopping biologics neither do they explicitly consider costs in their recommendations.

Table 16.5 shows a summary of ACR/SAA/SPARTAN and ASAS-EULAR recommendations for axSpA.[1,2]

CONCLUSIONS AND PERSPECTIVES

The treatment recommendations from ASAS-EULAR and ACR/SAA/SPARTAN provide clinicians with up-to-date, evidence-based guidelines for management of axSpA patients. There are some important differences that exist in their development process, although the treatment recommendations do not differ much. The framework of the ASAS-EULAR guidelines is intervention-focused and pays most attention to the musculoskeletal manifestations. Conversely, because ACR/SAA/SPARTAN has used GRADE methodology, treatment guidelines are focused on particular clinical scenarios. They also include recommendations specifically for extraarticular manifestations such as uveitis and IBD.

The current lack of evidence regarding management of some aspects of axSpA leaves a number of unanswered questions (see Table 16.6).[1,2] Both sets of recommendations recognize this and highlight the need for future research to guide the use of therapies. Another item on the future research agenda would be to implement the current guidelines in clinical practice and to determine if they improve patient outcomes.

Treatment recommendations need to be updated as new evidence is generated and new treatments are made available. Both sets of recommendations will therefore be updated at regular intervals. We hope that the current recommendations are useful for healthcare professionals taking care of patients.

TABLE 16.5
Comparison & Differences Between the ACR-SAA-SPARTAN and ASAS-EULAR aXSpA Management Guidelines

Feature	ACR/SAA/SPARTAN	ASAS-EULAR
Composition of committee	Physicians (rheumatologists and nonrheumatologists) and patients were involved in the development process	
	Most representation from North America	Representation from 14 countries across Europe, North America, and South America
Methodologies used to generate guidelines	GRADE methodology	OCEBM methodology and EULAR Standardized Operating Procedures (SOP)
General principles	Multidisciplinary approach, best possible care, and patient education	
	No mention of treat-to-target or cost-effectiveness	Treat-to-target and cost-effectiveness included
Outline of guideline	Separate recommendations for AS and nr-axSpA	AS and nr-axSpA clubbed into one set axSpA
Escalation of therapy	Based on active versus stable disease (patient's symptoms and clinical judgment of physician)	Based on disease activity measurements (ASDAS or BASDAI)
Nonpharmacologic therapy	Physical therapy recommended (active > passive)	
PHARMACOLOGIC THERAPY		
NSAIDs	Used as first-line treatment	
TNFi[a]	If 1-month trial of NSAIDs fails, axial disease continues to be active (no particular TNFi recommended)	
TNFi failure	Use alternative TNFi	Use alternative TNFi or IL-17i
TNFi toxicity	Use sulfasalazine or high-dose pamidronate (SAARD)	Use IL-17i

[a]IL-17i might be used as a first-line biologic under certain circumstances according to the ASAS-EULAR recommendations.

TABLE 16.6
Unanswered Questions in the Management of axSpA

Unanswered Questions in the Management of axSpA

1. Would combination treatment of traditional disease-modifying antirheumatic drugs (DMARDs) with TNFi help decrease antidrug antibody levels?
2. Would monitoring TNFi drug levels be useful?
3. Does alteration of the gut microbiome contribute to pathogenesis of axSpA and how can it be harnessed to discover new therapeutic modalities?
4. Can the differential response to the available biologic agents be predicted?
5. At what stage of the disease are the biologic agents most effective? Is there a therapeutic window?
6. Could MRI be used in monitoring disease activity?
7. Would regular monitoring of disease activity improve patient-related outcomes?
8. How does one define disease remission in axSpA?
9. Would TNFi be useful after failure IL-17i?
10. How to treat patients after failure of TNFi and IL-17i?
11. Is a combination therapy of TNFi and IL-17 inhibitors a treatment option in axSpA?

REFERENCES

1. Van Der Heijde D, Ramiro S, Landewé R, et al. 2016 update of the ASAS-EULAR management recommendations for axial spondyloarthritis. *Ann Rheum Dis.* 2017;76(6):978–991. https://doi.org/10.1136/annrheumdis-2016-210770.

2. Ward MM, Deodhar A, Akl EA, et al. American College of rheumatology/spondylitis association of America/spondyloarthritis research and treatment Network 2015 recommendations for the treatment of ankylosing spondylitis and nonradiographic axial spondyloarthritis. *Arthritis Rheumatol.* 2016;68(2):282–298. https://doi.org/10.1002/art.39298.

3. Guyatt GH, Oxman AD, Vist GE, et al. GRADE: an emerging consensus on rating quality of evidence and strength of recommendations. *Chin J Evid Based Med.* 2009;9(1):8–11. https://doi.org/10.1136/bmj.39489.470347.AD.

4. Van Der Heijde D, Aletaha D, Carmona L, et al. 2014 Update of the EULAR standardised operating procedures for EULAR-endorsed recommendations. *Ann Rheum Dis.* 2015;74(1):8–13. https://doi.org/10.1136/annrheumdis-2014-206350.

5. Bulstrode SJ, Barefoot J, Harrison RA, Clarke AK. The role of passive stretching in the treatment of ankylosing spondylitis. *Rheumatology.* 1987;26(1):40–42. https://doi.org/10.1093/rheumatology/26.1.40.

6. Kjeken I, Bø I, Rønningen A, et al. A three-week multidisciplinary in-patient rehabilitation programme had positive long-term effects in patients with ankylosing spondylitis: randomized controlled trial. *J Rehabil Med.* 2013;45(3):260–267. https://doi.org/10.2340/16501977-1078.

7. Figen A, Gecene M, Gunduz R, Borman P, Yorgancioglu R. Long-term effects of comprehensive inpatient rehabilitation on function and disease activity in patients with chronic rheumatoid arthritis and ankylosing spondylitis TT - Kronik romatoid artrit ve ankilozan spondilitli hastalarda kapsamli{dotless} yatan. *Turk J Rheumatol.* 2011;26(2):135–144. http://ovidsp.ovid.com/ovidweb.cgi?T=JS&CSC=Y&NEWS=N&PAGE=fulltext&D=emed10&AN=2011351201%5Cnhttp://lib.exeter.ac.uk:4556/resserv?sid=OVID:embase&id=pmid:&id=doi:10.5-152%2Ftjr.2011.020&issn=1309-0291&isbn=&volume=26&issue=2&spage=135&pages=135-144&date=20.

8. S S, T G. The effect of a home based exercise intervention package on outcome in ankylosing spondylitis: a randomized controlled trial. *J Rheumatol.* 2002;29(4):763–766. http://ovidsp.ovid.com/ovidweb.cgi?T=JS&PAGE=reference&D=emed5&NEWS=N&AN=2002138536.

9. Dagfinrud H, Hagen KB, Kvien TK. Physiotherapy interventions for ankylosing spondylitis. *Cochrane Database Syst Rev.* 2008;2008(1):CD002822.

10. Dundar U, Solak O, Toktas H, et al. Effect of aquatic exercise on ankylosing spondylitis: a randomized controlled trial. *Rheumatol Int.* 2014;34(11):1505–1511. https://doi.org/10.1007/s00296-014-2980-8.

11. van Tubergen A, Landewé R, van der Heijde D, et al. Combined spa-exercise therapy is effective in patients with ankylosing spondylitis: a randomized controlled trial. *Arthritis Rheum.* 2001;45(5):430–438.

12. Altan L, Bingöl Ü AM, Yurtkuran M. The effect of balneotherapy on patients with ankylosing spondylitis. *Scand J Rheumatol.* 2006;35(4):283–289. https://doi.org/10.1080/03009740500428806.

13. Gurcay E, Yuzer S, Eksioglu E, Bal A, Cakci A. Stanger bath therapy for ankylosing spondylitis: illusion or reality? *Clin Rheumatol.* 2008;27(7):913–917. https://doi.org/10.1007/s10067-008-0873-5.

14. Karapolat H, Eyigor S, Zoghi M, Akkoc Y, Kirazli Y, Keser G. Are swimming or aerobic exercise better than conventional exercise in ankylosing spondylitis patients? A randomized controlled study. *Eur J Phys Rehabil Med.* 2009;45(4):449–457.

15. Van Der Heijde D, Baraf HSB, Ramos-Remus C, et al. Evaluation of the efficacy of etoricoxib in ankylosing spondylitis: results of a fifty-two-week, randomized, controlled study. *Arthritis Rheum.* 2005;52(4):1205–1215. https://doi.org/10.1002/art.20985.

16. Dougados M, Béhier JM, Jolchine I, et al. Efficacy of celecoxib, a cyclooxygenase 2-specific inhibitor, in the treatment of ankylosing spondylitis: a six-week controlled study with comparison against placebo and against a conventional nonsteroidal antiinflammatory drug. *Arthritis Rheum.* 2001;44(1):180–185. https://doi.org/10.1002/1529-0131(200101)44:1<180::AID-ANR24>3.0.CO;2-K.

17. Barkhuizen A, Steinfeld S, Robbins J, West C, Coombs J, Zwillich S. Celecoxib is efficacious and well tolerated in treating signs and symptoms of ankylosing spondylitis. *J Rheumatol.* 2006;33(9):1805–1812.

18. Dougados M, Gueguen A, Nakache JP, et al. Ankylosing spondylitis: what is the optimum duration of a clinical study? A one year versus a 6 weeks nonsteroidal anti-inflammatory drug trial. *Rheumatology.* 1999;38(3):235–244. https://doi.org/10.1093/rheumatology/38.3.235.

19. Benhamou M, Gossec L, Dougados M. Clinical relevance of C-reactive protein in ankylosing spondylitis and evaluation of the NSAIDs/coxibs' treatment effect on C-reactive protein. *Rheumatology.* 2009;49(3):536–541. https://doi.org/10.1093/rheumatology/kep393.

20. Bao C, Huang F, Khan MA, et al. Safety and efficacy of golimumab in Chinese patients with active ankylosing spondylitis: 1-year results of a multicentre, randomized, double-blind, placebo-controlled phase III trial. *Rheumatology.* 2014;53(9):1654–1663. https://doi.org/10.1093/rheumatology/keu132.

21. Barkham N, Coates LC, Keen H, et al. Double-blind placebo-controlled trial of etanercept in the prevention of work disability in ankylosing spondylitis. *Ann Rheum Dis.* 2010;69(11):1926–1928. https://doi.org/10.1136/ard.2009.121327.

22. Van Der Heijde D, Dijkmans B, Geusens P, et al. Efficacy and safety of infliximab in patients with ankylosing spondylitis: results of a randomized, placebo-controlled trial (ASSERT). *Arthritis Rheum.* 2005;52(2):582–591. https://doi.org/10.1002/art.20852.

23. Calin A, Dijkmans BAC, Emery P, et al. Outcomes of a multicentre randomised clinical trial of etanercept to treat ankylosing spondylitis. *Ann Rheum Dis.* 2004;63(12):1594–1600. https://doi.org/10.1136/ard.2004.020875.

24. Braun J, Van Der Horst-Bruinsma IE, Huang F, et al. Clinical efficacy and safety of etanercept versus sulfasalazine in patients with ankylosing spondylitis: a randomized, double-blind trial. *Arthritis Rheum.* 2011;63(6):1543–1551. https://doi.org/10.1002/art.30223.

25. Gorman JD, Sack KE, Davis JC. Treatment of ankylosing spondylitis by inhibition of tumor necrosis factor α. *N Engl J Med.* 2002;346(18):1349–1356. https://doi.org/10.1056/NEJMoa012664.

26. Dougados M, Braun J, Szanto S, et al. Efficacy of etanercept on rheumatic signs and pulmonary function tests in advanced ankylosing spondylitis: results of a randomised double-blind placebo-controlled study (SPINE). *Ann Rheum Dis*. 2011;70(5):799–804. https://doi.org/10.1136/ard.2010.139261.

27. Brandt J, Khariouzov A, Listing J, et al. Six-month results of a double-blind, placebo-controlled trial of etanercept treatment in patients with active ankylosing spondylitis. *Arthritis Rheum*. 2003;48(6):1667–1675. https://doi.org/10.1002/art.11017.

28. Inman RD, Maksymowych WP. A double-blind, placebo-controlled trial of low dose infliximab in ankylosing spondylitis. *J Rheumatol*. 2010;37(6):1203–1210. https://doi.org/10.3899/jrheum.091042.

29. Van Der Heijde D, Kivitz A, Schiff MH, et al. Efficacy and safety of adalimumab in patients with ankylosing spondylitis: results of a multicenter, randomized, double-blind, placebo-controlled trial. *Arthritis Rheum*. 2006;54(7):2136–2146. https://doi.org/10.1002/art.21913.

30. Braun J, Brandt J, Listing J, et al. Treatment of active ankylosing spondylitis with infliximab: a randomised controlled multicentre trial. *Lancet*. 2002;359(9313):1187–1193. https://doi.org/10.1016/S0140-6736(02)08215-6.

31. Huang F, Gu J, Zhu P, et al. Efficacy and safety of adalimumab in Chinese adults with active ankylosing spondylitis: results of a randomised, controlled trial. *Ann Rheum Dis*. 2014;73(3):587–594. https://doi.org/10.1136/annrheumdis-2012-202533.

32. Hu Z, Xu M, Li Q, et al. Adalimumab significantly reduces inflammation and serum DKK-1 level but increases fatty deposition in lumbar spine in active ankylosing spondylitis. *Int J Rheum Dis*. 2012;15(4):358–365. https://doi.org/10.1111/j.1756-185X.2012.01734.x.

33. Dougados M, Van Der Heijde D, Sieper J, et al. Symptomatic efficacy of etanercept and its effects on objective signs of inflammation in early nonradiographic axial spondyloarthritis: a multicenter, randomized, double-blind, placebo-controlled trial. *Arthritis Rheumatol*. 2014;66(8):2091–2102. https://doi.org/10.1002/art.38721.

34. Haibel H, Rudwaleit M, Listing J, et al. Efficacy of adalimumab in the treatment of axial spondylarthritis without radiographically defined sacroiliitis: results of a twelve-week randomized, double-blind, placebo-controlled trial followed by an open-label extension up to week fifty-two. *Arthritis Rheum*. 2008;58(7):1981–1991. https://doi.org/10.1002/art.23606.

35. Barkham N, Keen HI, Coates LC, et al. Clinical and imaging efficacy of infliximab in HLA-B27-positive patients with magnetic resonance imaging-determined early sacroiliitis. *Arthritis Rheum*. 2009;60(4):946–954. https://doi.org/10.1002/art.24408.

36. Landewé R, Braun J, Deodhar A, et al. Efficacy of certolizumab pegol on signs and symptoms of axial spondyloarthritis including ankylosing spondylitis: 24-week results of a double-blind randomised placebo-controlled Phase 3 study. *Ann Rheum Dis*. 2014;73(1):39–47. https://doi.org/10.1136/annrheumdis-2013-204231.

37. Sieper J, Van Der Heijde D, Dougados M, et al. Efficacy and safety of adalimumab in patients with non-radiographic axial spondyloarthritis: results of a randomised placebo-controlled trial (ABILITY-1). *Ann Rheum Dis*. 2013. https://doi.org/10.1136/annrheumdis-2012-201766.

38. Migliore A, Broccoli S, Bizzi E, Laganà B. Indirect comparison of the effects of anti-TNF biological agents in patients with Ankylosing Spondylitis by means of a Mixed Treatment Comparison performed on efficacy data from published randomised, controlled trials. *J Med Econ*. 2012;15(3):473–480. https://doi.org/10.3111/13696998.2012.660255.

39. McLeod C, Bagust A, Boland A, et al. Adalimumab, etanercept and infliximab for the treatment of ankylosing spondylitis: a systematic review and economic evaluation. *Health Technol Assess*. 2007;11(28):1–158.

40. Machado MADÁ, Barbosa MM, Almeida AM, et al. Treatment of ankylosing spondylitis with TNF blockers: a meta-analysis. *Rheumatol Int*. 2013;33(9):2199–2213. https://doi.org/10.1007/s00296-013-2772-6.

41. Ren L, Li J, Luo R, Tang R, Zhu S, Wan L. Efficacy of antitumor necrosis factor(α) agents on patients with ankylosing spondylitis. *Am J Med Sci*. 2013;346(6):455–461. https://doi.org/10.1097/MAJ.0b013e3182926a23.

42. Lie E, Van Der Heijde D, Uhlig T, et al. Effectiveness of switching between TNF inhibitors in ankylosing spondylitis: data from the NOR-DMARD register. *Ann Rheum Dis*. 2011;70(1):157–163. https://doi.org/10.1136/ard.2010.131797.

43. Song IH, Heldmann F, Rudwaleit M, et al. Different response to rituximab in tumor necrosis factor blocker-naive patients with active ankylosing spondylitis and in patients in whom tumor necrosis factor blockers have failed: a twenty-four-week clinical trial. *Arthritis Rheum*. 2010;62(5):1290–1297. https://doi.org/10.1002/art.27383.

44. Lekpa FK, Poulain C, Wendling D, et al. Is IL-6 an appropriate target to treat spondyloarthritis patients refractory to anti-TNF therapy? A multicentre retrospective observational study. *Arthritis Res Ther*. 2012;14(2):R53. https://doi.org/10.1186/ar3766.

45. Sieper J, Porter-Brown B, Thompson L, Harari O, Dougados M. Assessment of short-term symptomatic efficacy of tocilizumab in ankylosing spondylitis: results of randomised, placebo-controlled trials. *Ann Rheum Dis*. 2014;73(1):95–100. https://doi.org/10.1136/annrheumdis-2013-203559.

46. Poddubnyy D, Hermann KGA, Callhoff J, Listing J, Sieper J. Ustekinumab for the treatment of patients with active ankylosing spondylitis: results of a 28-week, prospective, open-label, proof-of-concept study (TOPAS). *Ann Rheum Dis*. 2014;73(5):817–823. https://doi.org/10.1136/annrheumdis-2013-204248.

47. Song IH, Heldmann F, Rudwaleit M, et al. Treatment of active ankylosing spondylitis with abatacept: an open-label, 24-week pilot study. *Ann Rheum Dis*. 2011;70(6):1108–1110. https://doi.org/10.1136/ard.2010.145946.

48. Lekpa FK, Farrenq V, Canouï-Poitrine F, et al. Lack of efficacy of abatacept in axial spondylarthropathies refractory to tumor-necrosis-factor inhibition. *Jt Bone Spine.* 2012;79(1):47–50. https://doi.org/10.1016/j.jbspin.2011.02.018.

49. Maksymowych WP, Jhangri GS, Fitzgerald AA, et al. A six-month randomized, controlled, double-blind, dose-response comparison of intravenous pamidronate (60 mg versus 10 mg) in the treatment of nonsteroidal antiinflammatory drug-refractory ankylosing spondylitis. *Arthritis Rheum.* 2002;46(3):766–773. https://doi.org/10.1002/art.10139.

50. Clegg DO, Reda DJ, Weisman MH, et al. Comparison of sulfasalazine and placebo in the treatment of ankylosing spondylitis: a department of veterans affairs cooperative study. *Arthritis Rheum.* 1996;39(12):2004–2012. https://doi.org/10.1002/art.1780391209.

51. Kirwan J, Edwards A, Huitfeldt B, Thompson P, Currey H. The course of established ankylosing spondylitis and the effects of sulphasalazine over 3 years. *Br J Rheumatol.* 1993;32:729–733.

52. Richter MB, Woo P, Panayi GS, Trull A, Unger A, Shepherd P. The effects of intravenous pulse methylprednisolone on immunological and inflammatory processes in ankylosing spondylitis. *Clin Exp Immunol.* 1983;53(1):51–59.

53. Ejstrup L, Peters ND. Intravenous methylprednisolone pulse therapy in ankylosing spondylitis. *Scand J Rheumatol.* 1985;32:231–233.

54. Haibel H, Fendler C, Listing J, Callhoff J, Braun J, Sieper J. Efficacy of oral prednisolone in active ankylosing spondylitis: results of a double-blind, randomised, placebo-controlled short-term trial. *Ann Rheum Dis.* 2014;73(1):243–246. https://doi.org/10.1136/annrheumdis-2012-203055.

55. Mintz G, Enríquez RD, Mercado U, Robles EJ, Javier Jiménez F, Gutiérrez G. Intravenous methylprednisolone pulse therapy in severe ankylosing spondylitis. *Arthritis Rheumatol.* 1981;24(5):734–736.

56. Coombes BK, Bisset L, Vicenzino B. Efficacy and safety of corticosteroid injections and other injections for management of tendinopathy: a systematic review of randomised controlled trials. *Lancet.* 2010;376(9754):1751–1767. https://doi.org/10.1016/S0140-6736(10)61160-9.

57. Wallen MM, Gillies D. Intra-articular steroids and splints/rest for children with juvenile idiopathic arthritis and adults with rheumatoid arthritis. In: *Cochrane Database of Systematic Reviews.* 2006:CD002824. https://doi.org/10.1002/14651858.CD002824.pub2.

58. Metcalfe D, Achten J, Costa ML. Glucocorticoid injections in lesions of the Achilles tendon. *Foot Ankle Int.* 2009;30(7):661–665. https://doi.org/10.3113/FAI.2009.0661.

59. Crofford LJ. Use of NSAIDs in treating patients with arthritis. *Arthritis Res Ther.* 2013;15(suppl 3):S2. https://doi.org/10.1186/ar4174.

60. Loh AR, Acharya NR. Incidence rates and risk factors for ocular complications and vision loss in HLA-B27-associated uveitis. *Am J Ophthalmol.* 2010;150:534–542. https://doi.org/10.1016/j.ajo.2010.04.031.

61. Van Royen BJ, De Gast A. Lumbar osteotomy for correction of thoracolumbar kyphotic deformity in ankylosing spondylitis. A structured review of three methods of treatment. *Ann Rheum Dis.* 1999;58(7):399–406. https://doi.org/10.1136/ard.58.7.399.

62. Roldan CA, Chavez J, Wiest PW, Qualls CR, Crawford MH. Aortic root disease and valve disease associated with ankylosing spondylitis. *J Am Coll Cardiol.* 1998;32(5):1397–1404. http://www.ncbi.nlm.nih.gov/pubmed/9809954.

63. Van Der Heijde D, Sieper J, Maksymowych WP, et al. 2010 Update of the international ASAS recommendations for the use of anti-TNF agents in patients with axial spondyloarthritis. *Ann Rheum Dis.* 2011;70(6):905–908. https://doi.org/10.1136/ard.2011.151563.

64. Braun J, Van Den Berg R, Baraliakos X, et al. 2010 update of the ASAS/EULAR recommendations for the management of ankylosing spondylitis. *Ann Rheum Dis.* 2011. https://doi.org/10.1136/ard.2011.151027.

65. Rudwaleit M, Van Der Heijde D, Landewé R, et al. The development of Assessment of SpondyloArthritis international Society classification criteria for axial spondyloarthritis (part II): validation and final selection. *Ann Rheum Dis.* 2009;68(6):777–783. https://doi.org/10.1136/ard.2009.108233.

66. Sieper J, Listing J, Poddubnyy D, et al. Effect of continuous versus on-demand treatment of ankylosing spondylitis with diclofenac over 2 years on radiographic progression of the spine: results from a randomised multicentre trial (ENRADAS). *Ann Rheum Dis.* 2016;75(8):1438–1443. https://doi.org/10.1136/annrheumdis-2015-207897.

67. Van Der Heijde D, Lie E, Kvien TK, et al. ASDAS, a highly discriminatory ASAS-endorsed disease activity score in patients with ankylosing spondylitis. *Ann Rheum Dis.* 2009;68(12):1811–1818. https://doi.org/10.1136/ard.2008.100826.

68. Sieper J, Deodhar A, Marzo-Ortega H, et al. Secukinumab efficacy in anti-TNF-naive and anti-TNF-experienced subjects with active ankylosing spondylitis: results from the MEASURE 2 Study. *Ann Rheum Dis.* 2017;76(3):571–575. https://doi.org/10.1136/annrheumdis-2016-210023.

69. Baeten D, Sieper J, Braun J, et al. Secukinumab, an Interleukin-17A inhibitor, in ankylosing spondylitis. *N Engl J Med.* 2015;373(26):2534–2548. https://doi.org/10.1056/NEJMoa1505066.

70. Chen J, Lin S, Liu C. Sulfasalazine for ankylosing spondylitis. *Cochrane Database Syst Rev.* 2014;11:CD004800. https://doi.org/10.1002/14651858.CD004800.pub3.

71. Chen J, Veras MM, Liu C, Lin J. Methotrexate for ankylosing spondylitis. In: *Cochrane Database of Systematic Reviews.* 2013. https://doi.org/10.1002/14651858.CD004524.pub4.

72. Haibel H, Brandt HC, Song IH, et al. No efficacy of subcutaneous methotrexate in active ankylosing spondylitis: a 16-week open-label trial. *Ann Rheum Dis.* 2007;66(3):419–421. https://doi.org/10.1136/ard.2006.054098.

73. Sochart DH, Porter ML. Long-term results of total hip replacement in young patients who had ankylosing spondylitis. Eighteen to thirty-year results with survivorship analysis. *J Bone Joint Surg Am.* 1997;79(8):1181–1189. http://www.ncbi.nlm.nih.gov/pubmed/9278078.

74. Tang WM, Chiu KY. Primary total hip arthroplasty in patients with ankylosing spondylitis. *J Arthroplasty.* 2000;15(1):52–58. https://doi.org/10.1016/S0883-5403(00)91155-0.

75. Joshi AB, Markovic L, Hardinge K, Murphy JCM. Total hip arthroplasty in ankylosing spondylitis: an analysis of 181 hips. *J Arthroplasty.* 2002;17(4):427–433. https://doi.org/10.1054/arth.2002.32170.

76. Ramiro S, Van Der Heijde D, Van Tubergen A, et al. Higher disease activity leads to more structural damage in the spine in ankylosing spondylitis: 12-year longitudinal data from the OASIS cohort. *Ann Rheum Dis.* 2014;73(8):1455–1461. https://doi.org/10.1136/annrheumdis-2014-205178.

77. Smolen JS, Schöls M, Braun J, et al. Treating axial spondyloarthritis and peripheral spondyloarthritis, especially psoriatic arthritis, to target: 2017 update of recommendations by an international task force. *Ann Rheum Dis.* 2018;77(1):3–17. https://doi.org/10.1136/annrheumdis-2017-211734.

CHAPTER 17

Economic Evaluations in Axial Spondyloarthritis

ANNELIES BOONEN, MD, PHD • CASPER WEBERS, MD

The World Health Organization, and various organizations with them, defines quality of care across six pillars: effectiveness, safety, timeliness, patient centeredness, equitability, and efficiency.[1] When providing healthcare, clinicians traditionally account for effectiveness and safety, and more recently, timeliness, patient centeredness, and equitability receive attention. When it comes to efficiency, however, clinicians feel often a conflict of interest between optimal care for the patient and costs for society. Notwithstanding, healthcare budgets are deficient to cover all possible healthcare services or technologies. Although society is definitely willing to pay for health, society also has limits in what it can afford. It is therefore important to balance the potential health gains against the costs of various options when making choices for diagnostic, preventive, and treatment strategies.

Health Technology Assessment (HTA) is the research that provides information on benefits and harms (both in terms of health and costs), when evaluating technologies or services in healthcare and public health. In addition, it considers organizational, social, legal, and ethical aspects of decisions in the systematic evaluation of the relation between health and micro-, meso-, and macrolevel factors that affect health directly or indirectly.[2] A health economic evaluation is a method within HTA that allows to weigh health benefits against costs of healthcare interventions in a specific healthcare setting (Fig. 17.1). The main purpose is to inform decisions to improve the uptake of cost-effective new technologies and prevent the uptake of technologies that are of doubtful value for the health system.

The history of economic evaluations for specific diseases usually follows the discovery of new technologies for use in healthcare. The first mention of a cost-effectiveness analysis (CEA) in ankylosing spondylitis (AS) was made in a paper from 1975, which discussed the role of HLA-B27 (which had just been discovered) in diagnosing AS. The authors were

critical about the use of HLA-B27 in clinical care and suggested a CEA to inform a further decision on this issue.[3] Most cost-effectiveness evaluations in axial spondyloarthritis (axSpA), however, have been performed following the availability of biologic disease-modifying antirheumatic drugs (bDMARDs) in the beginning of the 21st century. Although major benefits on disease activity had been seen, the drug costs were 40–80 times higher than the alternative at that time (NSAIDs), initiating the discussion whether and for which patients these drugs would be affordable for society. Although initial studies compared bDMARDs with usual care (NSAIDs), a next generation of models addressed comparative cost-effectiveness of different bDMARD and strategies of sequential bDMARDs, as well as tapering of drugs. In the latter type of analyses, the question is addressed whether monetary savings might justify some (temporary) loss in health.

In this chapter, we will provide an overview of published costs-effectiveness studies in axSpA, while emphasizing sources of uncertainty around the estimate. Although uncertainty is inherent to (any) modeling, its informative value for decision-making and research is too often neglected. We will therefore elaborate how insight into uncertainty of economic evaluations in axSpA can contribute to an epidemiologic and clinical research agenda for axSpA. First, however, we provide an overview of the basic methodological aspects of an economic evaluation.

METHODOLOGICAL CONSIDERATIONS OF ECONOMIC EVALUATIONS IN AXSPA

An economic evaluation is performed to understand the relation between changes in health and costs of a new (or existing) technology against an alternative (Fig. 17.2). Such evaluations are typically of interest when benefits of a new technology or service are expected,

Axial Spondyloarthritis. https://doi.org/10.1016/B978-0-323-56800-5.00017-5

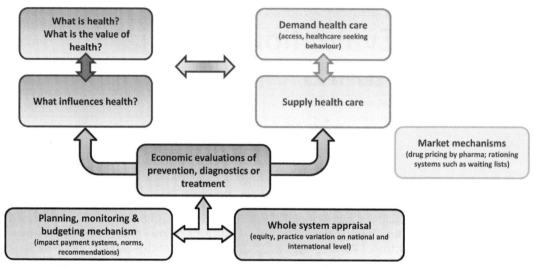

FIG. 17.1 Economic evaluations constitute an area of research within health technology assessment (HTA). Economic evaluations address the impact of new technologies or services on costs and health outcomes within an existing healthcare system (and thus represent a microeconomic evaluation).

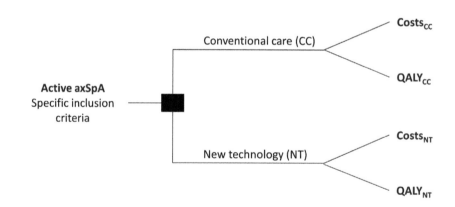

$$\text{Incremental cost-utility ratio (ICUR)} = \frac{\Delta \text{Costs}}{\Delta \text{QALY}} = \frac{\text{Costs}_{NT} - \text{Costs}_{CC}}{\text{QALY}_{NT} - \text{QALY}_{CC}}$$

FIG. 17.2 Simplified representation of an economic evaluation, clarifying that costs and effects over time of the intervention under evaluation are compared with conventional care (CC). The ratio between the differences in costs and in effects between options (treatment arms) is called the incremental cost-effectiveness ratio (ICER) and represents the additional costs (or savings) for extra gains (of losses) in health. When health gains over time are expressed in quality-adjusted life years (QALY), the cost-effectiveness ratio is specified as an incremental cost-utility ratio (ICUR).

but the technology is also costlier as compared with the best alternative in conventional care (CC).

Increasingly, cost-effectiveness studies are also informative when a strategy might result in some health loss but is less costly. An example could be

dose reduction of (costly) medication or active switching from original drug to a biosimilar. In the first approach, the technology under consideration is considered cost-effective if the ratio between cost and health gains is lower than a value considered

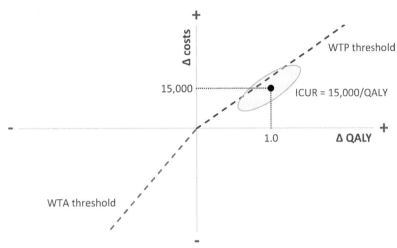

FIG. 17.3 The point estimate (*black dot*) and uncertainty around an incremental cost-effectiveness estimate (*light gray area*) are traditionally represented in a cost-effectiveness plane. The horizontal axis represents the differences in health benefits (usually QALYs) between new and conventional care, whereas the vertical axis represents the differences in costs. Point estimates in the north-east (NE) indicate the new strategy generates health gains but has extra costs. The willingness-to-pay (WTP) represents the threshold a specific society might be willing to pay for additional health and is represented by the line within the quadrant (*red dotted line*, NE quadrant). If the ICUR of a new technology is below the WTP threshold, this technology is generally considered cost-effective. Studies with a cost-effectiveness estimate on this line have a similar incremental cost-utility ratio (ICUR) but can differ in the absolute health gains or extra costs. The size and shape of the uncertainty cloud (often the 95% confidence interval) determine the likelihood a new strategy is cost-effective given a specific threshold. In the example, the uncertainty cloud crosses the WTP threshold, indicating it is not 100% certain whether the new technology would be cost-effective. Point estimates in the south-west (SW) quadrant indicate loss in health but savings in cost. The willingness-to-accept (WTA) refers to the amount of health forgone a society is willing to accept to save money (*blue dotted line*, SW quadrant). The WTA threshold is usually much higher than the WTP threshold.

acceptable for a specific jurisdiction or country to pay for a unit of health (willingness to pay). In the latter, the new approach/technology is acceptable if the ratio between costs and health gains exceeds value that is acceptable as monetary return for a unit of health forgone (willingness to accept) (Fig. 17.3).

Economic evaluations differ essentially from efficacy trials, in which they have to inform a decision-maker about the estimated cost-effectiveness of a new strategy in real clinical care.[2,4] On that line, several areas can be identified, which distinguish cost-effectiveness analyses from clinical trials:

- The perspective
  Although in efficacy studies, the benefits and harms are considered from the perspective of a patient (and sometimes of a caregiver), other perspectives are more relevant in economic evaluations, among which the societal perspective, the payer perspective, or the hospital perspective. The perspective has consequences on the choice of (health and cost) outcomes in the economic evaluation. For example,

a health outcome from a hospital perspective could be the "extra number of patients successfully discharged after a hip replacement," whereas from a societal perspective, the "extra health gained after hip replacement" would be the relevant outcome. On a similar note, from a payer perspective, the costs of a hospital day would be a tariff, whereas for a societal perspective, it would be a "true cost" estimate.

- The comparator
  As an efficacy study usually aims to provide evidence that a new technology has a strong influence on the outcome, a "next best" comparator that is ethically allowed is often chosen. In drug trials of bDMARDs in axSpA, this is often placebo (continuation of NSAID) or continuation of the ineffective bDMARD. In an economic evaluation, it is vital to compare a technology or service with the best available alternative in clinical care. For axSpA, this would be a head-to-head comparison of (a strategy of sequential) bDMARDs.

- The time horizon
  Although the duration of an efficacy study is usually chosen to ensure the maximal treatment benefit of the new technology can be reached, in an economic evaluation the long-term benefits and costs are relevant. In axSpA, a lifelong perspective has been recommended.[5] First, it is clear that short-term temporary improvements in health for persons with a chronic disease are less valuable than sustained improvements. Second, in axSpA the monetary (and health) benefits related to reduced need for joint replacement surgery or reduced chance for sick leave and work disability can only be seen in long-term time frames. The lifelong time horizon poses challenges as it requires data on long-term effectiveness of drugs and especially the course of disease in those that withdraw from drugs because of either lack of efficacy or side effects.
- The outcome: the cost-effectiveness ratio
  Typical for a full economic evaluation is that the outcome is a ratio. Importantly, the between group or incremental cost-effectiveness ratio (ICER) is what matters. The incremental ratio represents the average extra cost for one extra "unit of health" gained (or lost) per patient of the new opposed to conventional strategy. This incremental ratio is preferably based on the differences in the time-integrated costs and health benefits over the total lifespan of the patients.

- The health outcome: natural effect or utilities
  In a cost-effectiveness analysis, the health effect (denominator) is represented by a unidimensional natural clinical effect. Examples in axSpA would be the extra number of patients reaching remission in strategy A compared with B, the number of bleeding stomach ulcers avoided, the number of deaths avoided or even the (area under the curve of) units of disease activity gained. However, using natural units makes it difficult for decision-makers to compare between different innovations within a disease and even more so to compare efficiency of innovations between diseases. Moreover, the aim of medicine is to improve the overall health of persons, balancing all health domains (and effects and side effect). For this reason, the concept of utility has been brought forward. The utility is a type of health-related quality-of-life (HRQoL) measure, anchored between zero, equivalent to value of health equal to death, and 1, equivalent to a value of health equal to perfect health. This allows that the scores can be compared across diseases and interventions. The integration of utility over time (years) provides the quality-adjusted life year (QALY), a two-dimensional construct (Fig. 17.4). Important to the concept of utilities is its foundation in decision-making theory. In the setting of decision-making, a preference or value for a health state matters. On this line, choice-based experiments are required to elicit preferences or

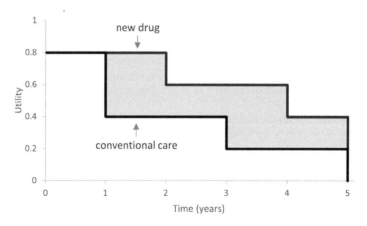

QALY (conventional care) = 1*0.8 + 2*0.4 + 2*0.2 = 2.0
QALY (new drug) = 2*0.8 + 2*0.6 + 1*0.4 = 3.2
Incremental QALY (grey area) = 3.2 - 2.0 = 1.2

FIG. 17.4 Calculation of QALY, a two-dimensional construct of time (x-axis) and utility (y-axis). *QALY*, quality-adjusted life year.

utilities for health. As such experiments are time-consuming, algorithms have been developed that allow to assess utilities using patient-reported HRQoL questionnaires (indirect utility). Although utilities are often generic, they might lack content validity and sensitivity to change. For this reason, disease-specific utilities are increasingly accepted in economic evaluations. In SpA, the Assessment of SpondyloArthritis International Society (ASAS) Health Index offers an algorithm to convert scores on the questionnaire into a utility. This improves comparison of QALYs among treatments or strategies, which is increasingly at stake in axSpA. Guidelines for economic evaluations recommend the use of the societal perspective in the main analysis. Persons from society are considered more objective, as they have not adjusted to the disease. Moreover, it is expected that persons from society have less self-interest, when it comes to distribution of resources across health states. Of note, when health effects are measured as QALYs, the economic evaluation is referred to as a cost-utility analysis (CUA). A CUA can be considered a special type of CEA, and the outcome is the incremental cost per QALY gained (incremental cost-utility ratio [ICUR]).

- The costs outcome (cost-of-illness)
  The costs-of-illness reflects all the costs resulting from the disease and its treatment. The types of costs that are relevant in an economic evaluation highly depend on the perspective from which the costs are calculated. In the societal perspective, two main cost categories are distinguished, the direct (healthcare and nonhealthcare) and indirect (or productivity) costs. The direct healthcare costs refer to all healthcare resources provided to and used by the patients (such as costs of care providers, technical procedures and medications, hospitalizations, formal care), whereas the direct nonhealthcare costs (also referred to as patient and family costs) refer to costs incurred by the patients but that are not reimbursed by the healthcare system (such as travel costs, costs of membership to a patient society, costs of informal care, costs of increased insurance premiums). The indirect or productivity costs reflect the costs to society because of loss of income for society because of sick leave and/or work disability. Although in a healthcare (payer's) perspective, only the direct healthcare costs are taken into account, in a societal perspective, all cost categories matter. The perspective of the cost-of-illness is not only relevant for the cost categories addressed but

also for the unit costs of the resources (of productivity). This is mainly an issue when it comes to the direct healthcare costs. In a healthcare (payers') perspective, these unit costs are usually tariffs. Tariffs are generally historical and/or negotiated and often do not reflect at all the true costs of the manpower needed or materials required. A typical example is diagnosis-related groups (DRGs), which reflect a payer's perspective but by no means the true costs. There is growing consensus that no distinction should be made between the costs related to the index disease and other disease or comorbidities, but that all cost of all health impairments (i.e., also other disease/comorbidities) should be considered.

- The setting: real life
  Economic evaluations aim to understand benefits and harms of innovations in real life and thus should account for case mix of patients such as age, gender, BMI, comorbidities/comedication, past history of drug interventions, risk for nonadherence, etc. For this reason, data from highly controlled (phase 3) trials and open-label extension studies might be considered less valid, and data from pragmatic trials (and meta-analyses of pragmatic trials) or registries with less stringent exclusion, less controlled treatment, and best alternative care in a comparator control group are preferred.

- Trial versus model-based evaluation and uncertainty
  Although an economic evaluation can be performed alongside a clinical trial, for reasons mentioned above, this is often less preferable. Therefore, often models are computed. However, models can be complex as often data to model short-, medium-, and long-term effects of drugs for different strategies are not available. Typically, multiple sources are needed to model health over time. Consequently, models are characterized by a more complex type of uncertainty. Similar as in trials, there is first-order uncertainty (variability around the estimates within the sample), but there is also second-order uncertainty because of heterogeneity among the different studies/data that provide data for the model. Of note, this uncertainty is often the consequence of lack of (good-quality) clinical or epidemiologic data. Fortunately, models nowadays can deal with uncertainty and can quantify the contribution of the different sources of uncertainty. These uncertainty analyses are therefore a great source to improve knowledge and estimates on real-life effectiveness and cost-effectiveness of medical care.

ECONOMIC EVALUATIONS IN AXSPA
Economic Evaluations of Non–Disease-Modifying Drug Interventions

The two first cost-effectoveness studies in axSpA considered the effect of exercise therapy.[6,7] Both studies were trial-based economic evaluations with a 9-month time horizon. In the first evaluation, supervised group exercise therapy in patients with AS required an extra cost of US\$409 per patient per year from the Dutch healthcare payer but resulted in a 5% additional increase in fitness, 7% additional improvement in mobility, and 28% difference in gain in overall global health.[6] Although extra benefits were small and no QALYs were provided, the extra costs were considered acceptable. The second analysis addressed persons with AS who suffered from limitations in physical functioning despite home or group exercise and revealed that spa exercise in Austria or in the Netherlands had an ICUR of €7465/QALY spa treatment in Austria and €18,575/QALY from a Dutch societal perspective when compared with continuation of CC.[7] Interestingly, when using the Short Form-6D (SF-6D) as an alternative utility to assess QALY in sensitivity analyses, the gain in health was smaller, making the ICUR less favorable but still acceptable for the Dutch healthcare system.[7,8]

When COX-selective NSAIDs proved more effective and safer, but also more costly than nonselective NSAIDs, a model with a 30-year time horizon was computed to evaluate the cost-effectiveness from a payer's perspective of etoricoxib relative to celecoxib and nonselective naproxen and diclofenac (all at recommended full doses) in the initial treatment of AS.[9] Patients who failed two NSAIDs were started on tumor necrosis factor alpha inhibition (TNFi). The efficacy of the different NSAIDs on AS symptoms and gastrointestinal as well as cardiovascular safety and mortality was modeled. Effect of drugs on BASDAI and BASFI was estimated with a mixed-treatment comparison meta-analysis of clinical trials and linked to QALY and disease-specific costs. Starting etoricoxib resulted in a small extra health benefit of 0.4 QALYs compared with the other strategies. The probability was above 99% that etoricoxib had the lowest cost. Etoricoxib was expected to save £13,620 relative to celecoxib, £9957 relative to diclofenac, and £9863 relative to naproxen. By having an improved safety profile and by postponing the start of TNFi, etoricoxib has a higher chance to be cost-effective for the UK payer. The model was repeated from the Norwegian perspective and provided similar results.[10] Of note, the manufacturer of etoricoxib was involved in the model and preparation of the manuscript.

Economic Evaluations of Biologic Disease-Modifying Drugs

The introduction of TNFi showed unprecedented improvement of function and health of patients with axSpA. However, TNFi and all other bDMARDs that became available afterward are costly, with annual costs between €12,000 and €18,000 per patient in Europe and 50%–100% more expensive in the United States of America (USA). To investigate whether bDMARDs would be cost-effective in clinical practice, several economic evaluations have been performed. These were primarily conducted in AS populations, as the concept of nr-axSpA was introduced later in time. Below, we summarize first the (short-term) cost-effectiveness studies of biologic treatments in axSpA to continue with the (long-term) models.

Incremental (short-term) cost-effectiveness analyses of bDMARD

Three cost-effectiveness studies on bDMARDs in axSpA are available, all with a short but variable time horizon and using observational or trial data of patients starting a TNFi. In a retrospective cohort study of patients with AS, psoriatic arthritis, or rheumatoid arthritis starting TNFi, it was found that drug costs to achieve a minimal clinically important difference (MCID) in HAQ-DI (0.2 points) were 49,000 Canadian dollars (CAD) and 36,000 CAD in the first and second year, respectively.[11] Especially in the second year, higher responder rates had been observed in AS compared with both other diseases, resulting in lower incremental drug costs per responder. In another study, using efficacy data from available RCTs on TNFi (etanercept [ETN], adalimumab [ADA], and certolizumab [CZP]) in persons with nr-axSpA, the drug costs per ASAS20/ASAS40 responder 1 year after starting TNFi were all upward of €40,000, but with the lowest number needed to treat and therefore lowest cost per ASAS responder for ADA.[12] More recently, a network meta-analysis of 15 RCTs in bDMARD-naive patients with AS was performed and used to calculate response rates for the different bDMARDs (infliximab (IFX), ETN, ADA, golimumab [GLM], CZP, and secukinumab [SEC]) compared with no bDMARD,[13] and it was found that the 12-week drug (and drug administration) costs to achieve an additional ASAS20 or ASAS40 response ranged from \$27,000 to \$76,000. Although IFX had the highest probability for response, treatment with ADA had the lowest costs and finally the most favorable cost per responder compared with no bDMARD. Extrapolating these data to annual costs is not possible, as the first 12 weeks of TNFi treatment has additional costs because of loading regimens for some of these drugs and as initial response does not equal sustained response.

Incremental cost-utility analyses of bDMARDs

Nineteen publicly available economic evaluations of bDMARDs in axSpA estimated the incremental costs per QALY, and 17 of them were long-term models (see Table 17.1). To understand a long-term economic evaluation in axSpA, it is important to realize that the start of any economic model is the representation of the course of the disease over time (Fig. 17.5). In all economic evaluations in axSpA, the course of BASFI and/or BASDAI (in the intervention and CC group) is the health outcome used to model the course of the disease. The initial values of BASDAI and/or BASFI, chance

TABLE 17.1

Main Characteristics and Results of the Studies Addressing (Long-Term) Cost-Utility of bDMARDs in axSpA

Author, Year Population	Comparison	Perspective, Country Currency, Price-Year	Time Horizon	Base-Case Results (ICUR, Unless Otherwise Stated)	Important Drivers[a]
Kobelt, 2004[14] AS	IFX vs. CC	Societal, UK British pounds, 2002	2 years (main) 30 years	Main model: £35,400/ QALY Long-term model: £9600/QALY	Perspective, horizon, dosing frequency IFX, discontinuation rate, BASFI progression on IFX
Boonen, 2006[15] AS	IFX, ETN vs. CC	Societal, the Netherlands Euros, 2002	5 years	IFX: €189,564/QALY ETN: €118,022/QALY	IFX/ETN cost
Kobelt, 2006[16] AS	IFX vs. CC	Societal & healthcare, Canada Canadian dollars, 2004	30 years	Can$37,491/QALY	Horizon, IFX cost, discontinuation rates
Botteman, 2007[17] AS	ADA vs. CC	Payer/NHS, UK British pounds, 2004	30 years	£23,097/QALY	Perspective, continuation after initial nonresponse, cost and utility estimation
Ara, 2007[18] AS	ETN vs. CC	Payer/NHS, UK British pounds, NR	25 years	£22,704/QALY	Estimated utility and costs, discontinuation rates
Kobelt, 2007[19] AS	IFX versus CC	Societal & payer, UK British pounds, 2005	Lifetime	Societal: IFX dominates Payer: £26,751–49,417/QALY	Perspective, horizon, IFX dosing regimen
McLeod, 2007[20] AS	ADA, ETN, IFX vs. CC	Payer/NHS, UK British pounds, NR	20 years	Long-term: ADA/ETN £98,910/ QALY IFX £175,000/QALY	Horizon, discontinuation rates, BASFI progression, sustained placebo response
NICE TA143, 2008[21] AS	ADA, ETN, IFX vs. CC	Payer/NHS, UK British pounds, NR	20 years	ADA/ETN £22,000–31,000/QALY IFX £49,000–65,000/ QALY	Differences in TNFi costs
Kobelt, 2008[22] AS	IFX vs. CC	Societal & healthcare, Spain Euros, 2005	40 years	Societal: IFX dominates Healthcare: €8866–22,520/QALY	Perspective, IFX dosing regimen, horizon, discontinuation rates
Fautrel, 2010[23] AS	IFX every 6 weeks vs. IFX on demand	Payer, France Euros, 2006	1 year	€50,760/QALY	NR

Continued

TABLE 17.1

Main Characteristics and Results of the Studies Addressing (Long-Term) Cost-Utility of bDMARDs in axSpA—cont'd

Author, Year Population	Comparison	Perspective, Country Currency, Price-Year	Time Horizon	Base-Case Results (ICUR, Unless Otherwise Stated)	Important Drivers[a]
Neilson, 2010[24] AS	ETN vs. CC	Payer & societal, Germany Euros, 2007	25 years	Payer: €54,815/QALY Societal: €22,147/QALY	Perspective, effectiveness ETN, discontinuation rates, estimated costs and utility
Tran-Duy, 2011[25] AS	Sequential treatment, TNFi included vs. TNFi excluded	Societal, the Netherlands Euros, 2010	Lifetime	€35,186/QALY	NR
Armstrong, 2013[26] AS	GLM vs. CC, ETN, ADA	Payer/NHS, UK British pounds, NR	Lifetime	GLM (and ADA) extendedly dominated by ETN ETN vs. CC £26,505/QALY	Response criterion
Tran-Duy, 2015[27] AS	Sequential treatment, TNFi included vs. TNFi excluded	Societal, the Netherlands Euros, 2014	20 calendar years (dynamic model)	€61,129/QALY	NR
Corbett, 2016[28] AS, nr-axSpA	ADA, CZP, ETN, GLM, IFX vs. CC	Payer/NHS, UK British pounds, 2014	60 years	AS: £19,240–66,529/QALY nr-axSpA: £28,247-35,290/QALY	TNFi cost (IFX vs. others), baseline and change in BASDAI/BASFI (AS), absence of placebo response on CC (nr-axSpA)
NICE TA383, 2016[29] AS, nr-axSpA	ADA, CZP, ETN, GLM, IFX vs. CC	Payer/NHS, UK British pounds, 2014	60 years	See Corbett, 2016 Biosimilar-IFX £36,751/QALY	See Corbett, 2016
Závada, 2016[30] AS	Reduced vs. standard TNFi dosing regimen	Societal, Czech Republic Euros, NR	1 year	Standard vs. reduced dosing €211,416/QALY	NR
Wolff, 2016[31] AS	TNF-naïve: SEC vs. ADA, CZP, ETN, GLM, IFX TNFi-experienced: SEC vs. CC	Payer/NHS, UK British pounds, NR	Lifetime	TNFi-naïve: £38,778–71,690/QALY for TNFi vs. SEC or SEC cost saving TNFi-experienced: £2223/QALY SEC vs. CC	Alternative effectiveness inputs bDMARDs (TNF-naïve); horizon, rebound (TNF-experienced)
Borse, 2017[32] AS	GLM vs. CC, ADA, CZP, ETN, IFX	Payer/NHS, UK British pounds, 2013	Lifetime	GLM vs. CC: £19,070/QALY GLM-dominated ADA/ETN	Long-term cost estimation, GLM cost

[a]As reported by authors of original publication or, if not stated by authors, based on the percent change in ICUR. Note that not all potential drivers have been investigated in each study.

ADA, adalimumab; *AS*, ankylosing spondylitis; *axSpA*, axial spondyloarthritis; *BASDAI*, Bath Ankylosing Spondylitis Disease Activity Index; *BASFI*, Bath Ankylosing Spondylitis Functional Index; *CC*, conventional care; *CZP*, certolizumab pegol; *ETN*, etanercept; *GLM*, golimumab; *ICUR*, incremental cost-utility ratio; *IFX*, infliximab; *NHS*, National Health Service; *NICE*, National Institute for Health and Care Excellence; *NR*, not reported; *nr-axSpA*, nonradiographic axial spondyloarthritis; *QALY*, quality-adjusted life year; *SEC*, secukinumab; *TA*, technology appraisal; *TNFi*, TNF inhibitor; *UK*, United Kingdom.

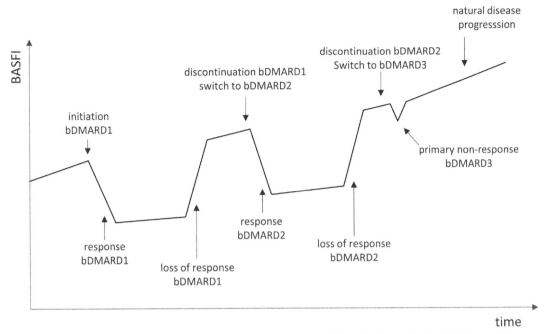

FIG. 17.5 The core of an economic evaluation is a disease model. In axSpA, usually the BASFI (or BASDAI in conjunction with BASFI) is the main measure used to represent the "severity" of disease over time. Usually, different sources are needed to model BASFI/BASDAI over time in those with and without the intervention. Essential elements of modeling health outcome are response to bDMARD (and values of BASDAI/BASFI before and after baseline in responders as well as nonresponders), short- and long-term drug discontinuation, and disease progression on different treatment strategies. *BASDAI*, Bath Ankylosing Spondylitis Disease Activity Index; *BASFI*, Bath Ankylosing Spondylitis Functional Index.

of response, and values after initial response are usually derived from trial data. The long-term evolution of BASFI/BASDAI with or without treatment is usually extracted from open-label or observational (registry) studies. Only in a next step, BASDAI and/or BASFI are linked to costs and utility. This latter relationship is often explored in data from (again) other observational studies, containing information on cost-of-illness studies and/or utilities in persons with axSpA.

Below, we summarize the CUAs following the chronology of publication, as this reflects nicely the increasing complexity of economic evaluations when more drug options become available, or when modeling improves because of more accurate clinical information on the disease course, more information becomes available to improve the disease model, or when new modeling methodology is introduced. The characteristics and results of the studies are summarized in Table 17.1.

The first economic evaluations compared (single or multiple) TNFi with CC without bDMARDs in

persons with active disease who had failed two NSAIDs (n = 12 studies). When more bDMARD became available, comparisons between bDMARDs were addressed (n = 2 studies), and two studies considered sequential use compared with no bDMARDs (n = 2). When IL-17 inhibitors became available as a new class of bDMARDs, economic evaluations were also performed in persons with axSpA that failed one or more TNFi (n = 1). Last but not least, to improve efficiency of bDMARD use, some studies addressed dose adjustments or tapering (n = 2).

Models comparing one bDMARD with care without bDMARD

Infliximab. Infliximab was the first bDMARD to be approved for AS, and in 2004 the first cost-utility of IFX compared with CC in AS was published.[14] Adopting a societal United Kingdom (UK) perspective and using IFX efficacy estimates from the fist RCT on IFX, the ICUR of IFX compared with CC was £35,000/QALY over a 2-year horizon. Despite substantial uncertainty regarding the long-term efficacy of IFX and the natural history of AS at that time, long-term cost-utility of IFX over 30 years was estimated at £10,000/QALY if IFX was assumed to have no effect on disease progression (BAS-FI). Uncertainty analyses showed that important drivers of long-term results were long-term IFX discontinuation rates, whether or not patients on IFX experienced disease progression (BASFI), cost (dosing) of IFX, and the study perspective (societal perspective being more favorable).

The model for this CUA has been adapted for three other CUAs.[16,19,22] In 2006, the ICUR of IFX compared with CC from a Canadian societal perspective using a 30-year horizon was CAD37,000/QALY in the main analysis.[16] The higher point estimate compared with the UK study might be explained by differences in resource use and unit costs between the countries as well as different discount rates. Again, drivers of results were disease progression while on IFX, long-term IFX discontinuation rates, and costs of IFX. In a second adaptation, the ICUR was again calculated for a lifetime time horizon from a societal UK perspective, but using drug effectiveness data from both pivotal RCTs on IFX.[19] Assuming IFX reduced or inhibited disease progression (BASFI) while on IFX, IFX dominated CC (i.e., had lower cost and more health benefits). Assuming IFX had no effect on disease progression, ICURs were between £12,000 and 15,000/QALY. In addition, ICURs were three to four times higher when adopting a payer's perspective (i.e., when excluding indirect costs). Further uncertainty analyses confirmed time horizon and IFX costs were relevant cost drivers. Finally, the latter model was used to explore ICU of IFX compared with CC from a Spanish societal perspective over a 40-year horizon.[22] In the main analysis, IFX dominated CC, regardless of the rate of disease progression while on IFX. From a payer's perspective, ICURs were between €15,000 and 32,000/QALY depending on assumed disease progression (BASFI) while on IFX. Again, important drivers of the point estimate were time horizon, long-term IFX discontinuation rates, and IFX cost.

Etanercept. In 2007 the first CUA of ETN versus CC from a UK payer's perspective over a 25-year horizon was published, using data from two RCTs as sources for efficacy.[18] With a main ICUR of £23,000/QALY (assuming no progression of BASFI while on ETN), ETN was considered cost-effective. Key drivers for the ICUR were the estimated health effects of ETN and mapping on utility, disease-related costs, and the long-term discontinuation rate of ETN. Using the same model in the German setting led to substantially different results (payer's perspective ICUR €55,000/QALY).[24] This

difference could largely be explained by differences in the acquisition cost of ETN between countries.

Adalimumab. Also in 2007, the cost-utility of ADA was modeled from a UK payer's perspective over a 30-year horizon, which revealed an ICUR of £23,000/QALY.[17] Uncertainty analyses indicated that the discount rates and estimates of cost and utility estimations through mapping on health outcomes (BASDAI and BASFI) were the most influential drivers of results. Two scenarios led to substantially different results: one adopting a societal perspective (ICUR around £5000/QALY) and one in which ADA was continued in all patients regardless of meeting response criteria (ICUR £63,000/QALY).

Models comparing different bDMARDs with care without bDMARDs. When evidence of efficacy of ETA and ADA in the treatment of axSpA became available, the cost-effectiveness of bDMARDs (IFX) was still questioned. Therefore, the economic evaluations of the new drugs still considered a treatment without a bDMARD as the conventional care comparator (see above). Notwithstanding, some studies (n = 5) performed evaluations of various TNFi in the same model, allowing some sort of comparative cost-utility.

The cost-utility of IFX and ETN, each compared with CC (no bDMARD) from a societal Dutch perspective over a 5-year horizon, was assessed in 2006.[15] ICURs in the main analyses were €180,000/QALY and €118,000/QALY for IFX and ETN, respectively. Models differed in initial efficacy of TNFi as revealed in available pivotal trials and in costs of both TNFi. As only two health states (BASDAI ≥4 or <4) were used to reflect short- and long-term efficacy and thus capture utilities and costs of AS, the opportunity to capture larger benefits of TNFi might have been missed. This explains partly why the incremental QALY gain was substantially lower compared with other studies.

To facilitate a decision on reimbursement of the different TNFi with proven efficacy in AS, the National Institute for Health and Care Excellence (NICE), the public body responsible for reimbursement recommendations in the UK, commissioned a CUA of IFX, ETA, and ADA compared with CC (no bDMARD) from a UK payer's perspective. In the publication from 2007, ICURs over a 20-year time horizon were estimated to be £99,000/QALY for ADA and ETN and £175,000/QALY for IFX.[20] Differences between drug costs, which were higher for IFX, explained mainly the differences between ICURs, as equal effectiveness and discontinuation rates for all TNFi were assumed. For each model, key drivers were long-term TNFi discontinuation rate, disease progression, and probability of spontaneous improvement in patients remaining on CC. In contrast to all earlier CUAs, ICURs in this study were increasing with longer time horizon, likely related to the assumptions on spontaneous recovery and further disease course of those treated or untreated. After consultation of clinical and modeling experts, reanalysis was requested by NICE.[21] This resulted in significantly lower estimates for all three TNFi (ICURs for ADA and ETN between £22,000 and 31,000/QALY; ICUR for IFX between £49,000 and 65,000/QALY) and resulted in NICE recommending ADA and ETN, but not IFX, as a cost-effective alternative treatment for AS in the United Kingdom in 2008 (NICA TA143). The large change in results after reanalysis was mainly attributed to differences in long-term progression of BASDAI and BASFI in the treatment opposed to CC strategy. A new CUA on a similar decisional question in 2014 investigated the incremental cost-utility of several TNFi (ADA, ETN, IFX, GLM, and CZP) for both AS and nr-axSpA. Synthesis of the literature on efficacy revealed slightly lower efficacy and more heterogeneity of results in nr-axSpA. Cost-utility estimates were £41,000–67,000/QALY, £22,000–37,000/QALY, £21,000–37,000/QALY, £21,000–37,000/QALY, and £19,000–34,000/QALY for IFX, ETN, ADA, GOL, and CZP, respectively, with ratios somewhat less favorable and more uncertain for nr-axSpA. The researchers identified a new factor of uncertainty, namely the differences in the baseline BASDAI/BASFI scores between TNFi responders and nonresponders.[28] Although seemingly self-evident, this had not yet been accounted for in previous models. Appraisal of these results by NICE (NICE TA383) in 2016, including additional analyses with biosimilar versions of IFX and ETN, resulted in NICE recommending all investigated TNFi as cost-effective alternatives for treatment of AS and nr-axSpA in the United Kingdom.[29] Of interest, although the model did not investigate cost-utility of sequential or intermittent TNFi treatment because of perceived lack of robust evidence, NICE considered sequential TNFi treatment a cost-effective alternative in the United Kingdom (based on the results from some RCTs and registries).

Models exploring cost-utility between bDMARDs and cost-utility in TNF-failing patients

Golimumab. By the time GLM became available in clinical care, TNFi was already part of CC in patients with active AS. On that line, NICE asked to appraise the clinical effects and cost-utility of GLM in comparison with no bDMARD and with ADA/ETN.[26] GLM was extendedly dominated (less cost-effective) by both ADA and ETN and thus not recommended as a cost-effective alternative. However, NICE still recommended GLM as a cost-effective alternative for AS in the United Kingdom. In 2017, an updated CUA (sponsored by GLM's distributor) reinvestigated the efficacy of GLM compared with other TNFi by a network metaanalysis. This resulted in a main ICUR of £19,000/QALY for GLM compared with CC without bDMARD from a UK payer's perspective over a lifetime horizon. When compared with ETA and ADA, GLM dominated both ETN and ADA.[32] Influential parameters were the estimation of long-term cost-of-illness, the cost of GLM, and the estimation of BASFI scores beyond the initial treatment period.

Secukinumab. With the aim to provide NICE guidance on the cost-utility of SEC, a new class of bDMARD drugs in the treatment of axSpA, a cost-utility evaluation of SEC in 2016 explored two scenarios. In the first scenario, SEC was compared with TNFi (as a class) in a TNFi-naïve population of persons with AS. In the second scenario, SEC was compared with CC (no bDMARD) in a TNFi-experienced population.[31] All analyses were performed from a UK payer's perspective and had a lifetime time horizon. In the first scenario, SEC generated somewhat less QALY but was also less costly, resulting in an acceptable appraisal. In the second scenario, the ICUR was also acceptable (£2223/QALY) from the UK perspective. NICE recommended SEC as an option for active AS in both patients who failed NSAIDs or TNFi.

Model addressing sequential bDMARDs compared with no TNFi and exploring dynamic population modeling. The first study addressing the cost-utility of sequential TNFi when compared with no availability of bDMARDs revealed that up to two consecutive TNFi were considered cost-effective (ICUR €35,000/QALY) over a lifetime time horizon from a Dutch societal perspective.[25] In a follow-up analysis with the same model, a dynamic population modeling approach was applied. In this analysis, the actual number of patients in a specific calendar year of a specific country/region is considered, and new patients diagnosed with AS and needing bDMARDs enter the model over calendar time. In this dynamic modeling, calibration between incidence of AS patients initiating bDMARDs and mortality is essential to maintain a correct number of patients (reflective of the true country prevalence) in the cohort. In contrast to a fixed cohort approach, as used in all other evaluations in axSpA, the dynamic population model has the advantage that

it provides the annual total (extra) costs and (extra) QALYs for the country/region.[27] ICURs in the dynamic model were higher (€61,000/QALY over a 20-year horizon) but still cost-effective for the Netherlands. The difference for the iCURs between both studies can partly be explained by the larger representation of new patients (which have higher costs in view of loading dose of TNF, also in view of nonresponders), inherent to the dynamic nature of this type of modeling. This might be further augmented by the different discount rates for costs and utilities. Of interest for this type of model, the availability of (a maximum of two consecutive) TNFi resulted for the Dutch society (17 million inhabitants) in an average increase in expenditures on drug costs of €168 to 205 million per year, but a decrease in the productivity costs of €13 and 31 million per year and of other healthcare costs of €7 to 12 million per year.

Models comparing different dosing regimens and tapering of bDMARDs. In view of the high costs per treatment and budget impact of bDMARDs, strategies have been developed with the main aim to reduce drug costs of treatment with bDMARDs. The cost-effectiveness and cost-utility of an on-demand versus a standard 6 weeks' dosing regimen of IFX was evaluated from a French societal perspective, using data from a 1-year randomized clinical trial. The additional direct and indirect costs to achieve one extra ASAS20 response or ASAS partial remission of the standard 6 weeks' dosing regimen were €16,000 and €23,000, respectively. The ICUR was €50,000/QALY. This paper raised ethical discussions, as the on-demand treatment resulted in a loss of 0.09 QALY, and questions at which conditions monetary returns can justify loss in QALY.[23]

Along a TNFi registry, cost-utility of standard versus (any) reduced doses of TNFi was investigated over a 1-year horizon from a Czech societal perspective.[30] Patients on reduced dose were matched to patients on standard dose by propensity score approach. All TNFi were pooled with regard to effectiveness and drug-associated costs. As costs-of-illness, with the exception of the costs of TNFi, were assumed to be equal in both groups, and the QALYs of standard dosing was only slightly higher (0.02 QALY) compared with reduced dosing, the ICUR of €211,000 gained for one QALY lost in case of reduced versus standard dosing was considered acceptable. Of note, within the short period of 1 year, already 21% of patients in the reduced dosing group required reescalation of TNFi treatment, and therefore the longer-term cost-effectiveness of reduced dosing remains uncertain.

INFLUENCE OF METHODOLOGICAL CHOICES AND ASSUMPTIONS ON (LONG-TERM) MODELS IN AXSPA

Fig. 17.6 visualizes the results of the 35 comparisons reported in the 17 published cost-utility studies of bDMARDs in axSpA compared with CC. As indicated above, the evaluations addressed five objectives or strategies: cost-effectiveness of single (n = 7), various (n = 5), or two (if needed) sequential (n = 2) bDMARDs to no bDMARD, cost-effectiveness between bDMARDs (n = 2), and cost-effectiveness of a new class of bDMARDs in TNFi-experienced patients (n = 1). All except one study addressed r-axSpA. Despite efforts to harmonize results by selecting point estimates based on similarity in parameter assumptions and by adjusting for differential timing and purchasing power parities between countries, results vary substantially and firm conclusions are not straightforward.

To gain insight into underlying reasons for these large differences within and between models, the model choices and parameter estimates that influence the ICUR in the uncertainty analyses within the studies and the main differences in model structure and assumptions across studies are discussed below. It is important to realize that several of the issues addressed are interrelated and that the magnitude of their effects on cost-utility estimates can be reinforced by each other.

Time Horizon

As specified in guidelines for economic evaluations, the time horizon should be of appropriate length, that is, long enough to capture differences in costs and effects between the alternatives. However, there are substantial uncertainties surrounding long-term disease progression of axSpA and how this is affected by short- and long-term treatment with bDMARDs.

Generally, a short horizon leads to higher costs per QALY.[14–20,22,24,26,27,31,32] Several factors account for the time influence. First, in the initial treatment period, both future responders and nonresponders receive an expensive bDMARD. These "up-front" drug costs (without health gain in a proportion of patients) drive cost-utility estimates.[17] Secondly, a shorter horizon excludes long-term benefits of the intervention, such as possible benefits of decreased structural damage on health utility or of reduced productivity losses on cost-of-illness. As indirect costs (of work disability) especially occur in the long term, this effect of time horizon is particularly relevant in a societal perspective. Thirdly, the relationship of BASFI with utility and costs is not linear[33]: higher BASFI scores tend to drive both costs and utilities to a greater extent than lower scores.[14,16] If two treatments differ in effect on BASFI and/or progression

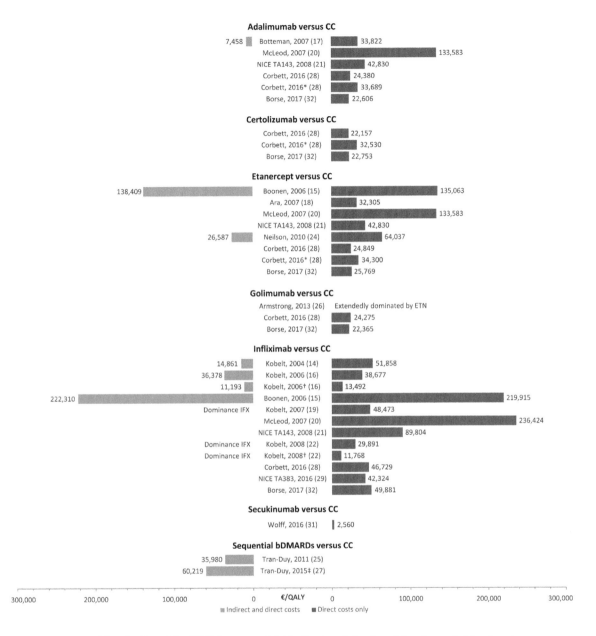

FIG. 17.6 Visualization of the ICUR from a societal (indirect and direct costs) and payer's (direct costs only) perspective of all published long-term cost-utility analyses of bDMARDs in axSpA. The point estimates were homogenized first by selecting from each study the results assuming 50% disease progression while on bDMARD (if available), and secondly by adjusting costs for differential timing and purchasing power parities across countries (updated to 2015 Euros). *CC,* conventional care; *QALY,* quality-adjusted life year; *Nr-axSpA population, †Reduced-dosing or flexible-dosing regimen, ‡Dynamic population study.

of BASFI over time, short-term models might miss potential benefits. Fourthly, assumptions on long-term effect of bDMARDs in terms of drug discontinuation and of BASFI progression after discontinuation have strong influence on treatment costs (which decrease) and benefits (maintained or lost depending in the assumptions) and can have a large (but difficult to predict) influence on the cost-utility ratio (see also later).

Finally, the effect of discounting is limited when the horizon is short.[19] These considerations partly explain differences in estimates between studies and within studies. For example, the difference in ICURs between the Dutch study on IFX and ETN with a 5-year horizon, and the UK studies on IFX with 30-year to lifetime horizon and ETN with a 25-year horizon, could partly be the result from the difference in horizon.[14,15,18,19] To illustrate how the horizon can affect results within a study, in the 2007 UK IFX study, changing the time horizon from lifetime to 10 years leads to a 63%–66% increase in ICUR.[19]

Perspective and Costs Considered

The context of the decision addressed in the economic evaluation defines which perspective is preferred. As for reimbursement and clinical decisions, the broad impact of the new technology on functioning and health, and the consequences on all type of costs are relevant, a societal perspective is recommended.[14,25] Cost-utility estimates of bDMARDs in axSpA from a societal perspective are expected to be more favorable compared with a healthcare perspective because benefits of bDMARDs also translate in decreased productivity losses, especially over a longer time horizon.[34,35] Higher medical costs of bDMARDs seem to be offset by reduced indirect costs. This is confirmed in most studies that provided scenario analyses for both perspective.[14–16,19,22,24] Switching from a payer perspective to a societal perspective could lead to a 6%–78% change in ICUR, or even change results from non-dominance to dominance. Current guidelines advise to present separate results of the direct and total (direct and indirect) costs, as both give different but complimentary information. This recommendation was clearly not systematically followed.

Costs of bDMARDs

Costs of bDMARDs have substantial effect on ICURs. The higher recommended dosing and therefore drug cost of IFX in axSpA generate higher ICURs compared with other bDMARDs, and this was particularly clear in the analyses in which the effectiveness and rates of discontinuation and adverse event rates of the various bDMARDs were assumed to be similar. The decision by NICE in 2008 to recommend ADA and ETN, but not IFX, for AS in the United States was largely driven by the differences in drug costs between IFX and the other bDMARDs.[21]

It is important to realize that price differences among bDMARDs can exist between countries (or even regions and hospitals).[36] Two studies on ETN illustrate the impact of such price differences on the cost-utility.[18,24] Both modeled cost-utility of ETN using a similar model, but one taking a UK and the other a German perspective. ICURs were substantially different, taking inflation and currencies into account: £23,000/QALY versus €55,000/QALY, respectively. Of note, ETN acquisition costs were over twice as high in Germany compared with the United Kingdom. When the German model was repeated using UK costs of ETN, the resulting ICUR (£19,000/QALY) was quite similar to ICUR in the (initial) UK analysis (£23,000/QALY). On this line, sensitivity analyses often showed that bDMARD cost was an important driver of results.[15,16,19,20,28,32] In the Dutch study on IFX and ETN, an 80% reduction of acquisition costs of IFX would reduce the ICUR in the societal perspective from €187,000/QALY to €21,000/QALY (90% change in ICUR).[15]

Initial Response: Criteria and Treatment Effect

The treatment effect of bDMARDs is a key driver of cost-utility estimates, and continuation of (costly) bDMARDs is conditional on treatment *response*. Except for the model that allowed sequencing of two bDMARDs, patients with axSpA and initial nonresponse convert to CC and do not reinitiate a second bDMARD therapy over time. Furthermore, the magnitude of the "initial response rate" is essential for appropriate modeling of disease (BASFI) over time. Model input for "initial response" is usually derived from RCTs, sometimes within the context of a (network) meta-analysis. However, primary outcome measures in trials can differ among each other and can differ from recommendations in clinical guidelines on how to assess response and thus decide on (dis)continuation. An example are the response criteria defined by the British Society for Rheumatology (BSR), which required either a 50% or ≥2 unit reduction in BASDAI, together with a ≥2 unit reduction in spinal VAS. Although some CUAs modeled initial response using these criteria, several other studies used only the 50% reduction in BASDAI as response criterion. The German study on ETN demonstrated how using these different response criteria could lead to change in ICUR greater than 30%.[24] The study investigating cost-utility of bDMARDs in nr-axSpA revealed how ICURs of TNFi compared with CC were affected when the treatment effect of TNFi was based on RCTs including both AS and nr-axSpA patients as opposed to those including only nr-axSpA patients. In this former scenario, ICURs were only slightly higher (approximately 2%) and more uncertain compared with the main analyses that included only nr-axSpA patients.[28]

Dealing With Spontaneous Recovery in the Conventional Care Group

One of the factors strongly influencing variation in ICURs between cost-effectiveness studies of TNFi compared with CC without TNFi can be found in the choice to include a spontaneous recovery in the CC group.[15,20] On the one hand, it is well known that persons included in RCTs, and even in cohorts, usually show an improvement in health, reflecting regression to the mean or a true placebo response. Ignoring this effect would likely be overly optimistic about the incremental effect of the new intervention. On the other hand, in longer-term studies, it is possible that part of the "placebo" effect in the CC would be temporary and thus the effect on the longer term will be attenuated. Extending this effect of spontaneous recovery to the intervention group signifies a small group continues treatment while spontaneous recovery had occurred. In clinical practice, medication might be tapered or stopped and thus reduce cost. Such real-life practice might counter (partly) overestimation of health gain resulting from spontaneous recovery in the non-bDMARD strategy. Although no clear recommendations exist on how to deal with this issue of spontaneous recovery (including placebo) effects, the effect is large. In two related models that compared ICUR of various TNFi with CC (without TNFi), assuming spontaneous recovery was possible leads to ICURs reduced by 30%–60%.[20,21]

Longer-Term Discontinuation Rate

It is important to distinguish between short-term and long-term bDMARD discontinuation. Short-term discontinuation (usually within the first 3 months) depends on inclusion of nonresponders, whereas long-term bDMARD discontinuation is defined as discontinuation beyond the period of initial response (usually beyond 3 months). Discontinuation can be caused by loss of initial response or development of adverse events. In most CUAs, long-term discontinuation rates are derived from open-label extension studies. Although registries could be an appropriate source for long-term discontinuation rates, these generally make no distinction between the initial 3-month period and subsequent periods, nor are they specific to responders. Interestingly, although the impact of long-term discontinuation rates on cost-utility can be large (more than 60% change in ICUR[24]), the direction of this impact can vary between studies. This is related to the balance between reduction in medication costs after discontinuation opposed to the level and duration of benefits of (past) bDMARD treatment on QALYs and to the effect on long-term disease costs (especially indirect

costs and costs of hospitalization). Generally speaking, incremental QALYs reported in cost-utility analyses are higher when discontinuation rates are lower and time on bDMARD increases.[16,24] Depending on the balance between the outcomes after discontinuation (variable loss in QALY, decrease in drug costs, but an increase in other costs), a higher long-term bDMARD discontinuation rate will affect the costs per QALY. Most studies in axSpA observe that lower discontinuation rates are favorable toward bDMARDs.[18,20,24] In some models, the opposite is observed. Note that these latter models were related.[14,16,19,22]

Long-Term Disease Progression

The long-term health consequences of axSpA, which are relevant for cost-of-illness and long-term utility, have been strongly associated with BASFI. BASFI scores reflect not only the reversible component of disease activity but also the disability related to structural damage.[37] Therefore, the course of health in economic evaluations of bDMARDs in axSpA is modeled using BASFI, and BASDAI plays a further role when linking BASFI to utility and cost-of illness. At least three groups of patients must be distinguished when considering disease progression: (1) patients on CC; (2) patients on bDMARD; and (3) patients who have discontinued bDMARD and switch to CC.

1. Patients treated by conventional care (no bD-MARDs) experience natural disease progression of axSpA. Patients on CC are usually assumed to have a constant annual rate of BASFI increase ("natural history"). This rate is derived from (a limited number of) cohort studies including bDMARD-naive axSpA patients with active disease. Whether disease progression in patients on CC would be equal to "natural history" remains uncertain, as conflicting evidence exists regarding an effect of NSAIDs on radiographic progression.[38,39] From a practical view, this does not matter for these analyses, as the patients in cohorts providing "natural history" progression estimates likely were treated with CC.

2. Disease progression in patients with axSpA treated with bDMARDs remains an important source of uncertainty in current economic modeling. Available economic evaluations assumed BASFI would either not progress at all, would progress at a lower rate, or progression would be equal to CC. In addition, some studies have assumptions on the timing of these effects. Examples are "delays" and "leveling-off" of bDMARD effects on BASFI progression.[26,28,32] On this line, recent data suggest that bDMARDs inhibit disease progression to some

extent, especially after a few years of bDMARD treatment.[40–42] Most studies have dealt with this uncertainty by exploring scenarios with varying BASFI progression, and results show that the rate of BASFI progression while on bDMARD can be an important driver of ICURs.[14,20] Obviously, assuming that BASFI progression is decreased (or even nonexistent) while on bDMARDs is favorable toward bDMARDs. As the difference in mean BASFI scores between those on bDMARD and those on CC increases over time, so does the difference in utility (derived from BASFI) and thus the amount of (incremental) QALY. The assumption of no BASFI progression at all while on bDMARD seems overly favorable toward bDMARDs. The within-study effect of assuming no BASFI progression while on bDMARD, compared with no effect of bDMARDs on progression at all, can vary from small (4% reduced ICUR) to substantial (60% reduced ICUR).[18,22]

3. Finally, disease progression after discontinuation of bDMARDs is even more uncertain. Most studies assume that disease progression postdiscontinuation is equal to progression in the CC population. Interestingly, none of the studies assumed that the disease would not progress after discontinuation (i.e., that the beneficial effect would be retained). However, some issues need careful consideration in relation to BASFI progression after bDMARD discontinuation. Response to bDMARD and loss of response after initial response are likely no random processes. In practice, those without initial response as well as those failing after initial response likely reflect a more severe disease phenotype, with different baseline characteristics and thus different BASFI progression. Also, it is likely that those discontinuing because of lack of response are phenotypically different from those discontinuing because of side effects, and could have different BASFI progression rates after discontinuation. The assumption of equal progression postdiscontinuation for all populations, regardless of responder status, is challenged by studies demonstrating that male gender and levels of acute phase reactants (both related to development and/or progression of structural damage) are predictors of bDMARD response.[43]

Rebound After Discontinuation

Independent of the challenges related to the long-term disease progression when failing bDMARDs after initial response, physical function (and disease activity) in axSpA is also expected to deteriorate as an immediate reflection of the loss of the drug's antiinflammatory effect. This effect is referred to as "rebound." In general, two different rebound scenarios are applied with regard to the increase in BASDAI and BASFI to a prespecified level ("rebound") after drug discontinuation (see Fig. 17.7).

1. Rebound to baseline (equal to gain): after bDMARD discontinuation, BASFI (and BASDAI) scores revert to pre-bDMARD (baseline) values and indirectly assume a lasting effect of bDMARDs on structural damage. In other words, those who withdraw from bDMARD after initial response restart progression from baseline but at a later moment. Their BASFI scores will never "catch" up with the CC population (when assuming equal progression rates after withdrawal as in CC).

2. Rebound to natural history (CC): after bDMARD discontinuation, BASFI (and BASDAI) scores revert to values as in the CC population at that time. This scenario assumes that after discontinuation of bDMARD, patients deteriorate to the point as if no initial response had occurred. In other words, the discontinuation group will "catch up" with the CC population. Obviously, this approach is less favorable toward bDMARDs.

An additional consideration related to the rebound scenario is the "speed" of rebound. Although some studies assume that rebound is instant, others assume that it takes 12–24 weeks to rebound after discontinuation.

As demonstrated in the UK model comparing various TNFi in AS and nr-axSpA compared with no bDMARD, the effect of the rebound scenario on results is difficult to interpret in isolation from other model parameters and assumptions.[28] ICURs for TNFi were more favorable (lower) for the AS population compared with the nr-axSpA population in the rebound equal to gain scenario. However, in the rebound to natural history scenario, the opposite was true. Factors driving this discrepancy were the differences between the AS and nr-axSpA populations regarding the size of the initial gain in BASDAI/BASFI and the BASFI progression (all were lower in the nr-axSpA population).

Although uncertainty regarding rebound remains, the rebound to baseline scenario is generally deemed a more plausible scenario by clinical experts.[29] In reality, the level of rebound probably lies somewhere in between both scenarios, which is why they are sometimes presented as "best" and "worst" case scenarios.[28] In the CUA comparing TNFi with CC in AS and nr-axSpA described above, assuming rebound to CC compared with rebound to gain leads to ICURs that were generally 70% (AS) and 18% (nr-axSpA) higher.

Influence of assumed 'rebound' scenario

Influence of both assumed 'rebound' scenario and assumed disease progression while on bDMARD

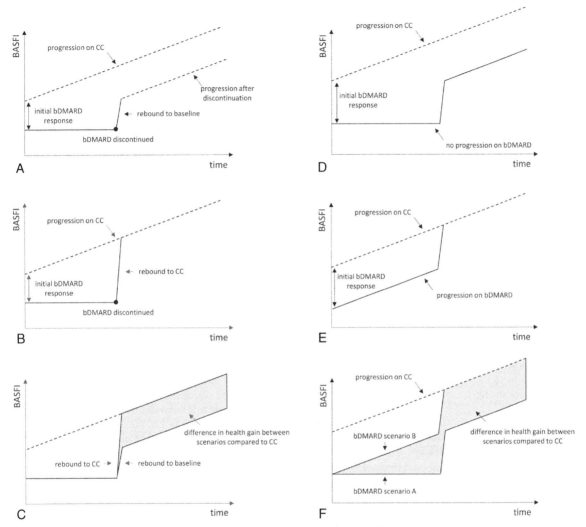

FIG. 17.7 The influence of rebound scenario **(A–C)** and combination of rebound scenario and disease progression assumptions while on bDMARD **(D–F)** on BASFI over time. As physical function (BASFI) is associated with health gain (QALY), assuming that patients after bDMARD discontinuation rebound to their baseline BASFI **(A)** or to the BASFI of the group not treated by bDMARD **(B)** will lead to different estimated health gain for patients on bDMARD compared with patients on conventional care (difference in estimated health gain marked as *gray area*, **(C)**). The same is true for the assumption regarding disease progression (BASFI) while on bDMARD. Assuming no disease progression while on bDMARD **(D)** or disease progression similar to those not on bDMARD **(E)** will lead to different estimated health gain for patients on bDMARD compared with patients on conventional care. In **(F)**, the difference in estimated health gain of bDMARD treatment compared with conventional care is depicted for the two most contrasting scenarios: no disease progression on bDMARD in combination with rebound to baseline after bDMARD discontinuation (scenario A, **(D** and **F)**) versus no inhibition of disease progression while on bDMARD and rebound to the conventional care population after bDMARD discontinuation (scenario B, **(E** and **F)**). *BASFI,* Bath Ankylosing Spondylitis Functional Index; *QALY,* quality-adjusted life year.

Clinical Practice

Although CUA models are an attempt to simulate "clinical practice," the data sources used to inform these models are often not congruent with clinical practice. Treatment efficacy is based on RCTs, which are known to include only certain subgroups of patients that might not represent the general axSpA population encountered in daily practice. The same holds true for discontinuation rates and adverse event rates in some models or for progression of BASFI in different relevant subgroups of patients. In addition, nondrug costs are often based on dated cohort studies, and results might not be transferable to other countries or settings. Even worse, guidelines used to inform model structure and key parameter inputs are not always adhered to in clinical practice. For example, to assess to which extent the UK guidelines on TNFi treatment for AS were followed in clinical practice, an audit was conducted in the United Kingdom in 2010.[44] The guidelines at the time recommended TNFi discontinuation at 12 weeks if response criteria were not met. This audit revealed that TNFi treatment was discontinued in *less than 20%* of the patients with inadequate response at 12 weeks. That continuation of bDMARD treatment in nonresponders can seriously affect cost-effectiveness of these drugs was demonstrated recently in a CUA using data from a prospective cohort of early SpA patients.[45] Whether these aspects of care should be incorporated in CUA can be debated, and doing so can be complex and time-consuming.

CONCLUSION, DISCUSSION, AND VIEW OF FUTURE DEVELOPMENTS

Knowledge on cost-effectiveness of managing patients with axSpA is mainly restricted to the cost-effectiveness of bDMARDs. Overall, available studies revealed large differences of cost-effectiveness not only between but also within studies. The majority of studies conclude that bDMARDs are cost-effective in the management of axSpA, especially when a longer time horizon and a societal perspective are considered. Few studies address sequential bDMARDs, but up to two bDMARDs seem favorable from an economic point of view. Essential to cost-effectiveness of bDMARDs is the drug price, and on this line, IFX (with higher dosing in axSpA) was less cost-effective and SEC (lower dosing in axSpA) was more cost-effective compared with other available bDMARDs. On the same line, the advent of biosimilars greatly improves the cost-effectiveness of bDMARDs.

It should be kept in mind that all cost-effectiveness studies were performed in wealthy countries, and mainly from a UK perspective. As shown in some papers considered in this chapter, transferability of economic evaluations in axSpA to other countries is mainly determined by the costs of drugs and of cost-of-illness of axSpA.[46] The latter is especially relevant when considering middle (or low-income) countries. Pricing of bDMARD drugs primarily follows market mechanism in the USA and Europe and is not adjusted to local purchasing power parities when made available in lower-income countries. This means that monetary returns by reduced hospitalizations/surgery or work disability are insufficient to offset the costs of bDMARDs, as the costs of hospitalizations and work productivity in relation to the cost of bDMARD are far lower than in wealthier Western countries. This results in unaffordable high cost-effectiveness of bDMARDs in the majority of countries worldwide. On the other hand, there is no evidence yet that the phenotype and (treated and untreated) course of axSpA differ between countries, which implies that the main structure of economic models (the course of health) would be worldwide applicable. Notwithstanding, increasing evidence reveals that the value patients or healthy persons attach to health states (utilities/QALYs) itself can differ between countries and is likely related to differences in culture and part of reference shift.[47] As "value for health" is a complex construct that is continuously evolving, but of key importance in healthcare decisions that aim to maximize health for all persons, the issue of measuring (value of) health across countries and the need to define a "global definition of health" merit far more attention. Last but not least, a major difference in the interpretation of the cost per QALY exists between countries. In the United Kingdom, a fixed willingness to pay threshold of £30,000/QALY is applied to decide whether an innovation in healthcare is cost-effective and can be reimbursed. In most other countries requiring cost-effectiveness analyses before deciding on reimbursement, the ICUR is appraised in the context of other factors, among which often the budget impact (not addressed in a cost-effectiveness analysis, which is a patient-level method). Although budgets are important, for a clinician likely the cost-utility should play a stronger role in decisions, as different compared with budget impact analyses, it ensures that resources are allocated to the innovations with the best balance between health and cost.

An interesting and important feature of health economic modeling can be found in the uncertainty analyses. Uncertainty around several parameters (additional to the perspective and costs of bDMARDs) was found in economic models in axSpA, and decisive changes in the point estimate of the ICUR were observed after uncertainty analyses. In view of the relevance of uncertainty, it is worthwhile to highlight the areas of uncertainty that are specific to modeling in axSpA, as they are actually related to clinical questions and require epidemiologic and outcome research in axSpA. The main clinical research questions essential for health economic modeling would be the following:

- What is severe axSpA? Is BASFI the best instrument to assess severe disease and disease progression? Is the ASAS health index and utility a better alternative to model health?
- What determines natural disease progression, are there subgroups of patients that should be distinguished?
- Are bDMARDs in clinical practice actually discontinued when initial response was not optimal?
- What is the rate of disease progression ("BASFI") while patients are on bDMARD, and is this depending on baseline patient characteristics?
- What are long-term discontinuation rates of bDMARDs after initial treatment response?
- What is progression of disease (BASFI) in those discontinuing bDMARD because of initial nonresponse and after loss of initial response? Is progression dependent on initial disease characteristics?
- What is the pattern of rebound of health (disease activity and physical function) after discontinuation, and how is rebound affected by treatment duration?
- How many sequential bDMARDs are (cost-)effective?
- Is a treat-to-low disease activity approach superior compared with an untargeted approach?
- What is the long-term effectiveness of tapering bDMARDs? Can we identify patients in which we can taper bDMARDs?
- Are the answers to the above questions different for AS and nr-axSpA?

To advance accuracy and standardization of health economic modeling, an open access model that is developed and updated in a Bayesian approach when new evidence becomes available, would be of great value. A nice example on open access modeling has recently become available for rheumatoid arthritis.[48] It is clear that such open available models will also save much research time, as the development of a disease model is extremely time-consuming.

Although it might be understandable that cost-effectiveness of bDMARDs received the greatest attention in economic evaluations in the past 15 years, several other areas in which cost-effectiveness would matter can be identified. Specifically with regard to costs-effectiveness of diagnostic or prognostic tools, economic evaluations can be informative. Early diagnosis of axSpA is a continuous clinical challenge, and new imaging and laboratory biomarkers are being developed. New classification criteria in which HLA-B27 and MRI play a key role have been developed to identify axSpA among low-back-pain patients. Several diagnostic algorithms have been proposed, which differ (among others) in the costs (MRI) and in accuracy (wrongly diagnosed patients will also be wrongly treated). It would be of interest to understand whether these different diagnostic algorithms differ in cost-effectiveness. A health economic model could further help to explore in which position of the current diagnostic algorithm, improvements in health because of better diagnosis can be maximized. Traditional clinical research on diagnostic accuracy does not account for the longer treatment effects, and thus ignores long-term health benefits and costs of diagnosis. Models allow to estimate this information and can reveal gaps in clinical and epidemiologic data, which are needed to provide more accurate estimates. On the same line, translational research on biomarkers to monitor disease, predict response, or predict successful tapering is growing. Again, modeling costs and benefits of biomarkers if implemented into current clinical criteria would offer the opportunity to understand the long-term impact on health and costs of improved patient selection. These so-called early technology evaluations can contribute to efficiency of research itself and should be a more natural part of translational biomarker (and drug) research!

When returning to the six pillars of quality of care, efficiency is perhaps the capstone of our healthcare system. Whether at the personal, payer, or societal level, at some point, resources will be finite. Only when resources are allocated efficiently, we can maximize the health gains for (all) patients.

REFERENCES

1. Institute of Medicine (IOM). *Crossing the Quality Chasm.* National Academies Press; 2001.
2. Drummond MF, Sculpher MJ, Claxton K, Stoddart GL, Torrance GW. *Methods for the Economic Evaluation of Health Care Programmes.* 4th ed. Oxford: Oxford University Press; 2015.
3. Kennedy GL, Wood PH. HL-A 27 and the diagnosis of back problems. *Rheumatol Rehabil.* 1975;14(3):168–172.
4. Husereau D, Drummond M, Petrou S, et al. Consolidated health economic evaluation reporting standards (CHEERS) statement. *BMJ.* 2013;346:f1049.
5. Bansback N, Maetzel A, Drummond M, et al. Considerations and preliminary proposals for defining a reference case for economic evaluations in ankylosing spondylitis. *J Rheumatol.* 2007;34(5):1178–1183.

6. Bakker C, Hidding A, van der Linden S, van Doorslaer E. Cost effectiveness of group physical therapy compared to individualized therapy for ankylosing spondylitis. A randomized controlled trial. *J Rheumatol.* 1994;21(2):264–268.

7. Van Tubergen A, Boonen A, Landewe R, et al. Cost effectiveness of combined spa-exercise therapy in ankylosing spondylitis: a randomized controlled trial. *Arthritis Rheum.* 2002;47(5):459–467.

8. Joore M, Brunenberg D, Nelemans P, et al. The impact of differences in EQ-5D and SF-6D utility scores on the acceptability of cost-utility ratios: results across five trial-based cost-utility studies. *Value Health.* 2010;13(2):222–229.

9. Jansen JP, Gaugris S, Choy EH, Ostor A, Nash JT, Stam W. Cost effectiveness of etoricoxib versus celecoxib and nonselective NSAIDS in the treatment of ankylosing spondylitis. *Pharmacoeconomics.* 2010;28(4):323–344.

10. Jansen JP, Taylor SD. Cost-effectiveness evaluation of etoricoxib versus celecoxib and nonselective NSAIDs in the treatment of ankylosing spondylitis in Norway. *Int J Rheumatol.* 2011;2011:160326.

11. Barra L, Pope JE, Payne M. Real-world anti-tumor necrosis factor treatment in rheumatoid arthritis, psoriatic arthritis, and ankylosing spondylitis: cost-effectiveness based on number needed to treat to improve health assessment questionnaire. *J Rheumatol.* 2009;36(7):1421–1428.

12. Olivieri I, Fanizza C, Gilio M, Ravasio R. Efficacy, safety and cost per responder of biologics in the treatment of non-radiographic axial spondyloarthritis. *Clin Exp Rheumatol.* 2016;34(5):935–940.

13. Betts KA, Griffith J, Song Y, et al. Network meta-analysis and cost per responder of tumor necrosis factor-alpha and interleukin inhibitors in the treatment of active ankylosing spondylitis. *Rheumatol Ther.* 2016;3(2):323–336.

14. Kobelt G, Andlin-Sobocki P, Brophy S, Jonsson L, Calin A, Braun J. The burden of ankylosing spondylitis and the cost-effectiveness of treatment with infliximab (Remicade). *Rheumatology (Oxford).* 2004;43(9):1158–1166.

15. Boonen A, van der Heijde D, Severens JL, et al. Markov model into the cost-utility over five years of etanercept and infliximab compared with usual care in patients with active ankylosing spondylitis. *Ann Rheum Dis.* 2006;65(2):201–208.

16. Kobelt G, Andlin-Sobocki P, Maksymowych WP. The cost-effectiveness of infliximab (Remicade) in the treatment of ankylosing spondylitis in Canada. *J Rheumatol.* 2006;33(4):732–740.

17. Botteman MF, Hay JW, Luo MP, Curry AS, Wong RL, van Hout BA. Cost effectiveness of adalimumab for the treatment of ankylosing spondylitis in the United Kingdom. *Rheumatology (Oxford).* 2007;46(8):1320–1328.

18. Ara RM, Reynolds AV, Conway P. The cost-effectiveness of etanercept in patients with severe ankylosing spondylitis in the UK. *Rheumatology (Oxford).* 2007;46(8):1338–1344.

19. Kobelt G, Sobocki P, Sieper J, Braun J. Comparison of the cost-effectiveness of infliximab in the treatment of ankylosing spondylitis in the United Kingdom based on two different clinical trials. *Int J Technol Assess Health Care.* 2007;23(3):368–375.

20. McLeod C, Bagust A, Boland A, et al. Adalimumab, etanercept and infliximab for the treatment of ankylosing spondylitis: a systematic review and economic evaluation. *Health Technol Assess.* 2007;11(28):1–158, (iii-iv).

21. National Institute for Health and Clinical Excellence. In: *Adalimumab, Etanercept and Infliximab for Ankylosing Spondylitis (TA143). May 2008.* London: NICE; 2008.

22. Kobelt G, Sobocki P, Mulero J, Gratacos J, Collantes-Estevez E, Braun J. The cost-effectiveness of infliximab in the treatment of ankylosing spondylitis in Spain. Comparison of clinical trial and clinical practice data. *Scand J Rheumatol.* 2008;37(1):62–71.

23. Fautrel B, Benhamou M, Breban M, et al. Cost effectiveness of two therapeutic regimens of infliximab in ankylosing spondylitis: economic evaluation within a randomised controlled trial. *Ann Rheum Dis.* 2010;69(2):424–427.

24. Neilson AR, Sieper J, Deeg M. Cost-effectiveness of etanercept in patients with severe ankylosing spondylitis in Germany. *Rheumatology (Oxford).* 2010;49(11):2122–2134.

25. Tran-Duy A, Boonen A, van de Laar MA, Franke AC, Severens JL. A discrete event modelling framework for simulation of long-term outcomes of sequential treatment strategies for ankylosing spondylitis. *Ann Rheum Dis.* 2011;70(12):2111–2118.

26. Armstrong N, Joore M, van Asselt T, et al. Golimumab for the treatment of ankylosing spondylitis: a NICE single technology appraisal. *Pharmacoeconomics.* 2013;31(5):415–425.

27. Tran-Duy A, Boonen A, van de Laar MA, Severens JL. Impact on total population health and societal cost, and the implication on the actual cost-effectiveness of including tumour necrosis factor-alpha antagonists in management of ankylosing spondylitis: a dynamic population modelling study. *Cost Eff Resourc Alloc.* 2015;13:18.

28. Corbett M, Soares M, Jhuti G, et al. Tumour necrosis factor-alpha inhibitors for ankylosing spondylitis and non-radiographic axial spondyloarthritis: a systematic review and economic evaluation. *Health Technol Assess.* 2016;20(9):1–334, (v-vi).

29. National Institute for Health, Care Excellence. In: *TNF-Alpha Inhibitors for Ankylosing Spondylitis and Non-radiographic Axial Spondyloarthritis (TA383). 1 February 2016.* London: NICE; 2016.

30. Zavada J, Uher M, Sisol K, et al. A tailored approach to reduce dose of anti-TNF drugs may be equally effective, but substantially less costly than standard dosing in patients with ankylosing spondylitis over 1 year: a propensity score-matched cohort study. *Ann Rheum Dis.* 2016;75(1):96–102.

31. Wolff RB N, Al M, Ryder S, et al. In: *Secukinumab for Ankylosing Spondylitis after Inadequate Response to Non-steroidal Antiinflammatory Drugs or TNF-alpha Inhibitors: A Single Technology Assessment. 15 April 2016 ed.* York: Kleijnen Systematic Reviews Ltd.; 2016.

32. Borse RH, Brown C, Muszbek N, Chaudhary MA, Kachroo S. Cost-effectiveness of golimumab in ankylosing spondylitis from the UK payer perspective. *Rheumatol Ther.* 2017;4(2):427–443.

33. Wailoo A, Hernandez M, Philips C, Brophy S, Siebert S. Modeling health state utility values in ankylosing spondylitis: comparisons of direct and indirect methods. *Value Health.* 2015;18(4):425–431.

34. van der Burg LR, Ter Wee MM, Boonen A. Effect of biological therapy on work participation in patients with ankylosing spondylitis: a systematic review. *Ann Rheum Dis.* 2012;71(12):1924–1933.

35. Gaujoux-Viala C, Fautrel B. Cost effectiveness of therapeutic interventions in ankylosing spondylitis: a critical and systematic review. *Pharmacoeconomics.* 2012;30(12):1145–1156.

36. Putrik P, Ramiro S, Kvien TK, et al. Inequities in access to biologic and synthetic DMARDs across 46 European countries. *Ann Rheum Dis.* 2014;73(1):198–206.

37. Machado P, Landewe R, Braun J, et al. A stratified model for health outcomes in ankylosing spondylitis. *Ann Rheum Dis.* 2011;70(10):1758–1764.

38. Sieper J, Listing J, Poddubnyy D, et al. Effect of continuous versus on-demand treatment of ankylosing spondylitis with diclofenac over 2 years on radiographic progression of the spine: results from a randomised multicentre trial (ENRADAS). *Ann Rheum Dis.* 2016;75(8):1438–1443.

39. Wanders A, Heijde D, Landewe R, et al. Nonsteroidal antiinflammatory drugs reduce radiographic progression in patients with ankylosing spondylitis: a randomized clinical trial. *Arthritis Rheum.* 2005;52(6):1756–1765.

40. Maas F, Arends S, Wink FR, et al. Ankylosing spondylitis patients at risk of poor radiographic outcome show diminishing spinal radiographic progression during long-term treatment with TNF-alpha inhibitors. *PloS One.* 2017;12(6):e0177231.

41. Haroon N, Inman RD, Learch TJ, et al. The impact of tumor necrosis factor alpha inhibitors on radiographic progression in ankylosing spondylitis. *Arthritis Rheum.* 2013;65(10):2645–2654.

42. Molnar C, Scherer A, Baraliakos X, et al. TNF blockers inhibit spinal radiographic progression in ankylosing spondylitis by reducing disease activity: results from the Swiss Clinical Quality Management cohort. *Ann Rheum Dis.* 2018;77(1):63–69.

43. Maneiro JR, Souto A, Salgado E, Mera A, Gomez-Reino JJ. Predictors of response to TNF antagonists in patients with ankylosing spondylitis and psoriatic arthritis: systematic review and meta-analysis. *RMD Open.* 2015;1(1):e000017.

44. Rees F, Peffers G, Bell C, et al. Compliance with NICE guidance on the use of anti-TNFalpha agents in ankylosing spondylitis: an east and west Midlands regional audit. *Clin Med (Lond).* 2012;12(4):324–327.

45. Harvard S, Guh D, Bansback N, et al. Access criteria for anti-TNF agents in spondyloarthritis: influence on comparative 1-year cost-effectiveness estimates. *Cost Eff Resourc Alloc.* 2017;15:20.

46. Welte R, Feenstra T, Jager H, Leidl R. A decision chart for assessing and improving the transferability of economic evaluation results between countries. *Pharmacoeconomics.* 2004;22(13):857–876.

47. Kiltz U, Essers I, Hiligsmann M, et al. Which aspects of health are most important for patients with spondyloarthritis? A best worst scaling based on the ASAS Health Index. *Rheumatol (Oxford).* 2016;55(10):1771–1776.

48. Incerti D, Jansen JP. A Description of the IVI-RA Model. http://www.thevalueinitiative.org/ivi-ra-value-model/. Last updated October 2017.

CHAPTER 18

Patient Education and Patient Service Organizations

CARLO V. CABALLERO-URIBE, MD • MUHAMMAD ASIM KHAN, MD, FRCP, MACP, MACR

INTRODUCTION

The word "doctor" is an academic title that originates from the Latin word that, according to Wikipedia, is an agentive noun of the Latin verb docēre [dɔˈkeːrɛ] "to teach." The earliest doctoral degrees (in theology, law, and medicine) reflected a historical separation of all university studies into these three fields. Doctor of philosophy (PhD) was originally a university degree granted to learned individuals who had achieved an approval of their peers by demonstrating a long and productive career in the field of philosophy (in the broad sense of the term, meaning the pursuit of knowledge). However, in the English language, the word *doctor* has long had a secondary meaning to indicate a physician.

A patient's trust and respect for his or her healthcare provider increases when being told the truth about the likely outcome of their disease process and any potential untoward effects of the prescribed treatment. Thus, it is imperative for physicians to educate their patients about their illnesses and address their concerns to enhance their understanding and compliance with the prescribed treatment. For that to happen, it must be understood that humans enjoy being around someone who will listen to their problems. Listening attentively to a patient's story without judgment helps a patient feel at ease. For patients with axial spondyloarthritis (axSpA), a chronic illness associated with pain and stiffness, the future is filled with uncertainty and the rheumatologist can play an important role in providing psychologic support through conversation that includes elements of empathy, honesty, and trust. Unfortunately, with the increasing use of electronic medical record systems, physicians are spending more time looking at their computer screens and clicking rather than looking at and conversing with their patients.

Dr. Lewis Nemes, PhD, who is a psychologist as well as a patient with ankylosing spondylitis (AS), advises that physicians should encourage their patients to be as actively involved in their treatment process as possible, and not simply be passive recipients of medical services. The rheumatologists and their patients form a team working toward the same goals: greater comfort, increased functionality, and improved quality of life. The rheumatologist should request an honest and accurate reporting of symptoms, medication effects, and relevant life circumstances to help establish the "team" philosophy. One should encourage and support active patients' involvement by asking what other ideas they might have to improve their physical and emotional health. A patient's trust and respect for his or her healthcare providers increases when being told the truth about the likely progression of the disease process and potential side effects of treatments. Dr. Nemes states, "unrealistic patient expectations should be addressed as soon as possible and as diplomatically as possible. Hope, realistic hope, for disease management is another way to build trust. Discussion about promising current treatments as well as new forms of treatment in development, with appropriate caveats, gives the patient something to hold on to." He emphasizes that we should encourage hope for better disease management and outcome by appropriate use of medications, diet, exercise, meditation, and cognitive/behavioral coping strategies. He stated that patients will lose confidence in their healthcare providers that "promise the moon but are unable to deliver." Providing realistic hope may help buffer the patient from unnecessary depression and anxiety.

The Concept of *Digital Health*

Digital health is an emerging field combining informatics to organize and improve health services through the Internet and related computer technologies, with emphasis on global, regional, and local healthcare perspectives.[1] In other words, it is simply medical treatment utilizing cyberspace and applying Internet and global communication networks to healthcare.

Axial Spondyloarthritis. https://doi.org/10.1016/B978-0-323-56800-5.00018-7

In this Internet age, younger generations are seeking knowledge about their health-related issues from "Dr. Google." This trend is fostered by several factors, such as (1) the availability of many information sources, (2) patients who are active in the search for medical knowledge, and (3) the changing role of healthcare professionals. Ready access to information also eases communication within different medical specialties. Modernization of the patient education and knowledge diffusion processes force health professionals to submit to this new way of approaching their role as healthcare givers and educators. Correct use of the new media in medicine will encourage acquisition of dynamic, practical, and accurate up-to-date medical knowledge, and also sharing of appropriate information with patients to establish a new form of communication and follow-up. As these new tools for acquisition and spread of medical knowledge become better understood by physicians and patients, the interest in their proper use will continue to increase. It would further improve the public health and also provide access to appropriate medical information to patients.[2]

E-patients and Social Media

Social media have encouraged patients to take on an essential role in their healthcare, and this has led to an important new concept called "E-patient."[3] One of the first authors to refer to E-patients was Ferguson, who in a seminal paper[4] referred to this kind of patient as the one who is proactive, properly educated in technology, actively involved in maintaining his or her own health, and interested in contributing to and investigating treatment of specific health conditions to improve medical care. A paper published in 2007 dealt with what we today call E-patients where the letter e refers to an equipped, enabled, engaged, empowered, and expert patient.[5]

The strategic use of social media seems to have multitude of benefits, such as keeping updated in a practical and dynamic manner, through sharing and spreading of relevant information quickly and efficiently, and to establish a new way of communication with patients and improving their medical follow-up. There are more complex relationships and interactions online between patients, physicians, and the general public, to the point that we could be discussing the emergence of safe or unsafe relationships and public and personal interactions, or combinations thereof. Some consider that the public nature of social networks hinders physicians' scope of work and affects the doctor-patient relationship. Medicine has traditionally valued privacy, confidentiality, one-on-one interaction, and formal conduct, whereas social media foster openness, outreach, connection, transparency, and informality that apparently seem to contradict the concept of medical professionalism.[6]

The American College of Physicians (ACP) recognizes that "emerging technology and societal trends will continue to change the landscape of social media and social networking, and how websites are used by patients and physicians will evolve over time," as well as the fact that "social media has transformed communication and is on its way to do so with healthcare. As clinical use grows, doctors must be aware of its implications for ethics, professionalism, relationships and the profession."[7] These recommendations not only acknowledge the importance of new media but also point out the absence of user policies or guidelines for better practices, including areas of concern (such as the use for matters not pertaining to clinical practice, implications for confidentiality, conflicts regarding use of social media as a tool for educating patients), and the way this could affect patients' trust in doctors or the doctor-patient relationship.[7–10]

VIRTUAL COMMUNITIES AND PATIENT ENGAGEMENT

The recent growth in online technology has led to a rapid increase in the sharing of health-related information globally. Health and social care professionals are now using a wide range of virtual communities of practice (VCoPs) for continuing professional education, knowledge management, and information sharing. There is some evidence that VCoPs can offer an informal method of professional and interprofessional development for clinicians and can decrease social and professional isolation.[11]

Social media can be the circulatory system of any society of knowledge and can act as a cornerstone of a vibrant community that interacts and grows. The digital communications strategy has proven to be efficient in disseminating information on specific topics by medical associations.[12] There is thus a need for professional societies and organizations of patients to be sources of reliable information in this "Dr. Google" era. For example, Pan-American League of Associations of Rheumatology (PANLAR) leadership has very recently made strategic improvement with specific objectives of working closely with health professionals and patients alike.[12–14] As a result, the PANLAR community has grown substantially, with over 25,000 "Likes" on Facebook page, over 3500 in Twitter, and also a growing presence in Instagram, LinkedIn, and YouTube.[12–14] PANLAR has also started inviting patients to its meetings to ensure their active participation in discussing issues that affect them.[15]

CONCLUDING REMARKS

There are many patient advocacy groups and scientific organizations listed below that provide very useful information to patients suffering from AS and related forms of spondyloarthritis.[16] There is a continued need for better education of patients and the community, in general, with regard to rheumatic diseases. It is important for medical organizations to use the new online ecosystem to achieve this goal.[17–21] Dr. Eric Topol, a famous physician and digital healthcare pioneer, challenged the medical establishment in his book *The Creative Destruction of Medicine*, to adopt technologies that will improve efficiency, lower costs, and make treatments more accessible and effective.[20] In his more recent book titled *"The Patient Will See You Now,"* he describes what he calls medicine's "Gutenberg moment" at present, giving the analogy of how the invention of the printing press in 1440 liberated knowledge from the control of an elite class.[21] He predicts that digital health technology is now going to do the same for medicine and explains its dynamic impact on the practice of medicine in the near and long term. The doctor is privy to much more medical knowledge, whereas the patient is the "single most unused person in health care" due, in part, to the inherent lack of parity in the doctor-patient relationship.

The need to understand the patient experience and perspective is highlighted by the results of the European Mapping of Axial Spondyloarthritis (EMAS) Survey of 2486 patients from 17 European countries living with axSpA that has very recently been presented.[22] The mean age of these patients was 44 years, and their mean age of symptom onset was 26.6 years. The mean diagnostic delay was 6.14 years in males and 8.24 years in females (p<0.001). Study of physical and psychological impact of axSpA found that 57.1% were at risk of psychological distress, 50.48% had sleep disorders, 38.6% suffered from anxiety, 33.87% had depression, 31.3% were obese or overweight, 28.19% had hypertension, 19.66% had hypercholesterolemia, 18.75% had serious infections requiring antibiotics, 16.98% had irregular heartbeat, 16.94% had psoriatic arthritis, and 16.94% had fibromyalgia. Approximately 70% of patients stated that their disease had limited their ability to carry out everyday activities. Roughly 74% of patients had difficulties finding a job, 44% required workplace adaptations, 40% stated that their illness influenced their job choice, and 28% moved to another job. Moreover, 20% of those employed or on sick leave feared losing their job or ability to work. Despite improvements in therapeutic management, there is still unacceptable delay in diagnosis, and impaired quality of life and professional opportunities that need solutions by shared decision-making and interaction of all the stakeholders in the care of these patients.

A LIST OF USEFUL WEBSITES
MedlinePlus
https://medlineplus.gov

MedlinePlus is the website of the National Institute of Health (NIH) for patients, family members, and the general public. It provides free, very reliable, and up-to-date information, videos, and illustrations, as well as links to the latest medical research and clinical drug trials. It is updated daily and carries no advertisements.

UpToDate
www.uptodate.com

UpToDate is a website that provides a very up-to-date information to healthcare providers. In addition, it offers them two types of patient education materials: "The Basics" and "Beyond the Basics." Physicians can search on "patient info" and print and share with their patients, or email the patient education information. The basic patient education material is written in plain language, providing an easy-to-read information about a given medical condition. Beyond the basic information is more sophisticated, and more detailed, written at the 10th to 12th grade reading level.

Ankylosing Spondylitis International Federation
www.asif.info/en

Ankylosing Spondylitis International Federation (ASIF) is a worldwide federation of voluntary nonprofit self-help patient societies and organizations that have been established in 1988 to raise awareness to public and healthcare providers of the needs of patients suffering from AS and related forms of SpA. It also assists in the formation of similar societies in other countries. The ASIF website provides a listing and web links for the various self-help societies and organizations worldwide; currently, 26 of them are in Europe, 9 in Asia/Australia, and 3 in the Americas. These societies actively advocate on behalf of patients and are active in educating the general public and the medical community. Many of them publish regular news updates, brochures, books, exercise videos, and online news magazines to educate the patient and their families, as well as the medical professionals and the general public. Three of the more important of these societies are listed below:

1. **National Ankylosing Spondylitis Society (NASS)**
   https://nass.co.uk
   NASS has the distinction of being the first nonprofit, self-help organization in the world to provide a wide range of comprehensive information about AS and related forms of SpA. It was established in 1976 at the Royal National Hospital for Rheumatic Diseases in Bath, UK. It is very active in advocating on behalf of patients and supports medical education and research. It also organizes and provides exercise therapy sessions supervised by physiotherapists.

2. **Schweizerische Vereinigung Morbus Bechterew (SVMB)** (Swiss Ankylosing Spondylitis Association)
   www.bechterew.ch
   This Swiss patient association, the second oldest, was established in 1978. It provides a wide range of information about the disease in German and French. It is very active in educating the general public and the medical community and also organizes physical therapy, swimming, and hydrotherapy sessions supervised by physiotherapists.

3. **Spondylitis Association of America (SAA)**
   www.spondylitis.org
   The SAA is a nonprofit patient organization that was founded in 1983 to advocate on behalf of patients suffering from AS and related forms of SpA in the United States. It has also been very active in educating the general public and the medical community and helping promote medical research.

Assessment of Spondyloarthritis International Society

www.asas-group.org

Assessment of Spondyloarthritis International Society (ASAS) is an international network of healthcare professionals dedicated to research and education in AS and related forms of SpA. Its mission is to support and promote the study of AS/axial SpA, and its excellent website provides extensive information and free teaching slides in various languages.

Spondyloarthritis Research and Treatment Network

www.spartangroup.org

Spondyloarthritis Research and Treatment Network (SPARTAN) is a network of healthcare professionals dedicated to research and education in SpA in North America. Its website provides useful information, such

as treatment guidelines for SpA developed in collaboration with ACR.

Group for Research and Assessment of Psoriasis and Psoriatic Arthritis

www.grappanetwork.org

The purpose of the Group for Research and Assessment of Psoriasis and Psoriatic Arthritis (GRAPPA) is to enhance research, diagnosis, and treatment of psoriasis and psoriatic arthritis.

It also facilitates sharing of information related to psoriasis and psoriatic arthritis, networking among different medical disciplines that see psoriasis and psoriatic arthritis patients.

American College of Rheumatology

www.rheumatology.org

The American College of Rheumatology (ACR) is committed to improving the care of patients with rheumatic disease and also provides information about AS and related form of SpA.

US Food and Drug Administration

www.fda.gov

The US Food and Drug Administration (FDA) provides indications for, usage of, and prescribing information for all drugs, including those prescribed for ankylosing spondylitis and spondyloarthritis.

National Institute for Health and Care Excellence

www.nice.org.uk

National Institute for Health and Care Excellence (NICE) provides evidence-based guidance for the diagnosis and treatment of ankylosing spondylitis and spondyloarthritis.

European Medicines Agency

www.ema.europa.eu/ema

The European Medicines Agency (EMA) is responsible for the scientific evaluation, supervision, and safety monitoring of medicines developed by pharmaceutical companies for use in the EU.

International League of Associations of Rheumatology

www.ilar.org

International League of Associations of Rheumatology (ILAR) is an international body of the associations of rheumatologists from around the world. It comprises partner organizations: EULAR (European League of Associations for Rheumatology), PANLAR (Pan American League of Associations for Rheumatology), APLAR (Asian and

Pacific League of Associations for Rheumatology), and AFLAR (African League of Associations for Rheumatology).

European League Against Rheumatism

www.eular.org

European League Against Rheumatism (EULAR) is an organization that represents the people with arthritis/rheumatism, health professionals, and scientific societies of rheumatology of all the European nations.

Pan-American League of Associations of Rheumatology

www.panlar.org

The Pan-American League of Associations of Rheumatology (PANLAR) integrates rheumatology scientific societies, health professionals related to rheumatic conditions, and rheumatic patient groups from all countries of the Americas.

Asian and Pacific League of Associations of Rheumatology

www.aplar.org

Asian and Pacific League of Associations of Rheumatology (APLAR) represents the people with arthritis/rheumatism, health professionals, and scientific societies of rheumatology of countries of Asia and the Pacific region.

African League of Associations of Rheumatology

www.aflar.net

African League of Associations of Rheumatology (AFLAR) is an international association that aims to promote rheumatology in Africa, by supporting interaction between African rheumatologists, to improve practice and education of rheumatology in African countries.

Ankylosing Spondylitis, Spondyloarthritis, and HLA-B27

www.spondyloarthritis-international.org

It provides clinical information about HLA-B27 and AS/axial SpA for patients and healthcare providers, and a glossary of medical terms used in the medical literature, and simple illustrations for lifelong exercises for patients. Some of the contents are taken from a book titled "*Ankylosing Spondylitis: The Facts*" that is written for patients, and another book titled "*Ankylosing Spondylitis - Axial Spondyloarthritis*" for allied health professionals [23,24].

ACKNOWLEDGMENTS

We are very grateful to Dr. Lewis Nemes, PhD (www. wellness.com), for his input.

REFERENCES

1. Van De Belt TH, Engelen LJ, Berben SA, Schoonhoven L. Definition of health 2.0 and medicine 2.0: a systematic review. *J Med Internet Res.* 2010;12(2).
2. Hughes B, Joshi I, Wareham J. Health 2.0 and Medicine 2.0: tensions and controversies in the field. *J Med Internet Res.* 2008;10(3).
3. Jadad A, Rizo C, Wenkin M. I am a good patient, believe it or not. *BMJ.* 2003;326(7402):1293–1295.
4. Ferguson T, Frydman G. The first generation of e-patients. *BMJ.* 2004;328(7449):1148–1149.
5. Ferguson T. *How the Can Help Us Heal Health Care.* E-patients. Available at: http://e-patients.net/e-Patients_White_Paper.pdf.
6. Caballero-Uribe CV. An education in digital health. In: Rivas H, Wac K, eds. *Digital Health. Health Informatics.* Cham: Springer; 2018.
7. Farnan J, Sulmasy L, Woster B, Chaudhry H, Rhyne J, Arora V. Online medical professionalism: patient and public relationships: policy statement from the American College of physicians and the federation of state medical boards. *Ann Intern Med.* 2013;158(8):620–627.
8. *American Medical Association's Opinion 9.124 – Professionalism in the Use of Social Media.* November 2010. Available at: http://www.ama-assn.org/ama/pub/physician-resources/medical-ethics/code-medical-ethics/opinion9124.page.
9. Moorhead A, Hazlett D, Harrison L, Carroll J, Irwin A, Hoving C. A new dimension of health care: systematic review of uses, benefits, and limitations of social media for health communication. *JMIR.* 2013;15(4):e85. Available at: http://www.jmir.org/2013/4/e85/.
10. Gholami-Kordkheili F, Wild V, Strech D. The impact of social media on medical professionalism: a systematic qualitative review of challenges and opportunities. *J Med Internet Res.* 2013;15(8):e184. Available at: http://www.ncbi.nlm.nih.gov/pmc/articles/PMC3758042/.
11. McLoughlin C, Patel KF, O'Callaghan T, Reeves S. The use of virtual communities of practice to improve interprofessional collaboration and education: findings from an integrated review. *J Interprof Care.* 2018;32(2):136–142. https://doi.org/10.1080/13561820.2017.1377692.
12. Caballero CV, Vecino-Moreno MJ, Arzuza J, Cecilia Rodriguez E, Stange L, Ferreyro L. Twitter, as an advocacy tool to Fight against rheumatic diseases. Poster # 279. *J Clin Rheumatol.* April 2018 (Book of Abstracts).
13. Caballero-Uribe CV, Vecino-Moreno1 MJ, Henriquez A, et al. Social networks as a tool for panlar to disseminate information about rheumatic diseases. Poster # 402. *J Clin Rheumatol.* April 2018 (Book of Abstracts).
14. Massone F, Martínez ME, Pascual-Ramos V, et al. Educational website incorporating rheumatoid arthritis patient needs for Latin American and Caribbean countries. *Clin Rheumatol.* 2017;36(12):2789–2797.
15. Richards T. Is your conference "patients included? *Blogs BMJ.* 2015. http://blogs.bmj.com/bmj/2015/04/17/tessa-richards-is-your-conference-patients-included/.

16. Feldtkeller E, Bruckel J, Khan MA. Scientific contributions of the ankylosing spondylitis patient advocacy groups. *Curr Opin Rheumatol.* 2000;12:239–247.

17. McGowan BS, Wasko M, Vartabedian BS, Miller RS, Freiherr DD, Abdolrasulnia M. Understanding the factors that influence the adoption and meaningful use of social media by physicians to share medical information. *J Med Internet Res.* 2012;14(5):e117.

18. Chetrien C, Azar J, Kind T. Physicians on twitter. *J Am Med Assoc.* 2011;305(6):566–568. https://doi.org/10.1001/jama.2011.68.

19. Choo EK, Ranney ML, Chan TM, et al. Twitter as a tool for communication and knowledge exchange in academic medicine: a guide for skeptics and novices. *Med Teach.* 2015;37(5):411–416.

20. Topol E. *The Creative Destruction of Medicine: How the Digital Revolution Will Create Better Health Care.* New York: Basic Books; 2012. ISBN: 9780465025503.

21. Topol E. *The Patient Will See You Now: The Future of Medicine Is in Your Hands.* New York: Basic Books; 2015. ISBN: 9780465054749.

22. Garrido-Cumbrera M, Poddubnyy D, Gossec L, et al. and on behalf of the EMAS Working Group. The European Map of Axial Spondyloarthritis: Capturing the Patient Perspective. *Curr Rheumatol Rep.* 2019 (in press): [Data Presented at ASIF 13th General Council Meeting, Guangzhou, China. October 11–12, 2018].

23. Khan MA. *Ankylosing Spondylitis.* New York; Oxford University Press, NY. 2009: 1–147.

24. Khan MA. *Ankylosing Spondylitis-Axial Spondyloarthritis.* Professional Communications, Inc. (PCI). West Islip, NY. November 2016: 1–333. ISBN: 978-1-943236-08-4

Index

(Note: Page numbers followed by "f" indicate figures, "t" indicate tables, "b" indicate boxes.)

Printed and bound by CPI Group (UK) Ltd, Croydon, CR0 4YY

03/10/2024

01040373-0001